M000032279

MANUAL OF EMERGENCY MEDICINE

6th Edition

Editor

G. Richard Braen, MD, FACEP

Professor and Chair, Department of Emergency Medicine, Assistant Dean,
Graduate Medical Education, School of Medicine and Biomedical Sciences,
State University of New York at Buffalo, Buffalo, New York

Editor Emeritus

Jon L. Jenkins, MD, FACEP

Former Chairman, Department of Emergency Medicine
Wakefield Hospital, Melrose, Massachusetts

Assistant Editors

Jeanne Basior, MD, FACEP

Associate Professor of Clinical Emergency Medicine, Assistant Residency Director,
Department of Emergency Medicine, School of Medicine and Biomedical Sciences,
University of Buffalo, Buffalo, New York

Samuel Cloud, DO, FACEP

Assistant Professor of Clinical Emergency Medicine, Assistant Residency Director,
Department of Emergency Medicine, School of Medicine and Biomedical Sciences,
University of Buffalo, Buffalo, New York

Christian DeFazio, MD, FACEP

Assistant Professor of Clinical Emergency Medicine, Residency Director,
Department of Emergency Medicine, School of Medicine and Biomedical Sciences,
University of Buffalo, Buffalo, New York

Robert McCormack, MD, FACEP

Associate Professor of Clinical Emergency Medicine, Department of Emergency Medicine
School of Medicine and Biomedical Sciences, University of Buffalo, Buffalo, New York;
Director, Department of Emergency Medicine, Buffalo General Hospital, Buffalo, New York

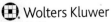 Wolters Kluwer | Lippincott Williams & Wilkins
Health

Philadelphia • Baltimore • New York • London
Buenos Aires • Hong Kong • Sydney • Tokyo

Senior Acquisitions Editor: Frances DeStefano
Product Director: Julia Seto
Vendor Manager: Bridgett Dougherty
Senior Manufacturing Manager: Benjamin Rivera
Senior Marketing Manager: Angela Panetta
Design Coordinator: Terry Mallon
Production Services: SPi Global

© 2011 by LIPPINCOTT WILLIAMS & WILKINS, a WOLTERS KLUWER business
Two Commerce Square
2001 Market Street
Philadelphia, PA 19103 USA
LWW.com

Printed in China

Library of Congress Cataloging-in-Publication Data
Manual of emergency medicine / editor, G. Richard Braen. — 6th ed.
    p. ; cm.
Includes index.
ISBN 978-1-60831-249-8
1. Emergency medicine—Handbooks, manuals, etc.   I. Braen, G. Richard.
[DNLM: 1. Emergency Medicine—Handbooks.   2. Emergencies —Handbooks. WB 39]

RC86.8.J46 2010
616.02'5—dc22

2010045968

To purchase additional copies of this book, call our customer service department at (800) 638-3030 or fax orders to (301) 223-2320. International customers should call (301) 223-2300.

Visit Lippincott Williams & Wilkins on the Internet: at **LWW.com.** Lippincott Williams & Wilkins customer service representatives are available from 8:30 am to 6 pm, EST.

CCS0411

10 9 8 7 6 5 4 3 2 1

*To our spouses from whom we get our love and support:
Kate, Brian, Heather, Marsilia, and Maria.*

Contents

Contributors

Jeanne Basior, MD, FACEP
Associate Professor of Clinical Emergency
*   Medicine*
Assistant Residency Director
Department of Emergency Medicine
School of Medicine and Biomedical Sciences
University of Buffalo
Buffalo, New York

Chapters 24 and 25

G. Richard Braen, MD, FACEP
Professor and Chair
Department of Emergency Medicine
Assistant Dean of Graduate Medical
*   Education*
School of Medicine and Biomedical Sciences
University of Buffalo
Buffalo, New York

Chapters 12 to 20, 24 to 51, 54
to 61 and 65

Samuel Cloud, DO, FACEP
Assistant Professor of Clinical Emergency
*   Medicine*
Assistant Residency Director
Department of Emergency Medicine
School of Medicine and Biomedical Sciences
University of Buffalo
Buffalo, New York

Chapters 1, 8, 9, and 11

Christian DeFazio, MD, FACEP
Assistant Professor of Clinical Emergency
*   Medicine*
Residency Director
Department of Emergency Medicine
School of Medicine and Biomedical Sciences
University of Buffalo
Buffalo, New York

Chapter 23

Christopher L. DeFazio, MD
(Deceased)
Clinical Instructor
Emergency Medicine
Tufts Medical School
Boston, Massachusetts
Chairman of Emergency Medicine
Melrose Wakefield Hospital
Melrose, Massachusetts

Chapters 1, 3, 4, 5, 6, 7, 8, 9, 10, 21, 23

David G. Ellis, MD, FACEP
Associate Professor of Clinical Emergency
*   Medicine*
Chief of Division of Tele-Informatics
Department of Emergency Medicine
School of Medicine and Biomedical Sciences
University of Buffalo
Buffalo, New York

Chapter 2

Christopher D. Gordon, MD
Medical Director and Vice President
Behavioral Health Advocates, Inc.
Framingham, Massachusetts
Assistant Clinical Professor
Department of Psychiatry
Harvard Medical School
Boston, Massachusetts

Chapters 66, 67, 68, 69

Christopher Jaksa, MD
Attending Physician
Walnut Creek Medical Center
Walnut Creek, California

Chapter 22

Jon L. Jenkins, MD, FACEP

Editor Emeritus
Manual of Emergency Medicine
Former Chairman
Department of Emergency Medicine
Wakefield Hospital
Melrose, Massachusetts

Chapters 12 to 20, 24 to 51, 54 to 61 and 65

Richard S. Krause, MD, FACEP

Associate Professor of Clinical Emergency Medicine
Department of Emergency Medicine
School of Medicine and Biomedical Sciences
University of Buffalo
Buffalo, New York

Chapter 62

Jonathan T. Lineer, MD

Attending Physician
Fairview Southdale Hospital
Minneapolis, Minnesota

Chapter 63

Deborah J. Mann, MD

Assistant Professor of Emergency Medicine
Department of Emergency Medicine
SUNY-Syracuse
Syracuse, New York

Chapter 34

Robert McCormack, MD, FACEP

Associate Professor of Clinical Emergency Medicine
Department of Emergency Medicine
School of Medicine and Biomedical Sciences
University of Buffalo
Buffalo, New York
Director
Department of Emergency Medicine
Buffalo General Hospital
Buffalo, New York

Chapter 18 and 19

Bruce Shannon, MD (Deceased)

Chapter 52, 53, 65

Alexander Walker, MD, FACEP

Attending Physician
Department of Emergency Medicine
Hallmark Health System
Melrose-Wakefield Hospital
Melrose, New York

Chapter 3

Preface

Since publishing the first edition of *Manual of Emergency Medicine* in 1986, we have consistently revised the text based on scientific and clinical advances in emergency medical care and changing patterns of practice. The current edition has been carefully reviewed and revised.

We believe the Manual provides a practical guide for the initial evaluation and management of both common and potentially life-threatening or limb-threatening conditions encountered in emergency medicine. We attempted to write and organize the Manual in a style and format that would be valuable to physicians at every level of training and experience.

This manual, because of size limitations inherent to the series, cannot provide the comprehensive or definitive standard of care for all patients. Additionally, the authors acknowledge that for many clinical problems in emergency medicine, there exist several, differing, acceptable, and appropriate management strategies, that medical opinions among experienced and thoughtful emergency physicians often diverge, and that few absolutes exist in medicine. Recommendations made in this edition, as well as in previous editions, must be interpreted in this context.

We are indebted to the many authors who contributed to this and past editions. Also, we are grateful for the numerous readers and reviewers who, over the years, have shared their comments and thoughts with us. We invite and appreciate your comments, thoughts, and suggestions.

G. Richard Braen

Editor's Note

In 1984, Drs. Jon Jenkins and Joseph Loscalzo felt that there was a need for a manual for emergency physicians, residents, and anyone who wanted to have a better knowledge of emergency medicine. The manual that they conceived was problem based, reflecting the chief complaints of patients who come to an ED for evaluation and care. The chapter headings for the medical problems included "shortness of breath," "chest pain," and "abdominal pain" as examples, instead of chapters on "congestive heart failure," "myocardial infarction," and "appendicitis." The authors wanted the manual to directly reflect the problems and thought processes that a practicing emergency physician would encounter and utilize. In 1986, the *Manual of Emergency Medicine* was first published. In addition to Drs. Jenkins and Loscalzo, there was one author, Dr. Bruce Shannon, who contributed multiple chapters. The book had 455 pages of text. In subsequent editions, additional authors were added. Dr. Loscalzo left the book after a few editions to become an editor for the *New England Journal of Medicine*.

For the third edition of the *Manual of Emergency Medicine*, Dr. Richard Braen was added as an author/editor. In the fourth and fifth editions, additional contributors were added, and now, in the sixth edition, four new assistant editors are added. The four are practicing and teaching emergency physicians and include Drs. Basior, Cloud, DeFazio, and McCormack.

Dr. Joseph Loscalzo is currently the physician and chief of Internal Medicine at the Brigham and Women's Hospital and is on the faculty of the Harvard Medical School. Dr. Jon Jenkins is a clinical instructor at Tufts University School of Medicine and is the president of Medical Reimbursement Systems, Inc., a specialized coding and billing company working with emergency physicians and hospitals.

Acknowledgment

Thanks to those from Lippincott Williams & Wilkins who made this book possible: Franny Murphy, Chitra Subramaniam, and Julia Seto.

PART 1

Cardiopulmonary Resuscitation

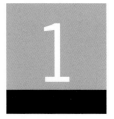

Cardiopulmonary Resuscitation

The techniques and strategies of cardiopulmonary resuscitation (CPR) have evolved over the years into an organized framework for the evaluation and treatment of patients with respiratory or cardiac arrest. It is reasonable for the emergency physician to consider these recommendations, based on currently available data, to be the best initial approach to most patients presenting with cardiorespiratory arrest; however, one understands that the recommendations evolve continuously and often dramatically change, suggesting that our understanding of the pathophysiology of this illness is partial at best and certainly not optimal. In the emergency department, basic CPR must proceed simultaneously with advanced resuscitation, the latter using medication and electrotherapy. This chapter thus deals with resuscitation by an emergency department team and does not cover the details of layperson and healthcare provider out of hospital CPR/advanced resuscitation.

BASIC CPR

- Focuses on the "ABCs," ensuring first that the airway is patent and adequate; second, that breathing is effective and results in appropriate air exchange within the chest; and third, that the circulation is restored.
- Recently minimally interrupted chest compressions have been emphasized as the most important aspect of CPR.

Airway

- In the obtunded or unconscious patient, the upper airway may become obstructed because of relaxation of muscle groups in the upper respiratory tract.
- Should upper airway obstruction by a foreign body be suspected, the airway should be cleared manually.
- When respiratory effort exists, airway patency can often be obtained by a variety of simple mechanical maneuvers that involve the mouth, chin, and mandible.

- When injury to the cervical spine is not present, simply tilting the head backward may be dramatically effective in opening the airway, and if so, signs of respiratory obstruction, such as stridor, may disappear.
- In some patients, the insertion of an oral or a nasal airway, provided that the former does not result in gagging or vomiting, followed by bag-valve–mask (BVM) ventilation as required, may provide adequate oxygenation while the physician attends to other aspects of CPR.
- In other patients with respiratory effort, the jaw thrust (which involves placing the fingers bilaterally behind the mandibular angles and displacing the mandible forward or anteriorly) or the chin lift may provide complete control of the upper airway.
- The jaw thrust, which results in little or no movement of the neck, is the preferred initial maneuver in patients with possible injury to the cervical spine.
- In all patients, supplemental oxygen should be administered.
- Despite respiratory effort by the patient, the use of supplemental oxygen, and the application of techniques to open the airway, the patient with persistent inadequate oxygenation will require establishment of a definitive airway.
- Rapid sequence endotracheal intubation is the preferred maneuver; relative contraindications include potential injury to the cervical spine, mechanical upper airway obstruction, severe restriction of cervical spine mobility, or severe perioral trauma.
- In some cases, nasotracheal intubation remains a valuable technique that may safely be used in the presence of contraindications to endotracheal intubation.
- Nasotracheal intubation should be avoided in patients with significant maxillofacial trauma, because intracranial penetration along fracture lines has been reported.
- Because of a variety of factors, in some patients, it may not be possible to obtain an airway by endotracheal or nasotracheal intubation. In these patients, BVM ventilation using an oral or a nasal airway (during which time the adequacy of oxygenation should be ensured by continuous pulse oximetry) should occur while one considers alternative techniques for airway control, including use of the laryngeal mask airway (LMA), or needle or surgical cricothyrotomy.
- The deflated LMA is inserted blindly into the hypopharynx, where cuff inflation produces an effective proximal and distal seal, with airflow then directed into the trachea. There is somewhat less airway protection from aspiration with the LMA; however, there is enthusiastic support for this device, particularly in settings associated with limited access to the patient, when possible injuries to the cervical spine preclude or complicate patient positioning for endotracheal intubation, or in situations in which early responders are untrained in endotracheal intubation. There is also significantly less risk of the "fatal error" associated with tracheal intubation (continuing to "ventilate" the patient after intubation of the esophagus).
- In patients without respiratory effort, immediate intervention is required to establish an airway and provide oxygenation. This should not interrupt chest compression whenever possible.
- Begin with BVM ventilation and 100% supplemental oxygen with the assistance of an oral or a nasal airway. When possible, evaluate oxygenation with pulse oximetry. Endotracheal intubation (or consideration of the alternative airway techniques, depending on the specific situation), as discussed, is then indicated, with needle or surgical cricothyrotomy considered alternatives for the patient who can be neither oxygenated nor endotracheally intubated.

Breathing

- Once airway patency is established, patients without adequate spontaneous respiratory effort require artificial ventilation.
- When available, a BVM with an oral or a nasopharyngeal airway and supplemental oxygen (100% FiO_2) is preferred to barrier devices and mouth-to-mouth ventilation, and it is more effective.
- Effective, sustained BVM ventilation is also preferable to the interrupted ventilation that can occur during multiple failed attempts at endotracheal intubation.
- The adequacy of ventilation is assessed by determining that breath sounds are present bilaterally, that an inspiratory increase in chest volume occurs with each inspiration, that skin color improves, and that arterial blood gases or pulse oximetry reflect appropriate oxygenation.
- It is also recommended that endotracheal tube (ET) placement be confirmed by nonphysical examination criteria such as capnography or color change CO_2 detectors.

Circulation

- The initial pulse check should take no longer than 10 seconds before initiating chest compressions.
- Precordial thumps are no longer recommended but are not discouraged in the patient with pulseless ventricular tachycardia (VT) or ventricular fibrillation (VF).
- Chest compressions should begin simultaneously with the establishment of an airway and the initiation of ventilation.
- Interruptions in chest compressions should be minimized at all costs.
- With the patient placed in a supine position on a hard surface, external cardiac compressions are initiated by placing the heel of one hand over the lower half of the sternum and the heel of the second hand on top of the first hand.
- Pressure over the xiphoid process should be avoided.
- With the elbows extended, rhythmic compressions should be provided by depressing the sternum 1.5 to 2.0 inches posteriorly in adults.
- Compressions should be smooth and should be performed at the rate of approximately 100/min.
- The efficacy of external compressions can be checked by palpating the carotid or femoral pulse.
- CPR cycles of 30 compressions to 2 breaths via a BVM should continue until the patient is connected to the defibrillator and an advanced airway is established.
- Ventilations should be given at a rate of 8 to 10/min during chest compressions once an advanced airway is established.

ADVANCED CARDIOPULMONARY RESUSCITATION

Early identification of the pulseless rhythm, minimally interrupted chest compressions, and early defibrillation of pulseless VT and VF are the initial goals of emergency department resuscitation in cardiac arrest.

Intravenous Access

- Initial venous access should be sought in a peripheral vein if possible (e.g., using veins in the antecubital fossa, generally the most accessible peripheral veins).

- Intraosseous (IO) access is an increasingly utilized modality in adults and should be considered in any patient in whom large bore peripheral venous access is difficult. This approach involves the use of a specially designed IO needle that is inserted into the proximal anterior tibial bone marrow; the distal femur, the proximal humerus, and distal tibia can also be used. If rapid volume expansion is needed, then fluids can be administered under pump pressure. The major complications of this procedure are tibial fractures, lower extremity compartment syndromes in the case of dislodged needles, and osteomyelitis.
- Central venous sites are avoided because of the increased time associated with their placement and the unavoidable interruption of CPR; hand and wrist peripheral IV sites are also less useful, as is femoral venous catheterization.
- One must remember that 1 to 2 minutes is required for medications administered at a peripheral site to reach the heart; this is true even when CPR is adequate.
- Drugs should be administered by rapid bolus and followed by a 20-mL bolus of fluid.
- When venous access is unobtainable, the following medications can be administered via ET tube: lidocaine, epinephrine, atropine, and narcan (LEAN), which are administered in approximately 2- to 2.5-times the recommended dose, first diluted in 10 mL of normal saline and then injected by passing a catheter beyond the tip of the ET.
- After injecting the medication, three to four forceful ventilations are provided.

Additional Recommendations

- In the past, the use of sodium bicarbonate was encouraged to treat acidosis associated with cardiac arrest; the use of sodium bicarbonate is now discouraged in routine CPR. The rationale for this change involves the lack of evidence supporting the use of this alkali in changing the outcome of routine CPR as well as a number of factors suggesting a negative effect. For example, bicarbonate (1) does not facilitate defibrillation or improve survival in laboratory animals in VF; (2) shifts the oxyhemoglobin saturation curve to the left, inhibiting the release of oxygen to the tissues; (3) produces a paradoxical acidosis in cells, which results from the ability of carbon dioxide, released from sodium bicarbonate, to diffuse freely into cells, depressing cellular function; (4) may inactivate administered catecholamines; and (5) induces a number of other adverse effects caused by systemic alkalosis produced from overvigorous administration. Bicarbonate is therefore not recommended in routine CPR.
- In certain specific circumstances, bicarbonate may be of use, but only when the diagnosis on which such therapy is based has been clearly defined. For example, patients with pronounced systemic acidosis associated with renal failure, patients with tricyclic antidepressant overdose, and patients with hyperkalemia documented before arrest may benefit from the prompt administration of bicarbonate.
- Bicarbonate can also be considered in patients with prolonged resuscitations, provided tracheal intubation and adequate ventilation have been provided (the administration of bicarbonate to patients with hypercarbic acidosis is harmful), and in patients with restoration of normal circulation after prolonged arrests.
- The routine administration of bicarbonate should otherwise, however, be avoided.
- Calcium should be used only in arrests associated with hyperkalemia, hypocalcemia, or calcium channel blocker toxicity.

- If possible, particularly in profoundly hypotensive patients who have regained pulses, bedside US may provide a clue as to the etiology of the shock (i.e., cardiac tamponade, free fluid in the abdomen suggesting intraabdominal aneurysm rupture, etc.).

Treatment of Rhythm Disturbances

Ventricular Fibrillation/Pulseless Ventricular Tachycardia

- The newest guidelines emphasize minimally interrupted CPR.
- Once diagnosed, it should be treated with immediate defibrillation using 120 to 200 J (biphasic device specific, 360 J monophasic device).
- Rhythm checks after defibrillation and stacked shocks are no longer recommended.
- Compressions should immediately follow defibrillation without a rhythm check for 2 minutes.
- After 2 minutes of CPR, the rhythm should be checked.
- If the VT/VF persists, then epinephrine (10 mL of a 1:10,000 solution or 1 mg) should be administered, either intravenously or, if venous access has not been obtained, by ET (2–2.5 mg is a reasonable adult dose).
- Then, the patient should be defibrillated again and CPR continued for another 2 minutes.
- If unsuccessful, the dose of epinephrine is repeated at 3- to 5-minute intervals, followed by repeated defibrillations at maximum joules, followed by 2 minutes of CPR as long as the patient remains in VT/VF.
- Vasopressin is an alternative to epinephrine in this setting; vasopressin is administered as a one-time intravenous (IV) dose.
- If these maneuvers fail, amiodarone should be administered in a 300-mg IV dose, followed by defibrillation and 2 minutes of CPR.
- A dose of amiodarone, 150 mg, may be repeated in 3 to 5 minutes.
- Lidocaine (1.5 mg/kg) is an alternative to amiodarone and is administered intravenously (or IO), after which defibrillation is repeated; additional doses of 0.5 to 1.5 mg/kg are administered up to a total dose of 3 mg/kg.
- Magnesium sulfate (1 to 2 g IV or IO) may be useful in torsade de pointes or in suspected hypomagnesemia.

Pulseless Electrical Activity

- In this disorder, there is ECG evidence of organized electrical activity but failure of effective myocardial contraction (absent pulses and heart sounds).
- Causes of pulseless electrical activity (PEA) to consider include the "5 Hs and 5 Ts": hypovolemia, hypoxia, hydrogen ion (acidosis), hyperkalemia, hypokalemia, hypothermia, tablets (overdose), tamponade (cardiac), tension pneumothorax, thrombosis (coronary), and thrombosis (pulmonary embolus).
- Treatment includes oxygenation; volume repletion; CPR; epinephrine (1 mg IV push every 3–5 minutes); atropine (1 mg intravenously, every 3–5 minutes up to a total of 0.04 mg/kg); rapid, empiric fluid challenge (in adults, 500 mL of normal saline recommended by some authorities); and consideration and correction of other causes of PEA.
- Bedside cardiac US can be very useful to confirm the absence of cardiac output and help to determine a correctable cause (cardiac tamponade, etc.).

Asystole

- Potential asystole may represent any one of three possible electrophysiologic events: extremely fine VF, pronounced bradycardia (supraventricular, junctional, or idioventricular), or true asystole.

- Therapy is predicated by one's inability to distinguish among these three causes using the electrocardiogram (ECG).
- At least two leads should be briefly analyzed before the diagnosis of asystole is made.
- One must remember that what appears to be a "flat line" may occur in several different settings, only one of which is true asystole.
- False asystole must be excluded by assuring that all connections/cables between the patient and the device(s) are intact and that the sensitivity or gain on the device is not too low or zeroed.
- When asystole is diagnosed, epinephrine (1 mg) and atropine (1 mg) should be concurrently administered along with minimally interrupted CPR.
- Rhythm checks are performed at 2-minute intervals.
- Atropine should be repeated at 3- to 5-minute intervals to a total dose of 0.04 mg/kg; epinephrine is also readministered at 3- to 5-minute intervals.
- Major causes for this dysrhythmia should be considered and include hypoxia, hyperkalemia, hypokalemia, preexisting acidosis, drug overdose, and hypothermia.
- If after treatment of asystole and any correctable known causes have failed, then the resuscitation may be terminated.

Bradycardias
- Bradycardias may be sinus, ectopic atrial, junctional, or idioventricular in origin.
- When associated with hypotension, clinical or ECG evidence of ischemia, or congestive heart failure, treatment should be initiated with atropine (0.5–1.0 mg IV, repeated as needed up to 0.04 mg/kg), followed by external or transvenous pacing, dopamine 5 to 20 μg/kg/min, or epinephrine 2 to 10 μg/min.
- Once a more rapid sinus or junctional rhythm is obtained (i.e., more than 60 beats/min), the presence of a pulse should be sought. If present, then blood pressure should be determined; if low, then volume repletion and vasopressors (dopamine 10 to 20 μg/kg/min or norepinephrine 16 to 24 μg/min) may be instituted.

Tachycardias
- Specific categories include atrial fibrillation/atrial flutter, narrow complex tachycardias stable wide complex tachycardias (unknown type), and stable monomorphic VT.
- In tachycardic patients, it should be established initially if the patient is stable or unstable (i.e., presence of chest pain or hypotension).
- If the patient is stable, then the rhythm should be determined and treated accordingly (see later).
- If the patient is unstable (diminished level of consciousness, hypotension, CHF, or acute coronary syndrome) and the accelerated rate appears to be a cause of the patient's symptoms, then the patient should be cardioverted.

Atrial Fibrillation/Atrial Flutter
- Rate control of rapid ventricular response with beta-blockers, diltiazem, or amiodarone (if the other two fail or are contraindicated) along with anticoagulation is the mainstay of therapy for most patients.
- In the patient with duration less than 48 hours or in the hemodynamically unstable patient, one may consider DC cardioversion or pharmacologic cardioversion with amiodarone, flecainide, or propafenone.
- If the duration is greater than 48 hours, then cardioversion (DC or pharmacologic) should be avoided due to the risk of cardiogenic embolization. Appropriate rate control and anticoagulation should be instituted.

- If more immediate cardioversion is required, then IV heparin should be administered, followed by transesophageal echocardiogram (to exclude atrial thrombus), prior to cardioversion. This is followed by 4 weeks of oral anticoagulation.
- In the patient with Wolff-Parkinson-White (WPW) syndrome who presents in rapid AF, AV nodal blocking agents (adenosine, diltiazem, digoxin) should be avoided in order to not enhance conduction via the accessory pathway. DC cardioversion or amiodarone (150 mg IV) should be utilized instead.

Regular Narrow-Complex Supraventricular Tachycardias

- These are of three types: paroxysmal supraventricular tachycardia (PSVT), multifocal atrial tachycardia (MAT), and junctional tachycardia.
- If the patient is unstable, DC cardioversion is the recommended initial treatment.
- If the patient is stable, then a 12-lead EKG should be obtained.
- Vagal maneuvers can be considered, followed by treatment with adenosine (which will convert PSVT, but is unlikely to convert MAT or junctional tachycardia).
- Adenosine is given as a 6-mg rapid IV push. Two more doses of 12 mg may be tried if the PSVT does not convert.
- For patients with PSVT in whom adenosine fails, AV nodal blockage (with diltiazem or beta-blockers) or DC cardioversion can be used; if these are unsuccessful, then amiodarone can be used.
- Adenosine and cardioversion are unlikely to convert patients with MAT and junctional tachycardia. These entities can be treated with diltiazem and beta-blockers.

Regular Wide-Complex Tachycardias

- These arrhythmias may represent either monomorphic VT or supraventricular tachycardia (SVT) conducted aberrantly; distinguishing between these two mechanisms is necessary for optimal treatment of the arrhythmia.
- Differentiation may not be possible in all cases.
- When patients are stable, a full 12-lead ECG is useful in attempting to differentiate these two rhythms.
- Table 1-1 lists the ECG features that may differentiate ventricular from SVT with aberrancy.

Table 1-1	Electrographic Features Differentiating VT from SVT with Aberrancy	
	VT	**SVT with Aberrancy**
QRS width	Often ≥0.14 s	Usually <0.14 s
QRS width, onset to S-trough	≥0.11 s	<0.11 s
Axis	Bizarre	Normal
V_1	Rs, RsR', Rsr'	rsR'
V_6	S wave present	S wave absent
Fusion beats	Present	Absent
AV dissociation	Present	Absent

VT, ventricular tachycardia; SVT, supraventricular tachycardia.

- It is important to note that the presence of a consistent relationship between P waves and QRS complexes does not exclude VT.
- In some patients with VT, the atria may be activated in a retrograde fashion producing a 1:1 relationship; in other patients, isorhythmic but independent depolarizations of the atria and ventricles occur and may artifactually appear as if the former were conducted.
- When hemodynamic stability is not present, DC cardioversion is the treatment of choice.
- If SVT with aberrancy is suspected, adenosine may be used.
- If the regular wide complex tachycardia is suspected to be VT (older patient, history of CHF/CAD) and the patient is symptomatic, DC cardioversion is recommended.
- If the patient is stable, amiodarone (150 mg IV bolus over 10 minutes repeated as needed to a maximum dose of 2.2 g in 24 hours) may be utilized. Procainamide and sotalol are alternatives.
- It should be noted that lidocaine and bretylium are no longer recommended in the wide complex tachycardia unknown-type protocol.

Irregular Wide-Complex Tachycardias
- This rhythm occurs in AF with aberrancy, AF in a patient with WPW, or polymorphic VT.
- AF with aberrancy and AF in the WPW patients should be treated as discussed in the AF section above.
- Polymorphic VT occurs when ventricular activation is variable.
- Torsade de pointes is polymorphic VT in a patient with a prolonged QT interval present in a baseline sinus EKG and is commonly due to drugs or cardiac ion channel abnormalities.
- Torsade de pointes is an unstable rhythm that can quickly degenerate to VF.
- Unstable polymorphic VT (including torsades) should undergo immediate DC cardioversion.
- If the patient is noted to have a prolonged QT during a sinus interval (torsades), magnesium 2 g IV over 5 to 10 minutes may be tried, provided the patient is stable.
- Isoproterenol and ventricular overdrive pacing have also been noted to be effective in patients with torsades. This effect is due to the natural shorting of the QT interval as the heart rate increases.
- Magnesium is unlikely to terminate polymorphic VT in the patient with a normal sinus QT interval.
- Amiodarone may be effective in terminating stable polymorphic VT in a patient with a normal sinus QT interval.

PEDIATRIC CARDIOPULMONARY RESUSCITATION

Resuscitation of the infant or child involves the same basic principles of airway management, circulatory assistance, and pharmacologic interventions discussed with respect to the adult, with a few specific differences.

Airway and Breathing
- Because children younger than 6 months are obligate nose breathers, obstruction of the nose, from whatever cause, can rapidly result in respiratory failure; because of this, nasogastric tube placement is generally deferred in the acute setting.

- In addition, the anatomy of the upper airway differs in the small child; the oral cavity is small, the tongue is relatively large, the larynx is anterior, and the trachea is short.
- These anatomic differences must be appreciated if the delivery of oxygen and intubation is to be successful and entry into the bronchi is prevented.
- In addition, during the administration of oxygen and in preparation for intubation, hyperextension of the neck, particularly in the infant, is to be avoided because the anatomic topography of the oropharynx is such that optimal airway patency is achieved with the neck held in the neutral position.
- With respect to intubation, for neonates and children younger than 2 years, the position of sniffing is most appropriate, whereas for older children, extension of the head will be helpful.
- Obstruction of the airway (e.g., secondary to foreign body, epiglottitis) remains an important cause of respiratory arrest in children and must be considered in all patients.
- Mouth-to-mouth, mouth-to-nose, and BVM ventilation of the infant and child, when successful, produce appropriate thoracic motion and auscultatory evidence of air exchange; these techniques may provide adequate oxygenation for prolonged periods and are preferable to multiple failed attempts at intubation, during which time oxygenation is interrupted.
- Ventilations should never provide excessive tidal volumes.
- In children 5 to 7 years old, teeth are easily avulsed and can then enter the trachea.
- Insertion of an oral airway, if necessary to improve oxygenation, should not be rotated into position in the usual manner but rather should be placed in the proper position under direct vision with a tongue blade.
- Surgical cricothyrotomy is rarely undertaken in the child younger than 12 years; needle cricothyrotomy followed by pressure insufflations is the initial procedure of choice when other routine and backup measures to establish an airway have failed.
- Approximate ET sizes can be estimated on the basis of the diameter of the child's fifth finger or the size of the external nare's.
- Another method to estimate the appropriate uncuffed tube size for an infant or small child is the formula: (age in years/4) + 4.
- For cuffed tubes: (age in years/4) + 3.

Age	Size (mm)
Premature to 3 mo	2.5–3.0
3–18 mo	3.5–4.0
18 mo–5 y	4.0–5.0
5–12 y	5.0–6.5
12 y and older	6.5–8.0

- The LMA has been approved for pediatric use. It is a tube with a mask-like projection on the end. It is introduced into the hypopharynx and a balloon cuff is inflated, securing the distal opening of the tube above the glottic opening. The LMA does not prevent aspiration and cannot be used in a child with an intact gag reflex, and medications cannot be given through the device.

Circulation

- Interruptions in chest compressions are once again to be minimized.
- In the infant and child younger than 2 years, chest compressions may best be accomplished using two hands, placing the thumbs over the sternum with the fingers curled around the child's back to stabilize the spine and the child during compressions. Allowing complete relaxation between compressions is essential to permit maximal filling of the ventricles.
- In infants, the sternum should be compressed to a depth of one third to one half the anterior-posterior diameter of the chest at a rate of at least 100/min.
- In children, chest compressions at 100/min are also recommended using a similar hand placement technique as with adult chest compressions.
- The chest compression should also depress the sternum one third to one half the anterior-posterior diameter of the chest.

Vascular Access

- It is most readily obtained by peripheral vein cannulation or IO access.
- IO access is a safe and rapid route to administer drugs, crystalloid, and blood.
- Central venous access is time-consuming and technically challenging and should not be the initial line of choice.
- The endotracheal route should be used when direct venous or IO access is not immediately available. Importantly, a 5-mL flush with normal saline and four manual ventilations should follow the administration of all medications.
- Shock in the child is initially treated with 0.9% saline or Ringer lactate and 20 mL/kg is administered over 10 minutes; an appropriate urine output is approximately 1 mL/kg/h. The fluid challenge may be repeated as necessary to sustain blood pressure, whereas other therapeutic maneuvers are undertaken based on specific cause.
- Type-specific blood, 20 mL/kg, or packed cells, 10 mL/kg, may be administered over 10 minutes in the case of hemorrhagic shock.

Pharmacologic Therapy

- Drugs used in pediatric CPR are essentially identical to those used for adults and are recommended for the same indications as discussed above. Dosages, of course, differ.
- Because of low glycogen stores, infants tend to become hypoglycemic when presented with shock, stress, and periods of high-energy use. Thus, glucose levels should be monitored and documented; hypoglycemia should be treated with glucose-containing IV infusions.
- It is important to note that epinephrine, atropine, naloxone, and lidocaine may be administered via ET if necessary.

Adenosine
- It is the drug of choice in SVT in children administered in a dose of 0.1 mg/kg, with a maximum dose of 6 mg. If the SVT persists, one may double the dose, with a maximum dose of 12 mg.

Amiodarone
- Dosage is 5 mg/kg over up to 1 hour. The dose may be repeated to a total of 15 mg/kg/d.

Atropine
- 0.02 to 0.03 mg/kg up to 0.5 mg in a child and 1.0 mg in an adolescent may be administered intravenously, intramuscularly, or by ET. The minimum dose is 0.1 mg.
- Calcium chloride, 10%, 0.1 mL/kg, or Calcium gluconate, 0.3 mL/kg, can be administered slowly intravenously over several minutes in documented hypocalcemia. Calcium chloride is preferred because of higher bioavailability.

Dextrose
- 5 to 10 mL/kg of $D_{10}W$ is administered intravenously.
- 1 to 2 mL/kg of $D_{50}W$.

Dopamine
- 2 to 20 µg/kg/min may be infused for pressor support.

Dobutamine
- 2 to 20 µg/kg/min.

Epinephrine
- 0.01 mg/kg (1:10,000 solution) IV or IO; or 0.1 mg/ kg (1:1000 solution) via ETT.
- For asystole or pulseless arrest, subsequent doses are 0.1 mg/kg (1:1,000) up to 0.2 mg/kg IV, IO, or by ETT.
- Maximum dose is 1 mg IV/IO, 10 mg via ETT.

Lidocaine
- It should be administered in no greater than a 1-mg/kg loading dose, generally implying 5 to 15 mg for infants and 20 to 50 mg for children, with a 20 to 50 µg/kg per minute continuous infusion as needed to suppress ectopy.

Naloxone
- For patients less than 20 kg: 0.1 mg/kg IV/IO/ETT.
- For patients greater than 20 kg: 2 mg IV/IO/ETT.

Procainamide
- 15 mg/kg over 30 to 60 minutes.

Sodium Bicarbonate
- 1 mL/kg of a 50 mEq/50 mL solution can be administered for prolonged arrests and in patients with an unstable hemodynamic status and documented metabolic acidosis.

Defibrillation
- It should be performed in children using 2 J/kg.
- AEDs may be used in children older than 1 year.
- Use a pediatric AED system, if available, in children in the 1- to 8-year age group.
- If a pediatric AED is not available, an adult AED device will suffice.

FORMAL ALGORITHMS FOR CARDIOPULMONARY RESUSCITATION

Algorithms for CPR as devised by the American Heart Association are reproduced in Figures 1-1 through 1-6.

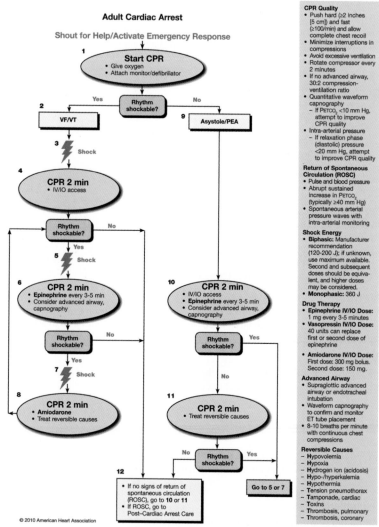

Figure 1-1. Adult cardiac arrest. (From Neumar RW, et al. Part 8: Adult Advanced Cardiovascular Life Support: 2010 American Heart Association Guidelines for Cardiopulmonary Resuscitation and Emergency Cardiovascular Care. *Circulation* 2010;122:S729–S767.)

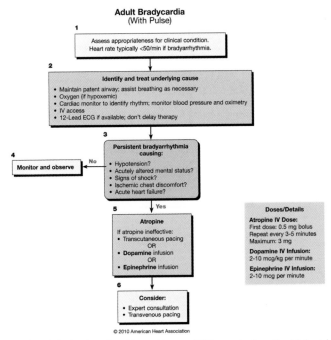

Figure 1-2. Adult bradycardia. (From Neumar RW, et al. Part 8: Adult Advanced Cardiovascular Life Support: 2010 American Heart Association Guidelines for Cardiopulmonary Resuscitation and Emergency Cardiovascular Care. *Circulation* 2010;122:S729–S767.)

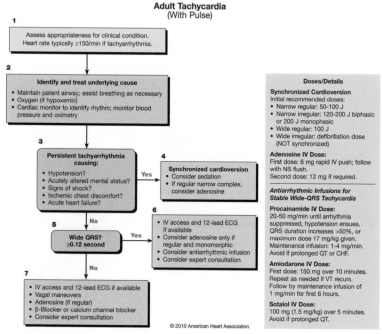

Figure 1-3. Adult tachycardia. (From Neumar RW, et al. Part 8: Adult Advanced Cardiovascular Life Support: 2010 American Heart Association Guidelines for Cardiopulmonary Resuscitation and Emergency Cardiovascular Care. *Circulation* 2010;122:S729–S767.)

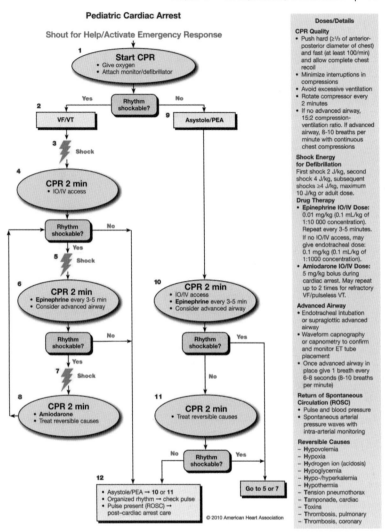

Figure 1-4. Pediatric cardiac arrest. (From Kleinman ME, et al. Part 14: Pediatric Advanced Life Support: 2010 American Heart Association Guidelines for Cardiopulmonary Resuscitation and Emergency Cardiovascular Care. *Circulation* 2010;122:S876–S908.)

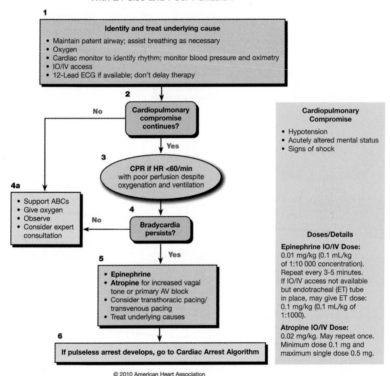

Figure 1-5. Pediatric bradycardia. (From Kleinman ME, et al. Part 14: Pediatric Advanced Life Support: 2010 American Heart Association Guidelines for Cardiopulmonary Resuscitation and Emergency Cardiovascular Care. *Circulation* 2010;122:S876–S908.)

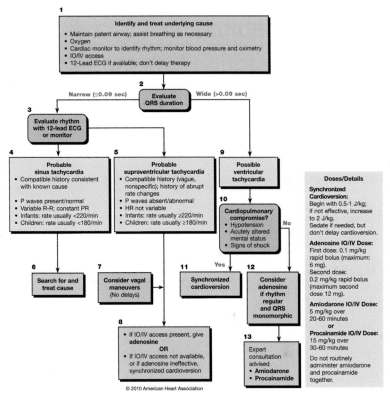

Figure 1-6. Pediatric tachycardia. (From Kleinman ME, et al. Part 14: Pediatric Advanced Life Support. 2010 American Heart Association Guidelines for Cardiopulmonary Resuscitation and Emergency Cardiovascular Care. *Circulation* 2010;122:S876–S908.)

2 Rapid Sequence Intubation

Optimal airway management may require rapid sequence intubation (RSI) using paralytic agents. The goal of this procedure is orotracheal intubation achieved by optimizing conditions for intubation and minimization of complications.

INDICATIONS FOR AGGRESSIVE AIRWAY SUPPORT

- Initial examination of patients presenting to the emergency department should include immediate assessment of the need for aggressive airway management (Table 2-1).
- A decreased level of consciousness is a key indicator of patients who may have inadequate ventilation, inability to protect their airway from aspiration, and upper airway obstruction (commonly the tongue).
- Measure the patient's response (eye opening, verbal response, motor response) after rapid delivery of a verbal or painful stimulus, and quickly calculate the Glasgow Coma Scale (Table 2-2).
- Useful guidelines include "less than eight, intubate," or intubation if ten or less in the trauma patient.
- Rapidly assess response to naloxone and flumazenil (if benzodiazepine overdose is suspected) and the glucose level (Dextrostix or glucometer).
- Early identification of patients with elevated intracranial pressure (trauma, decreased level of consciousness, papillary signs) may allow hyperventilation to produce immediate benefit before neurosurgical intervention.
- Hypoxemia may be rapidly identified by the presence of cyanosis; however, severely anemic patients may not show this important sign.
- Agitation, particularly in the elderly, may be an indicator of hypoxemia.
- Rapidly assess respiratory effort, including ventilatory rate, accessory muscle use, retractions, and sounds of small (wheeze) and large (stridor) obstructive airway disease.
- Monitor those individuals very closely, including the very young and the very old, who are not capable of maintaining the work of breathing given their reduced muscle mass and cardiac reserve.
- Anticipating airway obstruction and early intervention are crucial in the management of facial burns, inhalation injuries, and caustic ingestions.
- Attempt to locate family, surrogates, advance directives, or living wills in very elderly or debilitated patients to ensure that aggressive airway management is truly in the best interest of the patient and family.

B-A-S-I-C AIRWAY MANAGEMENT TECHNIQUES

- Before consideration of RSI, the airway management team (two to three persons) must achieve stabilization of the patient using basic airway techniques. This "buys time" for controlled preparation of equipment, pharmacologic agents, and definitive

Table 2-1	The Five Indications for Aggressive Airway Management

1. Inadequate ventilation
2. Inability to protect the airway
3. Upper airway obstruction
4. Elevated intracranial pressure
5. Hypoxemia

Table 2-2	Glasgow Coma Scale[a]

Best Motor Response

6	Obeys commands
5	Localizes to pain
4	Withdraws to pain
3	Abnormal flexion
2	Abnormal extention
1	No movement

Best Verbal Response

5	Oriented and appropriate
4	Confused conversation
3	Inappropriate
2	Incomprehensible sounds
1	No sounds

Eye-Opening

4	Spontaneous
3	To speech
2	To pain
1	No eye opening

[a]Glasgow Coma Scale score equals the sum of the scores from each of the three groups.

airway procedures. Basic airway control also reassures the clinical team and brings order to the chaos of early resuscitation. Failure to do so invites worsening hypoxemia, hypercarbia, aspiration, raised intracranial pressure, and cervical spine injury, and negates the benefits gained by early intubation.

• **B**reathe for the patient using a bag-valve–mask device. Mask designs using balloon or "jellyfish" design allow adequate sealing around the face and mouth with minimal operator effort, despite facial hair or an edentulous patient. Discriminating use of physical restraint in the combative patient may be essential to prevent further patient or staff injury.

• Provide an **A**irway for the patient using an initial jaw thrust or sniffing position if cervical spine injury is not suspected. An oropharyngeal or nasopharyngeal airway may be tolerated if the patient is significantly obtunded.

- **S**uction the patient to help prevent aspiration; the **S**elleck maneuver (cricothyroid cartilage pressure) may also prevent aspiration.
- Ensure that the oxygen tubing is attached and that the patient has high levels of **I**nspired oxygen saturation or FIO_2. This saturation and denitrogenation can be achieved by 4 to 5 minutes of breathing 100% oxygen via a nonrebreather facemask or four maximally deep breaths or bag-valve–mask ventilation. The pulse oximeter can be invaluable in assessing the adequacy of oxygenation and as reassurance of oxygen delivery during preparation and actual RSI procedure.
- Finally, protect the **C**ervical spine from further injury through cervical immobilization. First, use a cervical collar, followed by an assistant's using the forearms as a stabilizing bridge with elbows on the chest and hands on the occiput and zygoma during airway manipulation. If chest access is impossible from below the head, then apply the forearms to the parietooccipital skull with hands on the shoulders. Avoid in-line traction, which can lead to distraction of fractured cervical elements. Large clinical studies have shown orotracheal intubation with in-line immobilization to be safe and effective when used in the trauma patient with potential cervical spine injury.
- Emphasis must be placed on the ability to ventilate the patient adequately at this point before further intervention, particularly before the administration of paralytic agents. Ensure that the patient has cardiac monitoring and a functional, stable intravenous line.

OVERVIEW OF THE PROCEDURE OF RAPID SEQUENCE INTUBATION

- Eight words, all starting with "P," help to organize and summarize the RSI procedure.
  - **Prepare** the patient, medications, and equipment.
  - **Preoxygenate** the patient with 100% oxygen.
  - **Pretreat** to prevent bradycardia or rapid rise in blood pressure.
  - **Prime** the patient for sedation and amnesia.
  - **Paralyze** the patient for optimum intubating conditions.
  - **Pressure** is applied to the cricothyroid membrane to prevent aspiration.
  - **Place** the endotracheal tube, assisted by tracheal manipulation.
  - **Postintubation** care ensures proper positioning and ventilation.

Prepare Equipment and Support Team
- Evaluate the patient for potential difficulties in airway management.
- Have a kit or box made beforehand with all necessary equipment so that the intubator will not have to leave the patient's bedside to successfully complete the intubation.
- Select the appropriately sized endotracheal tube for patient size or age.
- Ensure that the laryngoscope light is intense and not yellow or absent.
- Use a stylet to maximize control at the tip during insertion.
- Mobilize respiratory therapy and ventilator availability.
- Prepare medications for pretreatment, sedation, and paralysis in well-marked syringes.
- Place a carbon dioxide detector in a convenient position for postintubation verification of proper tube placement.

Preoxygenate
- Preoxygenation with near 100% oxygen delivered by spontaneous breathing for 5 minutes through nonrebreather facemask or bag-valve–mask with high-flow

oxygen is required to ensure adequate oxygen reserve during RSI; preoxygenation occurs concurrently with the preparation phase.

Pretreat the Patient

- It is useful to give atropine (0.01 mg/kg, 0.6 mg is usual adult dose) to block bradycardia associated with succinylcholine in children or in already bradycardic adults.
- A nondepolarizing muscle relaxant administered in a small dose before paralysis, such as vecuronium (0.01 mg/kg, 1 mg usual adult dose) or low-dose succinylcholine (10 mg usual adult dose), may blunt the reflex tachycardia and hypertensive response from tracheal manipulation, which may lead, also, to an elevation in the intracranial pressure.
- Lidocaine (1.0–1.5 mg/kg, 70–100 mg usual adult dose) has become more controversial with little evidence to support its continued use to reduce intracranial pressure in head-injured patients.
- In emergency situations, pretreatment can be eliminated with minimal consequences for the patient if time is of the essence.

Prime the Patient for Sedation and Amnesia

- Sedative-hypnotic agents are useful adjuncts for sedation and amnesia.
- These include induction agents such as etomidate and propofol, the benzodiazepines (midazolam, diazepam), opioids (fentanyl, alfentanil) ketamine, and, less commonly in emergency settings, the barbiturates (thiopental, methohexital).
- Etomidate (0.3 mg/kg, usual adult dose 20 mg) is a nonnarcotic, nonbarbiturate, nonbenzodiazepine induction agent with rapid onset of action and brief duration of activity. This agent has little effect on the cardiovascular system, has a rapid onset of action and short duration of action, and is stable at room temperature. It remains a popular agent for RSI because of its applicability to a broad range of adult patients and brain-protective properties, particularly in trauma patients. Decreases in the production of cortisol and aldosterone reported in intensive care units during the 1980s do not appear to be of concern in the single-use, acute airway management setting.
- Benzodiazepines currently are a commonly used sedative-hypnotic agent in the emergency department. Midazolam (dosage 0.2 mg/kg, 14 mg usual adult dose) produces profound sedation, with a reliably rapid onset of action and 60-minute duration at this dosage and is preferred over diazepam. Use dosages of 0.1 mg/kg in the elderly or hemodynamically unstable patients. Benzodiazepines provide no protection against secondary brain injury in patients with head trauma or elevated intracranial pressure.
- Opioids such as fentanyl (dosage: pretreatment 1–2 μg/kg, 100 μg usual adult dose; induction 10–20 μg/kg, usual adult dose 1–2 mg) have a rapid onset of action and are effective in providing analgesia in addition to sedation and hypnosis. Opioids may protect against increases in intracranial pressure by blunting airway reflexes and decreasing the cerebral metabolic rate and blood flow. Precautions for fentanyl use include an association with bradycardia and muscular rigidity, which may impair ventilation with higher doses.
- Ketamine (1.5 mg/kg, usual 100 mg) is chemically related to phenylcyclohexyl piperidine, thus its association with emergence reactions, brain stimulation, and hypertension, which can be detrimental in brain injured patients. Its best application may be in patients with severe hypotension due to its effect on raising blood pressure and also in severe asthma and respiratory failure due to its bronchodilator effects.

- Propofol (1–2 mg/kg, usual 70–140 mg) is another agent that shares the properties of rapid onset, short duration, and neuroprotection with few aftereffects. It will, however, cause a predictable decrease in blood pressure, which can be severe in hypovolemic patients. Its primary use in the emergency department is in deep procedural sedation in patients with adequate volume status and stable hemodynamic systems.
- Barbiturates such as thiopental (3 mg/kg, usual 210 mg) have been pharmacologic mainstays of anesthesiologists and emergency physicians in the past. Ultrashort-acting barbiturates such as methohexital (1–1.5 mg/kg, usual 70–100 mg) provide effective anesthesia and cerebral protection with rapid recovery. A primary reason for lessened use of these agents in the emergency department is their effects as potent cardiac depressants, and they should be used with caution in patients with hypovolemia (trauma) and in hemodynamically unstable patients.

Paralyze the Patient to Accomplish Rapid, Controlled Intubation

- Relaxation with paralyzing muscle relaxants is crucial to the effective management of patients who present with extreme respiratory difficulty.
- The muscles of the mandible and pharynx must be relaxed to allow adequate visualization of the vocal cords.
- This is true particularly in the trauma patient in whom optimal intubating conditions on the first attempt are critical to success.
- Failure to relax the patient, or to attempt intubation with sedation only without paralysis, may create unacceptably high rates of first intubation attempt failures.
- The classic muscle relaxant for RSI remains the depolarizing muscle relaxant succinylcholine (1.5 mg/kg, usual 100 mg), which acts within 60 seconds.
- Despite some known contraindications and cautions, it is the primary agent for most RSI cases because of its rapid onset of action, short duration of action, superb intubating conditions, and low-volume dosing for the majority of patient weights.
- The intubating practitioner must be prepared to deal with the possibility of hyperkalemia (widened QRS or arrhythmias) or bradycardia.
- Avoid succinylcholine in patients with raised intraocular pressure, muscular dystrophies, and recent (7- to 10-day-old) burns.
- Pretreat with atropine in patients younger than 6 years of age to prevent bradycardia seen with succinylcholine.
- Nondepolarizing muscle relaxants are widely used in emergency medicine, with rocuronium (0.6–0.9 mg/kg, usual 40–63 mg) and vecuronium (0.2 mg/kg, usual 14 mg) as the agents of choice in this class.
- Nondepolarizing muscle relaxants such as rocuronium may challenge the rapid onset of action of succinylcholine, whereas vecuronium (0.15 mg/kg, usual 10 mg) is commonly used for maintenance of paralysis in the immediate postintubation period.
- Ensure adequate dosing in emergency conditions to achieve optimal intubation conditions, and inadequate paralysis should always lead to a check of the intravenous line to ensure that the medications are being delivered.
- Larger doses may result in prolonged (more than 2 hours) paralysis and the need for additional sedation.

Pressure Should be Applied to the Cricothyroid Cartilage (Selleck Maneuver)

- To prevent regurgitation and aspiration, particularly once the paralytic is administered.
- Pressure should be maintained until the balloon is inflated and the correct tube position is confirmed by objective method.

Placement of the Endotracheal Tube

- Placement of the endotracheal tube should be accomplished within a 45- to 60-second window of apnea time.
- It may be facilitated by using the BURP maneuver, which is backward upward rightward pressure to improve the alignment of the trachea for a right-hand–dominant intubator.

Postintubation Care

- Position the endotracheal tube for optimum safety and security.
- Unrecognized esophageal intubation is the most dangerous complication of endotracheal intubation, quickly leading to desaturation of the patient's blood oxygen levels.
- Emergency practitioners must use an objective method of confirming correct tube position in addition to visualization of the endotracheal tube passing through the vocal cords and larynx, which is the first step to ensuring proper placement.
- Novice intubators must not settle for less than full visualization of trachea and vocal cords to maintain appropriately high rates of first-pass success.
- Routine use of carbon dioxide detectors or end-tidal CO_2 monitoring can effectively eliminate esophageal intubation in the majority of RSI cases.
- These devices can be falsely negative in the cardiac arrest patient.
- Right mainstem intubation is the next most frequent complication of intubation.
- Overaggressive insertion of the endotracheal tube will place the tip of the tube below the carina of the lungs.
- Preferred adult positioning is typically achieved when the tube centimeter markings show 22 cm at the patient's teeth.
- In patients with obstructive lung diseases (COPD, asthma), the intubator must be wary of overzealous ventilation. In this subset of patients, the delivered breath, if not given adequate time to be exhaled, can cause breath stacking. This leads to a rise in intrathoracic pressure and decreased cardiac output, with subsequent hypotension.
- Tension pneumothorax must be suspected in the trauma patient with a decrease in blood pressure postintubation, with the intubator being prepared to place a large bore needle of adequate length in the second intercostal space, midclavicular line on the suspected side, followed by a chest thoracostomy tube.
- The endotracheal tube must be adequately secured with tape or a commercial tube securing device to ensure that it will not become dislodged during subsequent patient movement and diagnostic testing.

DIFFICULT INTUBATION

- Every clinician who undertakes RSI must anticipate problems with intubation and have a multiple option plan with readily available equipment before attempting the procedure.

Anticipate the Difficult Intubation

- The **3–3–2 Rule** may help predict an airway in which short anatomical distances increase the difficulty: if the patient's mouth does not open the distance of **3** finger breadths, if the distance from the tip of the mandible to the laryngeal cartilage is less than **3** fingers (anterior neck), and if the cephalocaudal distance from the floor of the mouth to the laryngeal prominence is less than **2** fingers, then the intubation may be difficult.

- The Mallampati score grades the potential for difficulty based upon the visible structures in the oropharynx when the patient opens the mouth and says "ah."
  - Class 1—The soft palate, fauces, uvula, and anterior and posterior pillars are visualized.
  - Class 2—Only the soft palate, fauces, and uvula are visualized.
  - Class 3—Only the soft palate and base of the uvula are visualized.
  - Class 4—Even the soft palate is not visualized.
- Other facial and physical features may portend a more difficult intubation through interfering with patient bagging or passing the endotracheal tube, including obesity, facial hair, facial burns, angioedema, a large tongue, buck teeth, facial fractures, limited neck mobility, and upper airway distortion or obstruction resulting from a tumor or trauma.

Stylet-Based Airway Adjuncts

- The elastic bougie is rapidly becoming indispensable for achieving high first-pass and second-pass success rates by allowing efficient cannulation of the trachea when only a small portion of the vocal cords, peritracheal muscle structure, or epiglottis is visible. This 60-cm 15-gauge flexible stylet with the angled tip is placed into the trachea, feeling for the "clicks" or hang-ups as it encounters the cartilaginous rings inside the trachea. In situations of laryngeal edema or burns, pressure on the chest may result in bubbles, which help guide placement of the stylet. A colleague can then slide an appropriately sized endotracheal tube down over the stylet, twisting as the tube is advanced through the trachea.
- The lighted stylet may also allow the tracheal location to be identified through the bright, anterior neck, midline glow created when the lighted tip is transilluminating the trachea.

Noninvasive Rescue Airway Adjuncts

- The laryngeal mask airway (LMA) with its oval flexible shape conforms to the internal shape of the pharynx, partially occluding the esophagus, and allows ventilation of the trachea to take place. Although it cannot totally prevent regurgitation and possible aspiration, its ability to be rapidly inserted and to quickly ventilate the patient in a failed intubation setting has made this device extremely valuable and popular to include in the airway armamentarium.
- A newer version of the device, the intubating LMA, allows an endotracheal tube to be inserted into the trachea through the LMA while in position, avoiding the risk of removal and aspiration.

Cricothyroid Membrane Airway Access

- In percutaneous transtracheal jet ventilation, a large-bore 14- to 16-gauge angiocath is inserted through the cricothyroid membrane, which is then connected to a high-pressure oxygen source with a jet injector valve to control gas flow. If all equipment is ready and in place, then this can be an extremely rapid, temporizing technique for insufflating oxygen into the trachea while more definitive measures such as orotracheal intubation or bronchoscopic-aided techniques can be performed. This technique oxygenates, but does not ventilate.
- Either the intubators themselves or the members of the team performing an RSI procedure must be capable of a surgical cricothyroidotomy if the patient is unable to be intubated through the mouth. It is performed by grasping the trachea from below, incising longitudinally across the cricothyroid membrane, and inserting and

lifting the thyroid cartilage upwards with a tracheal hook, so that a tracheal tube or No. 6 endotracheal tube can be inserted into the airway.

Other Techniques

• Video-assisted intubating devices (i.e., the Glidescope®) have come to the fore in the last several years.
• Endoscopic or bronchoscopic-assisted intubation may assist the intubator in identifying proper tracheal positioning without significant flexion or extension of the neck, which may be particularly useful in suspected cervical spine injuries. Retrograde intubation is performed by cannulating the cricothyroid membrane and then using a Seldinger technique to introduce a wire upward into the oropharynx where it is grasped, and an endotracheal tube is introduced into the trachea, following the wire below the vocal cords.

PART 2

Trauma

Initial Assessment of the Multiple Trauma Patient

TRIAGE

Triage is defined as the planning for care to patients on the basis of need or severity of illness. Although clear exceptions occur, patients with compromise of the airway should be seen and treated first because if the airway is inadequate, then survival is most immediately threatened. Second, breathing, or the adequacy of air exchange within the chest and oxygenation, must be ensured. Third, the circulation must be evaluated and restored and bleeding arrested. For most patients, these three priorities provide a reasonable initial basis for the determination of the urgency of care.

ASSESSMENT

Perhaps in no other clinical setting is the importance of a well-defined, rigorous strategy for patient evaluation more apparent than in the patient with multiple injuries. Begin the assessment with an initial evaluation using the mnemonic ABCDE; during this time, specific critical functions are sequentially evaluated, resuscitation is instituted, and life-threatening conditions are corrected. After the initial assessment and resuscitation, a more detailed secondary survey and a definitive care phase follow.

Primary Survey and Resuscitation

During the initial assessment, as one moves sequentially through the mnemonic, ABCDE, life-threatening conditions are diagnosed and corrected at each stage. This hierarchy of assessment and treatment should be strictly followed.

A: Upper airway is established and maintained with cervical spine control.
B: Breathing (or the adequacy of air exchange) is evaluated and established.
C: Circulation–blood pressure is evaluated and corrected, and bleeding is arrested.
D: Deficits of neurologic function are identified, and treatment is initiated.
E: Exposure is obtained by completely undressing the patient.

- **A: Upper airway is established and maintained along with cervical spine control.** All patients presenting with head, neck, or facial trauma, or neurologic symptoms, such as weakness or abnormalities of mental status after trauma, however subtle, must be assumed to have **injuries to the cervical spine**, and strict attention given to immobilization of the neck must be maintained. This is undertaken with a combination of a spine board, to which the patient's head must be secured, with the application of a rigid or semirigid cervical collar (not a soft collar) and manual maintenance of the head and neck in the neutral position.

  Airway intervention, if required, must proceed rapidly. Begin the assessment of the airway by determining whether the patient can speak normally; if so, a reasonable airway probably exists, and other priorities can be assessed. Patients without inspiratory effort and those with a Glasgow Coma Scale score of 8 or less require intubation to establish and secure a functional airway; while the neck remains immobilized, oral intubation should be undertaken as soon as possible. Patients with inspiratory effort but without adequate ventilation require a rapid and directed assessment of the pharynx to exclude local obstruction related to posterior movement of the tongue or the presence of swelling, bleeding, secretions, or gastric contents. Rigid suction and manual extraction should be used to clear the pharynx of any foreign material. Obstruction of the airway caused by posterior movement of the tongue is particularly common in lethargic or obtunded patients and may be quickly corrected by the insertion of an oral or nasal airway and/or the chin-lift or jaw-thrust maneuvers. Contraindications to the insertion of a nasal airway should be noted and include the suspicion or demonstration of a basilar skull fracture, cerebrospinal fluid otorrhea or rhinorrhea, or significant maxillofacial or perinasal injuries. The chin-lift and jaw-thrust maneuvers simply involve grasping the chin and angle of the jaw, respectively, and moving these structures anteriorly or upward in such a way that the tongue is displaced forward. Patients with extensive facial or neck injuries in whom intubation of the trachea is impossible require needle or surgical cricothyrotomy to secure the airway. When these techniques are unsuccessful, Ambu-bag–assisted ventilation with 100% oxygen and an oral or a nasopharyngeal airway may provide temporary oxygenation.

  There are a number of common, rapidly reversible causes of central nervous system or respiratory depression that commonly precipitate trauma by interfering with consciousness; these include hypoglycemia, opiate overdose, and Wernicke encephalopathy. These disorders must be considered and presumptively treated in all patients presenting with abnormalities of mental status after trauma, even when other explanations seem both obvious and adequate to explain the clinical presentation (e.g., head injury, alcohol ingestion, severe hypotension). Treatment includes the rapid intravenous administration of 1 ampule of 50% dextrose, 0.4 to 2.0 mg of naloxone, and 100 mg of thiamine; any response to the various agents should be carefully recorded. When improvement does occur, a variety of problems related to establishing or maintaining the airway, circulation, or both may be avoided.

- **B: Breathing (or the adequacy of air exchange) is evaluated and established.** After an airway is secured and ventilation with oxygen initiated, the adequacy of air exchange must be assessed. Bilateral and symmetric breath sounds (best heard in the axilla) should be present immediately after intubation or other airway establishment. Placement of the endotracheal tube in the esophagus is the most common cause of failure to ventilate the patient adequately after intubation, and this may be diagnosed by bedside capnography and auscultation over the stomach during ventilation. Failure to appreciate breath sounds on the left or reduced breath sounds on the left is often explained by the presence of the endotracheal tube in the right mainstem bronchus; this is easily corrected by deflating the cuff and then slowly pulling the tube back until bilateral breath sounds are heard. When these problems are excluded and ventilation or oxygenation remains inadequate, hemothorax, simple pneumothorax, and tension pneumothorax must then be considered and corrected if present. Flail chest, pulmonary contusion, and aspiration are additional diagnoses that may explain persisting hypoxia in the traumatized patient but initially remain diagnoses of exclusion.

- **C: Circulation–blood pressure is evaluated and bleeding arrested.** Evaluating the patient's pulse, skin color, and level of consciousness can be performed very quickly and provide a rapid bedside assessment of the adequacy of circulation.
  - **Control of bleeding**. External bleeding should be controlled by **direct pressure**. If an extremity is involved and direct pressure is unsuccessful, then elevation followed by the application of a proximal blood pressure cuff inflated above systolic pressure may be used temporarily while other care is rendered.
  - **Intravenous access** should be established with two 14- or 16-gauge short peripheral lines and normal saline or Ringer lactate solution and then rapidly infused.

    Central lines should not be used for initial fluid resuscitation because their placement, even in experienced hands, is more time-consuming, is associated with a higher rate of complications, and, most importantly, results in a dramatically reduced rate of fluid delivery as a function of catheter-induced resistance; a 16-gauge, 8-inch line, for example, delivers approximately half the fluid of a 16-gauge, 2-inch catheter per any unit of time.

  - **Initial fluid challenge**. Adults presenting with significant blood loss or established or evolving shock should be treated initially with 2 L of normal saline or Ringer lactate solution; this may be administered as rapidly as possible, usually over 5 to 10 minutes; and children may be administered 20 mL/kg over a similar interval.

  - **Blood replacement**. Although subsequent therapy will be dictated by the patient's response to the initial fluid challenge, most patients presenting with significant hypotension will require blood replacement, and a minimum of 4 U of packed cells should rapidly be made available. Although cross-matched blood is clearly preferable, its preparation requires between 50 and 70 minutes, and in many patients presenting with exsanguinating hemorrhage or severe hypotension, an abbreviated type and cross-match (which requires 15–20 minutes), type-specific blood (which requires approximately 10 minutes), or O-negative blood (which should be available immediately) should be transfused. Blood should be administered through macropore (160-μm) filters and, if possible, should be warmed before or during transfusion; warming is often impractical, however, because of the urgency of transfusion.

    Pressors have no role in the routine management of hemorrhagic shock; aggressive reexpansion of intravascular volume with crystalloid and/or blood remains the mainstay of initial treatment. Similarly, colloid solutions, including albumin, dextran, hetastarch, fresh frozen plasma, and plasma protein fraction (Plasmanate, Plasmatein), offer no particular advantage over normal saline or Ringer lactate in the initial management of the shock/trauma patient. The use of colloid solutions is also associated with markedly increased expense and some other disadvantages, that is, the risk of hepatitis with fresh frozen plasma and allergic reactions, renal damage, and increased bleeding tendency caused by decreased platelet adhesiveness with dextran.

- **Assessment of response to initial fluid challenge.** In general, patients who rapidly respond to the initial fluid challenge with a normal blood pressure and who remain stable may be assumed to have lost relatively little blood (<15%–20%) and will generally not require additional fluid challenges or blood replacement. Hospital admission for observation is required, and a minimum of 4 U of packed cells should remain available for emergency transfusion. Patients in whom only a transient increase in blood pressure is noted require rechallenge with normal saline or Ringer lactate solution and rapid blood replacement. If patients exhibit little or no response to the initial fluid challenge, then blood loss was either extensive or continuing, or the diagnosis of hypovolemic shock was in error. If the initial diagnosis is correct, then blood replacement must be aggressively undertaken and plans for possible surgical intervention pursued. Evidence of elevated right-sided pressures associated with systemic hypotension suggests that hypovolemic shock may have been at least an incomplete if not an incorrect diagnosis; one should immediately consider cardiac tamponade, tension pneumothorax, massive hemothorax, and congestive heart failure in these patients. These two groups may be differentiated by physical examination and by measurement of central venous pressure: If the diagnosis of hypovolemic shock is correct, then central venous pressure will be low, whereas if any of the other conditions exist, central venous pressures will be elevated.
- **Implications associated with massive blood transfusion.** Massive transfusion is defined as the replacement of half the patient's blood volume in a single hour or total blood volume replacement in less than 24 hours. Massive transfusion of packed red blood cells may result in hypothermia and occasionally both hypocalcemia and abnormalities of hemostasis. Hypothermia causes an increased affinity between oxygen and hemoglobin and interferes with the body's normal response to adequate resuscitation; efforts should be taken to prevent the development of hypothermia and to institute rewarming measures as early as possible. Coagulation factor depletion and thrombocytopenia secondary to dilution are typically not problems in the first hour of resuscitation but can become significant over the next 24 to 48 hours. Clotting factor replacement therapy should be considered in patients with 1.5 × total blood volume replaced, presenting hypothermia, liver dysfunction, or transfusion-induced hypothermia. One unit of fresh frozen plasma can be empirically administered for every 4 U of packed red blood cells and may prevent abnormalities of hemostasis caused by dilution. Alternatively, the need for treatment may be determined by frequent measurement of clotting parameters.

    Hypocalcemia is caused by chelation of intravascular calcium by the citrate preservative, and abnormalities of hemostasis are secondary to dilution of clotting factors. If more than 1 U of blood is transfused every 5 minutes, or in association with severe liver dysfunction, then hypocalcemia may become a problem; supplemental calcium can be administered slowly by separate intravenous line, if evidence of hypocalcemia (tetany, EKG changes) is noted.

    Hyperkalemia is usually seen only in patients massively transfused over a very short period of time. Transfused red blood cells take up potassium after becoming active, and hypokalemia can then occur. As with other electrolyte abnormalities in this setting, management, including replacement, is based on clinical evidence (e.g., EKG changes).

- **D: Deficits of neurologic function are identified, and treatment is initiated.** In general, during the initial assessment, the patient's overall neurologic status is grossly assessed and may simply be characterized as alert, responsive to verbal stimuli, responsive to painful stimuli, or unresponsive to all stimuli.

    Rapidly reversible causes of central nervous system depression, including hypoglycemia, opiate overdose, and Wernicke encephalopathy, must be considered and prophylactically treated. Similarly, seizure may have precipitated trauma, and the postictal state may produce persisting abnormalities of consciousness as well as focal neurologic findings. Persisting abnormalities of mental status at a time when blood pressure is normal or relatively normal should suggest cerebral injury.

    Injury **to the cervical spine** must be assumed to be present when consciousness is disturbed as a result of trauma, and 5% to 10% of such patients will be found to have a major cervical injury. Immobilization of the cervical spine is critical in patients presenting after trauma with even minor abnormalities of mental status, significant head or facial injuries, or other symptoms suggestive of cervical injury. Immobilization must be maintained until radiologic visualization of the proximal 8 vertebrae (C1-7 and T1) is complete and determined to be normal. Commonly, an initial view of the cervical spine demonstrates only the more proximal vertebrae. This must never be interpreted as a normal study, and an additional view must be taken while downward traction is applied to the forearms. If the distal vertebrae remain nonvisualized with this maneuver, then a swimmer's view should be obtained. Should any doubt exist as to the presence of a cervical injury, computed tomography (CT) scanning or MRI with neurosurgical or orthopaedic consultation is indicated, during which time immobilization and restriction of activity must be continued.

    Spinal shock, which must always be a diagnosis of exclusion (to the extent that the physician must prove that hemorrhage does not explain the patient's hypotension), may be noted immediately after injury to the spinal cord. Most patients present with systolic blood pressures in the range of 70 to 90 mm Hg and have warm extremities and a normal or only slightly elevated pulse, neither of which is an expected finding in patients with hemorrhagic shock. Additionally helpful findings include neck pain; flaccid areflexia, including the rectal sphincter; diaphragmatic breathing or apnea; priapism; a sensory level; and facial gesturing in response to painful stimuli above the level of the clavicles but not below them. The institution of pressors, if required, may be helpful and should be instituted in patients with spinal shock after blood loss is excluded or corrected.

- **E: Exposure is obtained by completely undressing the patient.** Patients must be fully undressed to allow a complete evaluation.

Secondary Assessment

After establishing a functional airway, ensuring appropriate gas exchange, and initiating fluid resuscitation, a more detailed evaluation of the patient may be undertaken. Begin at the head and move caudad. Patients without ventilatory insufficiency wearing motorcycle or football helmets should not have the helmets removed until the cervical spine is assessed. When the helmet must be removed, the neutral position of the head is first ensured by an assistant who stabilizes the helmet from the head of the bed. The opening of the helmet is then manually expanded, and it may then be gradually removed while the neck is immobilized in the usual manner.

Palpation of the entirety of the scalp, the facial bones, and a somewhat more detailed assessment of neurologic function should then be undertaken; asymmetry of the facial bones should be noted; and a gross assessment of vision may be undertaken in conscious patients. The presence of jugular venous distention and tracheal deviation must be noted; the posterior neck, back, chest, and abdomen are then inspected and palpated for local skin disruption or tenderness. Patients with gunshot or other penetrating injuries to the abdomen that are not superficial and patients with obvious intra-abdominal bleeding or injury require urgent laparotomy; preparations should be made early, concurrent with resuscitative efforts. Bilaterally equal breath sounds and heart sounds should again be evaluated. The genitalia are examined, and a rectal examination with particular attention to the position of the prostate, muscle tone, and the presence of blood is performed. The extremities are examined for evidence of hematoma, crepitus, deformity, and peripheral pulses; bleeding is controlled with direct pressure, and fractures are aligned and splinted.

At this stage in the examination, Foley catheter and nasogastric tube placement, if indicated, may be undertaken. A relative contraindication to Foley catheter placement includes suspected urethral disruption. Urethral injury is suggested by blood at the urethral meatus, gross hematuria, pelvic fracture, scrotal or perineal hematoma, and upward displacement of the prostate on rectal examination manifest as palpable emptiness, fluctuance, or hematoma in the usual area of the prostate. A rectal examination should, therefore, be undertaken in traumatized patients before Foley catheter placement when urethral injury is possible or suspected. When urethral injury is suspected, retrograde urethrography should precede catheter placement in stable patients. Patients requiring emergent treatment in the operating room may have the bladder decompressed at that time.

Relative contraindications to nasogastric tube placement include significant maxillofacial or perinasal trauma, the presence of cerebrospinal fluid otorrhea or rhinorrhea, or demonstrated fracture of the basilar skull relatively, because movement of the tube posteriorly into the brain along the fracture line may occur and has been reported. When the stomach must be emptied to prevent aspiration, passage through the mouth may be undertaken and the gastric contents removed.

In the special case of late second- or third-trimester pregnancy, the patient should be placed on the left side and assessment of fetal heart rate undertaken; rates between 120 and 160 are normal. An obstetrical consultation is recommended in pregnant patients with significant trauma.

RADIOLOGICAL STUDIES

Radiologic studies are obtained after the patient is stabilized. The cervical spine must remain immobilized until radiologic assessment of this area is complete. In addition, in the patient with multiple trauma, anteroposterior films of the chest and pelvis are obtained after stabilization.

The use of ultrasound in the emergency department (ED) by physicians is common. With the advent of portable ultrasound units, the use of this modality has increased dramatically, particularly in the assessment of the abdomen in blunt trauma. This examination has taken on the acronym of FAST, or the focused assessment by sonography in trauma. The primary goal of the examination is to identify intraperitoneal blood and secondarily to identify specific organ injuries. The examination can be performed in less than 3 minutes and has four primary views: subxiphoid, right upper quadrant, left upper quadrant, and suprapubic. The subxiphoid view is examined first for two major reasons. The first is to diagnose or exclude pericardial tamponade, which if present is treatable without having to move the patient to an operating room. The second is to identify blood within the left ventricle, which allows a standardization view of blood, thus helping the physician to positively identify blood when performing the other three views. The second or RUQ view evaluates the potential space between the liver and right kidney, known as Morrison pouch. In the supine patient with intra-abdominal trauma, a bleeding site above the pelvis will usually drain cephalad and bleeding below the pelvis will drain caudad; Morrison pouch (between the liver and right kidney) is the site of drainage for most patients with intra-abdominal injuries and can detect intraperitoneal blood in more than 50% of cases. The LUQ view attempts to visualize free fluid in the area of the left kidney and spleen, and the suprapubic view assesses the pouch of Douglas, where the initial signs of pelvic bleeding are often first noted. It is thought that this modality may decrease the need for other imaging modalities in the patient with blunt abdominal trauma before surgery. Technically what is required is a probe with a small footprint, 1 to 3 cm, and a range of 2.0 to 5.0 MHz. Potential negatives of this technique include extended training of personnel, failure to identify clotted blood, or misdiagnosing ascites for blood.

With the introduction and increasing availability of high-speed spiral CT, this modality has essentially become the imaging modality of choice in the patient with multiple trauma. The head, neck, chest, abdomen, and pelvis can be assessed, individually or together, literally in several minutes. In blunt abdominal trauma, an abdominal/pelvic CT is extremely sensitive and specific for liver and splenic injuries and for visualizing free intraperitoneal blood; the retroperitoneal space is particularly well visualized, and this modality has largely replaced the IVP for potential renal trauma. In addition, the study gives detailed and vital information to the trauma surgeon before surgical intervention. Diagnostic peritoneal lavage is still used, but typically when CT imaging is not readily available (Table 3-1).

OTHER CONSIDERATIONS

Trauma in the Patient with Hemophilia

Hemophilia A and B are sex-linked, recessive disorders resulting in defective coagulation of factors VIII and IX, respectively. Of the approximate 20,000 patients in the United States with hemophilia, 80% have factor VIII deficiency. In the general population, the range of normal factor activity varies from 50% to 200% (0.5–2.0 U/mL); the severity of hemophilia is quantified on the basis of the level of factor coagulant activity present. In all patients, 1% or less activity is considered severe, and these patients are subject to spontaneous bleeding; 1% to 5% activity represents moderate severity, with major bleeding primarily associated with trauma or surgery; and greater than 10% activity is considered mild, although bleeding after trauma and surgery similarly is noted. Bleeding may occur at multiple sites; however, recurrent hemarthroses with progressive joint destruction and intracranial bleeding remain the major causes of morbidity and mortality, respectively. Trauma remains a common and important precipitant of bleeding in all groups of patients.

A few general rules in regard to the evaluation and management of patients with hemophilia should be noted. Most patients presenting to the ED will be very familiar with their illness, including the severity of their disease (or percent factor level) and

Table 3-1	Revised Adult Trauma Score	
Criterion	**Points**	**Score**
Respiratory rate	>29	3
	Between 10 and 28	4
	6–9	2
	1–5	1
	0	0
Systolic blood pressure	>89	4
	76–89	3
	50–75	2
	1–49	1
	0 (no pulse)	0
Glasgow coma scale	13–15	4
	9–12	3
	6–8	2
	4–5	1
	3	0

Probability of survival by overall revised trauma score

12...0.995	8...0.667	4...0.333
11...0.969	7...0.636	3...0.333
10...0.879	6...0.630	2...0.286
9...0.766	5...0.455	1...0.250
		0...0.037

Revised trauma score (RTS) = 0.9368 GCS + 0.7326 SBP + 0.2908 RR.
It is heavily weighted to GCS to compensate for patients without multisystem injury or major physiological changes.
From Champion HR, Sacco WJ, Copes WS, et al. A revision of the Trauma Score. *J Trauma* 1989;29:623.

the various modalities of treatment. Many patients with moderate to severe disease will bring their own factor concentrate for replacement, and they should be allowed to use this in the ED. In all cases, immediate triage into the ED should occur, along with a very early consultation with the patient's hematologist. Intramuscular injections should be avoided; parenteral agents should be administered intravenously or subcutaneously. Ancillary studies and all invasive procedures should follow replacement therapy; replacement therapy should also be administered before transfer to another facility, if possible. Medications that interfere with coagulation or platelet aggregation should obviously be avoided.

The treatment of bleeding in **hemophilia A** involves the early and adequate administration of factor VIII as either concentrate (containing 200–1,500 U/20-mL bag—the actual number of units will be indicated on the bag) or cryoprecipitate (containing approximately 80–100 U/20-mL bag). At the current time, because concentrates can be subjected to virucidal treatments, these are considered safer and therefore preferred. It is important to remember that some patients with mild hemophilia A will respond to treatment with desmopressin (DDAVP), which is thought to act by stimulating release of factor VIII from body storage sites. Patients with factor VIII levels less than 10% are generally not considered candidates for treatment with DDAVP. DDAVP is the initial treatment of choice in patients with mild hemophilia A who have demonstrated a positive response to DDAVP infusion in the past, often via elective testing. The usual dosage of DDAVP is 0.3 μg/kg in 50 mL of normal saline administered over 30 to 40 minutes; a concentrated preparation, administered via nasal spray, is also under study. The treatment of **hemophilia B** requires replacement of factor IX with purified factor IX concentrates; cryoprecipitate is ineffective because of insufficient factor IX activity. Fresh frozen plasma can also sometimes be used in patients with mild factor IX deficiency associated with non–life-threatening bleeding; treatment options here are somewhat limited with fresh frozen plasma because of the low factor activity present and the consequently high volume of plasma required.

The primary goal of treatment for both hemophilia A and B is to achieve sufficient coagulant activity in the plasma to control or arrest bleeding. The amount of factor required is, therefore, based on the patient's basal factor activity level, which is relatively constant, and the potential severity of the specific bleeding episode. In general, minimum acceptable hemostatic levels for factors VIII and IX are as follows: for mild bleeding, 30%; for moderate bleeding, such as significant muscle or joint bleeding, 50%; and for severe or life-threatening bleeding episodes, 80% to 100%. It is important to remember that each unit of factor VIII infused per kilogram of body weight will raise the plasma factor VIII level by 2%; each unit of factor IX infused, because of a greater volume of distribution, will raise the plasma factor IX level by 1%. Therefore, 50 U/kg of factor VIII infused in a patient with severe hemophilia A should raise the plasma level of factor VIII to at least 100%; the infusion of 100 U/kg of factor IX in a patient with severe hemophilia B should produce a similar level. In patients with life-threatening bleeding, the basal factor activity level should be considered to be 0%.

Several examples of bleeding severity, as well as the recommended dosage of factor VIII replacement in each, follow. Conditions associated with mild bleeding require treatment with 10 to 25 U/kg of factor VIII. These include lacerations (single-day coverage is adequate), spontaneous epistaxis (may not require therapy if mild and controlled with pressure or other local measures), oral mucosal or tongue bites (may not require therapy), early hemarthrosis (usually single-dose therapy is adequate), and hematuria. Moderate bleeding requires treatment with 25 to 40 U/kg. These conditions include traumatic epistaxis (may require treatment for 5–7 days), lacerations of the tongue and oral mucosa and dental extractions (may require therapy for severe bleeding for several days), soft-tissue and muscle hematoma (may require treatment for severe bleeding for several days), and late or unresponsive hemarthroses (may require treatment for several days). Major or serious bleeding requires treatment with 50 U/kg and is seen after major trauma or surgery or in gastrointestinal, intracranial, retroperitoneal, or intra-abdominal bleeding. Bleeding in the neck and sublingual areas is also considered potentially severe. Treatment in this category should be continued for 3 to 5 days after bleeding stops. Patients with head injuries are considered at high risk for intracranial bleeding, are treated prophylactically (for severe bleeding), and require early CT scanning.

Once thawed, cryoprecipitate must be administered within 4 hours; cryoprecipitate should be ABO type–specific (a full crossmatch is not necessary) and should be administered through a blood filter or a platelet concentration infusion set (the latter contains a filter and allows cryoprecipitate to be administered by intravenous push).

Also, given that a number of other proteins are found in cryoprecipitate, patients may report itching, urticaria, and fever after its administration; these symptoms can be prevented or treated by administering diphenhydramine, 25 to 50 mg intravenously. Last, because the half-life of factor VIII is 8 to 12 hours, maintenance therapy includes administering one-half the above or initial dose at 8- to 12-hour intervals over the course of therapy. In regard to factor replacement with concentrate, once reconstituted, a vial should be administered; the entire contents of all vials should be administered, even though the calculated dose is somewhat exceeded.

Importantly, the emergency physician must maintain a very low threshold for recommending hospital admission for observation in patients with hemophilia, especially after trauma. The phenomenon of delayed bleeding, occurring up to 3 days after injury, should always be kept in mind. Observation is recommended for patients with blunt injuries involving the head, chest, back, or abdomen or occurring in areas where hematoma formation could be disastrous, such as the eye, mouth, or neck. As noted, patients with head injuries are at particularly high risk for intracranial bleeding and require early prophylactic therapy, admission for observation, and CT scanning.

The Emergency Department Management of Jehovah's Witnesses

Patients presenting to the ED who, based on particular religious convictions, refuse blood or blood component therapy pose complex ethical and medical concerns for the physician. Jehovah's Witnesses will not accept transfusion of whole blood, packed red blood cells, platelets, plasma, or white blood cells. The prohibition among Jehovah's Witnesses against accepting blood and blood component therapy derives from several Biblical mandates that, when violated, result in termination of the relationship between the Witness and God, excommunication, and loss of the prospect of everlasting life. Emergency physicians must understand this mandate and its consequences if treatment in the ED is to be sensitive, appropriate, and as medicolegally unencumbered as possible. Jehovah's Witnesses accept most other types of therapy, including surgery, the administration of medicines, and the infusion of nonblood fluids (e.g., crystalloids, nonblood colloid, dextrans, and other oxygen-carrying blood substitutes, such as perfluorochemical).

Recently, in the courts, there has been a tendency (when the interests of the state are not jeopardized) to allow the informed, competent adult to refuse lifesaving treatment for himself or herself. This right has included the refusal of Jehovah's Witnesses to accept transfusion based on religious grounds. Conversely, by virtue of the legal principle of *parens patriae* (the responsibility of the state to protect the health and welfare of its citizens), the right of parents to refuse potentially lifesaving therapy for their children, based on religious principles, is not absolutely ensured; in such cases, the courts have intervened and mandated that treatment be provided. Similarly, the courts have assumed an interest in the protection of the unborn child and mandated transfusion of the mother if required to prevent the child's death.

In the ED, one must remember that the individual who refuses to accept lifesaving treatment must be competent; such a refusal should not be followed in the case of an incompetent patient. The emergency physician must carefully assess and document the basis for diagnosing a patient incompetent. Abnormalities of vital signs, when significant, an altered mental status, and evidence of impaired cognition because of cerebral hypoperfusion, head injury, or drug or alcohol intoxication must all be assessed and may provide sufficient grounds for determining that the degree of competency required to make a lifesaving decision is not present and that such a decision need not be followed. As noted, most states have refused to allow parents to refuse lifesaving treatments for their children. In these cases, if time permits, hospital administration and hospital counsel must be contacted immediately to expedite issues related to the adjudication of competency, appointment of a temporary guardian, or permission to proceed with treatment. When treatment, in the judgment of the physician, is emergently required to save the life of a minor, then treatment must be provided, regardless of the parent's objection.

- **In summary,** the role of the emergency physician in the management of the Jehovah's Witness is complex. Several points should be emphasized:
  - The emergency physician must understand the consequences, for the Witness, of accepting blood or blood component transfusion.
  - The medical basis necessitating transfusion of blood or blood products must be explained to the patient in clear terms and documented in this manner in the records.
  - When a determination is made that the patient is not competent, the basis for this decision must be clearly formulated and documented in the record, after which treatment should proceed.
  - If refusal is by a competent adult, to whom the basis for recommending transfusion and the probable consequences of refusal of treatment have been made clear, that is, death, then the patient should not undergo transfusion.
  - Minors should receive treatment if required to save life or limb.
  - Generally, parents may not refuse, on behalf of their minor children, if lifesaving treatment is emergently required; again, the basis for which should be clearly discussed with the family and documented in the record. When some time exists, hospital counsel must be contacted to assist the physician as discussed.
- To assist the physician in this complex process, the following **protocol** is very useful and is reproduced with the authors' permission.

DIAGNOSE ACUTE MEDICAL AND SURGICAL EMERGENCIES AND INSTITUTE APPROPRIATE NONBLOOD THERAPY

Determine the nature and severity of the presenting clinical problem.
Evaluate the potential need for blood component therapy.
Institute treatment with crystalloids and selective plasma volume expanders.

DETERMINE THE INDICATION FOR BLOOD COMPONENT THERAPY

Establish the clinical indication for blood replacement in acute hemorrhage.
Establish the indication for transfusion of specific blood components such as platelets, granulocytes, cryoprecipitate, coagulation factor concentrates, plasma, and immune globulins.

DETERMINE THAT THE CLINICAL NEEDS OF THE PATIENT EXCEED THE RISKS OF TRANSFUSION

Evaluate the consequences of withholding blood component therapy.
When possible, obtain corroboration and concurrence by another physician (such as another emergency physician or consultant, such as a surgeon) regarding the indication for transfusion.

(Continued)

ASSESS THE COMMITMENT TO RELIGIOUS BELIEFS

Assess the commitment of the Jehovah's Witness to his or her religious beliefs as early as possible during treatment.

It is neither advisable nor productive to persuade the patient to abandon or violate his or her beliefs and consent to transfusion.

PERFORM AN ASSESSMENT OF COMPETENCE

The adult patient should be considered competent and may determine the course of treatment, provided the following requirements are fulfilled: normal vital signs, normal mental status, no evidence of toxins or intoxicants, demonstration of sound decision making and understanding, and absence of suicidal ideation.

Incompetent patients and minors must be considered unable to decide to refuse therapy, and a surrogate decision maker should be identified or appointed.

Rarely, formal psychiatric consultation and evaluation of competence are warranted.

COMMUNICATE OPENLY WITH THE PATIENT AND THE FAMILY

Provide direct, complete explanations and recommendations.

Respect the right of the patient and family to ask questions and to express their objections to transfusion.

In cases of incompetent patients or minors, describe surrogate decision making, explain the implications of court intervention and temporary guardianship, and discuss the possibility of legal proceedings.

Be prepared to address emotional responses (confusion, anger, loss of control, and sense of crisis) and conflicts in the patient and among family members that may arise from the objection to transfusion and the involvement of legal authorities.

OBTAIN INFORMED CONSENT (INFORMED REFUSAL)

Conduct a detailed informed consent discussion with the patient and family that involves all information that a responsible person would consider when deciding to accept or refuse blood component therapy, including the following: nature of the medical or surgical problem; purpose and indication of the proposed therapy; risks, consequences, benefits, and alternative treatment, if any, to the administration of blood component therapy; and consequences of withholding treatment.

In the competent patient who requires but refuses recommended transfusion, obtain a signed informed consent document that indicates refusal.

OBTAIN LEGAL CONSULTATION

Contact with the hospital attorney early in the course of management is essential for the following reasons: to help clarify liability issues for the hospital and the emergency physician and to facilitate efforts, should it become necessary, to contact the court for judicial resolution of a transfusion issue, an adjudication of competency, or the appointment of a temporary guardian.

DOCUMENT FINDINGS AND RECOMMENDATIONS

Documentation should include the following: vital signs; history and physical examination; mental status evaluation; evidence of intact or impaired thought processes; detailed information regarding competency determination; recommended medical therapy; reasons for the patient's refusal of therapy, along with the options, risks involved, and consequences; all explanations, recommendations, and informed consent information discussed with the patient and family; a copy of the executed informed consent and informed refusal documents, signed by the patient and family members; and any legal steps taken, such as contact with the hospital lawyer or administrators or with court authorities.

DEVELOP A POLICY AND PROCEDURE FOR MANAGEMENT

Develop a hospital policy and procedure for management *before* the Jehovah's Witness presents to the ED.

A document releasing the hospital, emergency physician, and all other physicians and hospital personnel from liability arising from following the competent patient's wishes should be developed in conjunction with hospital legal counsel.

Establish a specific protocol for linkage with the appropriate court and child protection workers so that a coordinated and timely response can be instituted when necessary.

Become familiar with the manner in which the local court will conduct a telephone hearing dealing with emergency care.

Become knowledgeable of the state and local legislation concerning Jehovah's Witnesses.

Reproduced from Fontanarosa GP, Giorgio GT. The role of the emergency physician in the management of Jehovah's Witnesses. *Ann Emerg Med* 1989;18:1089–1095, with permission.

4 Head, Neck, and Facial Trauma

STABILIZATION OF THE PATIENT

One of the most difficult problems in emergency medicine is the patient presenting with serious head or facial trauma, an altered mental status, and respiratory arrest or respiratory insufficiency requiring immediate airway intervention. In these patients, because of the abnormality of mental status (which may include frank coma), it is not possible before radiologic evaluation for the physician to exclude a potentially unstable injury to the cervical spine. For this reason, the neck must remain immobilized until such time when an injury is radiologically excluded. Immobilization is provided by a combination of a spine board (to which the patient's head and body should be secured), a rigid or semirigid cervical collar (not a soft collar), and an assistant who remains at the head of the bed and maintains the head in the neutral position; all movement of the neck is thereby prevented, and other diagnostic and therapeutic maneuvers may safely be undertaken.

After immobilization, patients who are unconscious without respiratory effort require intubation to establish a functional airway, and this must be a first priority. Laryngoscopically guided oral intubation is the technique of choice and must be undertaken without movement of the cervical spine; an assistant is essential in this regard and should remain at the patient's head providing constant, in-line stabilization. Patients with inspiratory effort may be nasotracheally intubated provided that significant maxillofacial, perinasal, or basilar skull injuries are not present; when present or suspected, nasotracheal intubation is relatively contraindicated.

In patients **with inspiratory effort** but without adequate ventilation, mechanical obstruction of the upper airway should be suspected and must be quickly reversed. The pharynx and upper airway must be immediately examined and any foreign material removed either manually or by suction. Such material may include blood, other secretions, dental fragments, and foreign body or gastric contents, and a rigid suction device or forceps is most effective for its removal. Obstruction of the airway related to massive swelling, hematoma, or gross distortion of the anatomy should be noted as well, because a surgical procedure may then be required to establish an airway. In addition, airway obstruction related to posterior movement of the tongue is extremely common in lethargic or obtunded patients and is again easily reversible. In this setting, insertion of an oral or a nasopharyngeal airway, simple manual chin elevation, or the so-called jaw thrust, singly or in combination, may result in complete opening of the airway and may obviate the need for more aggressive means of upper airway management. Chin elevation and jaw thrust simply involve the manual upward or anterior displacement of the mandible in such a way that airway patency is enhanced. Not uncommonly, insertion of the oral airway or laryngeal mask airway may cause vomiting or gagging in semialert patients; when noted, the oral airway should be removed and chin elevation, the jaw thrust, or the placement of a nasopharyngeal airway undertaken. If unsuccessful, patients with inadequate oxygenation require rapid sequence oral, or nasotracheal, intubation immediately.

If an airway has not been obtained by one of these techniques, Ambu-bag–assisted ventilation using 100% oxygen should proceed while cricothyrotomy, by needle or incision, is undertaken rapidly. In children younger than 12 years, surgical crico-thyrotomy is relatively contraindicated and needle cricothyrotomy (using a 14-gauge needle placed through the cricothyroid membrane), followed by positive pressure insufflation, is indicated. During the procedure, or should the procedure be unsuc-cessful, Ambu-bag–assisted ventilation with 100% oxygen and an oral or a nasal air-way may provide adequate oxygenation.

In addition, rapidly correctable medical disorders that may cause central nervous system and respiratory depression must be immediately considered in all patients and may, in fact, have precipitated the injury by interfering with consciousness. In all patients with abnormalities of mental status, but particularly in those with ventilatory insufficiency requiring emergent intervention, blood should immediately be obtained for glucose and toxic screening, and the physician should then prophylactically treat hypoglycemia with 50 mL of 50% D/W, opiate overdose with naloxone (0.4–2.0 mg), and Wernicke encephalopathy with thiamine (100 mg). All medications should be administered sequentially and rapidly by intravenous injection and any improvement in mental status or respiratory function carefully noted. Should sufficient improvement occur, other more aggressive means of airway management might be unnecessary.

After an airway is established and secured, a rapid focused examination of the patient should be performed. First, the adequacy of ventilation must be determined by careful assessment of the chest and specific interventions undertaken as indicated; replacement of intravascular volume and control of blood loss remain additional priorities.

Patients without shock but with persisting abnormalities of mental status unrespon-sive to the administration of dextrose, naloxone, and thiamine must be assumed to have significant head injuries, and treatment should be initiated as described in "Head Injury." Importantly, however, in patients with a serious head injury and established or evolving shock, the customary means of reducing intracranial pressure (restriction of fluids, the administration of furosemide, mannitol) must be abandoned and the more immediately life-threatening deficit in intravascular volume corrected aggressively. In any patient pre-senting with trauma, but particularly in the patient with an abnormal mental status, the possibility of occult chest or abdominal injuries (or both) must be carefully investigated and excluded. When injuries to these areas are noted and pose an immediate threat to life, the neck must remain immobilized while appropriate intervention is pursued.

CERVICAL SPINE INJURY

Approximately 5% to 10% of unconscious patients presenting as a result of a fall or motor vehicle accident have a major injury to the cervical spine. A number of findings may further suggest cervical spine injury; these include other associated injuries above the clavicle, diaphragmatic breathing or apnea, flaccid areflexia including a flaccid rec-tal sphincter, a sensory level as demonstrated by facial gesturing in response to painful stimuli above the clavicles but not below them, and hypotension associated with a normal heart rate and warm extremities (spinal shock). Priapism, although unusual, is further suggestive of spinal injury.

As discussed in "Stabilization of the Patient," absolute immobilization of the cervical spine using a combination of a spine board, to which the patient's head is secured, and a rigid cervical collar is required until such time when the entirety of the cervical spine is demonstrated to be normal radiologically. To this end, a lateral radiograph of the cervical spine must be rapidly obtained; downward traction on the patient's arms will facilitate visualization of the more distal vertebrae and should be undertaken initially.

Unfortunately, on the initial lateral view of the cervical spine, only the first five or six cervical vertebral bodies are typically identified. This must not be interpreted by the physician as a normal study. In fact, an initial view of the cervical spine in the injured patient that demonstrates only the more proximal vertebrae can be an important diagnostic clue to the presence of a distal (C6 or C7) cervical injury. The pathophysiologic mechanism explaining this is that injuries to the distal cervical cord leave the shoulder elevators unopposed; involuntary elevation of the shoulders in these patients thereby obscures radiographic demonstration of the more distal cervical vertebrae. Thus, the only acceptable initial study of the cervical spine is a lateral view in which all cervical vertebrae, including C7 and the C7-T1 interface, are well visualized. To this end, the x-ray technician frequently requires the assistance of the emergency department staff. Most often, if gentle but firm downward traction on the arms is applied, a satisfactory view may be obtained. If a second view is unacceptable, the swimmer's view should be obtained and will demonstrate the most distal vertebrae. When the initial portable lateral view is normal, an anteroposterior, lateral, and open-mouth odontoid view of the cervical spine should be obtained in stable patients; if this is normal, immobilization of the neck may be discontinued and further evaluation of the patient's injuries undertaken. When immediate surgical intervention for other injuries is not required and the above views of the spine are complete and normal, further radiologic assessment of the skull may proceed. The open-mouth odontoid view will significantly decrease the number of patients in whom the diagnosis of an important cervical injury is missed, and this should routinely be obtained before allowing unrestricted movement of the patient.

If any doubt exists after these initial studies as to the possibility of a significant cervical injury, or if a potentially unstable or significant cervical injury is demonstrated, immediate neurosurgical or orthopaedic consultation should be obtained. Computed tomography (CT) is another imaging modality that can be used; often, in the head-and-neck-injured patient, it is time-saving to scan rapidly through the head and neck. Recent studies have demonstrated there may be benefits of **methylprednisolone** in patients with acute spinal cord injuries; when this diagnosis is highly probable based on physical examination, patients presenting within 8 hours of injury may benefit from an initial intravenous bolus of 30 mg/kg, followed by 5.4 mg/kg/h for 24 hours. Patients treated in this manner may demonstrate improved neurologic status subsequent to the injury; patients presenting after 8 hours should be discussed with a neurosurgical or orthopaedic specialist. During this time, the patient should remain immobilized on a spine board to which the head has been secured utilizing a rigid or semirigid cervical collar (not a soft collar).

Serious injuries to the **neck in children** represent a difficult challenge for the emergency physician. Most cord injuries in children occur as a result of motor vehicle accidents or falls and are often associated with injuries to the head. The type of injury one expects is somewhat related to the age of the child. **In children younger than 7 to 8 years**, because of larger head-to-body ratio (relatively), there is increased ligamentous laxity and lack of vertebral ossification, and injuries to the upper cervical spine are most common. These are often subluxation injuries rather than actual fractures.

This often produces the **SCIWORA phenomenon**, or spinal cord injury without radiographic abnormality. The most common cause is a fall or motor vehicle accident; injury occurs as a result of transient impingement of unstable vertebral elements against the cord, which when spontaneously reduced appears radiologically normal. Some patients will report weakness, paresthesias, or pain in the neck or back; however, in some children, neurologic abnormalities may not be noted for several days. This diagnosis is important to consider in patients with symptoms suggesting possible spinal cord injury (paresthesias, transient weakness or referred pain, electric or shock-like symptoms in the neck or back, persisting pain), commonly associated injuries or findings (head injury, loss of consciousness, mental status abnormalities), or significant mechanisms of injury (falls, diving, deceleration or rotational injuries associated with motor vehicle accidents [MVAs]). Undiagnosed spinal cord injury associated with instability may result in additional injury to the cord. **Children older than 8 years** typically injure the lower cervical spine, and most injuries are visible by x-ray; there is significantly less concern regarding SCIWORA.

Patients in whom a spinal cord injury is suspected, based on history, examination, or radiologic findings, should remain strictly immobilized while emergent neurosurgical or orthopaedic assistance is obtained; particular attention should be directed to the patient's airway and overall respiratory status. Cervical injuries at or above the third cervical vertebra cause immediate loss of spontaneous respiration, whereas injuries somewhat below this level may also jeopardize adequate ventilation. The current recommendation regarding the **establishment of an airway** in patients requiring airway intervention after traumatic arrest is cautious orotracheal intubation with in-line immobilization; patients who are unconscious, but breathing, and who require airway intervention are best managed with cautious rapid-sequence orotracheal intubation. Both nasotracheal intubation and cricothyrotomy cause less movement of the cervical spine; however, both are technically more difficult and potentially more time-consuming, particularly cricothyrotomy.

In regard to **management**, all patients with neck symptoms, even if minimal, should remain immobilized and have plain cervical spine films performed; all seven cervical vertebrae should be visualized, including the C7-T1 interface. Because of the unreliability of negative plain films in **younger children**, all patients require a careful reevaluation in regard to developing symptoms and signs of spinal cord injury. Children with signs of neck injury, persisting or progressive symptoms, or specific symptoms suggestive of spinal cord injury (see previous) should have additional studies, including CT-enhanced or -directed imaging in selected or suspicious areas. MRI, if rapidly available, can also be useful in these cases in terms of directly assessing cord and ligamentous injuries, provided the patient is sufficiently stable. Additionally, in patients with a mechanism of injury associated with spinal cord injury, particularly in younger children, additional studies should be considered. **Older children** who remain completely asymptomatic and who have normal physical findings and a mechanism of injury unassociated with spinal cord injury can generally be discharged after a brief period of observation without ancillary studies. Any developing findings require CT tomography or MRI before discharge. Any positive or suspicious findings should be discussed with the orthopaedist or neurosurgeon.

HEAD INJURY

Skull roentgenograms will add very little to the patient's immediate management. In seriously injured patients, however, one must assume that injury to the cervical spine coexists and immobilization, as discussed in "Stabilization of the Patient," must be adequate.

A number of important historical features and physical findings may be present in patients with head injuries and should be investigated:

History

- Obtaining a history from relatives, observers, or friends is an essential aspect of the initial evaluation; specifically, any previous neurologic abnormalities, drug allergies, or medical problems should be identified. Details related to the injury should be ascertained; for example, what did police or emergency medical technicians estimate to be the speed of the vehicle or the distance of the fall? What was the condition of the automobile, steering wheel, and windshield? Was the patient noted to be initially conscious? What exactly did the patient fall on? Was the patient wearing a seat belt? Was an air bag deployed? Did the car rollover?

- If possible, the patient should be asked specifically about cervical area discomfort or related symptoms. Patients with abnormalities of mental status or reporting mild or vague discomfort or dysesthesias in the neck, shoulders, or upper extremities should have the cervical spine immobilized and a lateral cervical spine radiograph obtained to rule out any potentially important injury in this area.

- The patient should be asked to reconstruct the accident as well as events before and after the injury. Inability to do so suggests loss of consciousness or amnesia.

- Medical conditions that commonly precipitate trauma by interfering with consciousness should be carefully investigated. Chest pain or palpitations before or after the injury suggest cardiac-related disturbances in cardiac output, whereas anxiety or diaphoresis in the diabetic patient suggests hypoglycemia. Importantly in diabetics, hypoglycemia may have been corrected by stress or epinephrine-induced gluconeogenesis; therefore, a normal or relatively normal blood sugar after trauma should not be used to exclude preceding hypoglycemia. A history of seizure disorder, an aura before the injury, evidence of tongue biting or other intraoral injury, and loss of continence suggest seizure and, along with recent alcohol or drug ingestion, should be investigated. Specific neurologic symptoms occurring before the incident are helpful if recalled; a period of normal intellectual function after trauma followed by a deteriorating mental status or coma suggests epidural hemorrhage.

Physical Examination

- The most important guide to the management of the patient with head trauma is the mental status and its serial reevaluation (see Glasgow Coma Scale, Table 4-1). In patients with normal or relatively normal blood pressure and adequate oxygenation, significant abnormalities of mental status not responding to intravenous 50% dextrose, naloxone, and thiamine must be assumed to be secondary to injury to the brain and be treated as such. Mental status should be investigated in the usual manner, along with the routine neurologic examination, but the physician must recognize those subtle changes in personality reported by the family of the patient, such as combativeness or unusual aggressiveness. Also, subtle degrees of emotional lability may accompany important cerebral injuries and may be the first and often the only clue to their presence.

- Hypotension is not a usual finding in patients with isolated head injuries except when massive bleeding from the scalp occurs or as a terminal event; other injuries to the chest and abdomen must therefore be presumed to be present and excluded. Spinal shock may result in hypotension, although it is generally not profound, and this must remain a diagnosis of exclusion; when compared with hemorrhagic shock,

Table 4-1	Adult Glasgow Coma Scale	

Criterion	Score
Eye-opening response	
Spontaneous–already open with blinking	4
To speech–not necessary to request eye opening	3
To pain–stimulus should not be to the face	2
None–make note if eyes are swollen shut	1
Verbal response	
Oriented–knows name, age, etc.	5
Confused conversation–still answers questions	4
Inappropriate words–speech is either exclamatory or at random	3
Incomprehensible sounds–do not confuse with partial respiratory obstruction	2
None–make note if patient is intubated	1
Best upper limb motor response (pain applied to nail bed)	
Obeys–moves limb to command; pain is not required	6
Localizes–changing the location of the painful stimulus causes the limb to follow	5
Withdraws–pulls away from painful stimulus	4
Abnormal flexion–decorticate posturing	3
Extensor response–decerebrate posturing	2
No response	1

the extremities are warm and the pulse remains within the normal range. In these patients, other evidence of spinal cord injury is usually present, including flaccid paralysis, a flaccid rectal sphincter, a sensory level, apnea, or diaphragmatic breathing, and, occasionally, priapism.

- Ecchymosis and local swelling or hematoma that is overlying the area of the mastoid (Battle sign) suggest a temporal fracture, whereas medial orbital ecchymosis (raccoon eyes) suggests a fracture of the basilar skull. Blood behind the tympanic membrane (hemotympanum) or cerebrospinal fluid in the external auditory canal further supports the diagnosis of basilar skull fracture. A clear, watery nasal discharge in the traumatized patient that is determined to be of physiologic pH is characteristic of cerebrospinal fluid rhinorrhea and is also suggestive of fracture of the basilar skull.

- Papilledema is not an expected finding in the acutely traumatized patient because, in patients with elevated intracranial pressure, 10 or 12 hours is generally required for the development of this sign.

- A significantly dilated pupil, which may be initially reactive, is an important indicator of substantially elevated intracranial pressure and imminent transtentorial herniation; a contralateral or ipsilateral hemiparesis may be found as well. Emergency intervention as outlined in "Cerebral Contusion: Established Neural Dysfunction" is indicated acutely to reduce intracranial pressure.

Diagnostic Tests

As noted, skull radiographs add very little to immediate management. We suggest obtaining an immediate CT of the head without contrast in the following groups of patients:

- Patients with obvious focal neurologic deficits or an altered mental status
- Patients with a period of unconsciousness after the injury
- Patients with a palpable bony abnormality of the skull
- Patients in whom the history is unreliable or unobtainable because of age, intoxication, amnesia, or abnormalities of mental status
- Patients with penetrating trauma or injuries resulting from instruments or devices likely to depress the skull

General Principles of Management

Although patients presenting acutely with skull fractures must be managed on the basis of their individual clinical presentation and status, we believe that all such patients should be admitted to the hospital for observation. A small number of these patients with an initially normal neurologic examination and an unimpressive history will deteriorate and require urgent evaluation and care.

A few special injuries deserve additional discussion:

- Temporal fractures that cross the area of the meningeal artery are worrisome in that epidural hemorrhage related to arterial disruption may occur; careful in-hospital observation of these patients is therefore warranted.
- Depressed fractures often require operative elevation; therefore, admission and immediate neurosurgical consultation are appropriate.
- Basilar skull fractures, while producing a variety of clinical signs, may produce little in the way of radiologic findings; a diagnosis of "clinical basilar fracture" is therefore justified in patients with hemotympanum, cerebrospinal fluid otorrhea or rhinorrhea, or other clinical evidence of fracture despite normal roentgenograms.
- Compound fractures of the skull are managed as discussed in Chapter 10; aggressive irrigation, cleansing, and debridement are required and best performed in the operating room.

Conservative guidelines with respect to recommending admission for observation in selected patients with head injuries include

- Patients with significant amnesia
- Patients with focal neurologic findings
- Patients with skull fractures
- Patients with severe or progressive headache or vomiting
- Patients with abnormalities of mental status, particularly if progressive
- Patients with a potentially significant injury but without a competent adult to observe the patient after discharge

Specific orders for admitted patients depend on the physician's assessment of the extent of injury. Sleep medications are contraindicated during the initial period of observation, and aspirin should be avoided because of its effect on platelet function; headache should be treated initially with acetaminophen only, which may be administered by rectal suppository if necessary. In addition, narcotics should not be used during the initial period of emergency department observation because they may interfere with or make uninterpretable the sequential assessment of mental status during this period. Serial reassessment of neurovital signs is undertaken in all admitted patients, the frequency of which is determined by patients' clinical condition. Oral intake is generally restricted for the initial 24 hours, during which time isotonic maintenance fluids are administered intravenously.

SPECIFIC HEAD INJURIES

Concussion: Transient Neural Dysfunction

Concussion is classically defined as a transient episode of neural dysfunction resulting in temporary loss of consciousness after blunt trauma to the head.

- **Diagnosis.** At the time of examination, the mental status and general neurologic function are normal or rapidly improving; pathologically, simple concussion is not associated with any identifiable brain injury. Persisting abnormalities of consciousness, thought, speech, or the presence of other specific neurologic deficits imply cerebral contusion, which is discussed in "Cerebral Contusion: Established Neural Dysfunction." Although most physicians insist that a history of loss of consciousness be present before a specific diagnosis of "concussion" is justified, it is well recognized that a number of other symptoms may occur in association with or after head trauma and may imply an injury of similar severity. Amnesia, for example, suggests a significant concussive force. Other symptoms frequently reported in these patients include transient confusion, nausea and vomiting, light-headedness, vertigo, and a feeling of depersonalization.

  As noted, patients should specifically be asked to reconstruct the details of the accident, both before and after the specific injury; failure to do so suggests either loss of consciousness at the time of injury or amnesia. In addition, patients should specifically be questioned about discomfort in the cervical area, and if symptoms are reported in this area, if the history is unreliable or unobtainable, if abnormalities of mental status are present, or if an injury is suspected, then radiologic evaluation of the cervical spine should be obtained while the neck remains immobilized.

- **Treatment.** All patients with transient loss of consciousness, significant amnesia, or other severe or progressive central nervous system symptoms should have a CT scan of the head without contrast and cervical spine radiographs and be observed in the hospital.

- **Indications for emergency neurosurgical consultation and/or CT scanning** of the head include
  - Loss of consciousness (more than just seconds)
  - Antegrade amnesia over 5 minutes
  - Nausea or vomiting
  - Photophobia
  - Focal neurologic findings
  - Clinical evidence of skull fracture (including basilar skull fracture)
  - Penetrating head injury
  - Deteriorating mental status
  - New seizure
  - A headache that is becoming progressively worse
  - Head trauma involving significant acceleration/deceleration injury in those younger than age 2 and older than age 70* and in alcoholics*

---

*Between the ages of 30 and 70, the brain shrinks by 10%, making it easier for bridging veins to be injured, increasing the risk of a subdural hematoma. The same holds true for alcoholics, particularly those who are older than age 60.

Cerebral Contusion: Established Neural Dysfunction

Cerebral contusion is diagnosed on the basis of a persisting neurologic deficit after trauma to the head; this may include a reduced level of consciousness that is not rapidly improving, other abnormalities of thinking or speech, or other focal deficits.

Patients presenting to the emergency department after head trauma with any of the following signs or symptoms require urgent diagnostic evaluation and often the initiation of specific measures to lower intracranial pressure: mental status abnormalities, including a reduced level of consciousness, that are not rapidly improving; seizure activity; a focal or evolving neurologic deficit; and severe or worsening headache associated with evidence of increasing intracranial pressure.

The following recommendations are appropriate in these patients concurrent with CT and neurosurgical consultation.

- Intravenous access should be established and isotonic fluids administered at a keep-open rate to minimize fluid-induced cerebral edema.
- A number of additional disorders may mimic cerebral contusion and may have precipitated the accident initially by interfering with consciousness; 50 mL of 50% D/W, 0.4 to 2.0 mg of naloxone, and 100 mg of thiamine should be administered sequentially by rapid intravenous administration to all patients.
- Neurosurgical consultation should then be obtained as rapidly as possible; details related to the mechanism of injury and the patient's initial and present neurologic state described in descriptive terms are important observations and should be noted. How the patient appears and what the patient does in response to verbal and painful stimuli, whether any focal deficits are identified, and whether injuries to the cervical spine, chest, or abdomen coexist are important observations. When the patient last ate and any religious contraindications to treatment are additionally useful details if obtainable.
- The airway should be evaluated and protected.
- Patients who are unconscious or seize, or those whose mental status abnormalities are severe or progressive should be intubated and hyperventilated to maintain an arterial PCO_2 between 25 and 30 mm Hg. In addition, any patient with a significant head injury requiring emergency transfer for diagnostic or therapeutic intervention should be prophylactically intubated.
- A nasogastric tube should be carefully placed, provided contraindications do not exist (suspicion of basilar skull fracture or major perinasal or facial trauma), and the stomach contents emptied to prevent aspiration should vomiting occur.
- When injuries to the central nervous system are believed to be responsible for a persisting neurologic deficit, we recommend an immediate CT scan of the head should be obtained.
- Adults presenting with or developing seizures should be treated with phenytoin, which can be administered as rapidly as 50 mg/min (in normal saline) to a total of 1 g or 10 to 15 mg/kg in children administered not faster than 1 mg/kg/min. Persistent seizures associated with progressive acidosis or inability to adequately ventilate or intubate the patient may be terminated with diazepam, which may be administered to adults initially as 10 mg intravenous followed by 5-mg increments and to children in an initial dose of 0.1 to 0.25 mg/kg administered not faster than 1 mg/min to a maximum dose of 10 mg. A repeat dose may be given in 10 to 15 minutes if needed. Ativan may also be used in this setting. For adults, the initial dosage is 4 mg by slow intravenous push; this may be repeated once in 10 to 15 minutes. The dose of Ativan in children is 0.05 mg/kg by slow intravenous push, which may be repeated once as described.

• Patients demonstrating evidence of transtentorial herniation, who may present with a unilaterally dilated and often initially reactive pupil, must be aggressively treated. Ophthalmoplegia and contralateral or ipsilateral hemiparesis may be noted as well. Measures to decrease intracranial pressure along with urgent neurosurgical consultation should be immediately undertaken. When neurosurgical consultation is unavailable and deterioration is clear, emergency burr hole placement may be useful. A burr hole should be placed first on the same side as the dilated pupil, in the ipsilateral frontal, parietal, and then temporal areas. If this is unsuccessful, then similar contralateral placement may follow.

Acute Subdural and Epidural Hematoma

• **Acute subdural hematomas** may be either unilateral or bilateral and produce headaches, drowsiness, slowness in thinking, occasional agitation, or confusion, all of which may worsen progressively. A latent interval between the injury and the obvious progression to these symptoms may occur, lasting from several days to 2 weeks. Focal findings, including hemiplegia and aphasia, tend to occur late in the evolution of the process, being less prominent than the disturbances of consciousness noted in the disorder. Cerebral contusion is often associated with acute subdural hematoma, and the clinical distinction between these disorders is difficult, if not impossible, to make. Once frank coma has occurred, mortality approaches 50%. Temporal burr hole placement and clot evacuation are the essential therapeutic maneuvers. If herniation is imminent, emergency burr hole placement may be required.

• **Acute epidural hematomas** are typically caused by acute temporal or parietal bone fractures producing laceration of the middle meningeal artery and vein. In the classic presentation, the patient does not lose consciousness after the injury or is only momentarily unconscious. A latent period or "lucid interval" ensues, lasting from several hours to 2 days, after which increasingly severe headache, vomiting, drowsiness, confusion, seizures, and/or hemiparesis develop. Coma associated with findings suggesting markedly increased intracerebral pressure and imminent herniation may develop, often including pupillary dilation on the side of the hematoma, bradycardia, hypertension, and changes in the respiratory pattern. CT permits prompt diagnosis. Burr hole placement and clot evacuation are the essential therapeutic maneuvers; temporal or parietal burr holes may need to be placed emergently if temporal herniation is imminent. Operative results are generally excellent if delays in diagnosis and surgery are not unduly prolonged.

Penetrating Injuries to the Neck

Objects, usually knives, ice picks, or other instruments, located deep within the neck at presentation must be left in place and removed in the operating room. The object itself and surrounding hematoma may serve to tamponade lacerated vessels.

Given the extremely high density of vital structures within the neck (Fig. 4-1), combined with an increased prevalence of expanding and high-velocity bullets in civilian injuries, it is not surprising that mortality associated with such injuries is high. Furthermore, as missile velocity increases, damage to structures not directly in the trajectory of the bullet increases markedly. Therefore, in all but the most trivial of penetrating injuries, operative exploration of the neck may be required. Control of the airway by oropharyngeal or nasotracheal intubation or cricothyrotomy, if necessary, and fluid or blood resuscitation are obvious first priorities.

A variety of specific injuries may complicate the management of patients with penetrating injuries to the neck; these include massive bleeding and injury to the

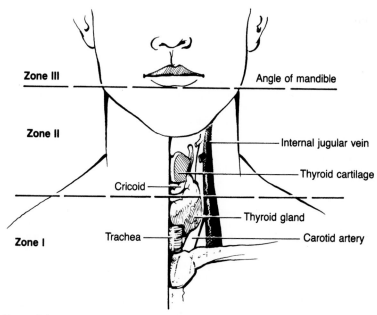

Figure 4-1. Anterior view of the neck. Significant structures and the zones of the neck are illustrated. (From Harwood-Nuss AL, Linden CH, Luten RC, et al., eds. *The clinical practice of emergency medicine*, 2nd ed. Philadelphia, PA: Lippincott-Raven, 1996:428, with permission.)

airway. Massive bleeding is associated with disruption of major, superficial venous vessels or the carotid. Bleeding should be treated initially with external, direct, manual compression only. Blind clamping or ligating of vessels and circumferential wraps are contraindicated, and in most patients, direct pressure alone will temporarily control bleeding. Neck wounds associated with bubbling or frothing suggest penetration of the airway; when noted, endotracheal tube passage and inflation distal to the site of presumed interruption are the treatment of choice before exploration (Table 4-2).

Laryngeal Injury

Blunt or penetrating trauma to the anterior or lateral neck may result in injury to the larynx; diagnostically, subcutaneous emphysema, crepitus, change or loss of voice, hoarseness, stridor, and local pain may all be noted. Lateral movement of the larynx may be associated with grating or crepitation in patients with cartilage disruption. In addition, when viewed from a lateral perspective, loss of the normally occurring cartilaginous landmarks may be apparent and may produce marked flattening of the neck. A vertical midline fracture of the thyroid cartilage is the most common laryngeal fracture.

Soft-tissue or xeroradiographic films of the neck and CT are helpful in confirming the nature and extent of injury as is fiberoptic laryngoscopy. Complete obstruction of the airway may occur in patients with significant crushing injuries or hemorrhage and may require emergent intubation, if possible, or tracheostomy. Early otolaryngologic consultation is advised when abnormalities of voice are noted after injury to the neck.

Table 4-2	Zones of the Neck

Three zones of the neck have been described. Injuries to each of these zones have different prognoses.

Zone I (top of the sternum to the cricoid cartilage)
Structures involved: thoracic outlet, great vessels, apices of the lungs, thoracic duct, thyroid gland, esophagus, airway
Management: often requires operative exploration
Mortality rates: very high because of operative difficulty

Zone II (cricoid cartilage to the angle of the mandible; accounts for up to 80% of penetrating neck injuries)
Structures involved: carotid artery, jugular vein, pharynx, larynx, esophagus, trachea
Management: bleeding control, exploration
Mortality rates: relatively low

Zone III (angle of the jaw to the base of the skull)
Structures involved: pharynx, mouth, carotid artery, jugular vein, parotid gland, cranial nerves, spinal cord, intracranial structures
Management: angiography necessary to evaluate distal internal carotid artery
Mortality rates: high morbidity due to difficulty of exposure

Facial Injury

Lacerations involving the face are discussed in Chapter 48. Facial trauma, although presenting dramatically, is rarely associated with mortality unless compromise of the airway occurs or other associated injuries threaten survival. The physician must recognize that important injuries to the head and cervical spine frequently coexist and must be suspected and diagnosed as early as possible. In addition, one must remember the overwhelming cosmetic and social importance of many facial injuries and the need for appropriate diagnosis and thorough treatment.

Nasal Fractures

Nasal fractures, although common, are clinically significant only if displaced, open, or associated with septal hematoma. Although radiologic assessment of the nasal bones may not alter immediate therapy, we generally recommend such assessment in patients with significant injuries to establish a diagnosis and thereby direct postinjury care.

Because the distal nose is entirely cartilaginous, it is radiolucent; obvious fracture deformities in this area, which will require definitive reduction, are therefore often not associated with any radiologic abnormality. In these patients with "clinically displaced nasal fractures," which is an appropriate diagnosis, and in other patients with radiologically demonstrated displaced fractures, either immediate or delayed reduction may be elected by the subspecialist. If delayed reduction is chosen, frequently 3 to 5 days after the injury, patients without head injuries may be administered an analgesic and instructed to apply a cold compress for 12 to 18 hours, to elevate the head on several pillows to reduce swelling, and to expect several days of posture-related changes in local swelling. Patients, and particularly parents, should be told that swelling increases with recumbency and improves during periods of activity simply because of the effect of gravity. Patients without deformity, displacement, or septal hematoma of the nose may be treated conservatively; however, follow-up in 4 to 5 days is recommended if the patient notes any cosmetic or functional defect. In addition, the symptoms and signs caused by the development of septal hematoma (increased pain, swelling inside the nose, obstruction of the naris, or a palpable hematoma involving the septum) should be discussed with the patient; if noted, immediate otolaryngologic or surgical consultation should be advised. Open or compound fractures are treated with thorough irrigation and cleansing, and patients should receive an appropriate antistaphylococcal antibiotic for 5 to 7 days. If a deformity is apparent, then the otolaryngologist or plastic surgeon may elect immediate reduction; therefore, consultation before discharge is appropriate.

As previously noted, in all patients with nasal fractures, hematomas of the septal area must be excluded and, if present, otolaryngologic consultation obtained; aspiration or incision and drainage of the hematoma will be undertaken. If undiagnosed, cosmetically devastating destruction of the superior portion of the nasal cartilage may result. Epistaxis may occasionally occur in association with nasal fractures and may be treated as described in Chapter 13.

Sinus Injury

With respect to the frontal sinus, it must be remembered that although radiologically depressed fractures may produce no cosmetically significant deformity at the time of injury, as local swelling subsides, a significant "indenting" type of defect may result. Otolaryngologic or plastic surgical referral is therefore appropriate 7 to 10 days after the injury, by which time local swelling will have subsided and the defect may be visualized and corrected if indicated. Fractures involving the posterior wall of the frontal sinus must be assumed to have torn the dura, and these patients should be treated with hospitalization, elevation of the head to 60 degrees if possible, and a course of antibiotics. Although the efficacy of antibiotics has not been clearly determined, most authors favor their use.

Ethmoid fractures are treated similarly. Cerebrospinal fluid rhinorrhea may occur and, if it does, confirms a dural tear. These patients require hospitalization, elevation of the head to 60 degrees, and a course of antibiotic therapy.

Maxillary Fractures

Maxillary fractures are produced by massive trauma to the face and have been classified by LeFort (Table 4-3). Waters radiologic view of the skull is the most sensitive plain film for identifying these injuries; however, CT is more sensitive. The clinical diagnosis is based on localized tenderness, malocclusion, and anteroposterior instability of the maxilla when the upper incisors and palate are grasped and force is exerted in the horizontal plane. Importantly, impacted fractures may not be associated with abnormal mobility, and in many patients, malocclusion will not be reported. In addition, in severely injured patients, posterior displacement of the maxilla may result in acute airway obstruction as local edema and hemorrhage evolve; in these patients, reduction of the fracture may be urgently required to establish an airway. Airway obstruction is possible with either a Le Fort II or Le Fort III fracture. The physician places the index and long fingers in the patient's mouth, "hooks" the palate, and pulls forward with some force, thereby accomplishing reduction.

Patients with maxillary fractures most often require hospitalization, observation, and, depending on the type of fracture, definitive surgical repair.

Table 4-3	Le Fort Fractures of the Maxilla	
Le Fort Class	**Area/Type**	**Airway Compromise**
I	Maxillary alveolar fracture (horizontal, crossing lateral wall of the maxillary sinus)	Rarely
II	Includes bony nasal skeleton and middle third of face; zygomas remain attached to base of the skull	Uncommonly
III	Facial bones in a block are separated from the base of the skull	Occasionally

Zygomatic Fractures

The zygoma, which forms the bony prominence of the lateral cheek, may be fractured as a result of a variety of insults. These include motor vehicle accidents, falls, and altercations. Patients report localized tenderness, and swelling is noted over the area of the fracture. A clinical diagnosis should be possible on the basis of a number of important findings: A "step-off" may be noted along the lateral or inferior orbital rim, trismus may be demonstrated in patients with fractures involving the area of the temporomandibular joint (TMJ), and diplopia, most often horizontal, may be noted in patients with lateral rectus damage or entrapment. Vertical diplopia suggests injury to and possible entrapment of the inferior rectus and/or inferior oblique muscles. In addition, anesthesia involving the territory of the infraorbital nerve (second division of cranial nerve V) and inferior displacement of the involved eye are important findings.

Waters projection and submental vertex views are useful radiographic studies in the demonstration of zygomatic fractures as is facial CT. Fractures that are displaced or rotated will generally require open reduction and fixation. Patients with disturbances of vision, as previously noted, require emergent ophthalmologic consultation.

Orbital Floor Fractures

Orbital floor or "blow-out" fractures typically occur as a result of blunt trauma to the eye or lids; these fractures may or may not be associated with injury to the eye itself and usually result from fist, ball, or other generally nonpenetrating contact. Sudden increases in intraorbital pressure result in a blow-out fracture (i.e., a fracture producing inferior displacement of the relatively weak orbital floor). The contents of the inferior orbit, particularly the inferior oblique and inferior rectus muscles, may herniate through the fracture site and, with evolving edema, may become entrapped and subsequently ischemic.

- The **diagnosis** of orbital floor fracture is frequently difficult, particularly when some delay occurs between injury and presentation; in these patients, local swelling may be marked. A history of blunt trauma to the eye is usually elicited, periorbital edema and ecchymosis, enophthalmos (backward displacement of the eye), infraorbital nerve anesthesia (upper lip, gingiva), and subconjunctival hemorrhage may be present. If inferior oblique or inferior rectus muscle entrapment exists, then limitation of eye movement may be noted. Diplopia associated with muscle entrapment may be elicited historically or may be demonstrated by the physician. Enophthalmos is a very important sign of orbital floor fracture, but it may be masked by local swelling and hemorrhage. Radiologic assessment of the orbit, including the Waters projection, should routinely be obtained when a diagnosis of orbital floor fracture is suspected. The Waters projection is particularly helpful, as is the orbital CT scan, in difficult or subtle fractures. Radiologic findings in patients with orbital floor fracture include clouding of the ipsilateral maxillary sinus (secondary to local hemorrhage or extrusion of orbital soft tissues into the sinus), fragmentation or disruption of the inferior orbital floor often with depression of bony fragments into the sinus, and infraorbital free air.

• **Treatment.** Patients with fractures of the orbital floor associated with diplopia or impaired extraocular muscle function require urgent ophthalmologic consultation because operative intervention may be required. In other patients, many authorities recommend a brief course of oral penicillin, Augmentin, or erythromycin and instructions to the patient to refrain from blowing the nose for 10 to 14 days, because this maneuver may introduce the contents of the sinus into the orbit through the fracture site.

Mandibular Fractures

Patients with fractures of the mandible present with localized pain and malocclusion. Panoramic or Panorex radiographic views, if available, are diagnostically more sensitive than routine radiographic studies for these fractures. Subjective dental malocclusion after trauma is a relatively specific symptom that should be radiographically investigated in all patients. It is important to remember that, although direct injury to the mandible may produce local fracture because of the topology of the mandible, an additional fracture is typically found elsewhere. Patients with mandibular fractures should generally be admitted to the hospital because fixation and a period of observation are usually indicated.

Dental Injuries

Teeth that are partially or completely avulsed from the socket can often be saved if appropriate treatment is instituted early. Partially avulsed teeth should be reseated and generally do well. Completely avulsed teeth may be reintroduced into the socket; this is preferably performed by the oral surgeon or dentist and must be undertaken early if teeth are to survive. When consultation would produce a delay of more than 30 minutes to 1 hour, reinsertion by the emergency physician may be undertaken and the tooth secured to adjacent teeth with suture material. Both en route to the emergency department with avulsed teeth and while in the department, teeth must be kept moist in a balanced, physiologic solution; saliva is appropriate en route (an awake, alert patient with no airway compromise can frequently hold the tooth in his or her mouth), and normal saline should be provided in the emergency department. Teeth that are completely avulsed and out of the socket for more than 18 to 24 hours generally do not survive, and reimplantation should not be attempted. Similarly, deciduous or baby teeth need not be reimplanted. Patients with partial avulsions, and particularly all patients with total avulsions, should be warned that the reimplanted tooth or teeth, because removed from the blood supply, might die. Discussion with and referral to an oral surgeon or dentist are appropriate.

Teeth that are fractured distally, if the detached fragment is recovered, can often be repaired or bonded to the remaining fragment; these should be retained and consultation obtained (Fig. 4-2).

Diagram of the Tooth Numbering System
(viewed as if looking into the mouth)

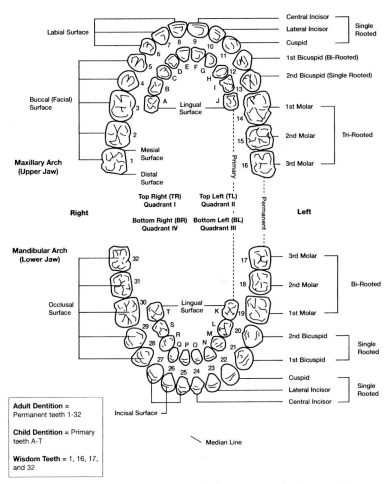

Figure 4-2. Dental anatomy. Common method of numbering teeth. (Courtesy of Ameritas Group, Lincoln, Nebraska.)

Avulsed or broken teeth may be aspirated and may occasionally enter coexistent intraoral or lip lacerations. In the patient with dental trauma in which teeth are fractured or avulsed and unaccounted for, a chest roentgenogram is usually advised to rule out occult aspiration. Lateral radiographic views of the lips or lateral "puff" cheek views are often helpful in patients with dental trauma and associated lip or intraoral injuries; previously unsuspected tooth fragments are often noted and of course must be removed before closure.

Temporomandibular Joint Dislocation

Dislocation of the TMJ may follow trauma to the face or may occur as a result of simply opening the mouth widely; yawning or chewing frequently precedes TMJ dislocation. Patients report severe discomfort, inability to close the mouth, and varying degrees of anxiety. Radiologic assessment of the mandible is indicated before attempts at reduction because condylar fractures are occasionally present and should be documented before manipulation. Bilateral dislocations often occur, and these should be treated as discussed.

- Importantly, **dystonic reactions to phenothiazine** may simulate TMJ dislocation, as well as a variety of other conditions. This phenomenon should be considered in all such patients and can usually be confirmed on the basis of history and treated with intravenous diphenhydramine, 50 mg in adults and 0.5 to 1.0 mg/kg in children. Adults may also be administered intravenous benztropine mesylate (Cogentin), 1 to 2 mg over 1 to 2 minutes.

- **Reduction.** Otolaryngologic or oral surgical consultation for reduction should be obtained in patients with coexistent condylar or other fractures. When coexistent fractures and acute dystonic reactions are excluded, reduction may be performed in the emergency department. Initial treatment begins by reassuring the patient and beginning a continuous infusion of 5% D/W. Although not always necessary, small intravenous doses of midazolam or diazepam are helpful in terms of relieving anxiety and eliminating local muscle spasm. A short-acting intravenous narcotic, such as fentanyl, may also be useful in this setting for reduction of pain and sedation. (Muscle spasm effectively acts to maintain the dislocation by exerting upward pull on the proximal mandible.) The patient should be placed supine on a stretcher with the head resting on a pillow. The position of the patient should facilitate downward pressure on the mandible; the physician must remember that dislocations occur superiorly. The physician should wrap padding around his or her thumbs before attempting a reduction. The physician places each padded thumb on top of the patient's posterior molars in such a way that the body of the mandible fits into the physician's palms and the fingers curl under the anterior mandible at or near the symphysis. Direct downward traction is gently applied to the mandible with slowly and gradually increasing force. In most patients, simply displacing the mandible inferiorly will result in spontaneous reduction. Occasionally, while downward traction is maintained on the mandible, gently elevating the symphysis with the fingers and pushing the mandible slightly posteriorly will be additionally required. Several attempts are occasionally required to relax or fatigue the musculature sufficiently. If reduction is not successful, then otolaryngologic or oral surgical consultation is indicated. Postreduction measures include a short course of analgesics for patients with significant spasm or discomfort and 3 to 4 days of soft foods with avoidance of widely opening the mouth.

Soft-Tissue Injuries of the Face

Lacerations involving the soft tissues of the face are discussed in Chapter 48.

- Lacerations occurring **between the tragus of the ear and either the corner of the eye or mouth** must be carefully examined to exclude injury to the facial nerve, parotid gland, and parotid duct. Motor function in the face, including eye closure, must be carefully assessed and noted. Lacerations involving these structures, particularly the proximal facial nerve or parotid duct, require plastic surgical or otolaryngologic consultation for repair.

• With its extensive and superficial distribution in the face and upper neck, the **facial nerve** is at great risk for interruption. Motor function in the face must therefore be carefully assessed in all patients before instrumentation or instillation of anesthetic agents. Patients with motor deficits require urgent subspecialty consultation because repair will be most successful if undertaken as soon as possible after the injury. Occasionally, with very peripheral interruptions, the consultant will elect not to repair or to defer the repair of these neural lacerations.

Traumatic Deafness

Hearing loss occurring after trauma is relatively uncommon; when noted, a slapping, diving, or blunt injury to the external ear or lateral head; an explosive injury; or actual fracturing of the skull has usually preceded the onset of symptoms. Injuries expected to produce conductive hearing deficits include perforation of the tympanic membrane, fracture or dislocation of the ossicles, obliteration of the patency of the external auditory canal, the presence of foreign material within the canal, hemorrhage into the middle ear, and, in patients with temporal skull fracture, actual tearing of the tympanic membrane. Fractures of the skull may result in sensorineural deficits because of direct crushing or disruption of the eighth nerve or organ of Corti. Patients exposed to explosive blasts, including the firing of handguns, may present with deafness caused by tympanic membrane or middle ear injury, or interference with cochlear hair cell function. Otolaryngologic consultation is advised for these patients.

5 Eye and Periorbital Trauma

The role of the emergency physician in the evaluation of patients with eye and periorbital trauma is to determine that visual acuity, extraocular muscle function, the corneal surface, and the fundus are normal. Limitation of extraocular movements or diplopia, for which all patients deserve careful evaluation, is an important finding and suggests the need for urgent ophthalmologic consultation. In addition, the importance of fluorescein staining of the cornea followed by examination under ultraviolet light cannot be overemphasized and must be routinely performed in all patients with ocular symptoms. The evaluation of patients with periorbital trauma should begin as soon as possible because local swelling, if marked, may interfere with ocular assessment.

Radiologic assessment should be considered in all patients with significant periorbital trauma because signs of ophthalmologic injury need not be present in patients with important fractures. The need for urgent consultation in patients with posttraumatic limitation of extraocular movement or diplopia is also important to emphasize because surgical intervention may be necessary.

BLUNT INJURIES TO THE EYE AND ORBIT

Blunt injuries to the eye and orbit may result in periorbital contusion ("black eye"), orbital or ethmoid fractures, corneal abrasions and/or foreign bodies, traumatic iritis, hyphema, dislocation of the lens, or actual rupture of the globe.

Periorbital Contusion

- Trauma to the periorbital structures may result in local blood vessel disruption and rapidly evolving, often extensive, swelling and ecchymosis; this reflects the relative distensibility of the periorbital soft tissues.
- Patients should be advised to avoid aspirin, to apply cold to the area (never a chemical ice pack, which may leak), and to expect swelling and ecchymosis to persist for several days to weeks.
- Elevating the head of the bed or using several pillows may somewhat impede gravity-induced nocturnal swelling.
- In patients with periorbital contusion, the eye itself must be carefully examined to exclude more significant injury.
- CT assessment of the orbit in patients with significant periorbital trauma is recommended (when available) because the classic signs of orbital fracture are frequently absent.

Orbital Floor Fracture

- Orbital floor or "blow-out" fractures typically occur as a result of blunt trauma to the globe; these fractures may or may not be associated with injury to the eye itself and usually result from fist, ball, or other generally nonpenetrating contact.

- Sudden increases in intraorbital pressure result in a blow-out fracture, that is, a fracture producing inferior displacement of the relatively weak orbital floor. Contents of the inferior orbit, particularly the inferior oblique and inferior rectus muscles, may herniate through the fracture site and, with evolving edema, may become entrapped and ischemic.

Diagnosis
- Diagnosis is frequently difficult, particularly when delay occurs between injury and presentation; in these patients, local swelling may be marked.
- A history of blunt trauma to the eye may be elicited; periorbital edema and ecchymosis, enophthalmos (backward displacement of the eye), infraorbital nerve anesthesia (upper lip gingiva), and subconjunctival hemorrhage may be present.
- If inferior oblique or inferior rectus muscle entrapment exists, then limitation of upward eye movement may be noted.
- Diplopia associated with muscle entrapment may be elicited historically or may be demonstrated by the physician.
- Enophthalmos is a very specific sign of orbital floor fracture, but it may be masked by local swelling and hemorrhage.
- Computed tomography (CT) assessment of the orbit (if available) should be routinely obtained when a diagnosis of orbital floor fracture is suspected.
- If CT is not available, facial x-rays including the Waters projection can be helpful in confirming the diagnosis.
- Radiologic findings in orbital floor fracture include clouding of the ipsilateral maxillary sinus (secondary to local hemorrhage or extrusion of orbital soft tissues into the sinus), fragmentation or disruption of the inferior orbital floor, often with depression of bony fragments into the sinus, and intraorbital free air.

Treatment
- Patients with fractures of the orbital floor associated with diplopia or impaired extraocular muscle function require urgent ophthalmologic consultation.
- Operative intervention may be required.
- Prophylactic antibiotics are controversial in orbital fractures.
- If used, they should cover sinus flora.
- Patients should be instructed to refrain from blowing the nose for 10 to 14 days, because this maneuver may introduce the contents of the sinus into the orbit through the fracture site.

Ethmoid Fracture
- Crepitus in association with trauma to the periorbital structures suggests an ethmoid fracture, which should be documented radiologically.
- Treatment is the same as for orbital floor fractures.

Traumatic Iritis
- Blunt trauma to the eye, if significant, is often associated with some degree of iritis. Patients report deep eye pain and photophobia, perilimbal conjunctival injection is noted (ciliary flush), the pupil is constricted, and "flare" is noted by slit-lamp examination representing inflammatory cells and exudate in the anterior chamber. Immediate ophthalmologic consultation is appropriate.
- Treatment includes topical steroids and cycloplegics.

Hyphema

- Injury to the iris and its associated vessels may result in bleeding that produces a meniscus or layering of blood along the lower anterior chamber in front of the iris.
- It is very important to remember that this sign may be absent unless the patient is examined after having been upright for 5 to 10 minutes; recumbency allows blood to layer within the eye uniformly, along the horizontal axis, making the hyphema difficult to detect.
- Patients may be totally asymptomatic, may report varying degrees of discomfort, or may be lethargic or vomiting as a result of acutely increased intraocular pressure. Because acute glaucoma may occur precipitously in patients with hyphema, immediate assessment of intraocular pressure is appropriate, and patients should be kept upright to prevent blood from obstructing the angle, which further increases intraocular pressure.
- Treatment includes patching of the affected eye, topical steroids, and cycloplegics.
- Antiplatelet analgesics such as aspirin and NSAIDs should be avoided.
- All patients with hyphema, and particularly those with elevated intraocular pressure, should be referred for immediate ophthalmologic consultation.

Dislocation of the Lens

- Dislocation of the lens is most commonly associated with blunt trauma to the eye, is frequently accompanied by other injuries, and often produces minimal symptoms and subtle findings. Patients may report only slightly blurred vision or, when complete posterior dislocation of the lens into the vitreous occurs, shadows moving across the visual field may be noted.
- Dislocations may be partial or complete and may be associated with secondary iritis or acute glaucoma; the latter occurs as a result of obstruction of the outflow tract of the anterior chamber.
- The diagnosis of lens dislocation should be suspected on the basis of a history of blunt trauma, subjective or objective evidence of reduced visual acuity, shimmering or quivering of the iris, or unevenness of the anterior chamber.
- Intraocular pressure should be measured in patients with lens dislocation; pressures of more than 40 mm Hg must be treated.
- Ophthalmologic consultation at the time of presentation is indicated.

Rupture of the Globe

- Rupture of the eyeball may occur as a result of blunt or penetrating trauma.
- Blunt trauma usually produces perilimbic or optic nerve area disruption.
- Vision is usually reduced, and the eye is soft to palpation.
- If this diagnosis is suspected, then manipulation should be minimal, the patient should be treated with systemic antibiotics that cover skin flora, antitetanus prophylaxis should be administered if warranted, and an eye shield should be gently applied.
- Emergency ophthalmologic consultation should be obtained.

Subconjunctival Hemorrhage

- After blunt trauma to the globe, coughing, vomiting, and other Valsalva-like maneuvers, bleeding into the bulbar conjunctiva may occur.
- The blood does not affect vision, and its distribution ends at the limbal margin.

- Patients should be advised to avoid aspirin and should be reassured that the blood and discoloration will resolve in 2 to 3 weeks.
- Patients using warfarin should be followed up closely by an ophthalmologist.

LACERATIONS AND PENETRATING INJURIES TO THE EYE

Lacerations Involving the Cornea and Sclera

- Antibiotics should be administered immediately, both topically (drops, not ointment) and systemically, and antitetanus prophylaxis administered as needed.
- The eye should be lightly patched with a protective shield.
- These lacerations require emergent ophthalmologic consultation.
- Complications of corneal lacerations include prolapse of the iris with production of a teardrop-shaped pupil. In addition, deep lacerations can lead to leakage of aqueous humor (detected by a fluorescein Seidel test).
- Based on the mechanism of injury, a retained intraocular foreign body should also be suspected; these are often best delineated with CT scanning.

Lacerations Involving the Lid Margins

- Those that involve the medial fifth of the lid and are more than superficial, those that obviously involve the lacrimal apparatus, and those that are "through-and-through" should generally be repaired by the ophthalmologist or plastic surgeon.
- Simple lid lacerations that do not involve the aforementioned structures may be primarily closed using a fine (6-0 or 7-0) nylon suture.

Conjunctival Lacerations

- If superficial, conjunctival lacerations need not be closed if they are smaller than 1 cm.
- Lacerations larger than 1 cm without underlying injury may be closed with 7-0 absorbable suture.

CORNEAL ABRASIONS AND FOREIGN BODIES

- Patients presenting to the emergency department reporting an ocular "foreign body" sensation will generally have either a corneal abrasion or a foreign body.
- It is necessary in such patients to obtain and record corrected (if possible) visual acuity in both eyes before treatment.
- Tetracaine should be instilled to facilitate the examination of the corneal surface. If a foreign body is noted, it may then be removed as outlined; frequently, however, the initial examination is unremarkable.
- It is imperative in these patients (and even when a single foreign body is identified and removed) that the upper and lower lids be everted and the respective cul-de-sacs closely examined.
- In all patients, the corneal surface should be examined under ultraviolet light after fluorescein staining to demonstrate any abrasions.
- Foreign material commonly becomes embedded under the lid, where, associated with eye movement, multiple, characteristic, vertically oriented abrasions involving the respective corneal surfaces are produced.
- When noted by fluorescein staining, this configuration should suggest a retained or fixed foreign body that may be visualized and removed after lid eversion.

- Many conjunctival or corneal foreign bodies can easily be lifted off the conjunctiva or cornea with a sterile, moistened, cotton-tipped applicator.
- A small-gauge needle or spud or burr may be required to remove the foreign body from the corneal surface.
- Foreign material that is deeply embedded in the cornea or is associated with a surrounding ring of rust requires treatment by the ophthalmologist.
- A 2- to 3-day course of a topically applied antibiotic ophthalmologic ointment should be provided.
- All patients should be examined in 24 hours to ensure that healing is complete and that infection has not occurred.
- Patients should be instructed to rest the eyes and to expect some return of discomfort as the topical anesthetic wears off.
- Patching is not generally required.
- Treatment should be provided for the patient's corneal abrasion (topical antibiotics, and consideration of cycloplegia and analgesics, if severe).
- Corneal ulceration may occur relatively rapidly around embedded corneal foreign material; this process produces a white or opaque discoloration of the cornea surrounding the foreign body. If this diagnosis is suspected, immediate ophthalmologic consultation is indicated before antibiotic instillation.

CHEMICAL EXPOSURE OF THE EYE

- Patients presenting to the emergency department with chemical exposure to the eye should be immediately triaged into the department.
- Bilateral pH determinations should be made and recorded, topical tetracaine should be instilled to achieve anesthesia, the lids should be everted, and irrigation with 1 L of normal saline should be initiated immediately. During this procedure, the patient should be asked to look to the four quadrants of gaze to ensure that all areas of the eye are irrigated and to facilitate entry of fluid into the cul-de-sacs.
- Lid eversion must be performed for upper and lower lids if the eye is to be adequately irrigated. Any solid material should be removed manually.
- The use of a Morgan lens will greatly facilitate irrigation. After 1 L of normal saline has been instilled, the pH should be rechecked, fluorescein staining of the eye should be performed, and visual acuity assessed.
- Patients suspected by history or by pH determination to have sustained alkaline exposure have the highest risk of permanent corneal damage.
- Alkali tends to penetrate corneal tissues by liquefaction necrosis and produces ongoing damage despite initial aggressive treatment. Such patients may require multiple liters of normal saline administered over several hours.
- Two or three liters is administered initially over 30 to 40 minutes, followed by a short waiting period, after which time the pH is checked and recorded; multiple additional irrigations may be required.
- Ophthalmologic consultation should then be obtained after alkali exposure or if after a nonalkali material exposure, ocular injury is demonstrated.

RADIATION AND LIGHT-INDUCED INJURIES

- Ultraviolet radiation emanating from welding arcs (flash burns or "arc eye"), short-circuited high-voltage lines, sunlamps, and bright, snow-covered environments may produce a superficial keratitis readily demonstrated by fluorescein staining of the cornea.

- Typically, a 6- to 12-hour symptom-free interval occurs after exposure (which may not be recalled) and the onset of symptoms.
- Patients report severe discomfort (which is usually superficially localized), photophobia, and blepharospasm.
- In many such patients, a horizontal band-like distribution of fluorescein will be noted, which reflects the shielding effect of the upper and lower lids.
- Treatment includes instillation of a local anesthetic, a mild cycloplegic to interfere with ciliary spasm, and systemic analgesics if needed. Patching the involved eye or eyes is helpful, and patients should be instructed to rest the eyes during the next 24 to 36 hours. Patients should be advised that some degree of discomfort will return after the local anesthetic wears off and before healing of the lesion has occurred, usually by 24 to 36 hours; systemic analgesics are useful for this reason.
- Ophthalmologic referral is appropriate at 24 hours should improvement fail to occur.

INTRAOCULAR FOREIGN BODIES

- Unfortunately, intraocular foreign bodies are not always recognized in the emergency department.
- Historically, the presence of such material should be suspected when patients report the onset of discomfort associated with the use or striking of metal on metal or the grinding of metal in some fashion.
- Patients may also report that vision is blurred.
- The lids, cornea, and conjunctiva must be closely examined for the presence of an entry wound; fluorescein staining followed by an examination under ultraviolet light will be helpful and may demonstrate a small puncture wound.
- Funduscopic examination should be undertaken and may allow definitive diagnosis; radiologic assessment of the orbit, although insensitive, is indicated after such an injury to demonstrate the presence of radiopaque material.
- CT of the orbit would be more sensitive for this, especially with metallic foreign bodies.
- Many foreign bodies are best left in place; however, a number of metals, such as copper and iron, should be removed because complications occur as they decompose.
- If an intraocular foreign body is suspected based on history or examination, ophthalmologic referral and consultation should be obtained in the emergency department.

6 Chest Trauma

The discussion of chest trauma is divided into two sections. The first deals with five conditions that may be rapidly fatal unless appreciated and therapeutic maneuvers instituted immediately; patients in this category will generally present with severe respiratory distress and/or evolving or established shock. The second section involves potentially serious or potentially fatal conditions, most of which will evolve less acutely and thus provide the physician with more of an opportunity for some degree of diagnostic evaluation. A number of relatively minor problems related to trauma to the chest and back are also discussed.

INITIAL ASSESSMENT

The initial assessment and management of the patient with serious chest trauma must include the early recognition of all of the following five conditions, any of which may be rapidly fatal unless appropriate therapeutic measures are instituted immediately. These include:
- Cardiac tamponade
- Tension pneumothorax
- Open or sucking pneumothorax
- Flail or unstable chest wall associated with respiratory insufficiency
- Massive hemothorax

Several general points relevant to the patient with serious chest trauma should be made:
- Establishing a patent airway, including intubation and ventilation in patients without appropriate ventilatory function, and ascertaining the adequacy of air exchange within the chest are initial priorities, as with all seriously injured patients.
- Two 14- or 16-gauge peripheral intravenous lines should be established immediately. Ringer lactate solution (or normal saline) is then infused. A central line should not be used initially for fluid resuscitation due to its length and narrow gauge.
- A portable roentgenogram of the chest should be obtained as soon as possible in all patients with severe chest injuries.
- The mechanism of injury is important to determine, because blunt and penetrating injuries to the chest are associated with specific disorders. For example, cardiac tamponade is unusual except in patients in whom penetration of the chest, back, or upper abdomen has occurred, whereas flail chest and pulmonary contusion occur most often in association with blunt trauma.
- There is often no correlation between the external appearance of the chest wall and the extent of intrathoracic injury; this is particularly true in young children who, because of an extremely compliant and resilient chest wall, may have severe compressive or crushing trauma producing devastating intrathoracic injury while the external chest remains normal.

- Many patients with serious trauma to the chest may have impressive or obvious extrathoracic injuries that are not life threatening; the acute treatment of these is obviously a secondary priority.

SPECIFIC DISORDERS

Cardiac Tamponade

Cardiac tamponade occurs in patients with lacerations or puncture wounds to the heart as a result of penetrating injuries to the anterior chest, upper abdomen, or back. The acute presentation of these patients is extremely variable and is determined by the extent and nature of the injury to the heart and to what extent bleeding is confined by the pericardium.

It is important to note that in patients with significant pericardial disruption, hemorrhage into the chest may occur, producing hemorrhagic shock and massive hemothorax; therefore, injuries to the heart should be suspected in patients presenting with hemothorax.

Frequently, pericardial continuity is sufficiently maintained to compromise the egress of blood from the pericardial sac, thereby producing cardiac tamponade. It is important initially to stress the following two points. First, progressive cardiac tamponade may be rapidly fatal unless treated in the emergency department with pericardiocentesis; and second, in patients with significant blood loss from whatever cause, many of the classic signs of tamponade will be absent or extremely subtle. The classic triad of Beck includes arterial hypotension, elevated venous pressure, and muffling of the heart sounds. It should be noted, however, that at least 30% of patients presenting with tamponade after penetrating injuries to the heart will *not* have initial evidence of increased venous pressure either clinically or by central venous pressure determination because of significant blood loss. Such patients will nevertheless manifest evidence of increasing venous pressure as fluid and blood replacement proceeds.

Diagnosis

Three very important diagnostic findings in patients with tamponade, which may also be seen in patients with tension pneumothorax, include tachycardia, hypotension, and a central venous pressure greater than 15 cm H_2O.

- Classically, patients with cardiac tamponade, if alert, report severe dyspnea, and many appear extremely anxious, restless, or agitated.
- Breath sounds are normal bilaterally unless significant hemothorax or pneumothorax coexists.
- Hypotension may be absent, mild, or marked as tamponade, bleeding, or both progress.
- A reduced pulse pressure may be noted transiently, and pulsus paradoxus may be noted (pulsus paradoxus is a decline of more than 10 mm Hg in systolic pressure associated with inspiration).
- Jugular venous distention, although frequently absent in volume-depleted patients, is an important finding if present, particularly when associated with hypotension. In addition, inspiratory filling of the jugular venous system or inspiratory increases in jugular venous pressure (Kussmaul sign) are additional findings.
- Muffling of the heart sounds may be noted on physical examination, and electrocardiographic evidence of reduced voltage or the finding of electrical alternans points toward a diagnosis of tamponade.
- Unless radiographs are available for comparison or hemothorax coexists, the chest roentgenogram is usually not particularly helpful.

- Emergency transthoracic echocardiography is the diagnostic procedure of choice, because it documents the presence of the pericardial effusion and signs of tamponade physiology (e.g., right atrial collapse). When as little as 200 mL of blood acutely enters the intact pericardial space, tamponade may occur, and this amount of blood will not significantly distort the cardiac silhouette.

Treatment

Once a diagnosis of acute cardiac tamponade is confirmed or suspected, emergency pericardiocentesis should be performed. In addition and importantly, because hemodynamic function of the ventricle can be improved in patients with cardiac tamponade by increasing right-sided filling pressures, the rapid administration of crystalloids or blood can be helpful.

- Have immediately available equipment for intubation and for cardiopulmonary resuscitation. Oxygen should be administered.
- Optimally, position patients on the stretcher with the head and thorax elevated at approximately 45 to 55 degrees.
- Prepare and drape the perixiphoid area.
- Immediately inferior and to the left of the xiphoid process, anesthetize the skin with 1% lidocaine.
- Connect a 16- or 18-gauge cardiac needle, 12 to 18 cm long, to a 50-mL syringe using a three-way stopcock.
- If ultrasound is available, this procedure is ideally done with ultrasound guidance.
- Alternatively, continuously record and closely observe a precordial or V-lead electrocardiogram while the needle is slowly advanced; this will signal cardiac penetration and prevent repeated cardiac puncture or laceration. If an alligator clip is available, this may be used to connect the pericardiocentesis needle to the V lead, which provides the most direct means of recording proximity to or contact with the epicardium during the procedure. If ventricular penetration occurs, then a typical "current-of-injury" pattern will be noted with elevation of the ST segment. If atrial penetration occurs, PR segment elevation may be noted. In addition, the occurrence of ectopic ventricular beats associated with needle advancement should also be noted and frequently signals cardiac penetration. When evidence of cardiac penetration occurs, the needle should be withdrawn several millimeters and this depth marked by attaching a snap or clip to the needle.
- The most common method is the paraxiphoid approach, with the needle angled down approximately 45 degrees and directed toward the medial left clavicle; the needle should be felt to move under the interior aspect of the ribs. Advance the needle carefully, gently aspirating, under ultrasound guidance or observing the heart monitor for the above-mentioned perturbations.
- One can occasionally feel the pericardium as it is entered, and if tamponade is present, blood is easily aspirated. As much blood as possible should be removed; however, clinical signs of improvement may occur after only a small volume is aspirated. Aspirated blood should be retained and, if it originates from within the pericardial space, may not clot. Blood that does clot may have originated from within the ventricle or atrium or, if from the pericardial space, may not have occupied that space for a long enough time for defibrination to occur.
- At the point of entry of the pericardial space or the point at which aspiration is most successful, a Kelly clamp or snap should be secured to the needle at the skin surface; this will stabilize its position during aspiration and will serve as a marker for subsequent aspirations, should they be necessary. Alternatively, a small plastic catheter may be inserted into the pericardial space should tamponade recur and reaspiration be required.

Other Measures

Patients with cardiac tamponade are considered candidates for thoracotomy, and appropriate preparations must be initiated early. In the patient with minimal benefit from initial pericardiocentesis, other treatable causes that may be rapidly fatal and produce findings consistent with tamponade should be reconsidered; these include tension pneumothorax and shock secondary to massive hemothorax. Importantly, all patients must be closely monitored for signs of recurrence of the cardiac tamponade. This should be readily demonstrated upon repeat ultrasound.

Tension Pneumothorax

Simple pneumothorax is complicated by tension when the chest wall or lung is disrupted in such a fashion as to allow air to enter the pleural space during inspiration but not escape during expiration. Progressively forceful inspiratory efforts then accumulate air under increasing pressure within the pleural space. Oblique or flap-type lacerations of the lung, for example, may be tethered in an open position during inspiration when intrapleural pressures decrease, only to become compressed during expiration. Eventually, as pressure increases, mediastinal displacement develops away from the involved side, thereby leading to compression and distortion of perimediastinal venous structures. Reduced venous return to the right side of the heart on this basis and marked compression of adjacent pulmonary parenchyma result in severe and progressive shunting and hypoxemia. If venous compromise and pulmonary compression are not corrected, then profound hypotension, hypoxemia, and death rapidly ensue.

Diagnosis

On arrival, patients generally report or have evidence of penetrating trauma to the chest, back, or upper abdomen.
- Evidence of ventilatory or circulatory compromise may be noted at the time of presentation.
- "Sucking" or open wounds of the chest may be noted (and should immediately be treated).
- The involved hemithorax may demonstrate decreased respiratory excursions, and breath sounds are generally reduced.
- Subcutaneous emphysema may be present.
- Deviation of the trachea away from the involved side and similar displacement of the cardiac apical impulse are late findings.
- Jugular venous distention and hyperresonance to percussion on the involved side are also late findings.
- A portable chest roentgenogram will demonstrate collapse of the involved lung with varying degrees of displacement of the mediastinal structures toward the opposite side. Tension pneumothorax should be a clinical diagnosis.

Treatment
- Immediate percutaneous needle puncture–aspiration using a 14- or 16-gauge needle is indicated.
- Place the needle in the second interspace along the midclavicular line.
- The diagnosis is confirmed when air rushes out of the chest.

Open Pneumothorax

Sucking chest wounds are easily diagnosed when one hears air rushing in and out of the wound.

Pneumothorax associated with open defects of the chest wall, the single or collective diameters of which approach the diameter of the trachea, will effectively compete with the trachea for airflow during inspiration. In patients with large open defects, shunting of air away from the trachea and alveoli may result in rapidly evolving respiratory failure unless airflow is redirected.

Treatment
- In patients with stable vital signs and adequate respiratory and circulatory function, the open wound should be covered with a sterile gloved hand, the surrounding area prepared in the usual sterile manner, and an occlusive dressing sterilely applied.
- Petrolatum-impregnated gauze is an appropriate dressing and should be applied, so it extends 2 to 3 inches beyond the wound edge in all dimensions; two layers may be required, and these must be secured to the chest wall on three sides with several layers of adhesive tape.
- A dry sterile dressing may then be applied. Occlusion of the dressing on three sides creates a flutter valve effect; closing the wound at all four sides could convert an open pneumothorax to a tension pneumothorax.
- After the wound is closed in the aforementioned manner, preparations for chest tube placement should be undertaken immediately. Should deterioration in respiratory or circulatory status occur during the procedure, tension pneumothorax should be suspected and the dressing removed or percutaneous puncture of the involved pleural space undertaken immediately.

Flail Chest

Three or more adjacent ribs, each fractured in two or more locations, may produce a localized section of chest wall that is unsupported and moves paradoxically during ventilation. Pathophysiologically, a chest wall segment that moves inward during inspiration interferes with normal ventilation to the extent that the adjacent lung is compressed and the normally occurring decrease in intrapleural pressure required to expand the lung during inspiration cannot occur. The extent to which ventilation is interfered with depends on the size and location of the "flail" or unstable segment and the presence or absence of previous pulmonary compromise.

Flail chest is primarily an anterior or anterolateral chest wall phenomenon because the posterior chest or back is well supported by overlying and associated musculature, thereby providing stability and minimizing paradoxical movement. In addition, patients with reduced respiratory effort from any cause and those with splinting of the involved hemithorax as a result of pain may not demonstrate paradoxical movement until deep breathing resumes or pain relief is obtained.

Diagnosis
- Diagnosis is based on a history of blunt trauma to the chest or back and inward or paradoxical movement of the injured chest wall segment during deep inspiration.
- Local pain on palpation and crepitus are frequently noted; early radiologic confirmation of fractures as well as the exclusion of simple pneumothorax, tension pneumothorax, pulmonary contusion, and significant hemothorax is indicated in all patients.

Treatment
- Administer oxygen.
- Venous blood gases and respiratory rate should be assessed frequently during the initial 48 hours of observation.

- Intubation for ventilatory assistance may be required for patients with progressive hypercapnia or irreversible hypoxemia.
- The development of significant dyspnea or fatigue remains an additional indication for intubation and assisted ventilation.
- In the emergency department, intubation should be strongly considered in patients with significant dyspnea, initial evidence of ventilatory insufficiency (manifest as hypercapnia or refractory hypoxemia), or progressive fatigue.

Massive Hemothorax

Blunt or penetrating injury to the chest may result in significant hemothorax.

Diagnosis

- Decreased breath sounds and percussion dullness over the involved hemithorax.
- Respiratory excursions may be decreased in patients with large effusions.
- An upright or semierect portable roentgenogram of the chest should be obtained; importantly, supine films, even if significant blood exists within the chest, may demonstrate only subtle degrees of uniform opacification that can be easily over-looked. In addition, pneumothoraces may be present as well, which are more reliably detected on upright films.
- CT may be helpful in making the diagnosis as well as identifying other intrathoracic injuries.

Treatment

- Reestablishment of normal intravascular volume and systemic arterial pressure is a first priority; hypoxia secondary to pulmonary compression can often be corrected initially by the simple administration of oxygen.
- After stabilization of the upper airway and blood pressure, a large-bore (36–42 French) chest tube should be placed in adults.
- In children, a 24 to 32 French chest tube should be used depending upon the child's size.
- The most common approach is the fifth intercostal space along the midaxillary line; the chest tube should be connected to 15 to 20 cm of H_2O suction in the usual manner and the hemothorax evacuated.
- Chest tube placement accomplishes several critical functions in patients with significant hemothorax: Lung re-expansion occurs and visceral and parietal pleural surfaces coapt, thereby minimizing bleeding; the probability of fibrothorax resulting from an organized, undrained hemothorax is reduced; and after determination of initial drainage, a record of continued drainage will indicate whether thoracotomy is required to control bleeding.
- Indications for thoracotomy include
  - Initial return of 1,000 mL of bloody drainage
  - Continuous bloody chest tube drainage of more than 200 mL/h for 4 hours
  - Persistent unexplained hypotension despite adequate volume replacement
  - The need for recurrent transfusions

Simple Pneumothorax

Injuries that have acutely but temporarily allowed air to enter the pleural space, have allowed the lung to collapse, and then have become stable are referred to as simple or, in some cases, closed pneumothoraces. These injuries may result from penetrating or blunt trauma and frequently involve trauma producing fracture and inward displacement of an overlying rib or ribs.

Diagnosis
- Pleuritic pain and dyspnea are reported by most alert patients.
- The physical examination may reveal crepitus or subcutaneous emphysema in association with rib fracture, evidence of chest wall penetration or contusion, decreased breath sounds, and hyperresonance to percussion, although the physical examination may be completely normal.
- Patients may appear acutely ill or may have minimal symptoms; signs and symptoms bear little relationship to the extent of collapse.
- An upright, posteroanterior, end-expiratory chest roentgenogram should be obtained and demonstrates peripheral absence of lung markings and the so-called pleural stripe, representing the visceral pleura separated from the chest wall; the latter should not be confused with the edge of the scapula.

Treatment
- Treatment depends on the symptoms, the extent of collapse, whether hemothorax coexists, and whether intubation and assisted ventilation or general anesthesia are required to intervene in other injuries.
- In all patients requiring intubation and assisted ventilation, general anesthesia, or air transport, chest tube placement is mandatory regardless of symptoms or extent of collapse.
- Bilateral pneumothoraces also require chest tube placement.
- A small, unilateral pneumothorax (<15%–20%) occurring in a healthy individual without severe symptoms may be closely observed within the ED without chest tube placement, provided that intubation and assisted ventilation or general anesthesia are not required for other injuries. All patients should be placed on 100% oxygen by nonrebreather facemask and monitored for several hours (some authorities advocate 6 hours, newer data supports 3 hours) whereupon a repeat chest x-ray is obtained. If the size of the pneumothorax increases or if symptoms worsen, then chest tube placement must be undertaken.
- Pneumothoraces greater than 15% to 20% generally require chest tube placement as described above.

Pulmonary Contusion

Pulmonary parenchymal hemorrhage and edema as a result of injury to the chest wall may be either localized to the area adjacent to the point of impact or generalized and involve the directly injured as well as the contralateral lung. Pulmonary contusion is most commonly caused by deceleration injuries; however, direct blows to the thorax, blast injuries, and high-velocity missiles may also produce severe pulmonary contusion. Whether localized or generalized injury occurs is a function of the severity of the initial insult. Importantly, initially even in patients in whom signs of extensive parenchymal pulmonary damage will develop over the ensuing several hours, symptoms may be minimal or totally absent, the physical examination may be unremarkable, and roentgenograms may be normal. For these reasons, in the evaluation of the acutely injured patient, pulmonary contusion is a diagnosis based on the physician's assessment of potential pulmonary injury. If such an injury is suspected, hospital admission for observation is indicated. The threshold for admission must be reduced in the pediatric patient, in whom unusual distensibility of the chest wall may produce no significant evidence of external injury despite major evolving parenchymal injury.

Diagnosis
- Dyspnea and a nonproductive cough are often the initial symptoms.
- A history of hemoptysis may be obtained in some patients.
- The physical examination reveals an increased respiratory rate, rales, or wheezes in the contused section of lung after the development of edema.
- The auscultory exam may initially be normal.
- As previously noted, radiographic assessment, if obtained soon after the injury, will generally be normal; subsequently, local or generalized consolidation of the involved lung may be seen.
- Scattered infiltrates are noted in some patients, and contralateral lung consolidation may follow in patients with extensive trauma.
- As noted, radiographic findings may lag behind clinical symptoms by several hours.

Treatment
- Use supplemental oxygenation as needed.
- Frequent assessment of the patient's respiratory rate, oxygenation, and level of respiratory fatigue will suggest the need for noninvasive (CPAP) or invasive respiratory assistance.
- Volume overload is to be avoided.
- Adequate pain control, either through the use of narcotics or through epidural analgesia, is a must.
- Deep breathing (via incentive spirometry) and frequent cough are encouraged.

Diaphragmatic Rupture

Blunt or penetrating trauma to the abdomen may result in clinically significant diaphragmatic tears. Most such injuries are associated with motor vehicle accidents producing severe pressure gradients across the diaphragm. The left hemidiaphragm is the site of injury 90% of the time. This injury is frequently complicated by serious intra-abdominal and intrathoracic injuries that often delay the diagnosis. Preoperative diagnosis of diaphragmatic rupture only occurs 50% of the time. Right-sided ruptures are almost never identified preoperatively.

Diagnosis
- When significant herniation of abdominal contents occurs into the chest, patients report chest pain, shortness of breath, and occasionally left shoulder discomfort, which is not affected by movement or palpation of the shoulder.
- Physical findings depend on the extent of herniation and are notable for displacement of bowel sounds into the appropriate hemithorax.
- In most patients, the diagnosis is made on the basis of radiographic assessment of the chest; however, rupture of the diaphragm is frequently unrecognized in patients with coexistent hemothorax.
- A repeat chest x-ray after the drainage of a hemothorax may reveal this injury.
- Radiologic findings include bowel in the chest, elevation of the involved hemidiaphragm, loss of the normal appearance or sweep of the hemidiaphragm, and coiling of the nasogastric tube in the chest.
- CT, especially thorax 3-D reconstructions, can be helpful in making this difficult diagnosis.

Treatment
- Nasogastric tube placement with continuous suction can afford considerable relief of pain in patients with distention-related discomfort and will effectively decompress the bowel.
- Surgical repair is always required and is generally undertaken as soon as possible. Even small tears will worsen and result in bowel herniation into the chest due to the parietoperitoneal pressure gradients.

Blunt Cardiac Injury

Contusion or blunt injury to the myocardium should be suspected in any patient with a significant anterior chest wall injury. The majority of patients with a cardiac contusion will have external signs of chest trauma. Although fracture or contusion of the sternum or anterior ribs may accompany this injury, these need not be present. Rapid deceleration in relatively high-speed motor vehicle accidents, producing steering wheel impact, remains the most common cause of this injury.

Diagnosis
- Examine patients with severe blunt chest trauma for cardiac chamber rupture (usually right sided) that can cause cardiac tamponade.
- This diagnosis is confirmed with the FAST exam.
- The initial absence of pain and a normal electrocardiogram (ECG) must not be used to exclude blunt cardiac injury, because most patients when first seen have normal ECGs, and discomfort may be delayed for several hours after the injury.
- The discomfort related to myocardial contusion is usually dull or pressure-like in character.
- The continuous nature of the pain may be diagnostically significant because most patients will have associated anterior chest wall injuries, the discomfort of which is often pleuritic in nature.
- Unexplained tachycardia is the most common finding in patients with blunt cardiac injuries.
- A typical pattern of ischemia or infarction may be noted in some patients, although nonspecific ST-wave and T-wave abnormalities are more common.
- Changes characteristic of pericarditis, a wide variety of conduction abnormalities, and dysrhythmias of all types, particularly ventricular premature beats, are commonly reported.
- Troponin T & I elevations (which often take several hours to occur) are highly specific for myocardial injury, and although their role is still unclear in blunt cardiac trauma, it appears that at least in some studies it is quite helpful as a screening laboratory test in establishing the diagnosis of more severe blunt cardiac injury.
- Transthoracic echocardiograms can show wall motion abnormalities.
- Admission is based on a high degree of suspicion in the appropriate patient.

Treatment
- Patients with evidence of hemopericardium need emergent operative care.
- Inotropic support may be needed for patients with severe myocardial contusion.
- Antiarrhythmia drugs may be used as appropriate.
- Uneventful recovery is the rule in most patients.
- Patients with previous cardiac disease, with ECG evidence of injury, or with new evidence of conduction abnormalities should be admitted to the intensive care unit.

Rib Fracture and Contusion

Blunt or penetrating trauma to the chest may result in single or multiple rib fractures or contusions.

Diagnosis

- Simple contusion to the rib or ribs is diagnosed on the basis of a history of trauma to the chest, localized discomfort in the area of injury or impact, and no radiographic evidence of bony injury.
- Rib fractures are associated with similar symptoms and signs; however, roentgenograms may be positive (although only in approximately 50% of patients with nondisplaced fractures), and local crepitus may be appreciated at or around the fracture site.
- Many patients with either contusion or fracture will report a pleuritic component to their discomfort and precipitation of severe or excruciating pain by sneezing, coughing, or sudden movement of the chest wall.
- In the emergency department, the physician must remember that occult visceral injury often coexists with "simple" rib contusion and fracture.
- These injuries are easily missed without a high index of suspicion.
- In addition, children, the elderly, and patients with preexisting pulmonary disease with rib fractures or contusions must be managed extremely conservatively if complications are to be avoided.
- It is well recognized that devastating intrathoracic and intra-abdominal injuries may occur in children without associated chest wall damage.
- This occurs because of the distensibility of the pediatric rib cage, which may be substantially deformed at the time of injury but show no evidence of external trauma at the time of the examination.
- All patients with suspected rib fracture should have a one-view chest x-ray to rule out pulmonic injury.
- All patients with significant contusion or bony injury overlying the kidney should have a urinalysis; hematuria in this setting must be considered to represent injury to the genitourinary system, the management of which is discussed in Chapter 9.
- Patients with concerning lower rib cage or abdominal symptoms after trauma to the thorax should have an abdominal and pelvic CT along with a more extensive diagnostic workup in line with advanced trauma life support (ATLS) recommendations to rule out serious coexisting pathology.

Treatment

- Elderly patients with severe pain, dyspnea, coexistent pulmonary or cardiovascular disease, or multiple fractures should be admitted for a period of observation and titration of analgesics.
- Hospital admission is particularly important for patients with previous disabilities or those living alone.
- Supplemental oxygen, encouragement of frequent voluntary cough and deep breathing, and attention to detecting early infection are also advised.
- The use of adhesive or other tapes or rib belts to stabilize such injuries should be avoided because many patients, particularly those with preexisting lung disease and the elderly, may have atelectasis and secondary pneumonitis as a result of mechanical interference with respiratory excursions and the clearing of pulmonary secretions.
- Deep breathing each hour, frequent forced cough, and the rapid resumption of normal activity will prevent the usual infectious complications of chest wall injury.

- Some authorities have reported symptomatic benefit from the use of a nonsteroidal anti-inflammatory agent, such as ibuprofen, 400 to 600 mg four times per day with food, in addition to a pure analgesic.
- Intercostal nerve block or an epidural block may be extremely effective for hospitalized patients and may eliminate the need for systemically administered analgesics; this may be extremely useful in the elderly patient, in the patient with pulmonary disease, and in patients with other injuries requiring serial reassessment.

First or Second Rib Fracture

Patients with first or second rib fractures must be considered to have experienced extraordinary chest trauma; coexistent injuries to the cervical spine, head, aorta, subclavian artery, and brachial plexus are common. A CT (preferably a CT angiogram) of the chest should be performed and the patient should be admitted for observation.

Esophageal Perforation

The esophagus may be perforated as a result of any of the following:
- Penetrating or blunt trauma to the neck, chest, or abdomen
- Instrumentation of the upper gastrointestinal tract
- Foreign body–related necrosis of the esophageal wall
- Caustic exposure
- Postemetic rupture (Boerhaave syndrome)

Diagnosis
- Patients report pain at the site of perforation and/or along the course of the esophagus.
- Pain is often increased by swallowing or inspiration and is often described as sharp and radiating toward the back or neck.
- Passive motion of the neck may increase pain when cervical esophageal perforation is present; subcutaneous air may be a prominent and important finding in these patients.
- As the gastrointestinal contents enter the mediastinum, mediastinitis evolves, producing varying degrees of dyspnea, fever, chest discomfort, and circulatory compromise; in many patients, sepsis evolves rapidly.
- Cervical subcutaneous emphysema or air, a "crunching" sound auscultated in association with systole (Hamman sign), and a nasal quality to the voice may be noted when mediastinal air is present.
- Early radiographic assessment of the patient with suspected esophageal perforation is mandatory.
- The classic chest x-ray findings include mediastinal or subcutaneous air, often associated with mediastinal widening, which may be subtle unless previous films are available for comparison.
- A "prevertebral shadow" may be noted on lateral views of the neck and cervical spine, which is manifest as an increased distance between the anterior edge of the vertebral bodies and the trachea.
- A pleural effusion or pneumothorax may be noted as well.
- A meglumine diatrizoate (Gastrografin) esophagography study is done initially, which, if negative, should be followed up by a conventional barium study (which has a higher sensitivity but is more toxic to the mediastinum).
- CT is recommended to identify other injuries and identify the extent of inflammation.

Treatment
- Treatment includes suspension of all oral intake and the administration of supplemental intravenous fluids, early surgical consultation, and appropriate intravenous antibiotics.

Subcutaneous Emphysema

Subcutaneous emphysema is a phenomenon occurring when air is allowed to enter the soft or subcutaneous tissues. A variety of both medical and traumatic conditions may produce or be associated with this finding:
- Pulmonary bleb rupture
- Breath-holding
- Emesis
- The Valsalva maneuver
- Gas-producing infections of the soft tissues
- Spontaneous esophageal rupture or perforation

Disruptions of the tracheobronchial tree that occur in extrapleural locations allow free air to enter the mediastinum and to track toward the anterior neck and face. In contrast, intrapleural disruptions are usually associated with pneumothorax and the development of chest wall air. The importance of recognizing subcutaneous emphysema in patients with chest or neck trauma is that significant tracheobronchial or pulmonary parenchymal injury is frequently associated with and specifically suggested by this finding. Subcutaneous emphysema is otherwise a relatively benign disorder.

Diagnosis
- The diagnosis of subcutaneous emphysema is usually straightforward, with clinical or radiographic evidence of soft-tissue air.
- Palpation produces a distinctive crepitation or crackling sensation.

Treatment
- Treatment includes a period of close observation and recognizing the frequent association in the traumatized patient between subcutaneous emphysema and injury to the tracheobronchial tree, lung parenchyma, and esophagus.

Scapular Fracture

Force sufficient to fracture the scapula must be considered significant, and coexistent injuries to the lung, shoulder, neck, and brachial plexus must be carefully considered. Neurovascular status in the extremity should be evaluated.

Treatment
- Treatment for most fractures involves a period of immobilization with a sling and swathe, analgesics, application of cold for 24 to 48 hours, and orthopaedic follow-up within several days.
- Early follow-up is recommended to institute appropriate range-of-motion exercises for the shoulder and elbow, because substantial disability may follow even a relatively brief period of immobilization.
- All patients should remove the sling for bathing and at bedtime.

Sternal Fracture

Sternal fracture results from direct, blunt trauma to the anterior chest, often associated with steering wheel impact. Sternal fractures are not in and of themselves dangerous but are a marker for other serious injuries. These injuries include esophageal and diaphragmatic injury, tracheobronchial tears, cardiac and pulmonary contusions, and injuries to the thoracic aorta.

Diagnosis
- Pain, often pleuritic, is reported at the site of fracture and may be confirmed by a lateral radiograph of the sternum or a CT of the chest.
- CT scans of the chest are usually warranted to identify associated injuries.

Treatment
- Treatment is aimed at other identified injuries.
- If other injuries are not identified after a careful history, physical, and radiographic examination and the patient is stable from a respiratory standpoint, discharge with close follow-up can be considered.
- Strongly consider admission of elderly patients with this injury for close observation.

Thoracolumbar Vertebral Injury

A variety of mechanisms, most often motor vehicle accidents or falls, may result in injury to the thoracolumbar spine. A hyperflexion hyperflexion injury produces compression of the anterosuperior portion of the vertebral body. Less often, a direct blow to the back results in fracture of a transverse process (or processes). A vertical compressive injury, such as that occurring in a fall, results in a bursting-type fracture of the vertebral body. Injuries associated with rotation typically cause a shearing or splitting-type fracture through the vertebrae; disruption of the posterior ligamentous elements of the column, resulting in instability, may be associated with such fractures. Because of the intrinsic stability and rigidity of the thoracic spine due to its connection to the rib cage, injuries are less common in this area; osteoporosis, however, markedly increases the tendency of all vertebral bodies to become compressed, and such fractures are noted incidentally throughout the spine. Coughing, sneezing, or simple lifting may result in compression in these patients. Fracture dislocation of the thoracolumbar spine is associated with major falls or deceleration injuries; the thoracolumbar junction is most commonly involved, and a teardrop or avulsing injury involving the inferior vertebral body is noted.

Diagnosis
- Diagnosis is made on the basis of the type of injury, physical examination, and a careful radiologic assessment of the spine.
- Plain films are the initial study of choice. If negative and the patient has significant thoracic pain, a CT of the thoracic spine is warranted.
- If a CT of the thorax is being performed, thoracic spine reconstruction can replace plain thoracic spine films.
- If a patient has neurologic symptoms with a negative CT of the thoracic spine, an MRI is warranted to evaluate for spinal cord injury.
- The posterior wall of the vertebral body and the associated posterior elements must be carefully examined for the presence of fracture or disruption.

Treatment
- Patients with injuries that are unstable or in whom a neurologic deficit is noted require immediate neurosurgical or orthopaedic consultation.
- Steroid infusion for has increasingly fallen out of favor in the treatment of significant spinal cord injuries.
- Mild therapeutic hypothermia for patients with evidence of significant spinal cord injury is recommended by some experts but is not fully validated.

Traumatic Asphyxia

Traumatic asphyxia is an uncommon condition resulting from acute and massive compression of the chest. Massive and instantaneous chest compression results in dramatic elevation of intrathoracic pressure with resultant retrograde flow through the right atrium, vena cavae, and associated venous structures draining the upper chest, head, and neck. Acute capillary distention, atony, and engorgement occur, followed by local desaturation of static blood. Patients often report loss of consciousness at the time of injury and present with facial edema, an unusual violaceous discoloration of the skin of the upper chest, face, and neck, and bilateral subconjunctival hemorrhages or petechiae.

If other chest injuries are absent, the condition is self-limited, usually resolves over 2 to 3 weeks, and requires no treatment other than reassurance. Unfortunately, as one would expect, associated injuries to the lung, heart, and chest wall frequently accompany traumatic asphyxia; for this reason, a period of in-hospital observation is usually advised.

Abstract: 7 Abdominal Trauma

The first concern for emergency physicians caring for patients with abdominal trauma is rapidly identifying and treating circulatory instability. Adhering to the "ABCs" of the initial trauma work-up and liberal use of the FAST exam will help to rapidly identify intra-abdominal injuries in at-risk patients.

INITIAL STABILIZATION

Control of Bleeding
• External bleeding should be controlled by direct pressure.

Intravenous Access
• Intravenous access should be established by two 14- or 16-gauge short peripheral lines through which, after insertion, blood may be drawn for type and cross-matching and other studies, and normal saline or Ringer's lactate solution rapidly infused if signs of hypovolemia are present.
• Central's lines should *not* be used for initial fluid resuscitation because their placement, even in experienced hands, is time consuming, associated with a higher rate of complications, and, most important, results in a dramatically reduced rate of fluid delivery as a function of catheter-dependent resistance. A 16-gauge, 8-inch line, for example, delivers approximately half the fluid of a 16-gauge, 2-inch catheter for any given unit of time.

Initial Fluid Challenge
• Adults presenting with hypotension or established or evolving shock should be treated initially with 2 L of normal saline or Ringer lactate solution; this may be administered to adults as rapidly as possible, usually over 5 to 10 minutes.
• Children may be administered 20 mL/kg over the same interval.

Blood Replacement
• Although subsequent therapy will be dictated by the patient's response to the initial fluid challenge, patients presenting with hypotension will require blood replacement, and a minimum of 4 U should be made available.
• Although cross-matched blood is clearly preferable, its preparation requires between 50 and 70 minutes, and in many patients presenting with severe hypotension or exsanguinating hemorrhage, an abbreviated cross-match (which requires 15–20 minutes), type-specific blood (which requires ~10 minutes), or O-negative blood (which should be available immediately) must be transfused.
• Blood should be administered through macropore (160 µm) filters and, if possible, warmed before or during transfusion; however, warming is often impractical because of the urgency of transfusion.

- Vasopressors have no role in the routine management of hemorrhagic shock; aggressive re-expansion of intravascular volume with crystalloid, blood, or both remains the focus of initial treatment.

Assessment of Response to Initial Fluid Challenge

- In general, patients who rapidly respond to the initial fluid challenge by relative normalization of blood pressure and who remain stable have lost relatively little blood (<15%–20%) and may not necessarily require additional fluid challenge or blood replacement; however, 4 to 6 U of packed red cells should be available for emergent transfusion.
- Patients in whom only a transient increase in blood pressure is noted require rechallenge with crystalloid and rapid blood replacement because greater initial blood losses have occurred or blood loss is continuing.
- Plans for definitive surgical intervention should be underway in these patients.
- If patients exhibit little or no response to the initial fluid challenge, then either the blood loss was extensive or continuing or the diagnosis of hypovolemic shock was in error.
- One should also immediately consider cardiac tamponade, tension pneumothorax, massive hemothorax, and congestive heart failure in patients with the appropriate physical exam and refractory hypotension.
- If the patient is truly hypovolemic, then blood replacement must be aggressively undertaken and plans for surgical intervention pursued immediately.

Hypocalcemia and Dilutional Coagulopathy

- Rapid, massive transfusion of packed red blood cells may occasionally result in hypocalcemia and abnormalities of hemostasis; hypocalcemia is caused by chelation of intravascular calcium by the citrate preservative, and abnormalities of hemostasis are secondary to dilution of clotting factors.
- It is recommended that calcium chloride, 0.2 g (2 mL of a 10% calcium chloride solution) be administered slowly through a separate intravenous line when multiple units of packed red blood cells are transfused at a rate that exceeds 100 mL/min.
- Doses greater than 1 g should generally not be administered unless objective serologic evidence of hypocalcemia is demonstrated.
- One unit of fresh frozen plasma can be empirically administered for every 2 to 3 U of packed red blood cells and may prevent abnormalities of hemostasis secondary to dilution.
- After 2 U of packed red cells, a platelet transfusion should also be considered.

Prophylactic Antibiotics

- When possible visceral or peritoneal penetration is suspected or has occurred, prophylactic antibiotics the cover skin and gut flora should be administered intravenously in the emergency department.

PENETRATING TRAUMA

Gunshot Wounds

- Patients who are hemodynamically unstable require operative intervention; plans for laparotomy should be initiated concurrently with initial fluid and blood resuscitation.

- Patients who are and remain hemodynamically stable in the ED are candidates for CT of the abdomen to ascertain the degree of intra-abdominal injury.
- Patients with isolated injuries to the liver or spleen without evidence of injury to an arterial or venous structure, hollow viscus or hemidiaphragm may be embolized or monitored depending on the severity of the injury.
- Most patients with a GSW to the abdomen will still require operative management.

Knife or Stab Wounds

- Patients with stab wounds to the abdomen, when hemodynamically stable, are usually managed selectively; patients who are hemodynamically unstable should undergo emergent laparotomy.
- Patients with peritoneal signs, exposed omentum, evisceration, implement in situ, evidence of diaphragm injury, or strongly positive FAST exam should also undergo operative exploration.
- A selective management strategy in the patients without the above findings is based on the fact that most patients with stab wounds to the abdomen do not have an intraperitoneal injury; in fact, only 50% of patients with intraperitoneal penetration have an intraperitoneal injury.
- Patients with an abdominal stab wound without the above signs or symptoms that mandate emergent exploration can proceed to CT or have their wound locally explored utilizing local anesthesia.
- If a wound is locally explored and found to have not violated the peritoneum, the patient can be discharged.
- If the peritoneum has been violated, or the physician chooses not to locally explore a wound, a CT with IV contrast can be obtained.
- If solid organ injury is found on CT, but the patient is hemodynamically stable, has a stable hemoglobin count, and does not develop symptoms of peritonitis, the patient may be managed without laparotomy.
- Certain centers with experience with intra-arterial embolization also can manage the patient with an actively bleeding solid organ injury (significant amount of hemoperitoneum, or a "blush" of contrast escaping from an active bleed seen on CT) and thus avoid laparotomy.

BLUNT TRAUMA

- Most often results in injury to the spleen and/or liver.
- Patients with evolving major intra-abdominal injuries may be relatively asymptomatic initially and may manifest minimal physical signs.
- Patients with intra-abdominal injuries and other distracting injuries (i.e., femur fracture, open fractures, etc.) may not have abdominal pain as their most pressing symptom.
- Physical findings in patients with blunt abdominal injuries, particularly those with coexistent neurologic injuries or alterations in cognitive function as a result of head trauma or alcohol or drug ingestion, may be misleading and may produce both false-positive and false-negative results.
- Patients with suspected intra-abdominal injuries should have a FAST exam.
- The abdomen should be inspected for seat belt signs, distention, and flank ecchymosis as these are signs that convey a higher risk of intra-abdominal injury.

- Criteria for emergency laparotomy include patients with free peritoneal fluid on FAST exam who also have hemodynamic instability not correctable with IV fluids or blood products.
- Patients who are initially hemodynamically stable or who stabilize with IV fluids and/or blood products are candidates for CT of the abdomen and pelvis with IV contrast.
- Unstable patients with abdominal injuries should never have a CT; they must either stabilize with the above interventions or have a laparotomy.
- PO contrast is not particularly helpful in identifying additional injuries and may be harmful (aspiration risk).
- Repeat FAST exams are useful for the patients who become unstable after an initial negative exam, patients with initial mildly positive exams, or patients who are delayed in going to CT.
- Nonoperative management of solid organ injury in blunt abdominal trauma has revolutionized the care for these patients.
- Most solid organ injuries that remain hemodynamically stable can be managed nonoperatively.
- Even significantly damaged solid organs can be managed without laparotomy in centers with experience in nonoperative management of solid organ injury, and who have the ability to perform intra-arterial embolization.
- Patients who remain hemodynamically unstable despite intervention, patients who have a strongly positive FAST exam (at least a centimeter-wide fluid stripe in Morrison pouch), patients who have diaphragmatic injury, and patients with hollow viscous perforation need emergent laparotomy.

8 **Pelvic Trauma**

Injuries to the pelvis can range from isolated pubic rami fractures with little debilitation, to life-threatening pelvic hemorrhage. Thus, careful attention must be paid to a patient's vital signs and physical exam, as severe injuries can often initially be occult.

INITIAL ASSESSMENT

- The "ABCs" of trauma apply.
- A portable AP pelvis radiograph should be obtained in a seriously injured trauma patient.
- Realize that patients with significant pelvic injuries often have injuries in other body systems.
- Realize that patients with pelvic bleeding can rapidly exsanguinate.
- Realize that pelvic (retroperitoneal) bleeding is not demonstrated by the FAST exam.

SPECIFIC DISORDERS

Pelvic Fractures

- Present with pain in the groin (pubic rami fracture), hip (acetabular or iliac fracture), or back (sacral fracture).
- The pelvis should be gently assessed for stability and pain by applying a compressive force across the hips and then downward with both hands on the anterior iliac wings.
- The perineum should be carefully inspected for scrotal, labial, and suprapubic hematomas.
- A rectal should be performed to assess for rectal lacerations or a high-riding prostate, which indicates urethral disruption (this finding is, however, insensitive).
- In women with pelvic fractures, a pelvic examination should be performed to rule out vaginal lacerations.

Diagnosis

- A portable AP pelvis radiograph should be obtained in the trauma bay.
- This can be especially useful in a patient with vital sign instability to rule-in a pelvic fracture and thus raise the suspicion of a retroperitoneal hemorrhage.
- In patients stable enough to have one, a CT of the pelvis (with fine cuts) has become the diagnostic study of choice to evaluate the bony pelvic structures for fracture. It is especially helpful to identify acetabular and sacral fracture that can be subtle.
- There are multiple classification systems for pelvic fractures that are complex and beyond the scope of this book and thus not included.

Treatment
- Hypotensive patients in whom an unstable pelvic fracture (i.e., "open-book" pelvis) is suspected or confirmed by portable pelvis radiograph should have a commercially available pelvic binder applied, or if this device is not available, a sheet can be wrapped tightly across the upper hips. This can cause a pelvic hematoma to tamponade itself.
- Simple pelvic fractures such as nondisplaced pubic rami fractures, an iliac wing fracture, or a simple sacral fracture are managed with a toe-touch weight-bearing strategy and gait advancement as tolerated.
- More serious pelvic injuries such as acetabular fractures, displaced pelvic fractures, and open-book pelvis injuries are managed with orthopaedic consultation and often surgical intervention.

Pelvic Hematomas
- As discussed previously, patients with retroperitoneal bleeding from a serious pelvic injury can rapidly exsanguinate.

Diagnosis
- This entity should be highly suspected in the patient who is hemodynamically unstable with a pelvic injury but without an external source of bleeding and with a negative FAST exam.
- In a patient stable enough, obtaining a CT will demonstrate this entity.
- A blush of contrast implies arterial bleeding.

Treatment
- In patients with venous and osseous bleeding associated with a pelvic fracture, a pelvic binder and, if necessary, surgical stabilization of the pelvis will cause tamponade of the pelvic hematoma.
- Patients with arterial bleeding can undergo an angiogram with embolization. This has become the procedure of choice in many trauma centers.
- Patients with other solid organ injury requiring surgical exploration with associated pelvic venous or arterial injury can be managed in the OR.

Genitourinary Trauma

INTRODUCTION

- The "ABCs" of trauma should be followed prior to investigation of a specific GU injury.
- Injuries to the genitourinary system may be associated with blunt or penetrating trauma to the flank, abdomen, or pelvis, or they may occur as a result of rapid deceleration, such as a fall from a significant height.
- Trauma involving the ribs and pelvis may be associated with important injuries to the kidney and bladder, respectively, and these may be occult on initial presentation.
- A spontaneously voided specimen of urine should be obtained from all patients with blunt or penetrating injury to the pelvis, abdomen, or flank.
- Patients unable to provide a specimen should be catheterized, *unless* urethral injury is suspected.

SPECIFIC DISORDERS

Urethral Injuries

- Urethral injuries occur much more frequently in men, and the treatment is more complex, so this section focuses on men with urethral injury.
- Urethral injuries can be split into two groups: anterior and posterior injuries.
- Posterior urethral injuries are the more serious of the two and occur in the membranous or prostatic portion of the urethra.
- Posterior urethral injuries usually occur as a result of major trauma that causes pelvic fractures.
- Anterior urethral injuries commonly result from a direct blow to the perineum, such as a straddle injury.
- The following signs suggest urethral injury:
  - Spontaneous oozing of blood from the distal urethra (implying that injury is below the urethral sphincter)
  - Scrotal, perineal, or anterior abdominal swelling secondary to extravasated blood and urine
  - A superiorly displaced prostate or a pelvic hematoma on rectal examination
  - Significant perineal or external genitalia trauma, suggesting a "straddle type" injury

Diagnosis
- If a urethral injury is suspected, then an emergency retrograde urethrogram should be obtained before instrumentation (Foley catheterization) of the urethra and will demonstrate extravasation of dye if urethral disruption or laceration is present.

- This is performed by injecting 10 mL of water soluble contrast into the urethral meatus and then obtaining radiographs to determine if extravasation is present.
- Catheterization may be performed after a normal urethra is visualized.

Treatment
- Urology consultation for placement of a Foley in patients with an anterior disruption or a suprapubic catheter in a patient with a posterior disruption or a significant anterior disruption.
- Anterior disruptions usually heal nicely with just a Foley (but they are at risk for urethral strictures in the future).
- Posterior urethral tears are usually repaired several days or a couple of weeks after the initial injury.

Bladder Injuries
- Bladder injuries can occur in blunt and penetrating trauma.
- Rupture is related to the volume of urine in the bladder.
- Extraperitoneal bladder ruptures account for two thirds of this entity.
- Bladder injuries caused by blunt force trauma are nearly always associated with pelvic fractures.
- Only the dome of the bladder is covered by peritoneum and at risk for intraperitoneal rupture.
- Associated bowel and vascular injuries occur in the majority of patients with a penetrating bladder injury.

Diagnosis
- Cystography should be performed in all patients with suspected bladder injuries.
- The traditional method is to instill approximately 350 mL of diluted IV contrast in saline into the bladder via gravity through a Foley catheter.
- Radiographs are taken at intervals during the instillation to evaluate for extravasation.
- A postvoid radiograph is then taken after drainage to look for subtle extravasation.
- Computed tomography (CT) cystography has largely replaced the traditional method in trauma centers.
- It is performed in much the same way, but with a pelvis CT done after contrast instillation.

Treatment
- Foley catheters are left in place in patients with bladder ruptures.
- Intraperitoneal ruptures require surgical management.
- Most extraperitoneal ruptures heal within a couple of weeks, and Foley catheter drainage is all that is required.

Renal Injuries
- Renal injuries occur as a result of penetrating or blunt injuries.
- Renal injuries that are severe can cause brisk retroperitoneal bleeding that will not be detected as free fluid on the FAST exam.
- Renal injuries should be suspected in any patient with flank pain or penetrating injury.

Diagnosis
- Renal injury may be noted first on the FAST exam as a parenchymal injury or perinephric hematoma.

- The test of choice is CT of the abdomen and pelvis.
- Approximately 30% of patients with significant penetrating trauma to the kidney will fail to demonstrate hematuria, as may patients with complete ureteral disruptions; therefore, the absence of hematuria cannot always be used to exclude renal or ureteral injury when such injuries are clinically suspected.
- Most patients, including those with brisk, impressive hematuria, may be transfused and stabilized while appropriate studies are obtained; it is particularly important to demonstrate a contralaterally present kidney with normal renal function, because an absent or nonfunctioning contralateral kidney will clearly influence operative management.
- The renal injuries demonstrated by CT scan may be categorized as follows:
  - Grade I—Renal contusion limited to a small subcapsular hematoma or less
  - Grade II—Parenchymal laceration less than 1.0 cm deep without an expanding hematoma
  - Grade III—Parenchymal laceration more than 1.0 cm deep without urinary extravasation
  - Grade IV—Parenchymal laceration extending into the collecting system and/or segmented renal artery thrombosis
  - Grade V—Thrombosis of the main renal artery, avulsion of the pedicle, and/or shattered kidney with poor visualization

Treatment
- Many trauma centers undertake emergency renal angiography to assess regional blood flow to the affected kidney if therapeutic embolization is being considered.
- Management will depend on the extent of extravasation and the structure involved. Some controversy exists as to whether all patients, even those with minor degrees of extravasation, should be explored; this decision will be made by the consulting subspecialist.
- If extravasation occurs as a result of penetrating trauma, then most authorities recommend early exploration.
- Grades I, II, and III renal injuries are treated with conservative management and observation.
- Vital signs, hematocrit, and degree of hematuria are followed; if they remain stable, patients can avoid operative management.
- Most of these injuries heal spontaneously and rarely require radiological selective embolization.
- Grades IV and V require embolization and/or more aggressive surgical interventions.

10 Extremity Trauma

FRACTURES: GENERAL PRINCIPLES

The emergency physician must be thoroughly familiar with a variety of descriptive orthopaedic terms, which, when appropriately used, will greatly facilitate the care and disposition of patients with fractures. Because most significant bony injuries should be discussed with the orthopaedic surgeon and such discussion and any recommendations documented, the importance of precise anatomic location and description of the fracture cannot be overemphasized.

- It is important for the emergency physician to communicate to what extent, if any, the previously normal appearance of the bone is now distorted by the fracture. This is performed by describing the position of the distal fragment in relation to the proximal fragment.
- Fractures are said to be complete when both cortices are broken; incomplete fractures involve only one cortex.
- Comminution occurs when more than two bony fragments are produced.
- Fractures must always be defined as closed or open.
- Two terms are used to describe any abnormalities noted: displacement and angulation.
- Displacement occurs when the distal fragment moves laterally away from the proximal fragment but maintains alignment along the long axis. The extent of displacement is described in terms of the percent or fractional diameter of the distal fragment.
- Angulation occurs when normal orientation of the long axis of the bone is deranged. With the patient in the anatomic position, the axis of the distal fragment with respect to the proximal fragment is noted. The amount of angulation, expressed in degrees, and the direction with respect to the proximal fragment are described.
- It is important to note whether fractures enter the joint or involve the articular surface. If so, precise or anatomic reduction is usually required, and consultation should be obtained before disposition.
- "Greenstick" and buckle (or "torus") fractures, both of which are particularly common in children, are examples of incomplete fractures. A greenstick fracture occurs when stress is applied to a long bone in such a way that bowing or angulation persists in association with cortical disruption or breakage on one side. Such fractures often require manipulation, including fracture of the contralateral cortex, to restore normal realignment; consultation is therefore indicated in all patients.
- Buckle (or "torus") fractures are extremely common and, because of often subtle radiologic and physical findings, are often unrecognized in the emergency department (ED). If all cortical contours of the involved area are carefully examined, then point irregularity, notching, discrete wrinkling, or a subtle abnormality will be detected in patients with such fractures.

- Fractures are described as transverse when cortical disruption occurs perpendicular to the long axis of the bone.
- Spiral fractures occur in association with rotational stress and are seen to spiral down the shaft of the long bone.
- Open or compound fractures occur when any actual or potential communication, however subtle, exists between the fracture and the outside environment.
- Avulsion fractures imply that the bony attachment of ligaments or tendons has been pulled off as a result of excessive force applied to that attachment.
- Impaction occurs when bone collapses into or onto bone. The proximal humerus is the bone most often described as impacted; however, depression of the tibial plateau and compression of vertebral bodies are other examples of impaction-type injuries.
- In patients who may require manipulation or operative reduction, the patient's history of allergies and anesthesia; the presence of other injuries, particularly involving the head, neck, chest, or abdomen; when the patient last ate; and whether religious or other reasons might prevent treatment in the usual manner are significant historic facts that should be obtained before orthopaedic consultation.

Common Errors in the Management of Patients with Fractures

- Failure to provide treatment "as if a fracture were present" in patients with significant physical findings but "normal" x-ray results
- Failure to immobilize the fracture with a sling or splint or to provide or recommend crutches to patients with significant soft-tissue injuries
- Failure to arrange and document appropriate follow-up at an appropriate interval
- Failure to examine and document neurovascular status in patients with proximal fractures
- Failure to diagnose "clinical fracture of the navicular" in the presence of appropriate clinical findings but normal roentgenograms
- Failure to diagnose "clinical fracture of the radial head" in the presence of appropriate clinical findings but normal roentgenograms
- Failure to appreciate by physical examination subluxation of the radial head in children with normal roentgenograms
- Failure to diagnose posterior dislocation of the shoulder
- Failure to diagnose tibial plateau fracture
- Failure to diagnose fractures of the fibula in patients with unimpressive histories and subtle findings

Consultation and Documentation

- Because management differs significantly for a number of common fractures, we generally recommend orthopaedic consultation in fractures seen in the ED.
- This ensures that the initial management and follow-up interval will be consistent with the wishes of the individual physician who will be responsible for the long-term care of the patient.

Neurovascular Status

- Normal neurovascular status (specifically a statement noting the presence of normal motor, sensory, and vascular integrity) should be demonstrated and documented in all patients with proximal fractures.
- If compromise of these functions is suspected or diagnosed, then immediate orthopaedic, neurosurgical, or vascular consultation should be obtained.

Open or Compound Fractures

- Open fractures occur when a potential or actual communication exists between the fracture and the external environment.
- Treatment must be individualized according to the bone involved, the nature of the fracture, and the extent of contamination; orthopaedic consultation should be obtained and documented in all such patients.
- Many open fractures will be best treated in the operating room; these generally include proximal fractures; fractures with significant contamination; fractures entering joints; fractures requiring manipulation, reduction, or both; and fractures associated with tendinous or neurovascular injury.
- Patients should not be allowed to eat or drink until the orthopaedic surgeon has determined whether definitive operating room, general anesthetic care will be required.
- Open wounds, including protruding bone, should be covered with a sterile saline dressing. When operating room care will be required, irrigation should generally not be undertaken in the ED because surface organisms may be introduced further into the wound and adjacent tissues.
- Protruding tissues, including bone, should be covered and left in place.
- Externalized material should not be placed back into the wound because contamination has probably occurred and intraoperative debridement will be necessary.
- Neurovascular status should be assessed and documented.
- Patients with any compromise should be immediately discussed with the appropriate subspecialist.
- Prophylactic antibiotic therapy is recommended in all patients with open fractures and should be instituted early and intravenously.
- Establishment of bactericidal antibiotic levels in the fracture hematoma is the goal of prophylactic therapy.
- Administer cefazolin (alternative: clindamycin 900 mg), 1 g, in the ED; an alternative is nafcillin, 1 g intravenous. Gentamicin, 1.5 mg/kg, should be added in contaminated open fractures.
- Antitetanus prophylaxis should be administered as appropriate.
- Analgesics should be administered in the ED unless a compelling contraindication (i.e., altered mentation) exists.

Stress Fractures

- Stress fractures are frequently misdiagnosed as shin splints or soft-tissue injury.
- The practitioner must recognize that stress fractures occur in the absence of significant trauma, frequently produce more chronic and less impressive symptoms, and often produce no radiologic abnormalities when the patient is first seen in the ED.
- Definitive diagnosis is therefore extremely difficult; however, an appropriate history should provide grounds for a tentative or clinical diagnosis and the institution of appropriate therapy.
- Most stress fractures occur in the lower extremity and under circumstances of recently initiated or accelerated activity.
- A runner, for example, may have recently increased his or her distance or reinstituted an exercise program after a period of relative inactivity.
- Common locations include the distal fibula, tibia, the metatarsals, and the femoral neck.

- Discomfort with palpation over the fracture site is often present; however, swelling, if noted, is minimal.
- Roentgenograms are initially normal, but if repeated 8 to 10 days after the onset of symptoms, they will often show evidence of periosteal reaction and bony sclerosis adjacent to the fracture site.
- A radionuclide bone scan will be positive at 4 to 6 days and may be helpful in selected patients to confirm the diagnosis somewhat earlier.
- Patients with suspected fractures should be provided with crutches, and a provisional diagnosis of stress fracture should be made.
- The use of the involved extremity should be minimized until a definitive diagnosis is clear.

Buckle and Greenstick Fractures

- Buckle fractures are separately discussed to emphasize the often subtle radiologic and clinical findings seen with these fractures, most of which occur in children.
- Such fractures are infrequently displaced or angulated and are diagnosed on the basis of subtle wrinkling or notching of one side of the cortex; treatment, when a single bone is involved, is most often symptomatic and supportive.
- Greenstick fractures occur when stress is applied to a long bone in such a way to produce persistent bowing or angulation; cortical breakage on one side is noted.
- Angulation, which may be significant, requires reduction.
- Radiologic findings in both groups of patients, particularly those with buckle fractures, may be subtle and are frequently overlooked.
- A careful tracking of the cortical outline, which should define a smooth, gentle, uninterrupted curve, will disclose the site of fracture.

Other Fractures in Children

- In addition to buckle and greenstick fractures, injuries involving the epiphysis, the cartilaginous, radiolucent area at or near the end of long bones from which future growth occurs, are common and must be accurately diagnosed (Fig. 10-1).
- A high degree of suspicion regarding epiphyseal injury should be maintained, and when diagnosed, a conservative approach to treatment is appropriate; unfortunately, significant abnormalities of growth involving the injured epiphysis develop in approximately 10% of patients with epiphyseal fractures.
- The most commonly involved areas, in decreasing order of frequency, are the distal radius, distal tibia, phalanges, and proximal humerus.
- The peak age of occurrence is 12 years, and most patients are male.
- Radiologic assessment of the involved area will allow a definitive diagnosis.
- Salter and Harris have classified these fractures into five distinct categories:
  - Class 1: No bony disruption occurs, but slippage or separation of the epiphysis from the metaphysis is noted. Closed reduction is the treatment of choice.
  - Class 2: Separation through part of the epiphyseal plate occurs and a metaphyseal fracture is associated; treatment is by closed reduction.
  - Class 3: A fracture is noted extending from the joint space to the epiphyseal plate and then laterally to the periphery; treatment may be either open or closed reduction.
  - Class 4: These fractures extend from the articular surface through the epiphyseal plate and across the metaphysis; open reduction is usually required.
  - Class 5: These injuries involve severe crushing of the epiphyseal plate; displacement is unusual, and frequently these injuries are unappreciated. Growth disturbances are commonly associated with this type of fracture.

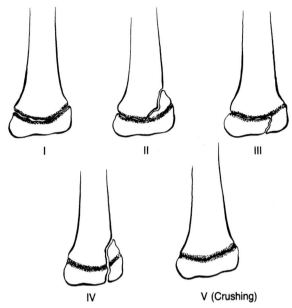

Figure 10-1. Nomenclature of representative fractures involving the growth plate in children. (From Harwood-Nuss AL, Linden CH, Luten RC, et al., eds. *The clinical practice of emergency medicine*, 2nd ed. Philadelphia, PA: Lippincott-Raven; 1996:1213, with permission.)

AMPUTATION AND REPLANTATION

- Recent advances in replantation surgery dictate that most extremity amputations and thumb and multiple digit amputations are initially considered replantable and that attempts are made to preserve viable tissue.
- The actual decision to proceed with replantation should be made after consultation by the emergency physician directly with the regional replantation team or surgeon.
- Pertinent details include associated major injuries to the head, neck, chest, or abdomen; clear medical contraindications to transport or prolonged surgery; and whether fractures, extensive crushing, or other injuries involve the amputated part.
- When these exist, when a single finger or the lower extremity is involved, when the patient is elderly, when extensive bacterial contamination is present, when a prolonged period of time between the injury and the institution of cooling has elapsed (i.e., more than 6 hours in the proximal arm and leg or more than 12 hours in distal amputations), or when severe degloving or avulsing is the mechanism of injury, the success of replantation is unlikely.
- Conversely, patients with multiple digits amputated, particularly the thumb, amputations occurring in children, and those associated with a short period of warm ischemia, minimal bacterial contamination, minimal crushing of the amputated part, and no significant other major trauma are generally considered the best candidates for replantation.

- These factors will be carefully considered by the transplant team. A general approach to initial treatment follows:
  - Initially, all amputations should be considered replantable and efforts made to preserve all tissue.
  - Given that bacterial contamination by hospital personnel is relatively common, sterile gloves should be worn when examining the patient and handling the amputated part.
  - Extensive bleeding, even with proximal amputations, is uncommon. Elevation of the stump and direct pressure, followed by a pressure dressing, are sufficient to arrest hemorrhage in virtually all patients. Blind clamping or ligating of vessels is to be avoided. When bleeding is extensive and uncontrolled by these measures, a proximal tourniquet or blood pressure cuff may be applied briefly.
  - Both wounds should be irrigated gently with Ringer lactate or normal saline solution; 250 mL to each site is adequate unless extensive contamination is present. More extensive irrigation and debridement should be deferred in most patients. The use of antiseptic solutions is discouraged.
  - The amputated part should be handled in a sterile manner and a sterile sponge dampened with Ringer lactate or normal saline solution applied to the wound. The part should then be wrapped in moist sterile towels and placed in a plastic bag; the bag should then be put in ice. Dry ice should never be used.
  - One gram of cefazolin, or a comparable agent, should be administered intravenously to adults and antitetanus prophylaxis should be administered if needed.
  - Analgesics may be administered, provided other injuries requiring frequent reassessments are not present.
  - Intravascular volume should be assessed and corrected if required.
  - A roentgenogram of the amputated part, particularly when crushing is the mechanism of injury, may be useful in estimating viability.
  - The replantation team should be contacted to discuss the feasibility of transport and replantation.

WRINGER-TYPE OR ROLLER-TYPE INJURIES

- In the past, wringer washing machines accounted for the majority of wringer-type or roller-type injuries; however, today, machinery using closely approximated rollers is responsible for most such accidents.
- Classically, the hands or fingers are involved and, importantly, the true extent of the injury is frequently underestimated at the time of presentation.
- A conservative approach to the disposition and treatment of these patients is therefore warranted.
- A variety of mechanisms may be associated with wringer-type trauma; these include heat injury, contusion, shearing or separation of tissue and tissue planes resulting in deep hematoma formation, peripheral nerve damage, avulsing or degloving of soft tissues, and fracture.
- Information should be obtained as to the temperature of the machine, the mechanism of extrication, the actual width between the rollers, and the duration of contact.
- Complete sensory and motor testing of the involved extremity should be undertaken initially.
- Although sensory abnormalities are frequently neuropraxic in type and therefore recovery is expected, they cannot be assumed to be so at presentation.

- Enhancement of discomfort or elicitation of pain with passive extension of the fingers or toes suggests injury to deep tissues and may represent or predict a future compartment syndrome.
- Roentgenograms should be obtained to exclude associated fracture.
- The treatment of patients with suspected or evolving significant injuries consists of in-hospital observation for 24 to 48 hours, meticulous irrigation and cleansing of open areas, strict elevation of the extremity, and early drainage in the operating room of subcutaneous or subfascial hematomas. Vascular status must be reassessed frequently to detect evolving ischemia.
- Administer antitetanus prophylaxis as needed, and if injuries are open and extensive or if bacterial contamination is likely, then prophylactic antibiotics should be administered.
- An appropriate antibacterial ointment may be applied to abraded areas.
- Grafting should usually be deferred until local swelling has resolved.

PRESSURE OR GREASE GUN INJURIES

- Devices generating high pressures to expel paint, grease, or other materials are now commonly used in the industry and may result in injury.
- The hand is often involved, and the extent of injury is often underestimated at the time of presentation.
- This occurs because the entry site associated with such injuries is often minor, and at presentation, patients may be minimally symptomatic.
- Occasionally, if the material is radiopaque, a radiograph may demonstrate tracking of the material along the fascial planes.
- Admission is recommended for observation, elevation, and early operative exploration and irrigation.
- Patients presenting with established swelling, tenderness, or erythema along the tendon sheaths or fascial planes are candidates for admission, intravenous antibiotics, and early exploration and irrigation.

COMPARTMENT SYNDROMES

- Crushing or penetration of tissues with resultant local hemorrhage and swelling may result in compromise of neural and vascular function; this may occur in open and closed injuries, although it is more common in the latter, in which case intact fascial planes operate to prevent expansion or decompression.
- Most commonly, compartment syndromes occur in the forearm and the lower leg; however, the hand, fingers, and foot may become involved as well.
- Penetrating injuries may result in compartment syndromes secondary to progressive hemorrhage that remains similarly confined.
- Compartment syndromes are diagnosed on the basis of a high degree of suspicion and frequent reassessment of distal vascular and neural function.
- Importantly, even in patients with evolving ischemia, distal pedal pulses may be present, and this must therefore not be used to exclude compartment syndrome; similarly, determination of flow by Doppler analysis does not exclude evolving vascular compromise.
- The diagnosis is definitively made by directly measuring the pressure of the affected compartment.

- There are many methods to accomplish this, but basically, a catheter and a pressure transducer are introduced into the suspected compartment, and measurements are made directly from this.
- A resting pressure of 30 mm Hg is diagnostic of compartment syndrome.
- When a significant proximal injury is associated with distal symptoms suggestive of neural ischemia (numbness, paresthesias, or pain) or when clinical evidence of vascular insufficiency exists (i.e., coolness, pallor, or reduced capillary filling), measures must be immediately undertaken to reduce local pressures.
- A workup for rhabdomyolysis should be considered, especially if larger muscle compartments are involved.
- Any restricting devices, such as wraps, casts, or splints, must be removed immediately; the extremity elevated; and emergency general or vascular surgical consultation for fasciotomy obtained.
- If it is not immediately available and if ischemia is severe, then fasciotomy in the ED may be required to prevent necrosis.

SPECIFIC INJURIES OF THE UPPER EXTREMITY

Clavicle Fracture

- Most clavicle injuries occur from a direct fall on the lateral shoulder or onto an outstretched hand.
- Very young children who are unable to localize their discomfort are brought to the ED by parents because the child will not or cannot use the involved extremity.
- The treatment of clavicular fractures is determined by the location of the fracture and, in the case of distal fractures, whether displacement is noted.
- Fractures are of three types:
  - Group 1: Fractures involving the medial third of the clavicle
  - Group 2: Fractures involving the distal third of the clavicle
  - Group 3: Fractures involving the proximal third of the clavicle
- Each group is made up of multiple subtypes depending on the fracture pattern.

Treatment

- Treatment for group 1 and 2 clavicle injuries includes a simple sling for support and analgesics for comfort. Figure-of-eight slings are no longer widely employed for these fractures.
- Patients with group 3 fractures may require operative reduction and internal fixation; definitive treatment should be discussed with the orthopaedic surgeon at the time of presentation.
- Importantly, all patients receiving a sling should be instructed to remove the sling once each day and to fully rotate and extend the elbow; this is particularly true in elderly patients.

Sternoclavicular Injuries

- Injury to the sternoclavicular joint may produce a simple sprain (first degree), subluxation (second degree), or actual dislocation (third degree).
- Dislocation may be anterior or posterior and is associated with complete rupture of the sternoclavicular and costoclavicular ligaments.
- Subluxation or second-degree sprain results from rupture of the sternoclavicular ligament; a partial tear of the costoclavicular ligament is also present in most patients.

- Oblique views of the sternoclavicular area may demonstrate displacement in patients with subluxation or dislocation.
- First-degree and second-degree sprains of the sternoclavicular joint require only supportive or symptomatic therapy and the avoidance of strenuous activity for 3 to 5 days.
- Anterior dislocations should generally be treated conservatively initially, followed by resection in persistently symptomatic patients.
- Posterior dislocations of the medial clavicle are important for the emergency physician to appreciate because they acutely require reduction if compression of the trachea, great vessels, or other vital mediastinal structures occurs.
- In these patients, one or two sandbags or rolled towels should be placed in the middle of the back and the shoulders retracted posteriorly against the stretcher; this maneuver allows the medial clavicle to disengage itself from the sternum and move anteriorly. If reduction does not occur, then while the shoulders remain retracted, the lateral end of the clavicle must be pushed posteriorly in an attempt to lever the medial clavicle anteriorly. If this is unsuccessful, then after locally anesthetizing the overlying skin and medial clavicle (including the periosteum), the bone should be grasped with a towel clip and elevated into position; a figure-of-eight splint should then be applied, followed by orthopaedic consultation.
- Patients without life-threatening symptoms related to mediastinal compression should be discussed with the orthopaedic surgeon, who may elect either operative or nonoperative reduction.

Acromioclavicular (AC) Injuries

- Most such injuries occur when force is applied to the lateral or superior aspect of the acromion.
- Injuries are graded as type I to VI.
- Types IV to VI are rare and will not be discussed in detail.
- Standard shoulder radiographs are usually adequate in confirming the diagnosis, but weight-bearing views should be employed in questionable cases.
- Type I injuries are caused by a sprained AC and coracoclavicular (CC) ligaments and are diagnosed on the basis of tenderness over the AC joint. Minor swelling may be noted as well. Weight-bearing views of both AC joints are normal and symmetric.
- Type II injuries are caused by torn AC ligaments but the CC is intact. They are diagnosed on the basis of tenderness, significant swelling, and mild deformity at the AC joint. If needed, weight-bearing views will demonstrate upward displacement of the lateral clavicle by not more than the diameter of the clavicle at that point.
- Type III injuries are diagnosed on the basis of tenderness, swelling, and an obvious deformity at the AC joint; radiologically, weight bearing produces marked upward displacement of the lateral clavicle and an increased distance between the coracoid process and the clavicle.
- Type I and II should be treated conservatively with a sling and analgesics as required. In these patients, early orthopaedic referral is recommended, primarily to institute a physical therapy program and to assess the patient's progress. Patients may remove the sling for bathing and at night if symptoms are not excessive.
- Type III injuries should be discussed with the consultant at the time of presentation because open reduction and internal fixation are often required for definitive repair.

Fractures of the Scapula

- The scapula is fractured by direct blows and major torso trauma; thus, significant force has been exerted to the back, and concomitant injuries to the shoulder, neck, kidney, lung, and mediastinal structures must be considered.
- Liberal use of chest CT (with fine cuts through the scapula to aid in surgical operative planning) is warranted.
- Treatment depends on the severity of the fracture and ranges from a sling, analgesics as required, and early referral to institute a program of shoulder mobilization exercises to operative fixation.
- Orthopaedic consultation in the ED is required.

Fractures of the Proximal Humerus and Shaft

- Most fractures of the proximal humerus occur in elderly patients and are nondisplaced or minimally displaced fractures of the neck.
- These may easily be treated, after orthopaedic consultation and demonstration of normal neurovascular function, with a simple sling, Velpeau bandage, or a commercial collar cuff and swathe. Analgesics and early orthopaedic to institute range-of-motion exercises are advised.
- Patients with displaced or comminuted fractures, fracture dislocations, fractures involving the articular surface, and fractures occurring in the younger patient require consultation at the time of presentation because operative treatment may be elected.
- Shaft fractures, particularly those that are distal, must be evaluated carefully because injury to the radial nerve may be associated. The patient should be evaluated for evidence of wrist drop, that is, inability to extend the wrist, fingers, or thumb.

Dislocation of the Shoulder

- Ninety to ninety-five percent of glenohumeral dislocations are anterior, present with severe pain and immobility of the shoulder, and may be easily reduced by the emergency provider.
- Posterior dislocations are uncommon; they occur in association with direct trauma, seizure, or electrocution; and present similarly to anterior dislocations.
- Inferior dislocations (luxatio erecta) are extremely uncommon and present with the patient's arm in full abduction with the humeral head against the axillary rib cage. This entity needs immediate orthopaedic consultation.
- Because of deceptively normal anteroposterior views of the shoulder, posterior dislocations are undiagnosed in the ED in approximately 50% of patients. This is readily explained because pure posterior movement of the humeral head, if unassociated with displacement in any other direction, will appear relatively normal on routine anteroposterior views. However, slight lateral displacement of the humeral head, which radiologically produces less than the expected amount of overlap between the humeral head and the posterior rim of the glenoid fossa, is a clue to the presence of a posterior dislocation.
- For this reason, anteroposterior, lateral, and axillary views of the shoulder are always indicated in patients with suspected shoulder dislocations.
- Prereduction radiographs may not be needed if the patient has experienced repeated dislocations.
- Radiographs should be done with adequate analgesics as acquiring these films can be quite painful. If severe pain and immobility persist, despite normal-appearing radiographs, a CT of the shoulder will disclose occult dislocations.

- Shoulder dislocations are associated with severe discomfort, and most patients resist any movement of the extremity, particularly abduction.
- Anterior dislocations typically produce a "square" shoulder when viewed from an anteroposterior perspective and a palpable, but often not visible, "step-off" below the now more prominent acromion.
- Posterior dislocations produce palpable emptiness of the anterior compartment of the shoulder and a fullness posteriorly with prominence of the coracoid process.
- The treatment of anterior dislocations follows; posterior and inferior dislocations may require reduction under general anesthesia, and therefore, prompt orthopaedic consultation is appropriate.
- Coexistent fractures of the humeral head or glenoid are not uncommon and should be excluded radiologically before any attempt at reduction is made. When present, orthopaedic referral should be obtained.
- Assessment and documentation of neurovascular status are important and should be performed before and after reduction in all patients.
- Axillary nerve function should be evaluated in particular.
- The treatment of anterior dislocations with respect to the method of reduction is highly variable.
- Most reductions require procedural sedation for the patient to tolerate.
- Traction-countertraction is the most widely employed technique but is falling out of favor for less traumatic reduction techniques. A sheet is placed around the supine patient's thorax and held by one practitioner. A second practitioner grasps the affected slightly abducted arm with the elbow held in 90 degrees of flexion while providing traction and internal or external rotation until a clunk is felt as the shoulder is reduced.
- The Stimson technique requires that the patient be placed prone while holding a 10-lb. weight. Reduction may take up to 30 minutes.
- An increasingly popular variation of the Stimson technique is called scapular manipulation. This calls for the same weight-bearing, arm-hanging technique as in the Stimson's, while a practitioner gently rotates the tip of the scapula medially using his or her thumbs.
- External rotation is a technique employed with the patient in the supine position with the affected arm fully adducted. The elbow is flexed to 90 degrees and the arm is slowly externally rotated without traction.
- If reduction is not successful, orthopaedic evaluation is mandatory.
- Occasionally, general anesthesia will be required to achieve sufficient sedation and pain relief to overcome local muscle spasm and effect reduction.
- A postreduction roentgenogram should be obtained and neurovascular function reassessed.
- Significant tears of the rotator cuff may complicate dislocation; initiation of abduction should be demonstrated after reduction to exclude this injury.
- Post-reduction treatment includes a sling and swathe, a short course of analgesics, and early orthopaedic follow-up in approximately 3 to 5 days to institute range-of-motion exercises.

Tears of the Rotator Cuff

- The rotator cuff is made up of four muscles, which attach to the greater and lesser tuberosities of the humerus.
- These include the supraspinatus (the most frequently torn of the muscles), subscapularis, infraspinatus, and teres minor.

- Typical mechanisms that result in this injury include a fall on the outstretched arm, direct fall on the shoulder, or heavy lifting.
- On examination, there is tenderness to palpation at the tuberosities, and abduction of the arm, particularly its initiation, is weak and elicits discomfort.
- Roentgenograms are normal or may rarely demonstrate an avulsion-type injury to the tuberosity.
- Definitive diagnosis is made by MRI.
- Treatment is somewhat dependent on the patient's age, lifestyle, and extent of disability present.
- In the young patient with a large tear or an associated avulsion fracture, the threshold for early repair is reduced, whereas a period of observation is generally elected for the older patient.
- Orthopaedic outpatient follow-up is appropriate for such patients.

Radial Nerve Palsy

- Penetrating trauma to the axilla, dislocation of the shoulder, humerus fracture, and pressure neuropathies may all produce radial nerve palsy.
- Pressure neuropathies may result from crutches that are too long for the patient, placing undue pressure in the axilla. The so-called Saturday night palsy results from the arm being hung over a chair during alcohol-induced sleep.
- The radial nerve can also be injured when medications are injected into the posterior portion of the upper arm.
- Signs of radial nerve impairment include loss of wrist extension, loss of finger and thumb extension, and weakness of both elbow flexion, caused by brachioradialis impairment, and supination.
- Very proximal lesions may also produce loss of elbow extension secondary to triceps paralysis.
- Sensory loss is most consistently noted to involve the dorsal aspect of the hand.
- Treatment includes orthopaedic or neurologic referral, physical therapy, and the application of a wrist splint in the position of function.

Biceps Brachii Rupture

- Rupture of the biceps may occur distally in the biceps tendon, in the bulk of the muscle, or in the tendon of the long head of the biceps.
- Most ruptures occur traumatically when excessive or sudden stress is applied across the bicep.
- The diagnosis is based on this history, and most patients report an audible or palpable "snap" or the sudden sensation that the muscle has given way or is weakened at the time of rupture.
- This sensation is followed by local discomfort, a palpable defect or step-off along the bicep, or a proximally bulging or "Popeye-"type muscle.
- An acute rupture of the distal tendon is treated surgically, whereas muscle and long tendon ruptures are most often treated conservatively with an initial period of cold application, analgesics as required, and restriction of activity.
- A sling is recommended for several days, to be removed at night, and orthopaedic follow-up in 3 to 5 days is advised.

Injuries to the Elbow

- To the nonradiologist, the bones of the elbow, particularly in the child with incomplete ossification, represent an extremely difficult area.

- Because of this and because some fractures may not be apparent on initial views, a very conservative approach to the treatment of elbow injuries, particularly in children, is warranted.
- A relatively low threshold for obtaining consultation or requesting contralateral views of the uninjured elbow for comparison should be maintained.

Fractures
Proximal Radial Head and Neck
- Patients with fractures involving the radial head or neck, often occurring as a result of trivial trauma, present with often poorly localized discomfort to the area of the proximal radius.
- Because initial roentgenograms may be normal despite the presence of a fracture, the physician must be aware of the important clinical signs suggesting this injury; these include accentuation of discomfort with rotation of the forearm and with hyperflexion and hyperextension of the elbow.
- When these signs are present despite a normal initial study, a diagnosis of "clinical or occult fracture of the radial head or neck" is justified.
- The diagnosis is further suggested when the so-called posterior fat-pad sign is present; this is seen as a radiolucent area posterior to the distal humerus on the lateral view of the elbow and suggests intra-articular bleeding.
- The anterior fat-pad sign, or sail sign, is not as diagnostic of injury when small, because this can be a normal finding.
- When an occult or clinical fracture is diagnosed on the basis of clinical signs (and negative x-rays), patients should understand that although a possible fracture exists, it cannot be definitely diagnosed until a healing line is noted in approximately 10 to 12 days.
- CT in equivocal cases can also demonstrate the fracture.
- Treatment includes a sling, analgesics, and orthopaedic follow-up in 10 to 12 days to reevaluate the elbow radiologically (and thereby exclude a fracture) and to institute a program of range-of-motion exercises.
- Patients who are minimally symptomatic should remove the sling each day for 20 to 30 minutes while they bathe, and all patients should be instructed to remove the sling at night so as to prevent the development of elbow and shoulder stiffness.
- Patients with displaced or comminuted fractures of the radial head or neck require additional therapy (i.e., reduction, fixation, or occasionally excision); consultation at the time of presentation in these patients is therefore indicated.

Supracondylar Fractures
- Supracondylar fracture is an injury often seen in children and the elderly.
- The injury commonly results from a fall on an extended, outstretched arm.
- This injury is associated with a relatively high degree of neural and arterial injury owing to the proximity of the ulnar, median, and radial nerves and brachial artery to the elbow.
- A low threshold for angiogram must be maintained if vascular injury is suggested by the physical exam (i.e., diminished pulses, poor capillary refill, etc.).
- Conscientious determination of neurovascular function in the forearm and wrist and orthopaedic consultation are indicated early in the management of these patients.
- Most of these injuries need urgent operative management.

Intra-articular Fractures Involving the Elbow
- Intra-articular fractures involving the elbow should be evaluated by the orthopaedic surgeon at the time of presentation; frequently internal fixation after reduction is required.

Olecranon Fractures
- Olecranon fractures may be complicated by displacement, comminution, injury to the ulnar nerve, and rupture of the triceps mechanism at the elbow.
- Ulnar nerve injury is suggested by numbness or paresthesias involving the fourth and fifth fingers; triceps rupture is diagnosed on the basis of the patient's inability to extend the elbow against gravity.
- Undisplaced fractures are generally treated with a posterior splint with the elbow flexed at 90 degrees and early institution of range-of-motion exercises and follow-up in 3 to 4 days.
- Patients with triceps rupture, ulnar nerve injury, or displaced (>2 mm) or comminuted fractures require orthopaedic evaluation, because operative repair, stabilization, or both are often required.

Dislocation of the Elbow
- Differentiated from supracondylar fracture by the disappearance of the normally present triangular configuration of the posterior elbow represented by the epicondyles superiorly and the olecranon inferiorly; this equilateral relationship is generally maintained in patients with fractures but distorted in patients with dislocation of the elbow.
- Radiologic assessment will further clarify the nature of the injury.
- Treatment involves rapid assessment of neurovascular status; thereafter, orthopaedic consultation for reduction should be obtained as soon as possible.
- Fractures of the elbow are found concomitantly in 30% to 40% of cases. Injuries to the ulnar nerve, median nerve, and brachial artery may occur.
- Because extraordinary opposing forces operate to maintain or stabilize the dislocation, sedation is virtually always required.
- Without adequate relaxation of surrounding muscle groups by appropriate sedation and analgesia, reduction is impossible, and in some patients, reduction in the operating room under general anesthesia may be elected.
- Most dislocations are posterior and reduction is straightforward. An assistant stabilizes the distal humerus, and traction is applied along the axis of the forearm until the elbow can be brought into flexion. At this time, traction is continued at the wrist and forearm while posterior countertraction, which must be forceful, is applied at the distal humerus. Reassessment and documentation of neurovascular function must follow reduction along with radiologic reassessment.

Subluxation of the Radial Head (Nursemaid's Elbow)
- This is a relatively common cause of elbow pain in children (usually between the ages of 1 and 5 years) who typically are brought to the ED because of failure to use the extremity.
- The history, if complete, will usually include the acute onset of pain or immobility associated with longitudinal traction on the outstretched arm.
- The child cries irritably, often supports the arm, and refuses to use the injured arm.
- Most patients will present with the forearm pronated and the elbow extended. In somewhat older children, discomfort may be localized to the elbow.
- Mild tenderness to palpation is generally noted over the proximal radius, and this is clearly accentuated by rotation, particularly supination, of the forearm.
- Swelling and deformity are not expected findings in patients with simple subluxation; when present or when the history of the injury is unclear or involves direct

trauma, radiologic assessment of the elbow should be obtained before manipulation to exclude fracture or dislocation.

- If fracture or dislocation of the elbow is noted, orthopaedic consultation should be obtained.
- Reduction is simple and straightforward; the physician places the thumb of one hand against the proximal radial head, grasps the wrist and forearm with the other, and simply flexes the elbow to approximately 90 degrees while supinating the forearm.
- When reduction is successful, a palpable but subtle "click" is often noted, indicating that the radial head has been repositioned within the annular ligament.
- In some patients, reduction is immediately associated with the resumption of normal use of the extremity and the total disappearance of pain; the diagnosis is then clear and roentgenograms are unnecessary.
- Often, within 20 to 30 minutes, a complete return of full range of motion unassociated with discomfort will be noted.
- Such patients may be discharged with pediatric or orthopaedic follow-up as required.
- The mechanism of injury, that is, pulling on an outstretched arm, should be explained to the parents to prevent future subluxations.
- In patients with persisting discomfort or when the patient persistently refuses to use the extremity, radiologic assessment of the extremity and clavicle should be obtained.
- If this is normal, and if localization of discomfort to the elbow is convincing, a repeated attempt at reduction is indicated, which, if unsuccessful, should be followed by orthopaedic consultation.

Nerve Disruption or Compression

Precise motor and sensory testing and its documentation must be undertaken in all patients with appropriate injuries involving the upper extremity. Patients with penetrating injuries involving the upper arm, forearm, and wrist must be carefully assessed with respect to these functions; motor and sensory functions related to median, ulnar, and radial nerves (Fig. 10-2) are briefly reviewed.

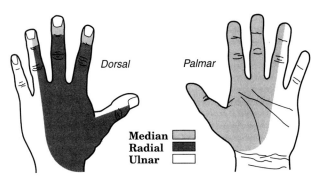

Dorsal   *Palmar*

Median ☐
Radial ■
Ulnar ☐

Figure 10-2. Hand sensory nerve innervation.

Median Nerve
- **Sensory:** Tip of index finger (particularly) and palm radially
- **Motor:** Wrist, index finger, thumb, and long finger flexors
- **Examination:** Loss of sensation involving the tip of the index finger and radial side of the palm; the ability to oppose the tip of the thumb to the tips of the other fingers is impaired, and with the patient's palm up, the thumb cannot be pointed directly toward the ceiling. Weakness of the thumb, index, and long finger flexors is noted. If interruption is proximal, wrist flexion is impaired.

Ulnar Nerve
- **Sensory:** Fifth finger, ulnar side of fourth finger, and ulnar side of hand
- **Motor:** Fourth and fifth distal interphalangeal (DIP) flexors, finger spreaders, and thumb adductor
- **Examination:** Loss of sensation as listed and inability to spread the fingers against resistance when fully extended; flexion at the DIP joint of the fourth and fifth fingers is impaired. Patients cannot hold a piece of paper against resistance in the web space between the thumb and index fingers and have difficulty forming a perfect "O" with the thumb and index finger.

Radial Nerve
- **Sensory:** Majority of the back of the hand
- **Motor:** Wrist extensors, proximal phalanx extensors, thumb extensor, and abductor
- **Examination:** Sensory loss to the back of the hand, and wrist drop is noted with proximal injuries, as is absence of the brachioradialis reflex. The proximal phalanx cannot be extended, nor can the thumb be abducted or extended.

Lateral Epicondylitis (Tennis Elbow)
- Patients with lateral epicondylitis usually provide a history of repetitive or excessive use of the muscles of the wrist or forearm; however, often, no such history is present.
- It is a tendenosis (microtears in a tendon) that involves the origin of the extensor carpi radialis brevis muscle.
- On examination, tenderness of the lateral epicondyle is noted with palpation, which is accentuated by extension of the wrist, particularly against resistance.
- Passive range of motion of the elbow is normal.
- Treatment involves limiting maneuvers resulting in repetitive use of the forearm and wrist extensors, providing a sling, and instituting a course of oral nonsteroidal anti-inflammatory agents.
- A variety of splint-type devices are available (these are referred to as "tennis-elbow bands" or "wraps") that when applied result in mild compression of the muscles of the forearm, in this case the forearm extensors, thereby reducing transmitted force to the epicondyle.
- Although the local injection of corticosteroids is effective, this treatment should probably be reserved for patients not responding to more conservative therapy.
- Only 10% of patients eventually require surgery.

Medial Epicondylitis (Golfer's Elbow)
- Patients with medial epicondylitis present with discomfort localized to the medial epicondyle, clearly accentuated by valgus stress applied to the elbow joint.
- The origin of the pain is a tendenosis most commonly of the pronator teres and/or flexor carpi radialis.

- Ulnar nerve irritation is commonly associated with this entity.
- Treatment includes avoiding activities that reproduce the pain, stretching and strength improvement regimens, and use of an anti-inflammatory agent.
- A variety of splint-type devices are available that when applied result in mild compression of the muscles of the forearm, in this case the forearm flexors and major pronator, thereby reducing transmitted force to the epicondyle.
- Local injection with a corticosteroid may also be recommended in particularly refractory or symptomatic cases but must be undertaken with caution because of the proximity of the ulnar nerve.
- Surgical therapy is needed in a minority of cases.
- These patients should be referred to an orthopaedic surgeon for follow-up.

Olecranon Bursitis
- Patients present with pain overlying the olecranon, and a history of chronic or acute injury to the area is frequently present.
- The posterior elbow is tender to palpation, often markedly inflamed with increased warmth and erythema, and the thickened, fluid-filled or "boggy" olecranon bursa is easily appreciated.
- The differential diagnosis of olecranon bursitis includes crystalline synovitis (gout, pseudogout) and septic bursitis.
- Septic bursitis must always be considered and excluded, especially when penetrating trauma has preceded the onset of symptoms or when evidence of systemic infection is present. Under these circumstances, sterile aspiration of the bursa is indicated in all patients.
- Treatment includes a sling, and the administration of a nonsteroidal anti-inflammatory agent.
- Patients should be advised that if symptoms have not improved in 5 to 7 days, aspiration and possible steroid injection may be required; orthopaedic follow-up at this time is therefore advised.
- Analgesics are often required during the initial 2 to 3 days of treatment and should be provided.
- An occasional patient with chronic or refractory symptoms will require eventual excision of the bursa.

Ulnar Nerve Compression
- The ulnar nerve may be compressed or injured at a number of sites along its path.
- This may occur chronically or acutely, and most commonly, entrapment or injury occurs at the wrist or elbow.
- A history of trauma frequently precedes the onset of symptoms, and in these patients, radiologic assessment of the involved area is recommended.
- Some patients will report the subacute onset of symptoms after maneuvers that repetitively contuse or stretch the nerve; these may involve simply leaning on the elbow, allowing the elbow to rest on the window, door frame, or center console while driving; lifting weights (e.g., repetitive curls); or operating machinery resulting in excessive wrist motion.
- A relatively common presentation involves striking the area of the ulnar groove at the elbow followed by the immediate onset of local discomfort, numbness, and tingling involving the ulnar side of the palm and fourth and fifth fingers.
- Motor loss is not uncommon and is manifest as finger clumsiness in undertaking fine or precision-type manipulations, weakness of the finger spreaders, and all motor

functions of the fifth finger; eventually, if compression is not relieved, atrophy or asymmetry of the hypothenar eminence may be noted.

- Treatment is dependent on the extent of symptoms and whether motor involvement is present and to what extent. Colles or Smith fracture of the wrist and fractures of the elbow should be excluded when trauma has preceded the onset of symptoms. Some patients, as a result of significant symptoms or progressive motor loss, will require decompression; orthopaedic consultation should therefore be obtained in patients presenting with evidence of motor loss. Other patients with mild symptoms and no evidence of motor loss may be treated with a nonsteroidal anti-inflammatory agent and avoidance of positions or maneuvers that repetitively stretch or contuse the ulnar nerve.
- Patients should be advised to avoid excessive flexion of the elbow because this may further compress the nerve at the ulnar groove; pronation has a similar effect.
- A sling is generally not advised; patients with refractory symptoms may require local steroid injection after a period of conservative treatment has failed.

Shaft Fractures of the Radius and Ulna

- When a significant injury to the forearm is noted, involving either one or both bones, it is critical that the physician carefully evaluates, both by radiologic and physical examination, the elbow and wrist.
- Monteggia (proximal one third ulnar shaft fracture and dislocation of the radial head) and Galeazzi (distal radial fracture and dislocation of the distal radioulnar joint) fractures will not be missed if this rule is followed.
- Greenstick fractures in children involving either one or both bones should be discussed with the orthopaedic surgeon; particular attention should be directed toward any angulation produced by the fracture.
- Frequently, closed reduction and, if significant angulation is present, fracture of the contralateral cortex under general anesthesia will be required to establish realignment; plaster immobilization will then be undertaken.
- Buckle fractures frequently involve the forearm, and when a single bone is involved, a simple splint is usually sufficient provided that angulation is absent; buckle fractures involving both bones should be discussed with the orthopaedic consultant as to definitive treatment.
- In adults, nondisplaced fractures involving both bones are generally treated with plaster immobilization, while closed reduction or operative intervention may be required for patients with displacement or abnormalities of alignment.

Fractures of the Wrist

- Injuries to the epiphyseal plate must be considered in all children presenting with injuries to the wrist; suspected or demonstrated fractures should be discussed with the orthopaedic surgeon.
- In adults, Colles classic wrist fracture involves a fracture through the distal radius with dorsal displacement of the distal fragment; approximately 50% of patients present with an associated fracture through the base of the ulnar styloid.
- Carpal fractures or fracture dislocations and injuries to the hand, forearm, and elbow can coexist and should specifically be considered and excluded by careful palpation and radiologic assessment.
- In patients with Colles fractures, minor amounts of displacement can usually be tolerated without intervention; however, restoration of normal function is enhanced by a more precise reduction.

- As previously noted, neurovascular compromise requires urgent orthopaedic consultation and reduction.
- When neurovascular compromise is not present and when insignificant displacement and no dorsal angulation are present, after consultation, splinting, ice, analgesics, and elevation may be elected. Plaster splinting is often performed initially, with a cast placed when some of the swelling has subsided.
- Less commonly, volar displacement of the distal segment occurs, resulting in a so-called Smith fracture. Smith fractures are classically considered unstable, and for this reason, orthopaedic consultation at the time of presentation is recommended; open reduction and internal fixation will often be elected.
- All patients with wrist fractures obviously require careful assessment of neurovascular function; specific attention must be directed to median nerve function, which may be altered as a result of compression or transection.
- Neurovascular status, as always, should be documented in the involved extremity, as should orthopaedic consultation.

Scaphoid Fractures

- These injuries are unfortunately commonly missed and therefore inappropriately treated.
- Importantly, initial roentgenograms, if obtained within several days of the fracture, may be normal unless displacement or separation of the fracture fragments is present.
- The clinical diagnosis of occult or clinical scaphoid fracture is therefore warranted when the clinical findings suggest this diagnosis.
- Scaphoid injuries most often occur when the wrist is hyperextended; patients report falling on the hand with the wrist in extension.
- Physical findings may be subtle; however, tenderness to palpation is present overlying the scaphoid, in the area of the so-called anatomic snuffbox.
- When tenderness is present in this location despite normal roentgenograms, a clinical diagnosis of fracture should be made.
- Importantly, well-recognized complications of failure to diagnose this fracture include avascular necrosis and nonunion of the scaphoid.
- Patients with tenderness over the scaphoid, particularly when a hyperextension injury is reported, without a roentgenographically demonstrable fracture should be given a clinical diagnosis of occult or clinical fracture of the scaphoid and splinted for 2 weeks.
- A repeat roentgenogram at 10 to 12 days should demonstrate or exclude a fracture, but if pain persists and a fracture is not demonstrated, a bone scan or CT can be utilized to exclude scaphoid fracture.
- Demonstrated fractures require plaster immobilization for up to 12 weeks.

Other Carpal Injuries

- Although carpal fractures are relatively uncommon, failure to recognize them and provide immobilization may result in prolonged symptoms and significant morbidity.
- Carpal fractures that are displaced should be corrected and neurovascular status carefully assessed.
- Dorsal wrist trauma can result in minor chip fractures; these are most often treated symptomatically with ice, elevation, analgesics as required, and splinting.

- Volar dislocation of the lunate, although uncommon, should be diagnosed on the basis of a history of wrist hyperextension followed by volar pain, fullness with palpation, loss of wrist flexion, and volar displacement of the lunate (no longer appearing under the capitate) on the lateral view of the wrist.
- Treatment includes orthopaedic consultation and closed reduction followed by plaster immobilization.
- Fracture of the lunate, similar to that of the navicular, may be radiographically occult and is diagnosed on the basis of local tenderness; treatment generally involves plaster immobilization.
- Perilunate dislocation is diagnosed on the basis of a lateral view of the wrist, where the normally present vertical relationship between the "cup" of the radius (in which is found the lunate, above which is noted the capitate) is distorted. Specifically, the capitate is noted to be dislocated dorsally; a fracture of the navicular is frequently present as well. Reduction and splinting are necessary. Orthopaedic consultation before disposition is advised.

Metacarpal Fractures

Metacarpal Neck Fractures
- Metacarpal neck fractures, particularly the fifth and fourth, are common in the ED; fractures of the fifth metacarpal neck are referred to as boxer fractures and often result from striking an object with the fist.
- Volar displacement of the distal fragment is the rule.
- A patient with fourth or fifth metacarpal neck fractures can generally be splinted if less than 45 degrees of volar angulation is present (necessitating closed reduction).
- Splints for metacarpal fractures are forearm based; keep the wrist in 20 to 30 degrees of extension and provide 70 to 90 degrees of flexion at the metacarpophalangeal (MCP) joint, extending to the interphalangeal joint (IP). Buddy taping the affected digit can aid with rotational deformities.
- Fractures involving the neck of the index and long fingers require almost perfect reduction (<15 degrees of angulation) to ensure normal function, unlike the fourth or fifth metacarpal neck fractures in which angulation is better tolerated. These fractures must be splinted and eventually casted to maintain the reduction.
- When an open injury has resulted from striking teeth, it must be treated aggressively as a human bite.

Metacarpal Shaft Fractures
- These injuries must be carefully assessed to exclude rotational deformity, and unlike metacarpal neck fractures, less angulation of the shaft can be tolerated without eventual deformity and loss of function. The general rule for degree of displacement for metacarpal shaft fractures is 10 degrees for the second and third metacarpals, 20 degrees for the fourth, and 30 degrees for the fifth metacarpal.
- Importantly, to assess the extent of functional rotation, the hand should be examined with the palm up and the fingers in flexion; this simple exercise often makes otherwise subtle rotational deformities obvious.
- If displacement is present, closed reduction and splinting should be performed.
- In patients with displacement or when more than one fracture exists, orthopaedic consultation is warranted.

Metacarpal Base Fractures
- These injuries require reduction if more than 2 mm of articular surface disruption is present, if more than minimal angulation is present, or if there is a dislocation of

the carpometacarpal (CMC) joint. After reduction, a forearm-based splint is applied as described above.
- The thumb is an exception. Metacarpal fractures involving the base of the thumb are often both intra-articular and dislocated (Bennett fracture, Rolando fracture). Reduction must be precise, and orthopaedic consultation is required.

Gamekeeper Thumb

- Gamekeeper thumb is a term denoting rupture of the ulnar collateral ligament of the MCP joint of the thumb; ligamentous strain may also occur.
- The name is derived from the Scottish gamekeeper, who would break the neck of a hare by holding it between the thumb and index finger, resulting in chronic ligamentous laxity or rupture.
- Injury to the ligament usually follows the application of a radial moving force across the MCP joint. In all injuries involving the proximal thumb, ligamentous stability should be demonstrated by reproducing this stress across the MCP joint.
- Rupture of the ligament, diagnosed on the basis of finding significant laxity or that the joint appears to "open" when stress is applied across it, requires operative repair.
- Incomplete tears require splinting and orthopaedic referral; a spica cast will generally be applied for 6 to 8 weeks.

Proximal and Middle Phalanx Shaft Fractures

- Nondisplaced, nonangulated fractures that do not have a rotational component and do not involve the articular surface of the joint may be treated simply with a protective splint or stabilization by taping to the adjacent, larger finger.
- Three weeks of splinting is usually required for proximal fractures, whereas 12 to 14 days is adequate for those involving the middle phalanx.
- Elevation of the hand, the intermittent application of cold for 24 hours, analgesics as required, and early orthopaedic follow-up to institute active range-of-motion exercises are advised.
- Commonly, significant angulation or displacement is present; these injuries are best considered unstable, even after reduction, and should be discussed with or evaluated by the orthopaedic or hand surgeon, who may elect internal fixation.
- As noted, fractures complicated by involvement of the joint space should be evaluated by the consultant as well because precise reduction is essential.
- It is important to note that rotated proximal and middle phalanx fractures may result in significant morbidity and loss of function.
- A surprising degree of rotation may exist in patients with very benign-appearing roentgenograms; this is even true in children with otherwise simple buckle fractures.
- To assess rotation, one simply examines the hands simultaneously, palms up, with the fingers in first semiflexion and then in full flexion. Fractures associated with significant rotation produce varying degrees of overlapping of the fingers and the tendency of the fingers to point along different lines.

Intra-articular Fractures

- The generally accepted rule that fractures involving the joint surface require precise or anatomic reduction is particularly true with respect to finger fractures.
- Such fractures involving the joint should be discussed with the subspecialist. A few special fractures that are particularly common are noted.

Fractures Involving the Volar DIP Joint

- This benign-appearing but often serious intra-articular fracture occurs when the distal insertion of the flexor tendon of the DIP joint avulses a portion of the articular surface.
- Fractures involving greater than 15% of the joint surface at this point should be considered complex to the extent that subluxation of the joint with resultant chronic disability is relatively common; such fractures should usually be treated with open reduction and internal fixation.
- Fractures involving less than 15% of the joint surface can usually be treated with 4 weeks of immobilization; consultation in either case is advised.

Avulsion Fracture Involving the Distal Phalanx at the Insertion of the Extensor Tendon

- Fractures involving less than 25% of the joint surface may be treated with simple splinting to result in DIP hyperextension; the proximal interphalangeal (PIP) joint should not be immobilized.
- Fractures involving more than 25% of the joint surface require open reduction and internal fixation.
- Extensor tendon avulsion frequently coexists and, in the absence of joint involvement of less than 25%, is treated by simple DIP hyperextension without PIP immobilization.
- Rupture of the central slip of the extensor apparatus at the PIP commonly coexists and allows the extensor mechanism to migrate volarly, resulting in fixed PIP flexion; treatment is surgical repair.

Fractures of the Distal Phalanx

- Fractures of the most distal phalanx or tuft are extremely common and may most often be satisfactorily managed in the ED.
- Frequently, however, such fractures are complicated by more significant injury to the soft tissues of the distal finger.
- Distal tendon disruption must always be considered and excluded.
- Subungual hematoma frequently coexists, implies the presence of a badly contused or lacerated nail bed, and may simply be drained by placing a small hole over the collection, thereby allowing the blood to drain. This is easily accomplished with the use of commercially available drills or hot cautery; a dry dressing is then applied.
- In most patients, simple tuft fractures can be treated with a distal splint (which does not restrict mobility of the PIP joint) applied loosely for protection and analgesics as required.
- Fractures of the distal phalanx are typically painful, and a narcotic analgesic should be provided to symptomatic patients.
- Orthopaedic follow-up should be recommended in 12 to 14 days, and patients should be instructed to remove the splint each day to prevent stiffness of the distal joint and to cleanse the skin. If significant crushing has occurred in the area of the proximal nail bed, patients should additionally be warned regarding the possibility of permanent nail loss.
- Transverse fractures that are proximal and angulated may require definitive reduction and internal fixation; orthopaedic consultation is therefore advised at the time of presentation.
- Similarly, fractures that enter the joint space should be discussed with the subspecialist, because precise alignment of the fracture site is needed to restore and ensure full recovery.

Metacarpophalangeal Dislocations

- Dislocation at the MCP joint may be either dorsal or volar and may involve either the fingers or the thumb.
- Although any of these dislocations may be reduced in the ED, interposition of soft tissue is common and effectively operates to prevent reduction; such patients will require open reduction.
- As with any dislocation, radiologic assessment of the area before manipulation is indicated to demonstrate coexistent fracture.
- In patients with dorsal dislocations after digital block proximal to the injury with 1% or 2% lidocaine, the joint may be reduced by hyperextending the finger or thumb, applying traction along the line of dislocation, and simultaneously placing downward pressure on the proximal aspect of the dislocated fragment.
- Unfortunately, as previously noted, interposition of soft tissues is common and is suggested by resistance or the initial failure of reduction; prompt orthopaedic consultation is then indicated.
- In other patients, marked palmar displacement of the metacarpal head should be obvious by examination and implies herniation of the metacarpal through the flexor apparatus; this will frequently make reduction in the ED impossible. Early consultation is appropriate.
- Postreduction treatment when normal motor and collateral ligament function is demonstrated involves a volar splint with the MCP joint fixed in 30 degrees of flexion; early orthopaedic follow-up is again appropriate to institute range-of-motion exercises.

Interphalangeal Dislocations

- These injuries are usually easily reduced.
- Phalanx fractures and ligamentous injuries, however, can coexist and must be considered; phalanx fractures should be documented radiologically before manipulation.
- Careful testing of motor function and collateral ligament function after reduction should be undertaken in all patients.
- A digital block with 1% or 2% lidocaine may be indicated in particularly anxious or symptomatic patients but is often unnecessary, particularly in patients with dorsal dislocations.
- Reduction is usually straightforward and involves stabilization of the proximal segment and longitudinal traction placed on the distal segment along the line of dislocation, followed by definitive reduction.
- Full motor function should then be assessed and documented and collateral ligament stability determined.
- If abnormalities of motor function are present suggesting tendon avulsion or if stress testing of the joint discloses collateral ligament laxity or disruption, orthopaedic or other subspecialty consultation should be obtained for possible repair.
- The emergency physician must not be too aggressive with failed reductions because failure of an initial attempt often suggests interposition of soft tissues (i.e., tendon).
- In these patients, closed reduction will be impossible without damage to these tissues. Open reduction often will be required.
- Postreduction treatment, after determination of normal motor function and collateral ligament integrity, involves the use of a volar splint with the PIP joint fixed in approximately 15 to 20 degrees of flexion; early follow-up is indicated within 3 to 5 days to institute range-of-motion exercises.

Tendon Rupture

- A common injury involves rupture of the extensor tendon at its insertion on the dorsal distal phalanx, producing a so-called "mallet finger."
- The usual precipitating event is forced and violent flexion when the finger is extended; this is a common baseball injury.
- Radiologically, approximately 25% of patients have an associated avulsion or chip fracture of the dorsal proximal distal phalanx.
- When such fractures involve more than 25% of the articular surface, open reduction and internal fixation may be required, and orthopaedic consultation should be obtained.
- On examination, extension of the DIP joint is impossible, there is usually slight flexion of the finger at rest, pain is minimal to moderate, and the finger is often said to be "floppy."
- Treatment involves splinting the DIP joint in hyperextension and recommending orthopaedic follow-up in 5 to 6 days.
- Importantly, only the DIP joint should be immobilized, and devices that interfere with motion of the other fingers or other joints of the involved finger should strictly be avoided.
- Another common injury involves rupture of the central slip of the extensor mechanism near the PIP joint; this allows slippage or volar movement of the lateral bands of the tendon such that flexion at the PIP joint and extension at the DIP joint are produced. The PIP joint in such patients cannot be extended. Treatment involves orthopaedic consultation for possible repair. Again, a fracture may complicate this injury.
- Rupture of flexor tendons occurs when the finger is forcibly hyperextended while flexed. Operative repair is indicated and therefore consultation should be sought at the time of presentation.
- Rupture of the flexor digitorum profundus from its insertion on the volar distal phalanx, which results in loss of flexion at the DIP joint, is not an uncommon injury and is often missed in the ED. To assess the integrity of this tendon, both the MCP and PIP joints must be held in extension to eliminate recruitment of other DIP flexors.
- Rupture of the extensor pollicis longus may result from acute flexion injuries of the DIP joint of the thumb or may occur in association with wrist trauma, most often a Colles fracture. Inability to extend the DIP joint of the thumb and partial weakness of the more proximal extensors are noted. Orthopaedic or other subspecialty consultation should be obtained when the diagnosis is suspected because definitive repair will be required in most patients.

Tendon Lacerations

- The diagnosis of tendon interruption should always be made on clinical grounds despite nonvisualization of the severed tendon.
- It must be remembered that the skin laceration may be far removed from the location of the tendon interruption; this occurs because after transection, retraction of the tendon occurs, essentially pulling the severed ends out of or away from the wound.
- Extensor tendons are routinely repaired in the ED, whereas flexor tendon repairs are undertaken in the operating room.
- Antibiotics covering skin flora are frequently employed, but the data regarding their effectiveness at infection prevention are lacking.

SPECIFIC INJURIES OF THE LOWER EXTREMITY

Pelvic Fractures

- Although often associated with severe trauma, pelvic fractures may occur as a result of minor falls or motor vehicle accidents.
- Many patients with fractures not involving the major weight-bearing structures of the pelvis will be ambulatory when first seen, and if other associated injuries are more symptomatic or obvious, pelvic symptoms may initially be trivialized or unrecognized.
- Patients with pelvic fractures may report discomfort, which is often described as a mild ache, localized to the general area of the bony pelvis or hip.
- Localization of pain along the inguinal ring or crease is suggestive of anterior pelvic disruption and is commonly reported by such patients.
- Bilateral downward pressure applied to the anterior iliac crests often produces pain or crepitus in patients with such injuries and must be performed cautiously.
- The definitive diagnosis requires radiologic assessment in all patients with pelvic symptoms after lower abdominal or pelvic trauma.
- An initial anteroposterior pelvic view should be obtained, followed by specific views to assess symptomatic areas—sacrum, coccyx, and posterior acetabulum.
- CT may be required for a full assessment of the fracture(s) and in the patient with persistent pain and negative films.
- With respect to serious pelvic injuries, the following general points should be considered:
  - A significant number of patients presenting to the ED with a pelvic fracture will be hypotensive with evidence of evolving or established shock; reestablishment of normal intravascular volume and stabilization of bleeding are obviously first priorities in such patients.
  - Some patients admitted to the hospital with initially uncomplicated fractures will develop evidence of shock or peritonitis as bleeding continues around the fracture site or in association with unrecognized or asymptomatic pelvic or abdominal visceral trauma.
  - Retroperitoneal bleeding may occur in association with pelvic fractures, may be brisk, and may be accompanied by minimal symptoms; backache, which may be mild, paralytic ileus, vomiting, nausea, loss of asymmetry of the normally present psoas shadow on plain roentgenograms of the abdomen, and occult shock should all suggest this complication.
  - Injuries to the genitourinary system frequently coexist in patients with pelvic injuries.
  - A normal urinalysis is helpful in excluding such injuries in most patients; however, extensive damage to the kidney may not be associated with hematuria, a finding especially true in patients with penetrating injuries and those with complete ureteral disruption.
  - Hematuria in association with pelvic trauma or fracture suggests the possibility of a major genitourinary injury, the management of which is discussed in Chapter 9.
- The treatment of patients with pelvic fractures includes the following:
  - Patients with significant pelvic trauma or pelvic fractures involving the pelvic ring should be admitted to the hospital for observation, stabilization, and possible definitive reduction.

- Patients with hematuria or symptoms suggestive of genitourinary injury will require additional urgent evaluation; specific evaluation and management are discussed in Chapter 9.
- Patients with minor pelvic fractures not involving the pelvic ring, minimal symptoms, and no other associated injuries may be discharged with the advice to bear weight as tolerated.
- A short course of analgesics and appropriate orthopaedic follow-up should be provided; in other patients, as noted, admission is strongly recommended.

Fractures of the Coccyx

- Fractures of the coccyx are relatively common, occur most often as a result of direct trauma, may involve displacement of the coccyx as well as fracture, are generally unassociated with other injuries, and are most often treated symptomatically.
- Rarely, coccygeal fractures produce rectal laceration or local soft-tissue hemorrhage that may encroach significantly on the rectal outlet.
- For this reason, a digital examination with guaiac testing for occult blood must be performed in all patients with significant coccygeal injuries.
- Admission is generally not required in patients with uncomplicated injuries.
- Generally, sitz baths, nonsteroidal anti-inflammatory agents such as ibuprofen taken with food, and the so-called donut for use in the sitting position are additionally helpful.

Avulsion Fractures Involving the Trochanters

- In children and adolescents, isolated avulsion fractures of the lesser trochanter are not uncommon.
- Fractures displaced less than 2 cm may be treated symptomatically with crutches, analgesics, and several days of bed rest.
- Fractures displaced more than 2 cm require internal fixation, and orthopaedic consultation should therefore be obtained.
- In older patients, avulsion fractures involving either trochanter, if displaced more than 1 cm, generally require internal fixation; those with lesser amounts of displacement may be treated symptomatically.

Fracture of the Hip and Femur

- Because management of femoral fractures is complex and mostly operative, orthopaedic consultation should be obtained as soon as the diagnosis is made.
- In patients with shaft fractures, a splinting device (e.g., the Hare traction splint) should be applied to try to achieve anatomic alignment and decrease hematoma formation.
- In patients with shaft fractures, soft-tissue injury is often extensive and blood losses of greater than 2 U are not uncommon.
- Neurovascular status in the distal leg must be assessed immediately at presentation.

Dislocation of the Hip

- Because of the size and structure of the hip joint and its inherent stability, major force is required to dislocate it; it is therefore not surprising that other injuries frequently coexist.
- Hip dislocations are frequently associated with acetabular and femoral fractures, and concomitant injury to the ipsilateral knee is common.

- Statistically, most dislocations occur posteriorly and present with severe discomfort localized to the hip and buttock, where the femoral head may often be palpated; shortening of the extremity, flexion at the hip, and internal rotation are noted and may simulate simple fracture of the hip.
- Sciatic nerve injury can occur in association with posterior dislocation and should be considered.
- Patients with less common anterior dislocations report anterior and often medial discomfort; the femoral head may be palpated in this location.
- Pulses and neurologic status should be evaluated immediately.
- Dislocation of the hip represents one of the true orthopaedic emergencies, and reduction should proceed as soon as possible; emergency orthopaedic consultation should therefore be obtained.
- The reduction should proceed utilizing monitored procedural sedation.
- The pelvis should be stabilized by an assistant; traction is applied to the femur along the line of displacement.
- When lengthening is noted, which requires some force, small degrees of internal and external rotation will most often result in reduction.

Slipped Capital Femoral Epiphysis

- Slipped capital femoral epiphysis is found most commonly in obese children and adolescents who, after minor or unrecalled trauma, present with hip or knee pain or limp.
- Discomfort is expected to be increased with internal rotation of the hip.
- Typically, the femoral epiphysis is displaced posteriorly and inferiorly and is so observed radiologically by anterior and lateral views of the pelvis and hips; lateral views are taken in the frog-leg position with the hips flexed 90 degrees and abducted 45 degrees.
- Complications include avascular necrosis of the femoral head and premature fusion of the epiphyseal plate.
- Prompt orthopaedic consultation is appropriate in such patients.

Transient (Toxic) Synovitis of the Hip

- Toxic synovitis of the hip is a transient, self-limited phenomenon occurring primarily in children, mostly boys, between the ages of 5 and 10 years.
- Patients with toxic synovitis of the hip present with hip or knee pain and limp.
- Pathophysiologically, toxic synovitis of the hip is not well understood, although occasionally minor trauma or febrile illnesses precede or accompany the onset of symptoms.
- Low-grade fever, limitation of motion as a result of local muscle spasm, accentuation of discomfort with movement of the leg, and minor joint swelling may be noted; the extremity is most often internally rotated, adducted, and somewhat flexed.
- The differential diagnosis in these patients should include septic arthritis, osteomyelitis, slipped capital femoral epiphysis, and early Legg-Calvé-Perthes disease.
- Radiologically, the involved hip is normal.
- Severe pain, fever, elevated WBC, and an elevated ESR (>20) suggest septic arthritis. US demonstrating an effusion that then needs arthrocentesis will differential between these two diagnoses.
- Treatment, when septic arthritis and osteomyelitis are unlikely or excluded, involves several days of bed rest, acetaminophen for discomfort, and orthopaedic follow-up in 3 to 5 days if symptoms are not resolving.

Adductor Muscle Strain

- Forceful or exaggerated abduction of the upper leg is the usual mechanism of adductor muscle strain and is common in gymnasts and cheerleaders; the so-called splits are a common precipitant in such patients.
- Pain, which is made worse by adduction of the leg against resistance, is an expected finding; pain at rest is usually reported along the inguinal crease or medial, proximal thigh.
- Avulsion fractures of the femur, often resulting from similar maneuvers, should be excluded radiologically.
- Treatment in patients with simple muscle strain includes ambulation as tolerated, the application of cold, proscription of activities resulting in discomfort for 7 to 10 days, crutches, and follow-up as required.

Rupture of the Quadriceps Tendon

- Rupture of the quadriceps tendon usually occurs when extreme force is applied while the knee is flexed; elderly persons are most often affected.
- Local tenderness is noted along the quadriceps tendon, which is often retracted; distal displacement of the patella, absence or weakness of extension of the knee against gravity, and a palpable defect proximal to the patella are also seen.
- Swelling and ecchymoses may evolve relatively rapidly.
- Rupture of the patellar tendon and fracture of the patella may produce similar symptoms and must be considered in the differential diagnosis.
- Complete tears are repaired surgically, whereas lesser injuries should be discussed with the consultant; conservative treatment is usually indicated to prevent completion of the injury.

Fracture of the Patella

- For a complete evaluation of the patella, anteroposterior, lateral, intercondylar notch, and sunrise views should be obtained when a high degree of suspicion regarding patellar fracture exists.
- It must be remembered that approximately 2.5% of the population possess bilaterally bipartite patellae, which may easily be confused with fracture. A contralateral view will show the same abnormality and should be obtained when any doubt exists.
- Nondisplaced fractures can be managed with casting and modest weight bearing.
- Displaced, comminuted, or open fractures need emergent orthopaedic consultation for ORIF.

Dislocation of the Patella

- The patella most often becomes dislocated laterally and may either reduce spontaneously or present with severe pain and deformity of the knee.
- Reduction occasionally occurs spontaneously but may be accomplished by exerting pressure on the lateral patella while extending the knee.
- This maneuver usually produces prompt restoration of full passive range of motion.
- Radiographs of the knee should be obtained to rule out any bony injury.
- In patients who are extremely uncomfortable or anxious, monitored procedural sedation will facilitate the reduction.
- Knee immobilization and crutches are recommended.

Fractures of the Proximal and Mid Tibia and Fibula

- Fractures of the tibia require careful assessment of neurovascular function and prompt orthopaedic consultation.
- Compartment syndrome can occur in severe tibial fractures and needs to be watched for.
- Tibial plateau fractures represent a relatively commonly overlooked injury, and special attention should therefore be directed to this area.
- Although many fibular fractures may satisfactorily be treated with symptomatic measures, subspecialty management is variable enough to seek consultation from the physician who will ultimately follow-up the patient.
- Dislocation of the head of the fibula should be considered in patients with local pain or prominence of the proximal fibula; fractures of the fibula may be associated with perineal nerve injury that must be assessed.

Dislocation of the Knee

- Traumatic dislocation of the knee is uncommon. When it occurs, however, extensive damage to the surrounding periarticular structures should be anticipated.
- Injuries may involve posterior movement of the tibia on the femur (posterior dislocation), anterior movement of the tibia (anterior dislocation), or lateral movement, and all may involve significant rotation.
- In patients with complete dislocation, rupture of collateral and cruciate ligaments and tearing of the joint capsule are expected.
- In patients with posterior dislocations, damage to the common peroneal nerve and popliteal artery is common.
- In patients with lateral dislocations, reduction is usually undertaken under general anesthesia in the operating room; frequently, attempts at closed reduction in these patients are unsuccessful because of interposed soft tissues.
- In all patients, emergent reduction should be undertaken, and immediate orthopaedic consultation is advised to assist with this procedure.
- Monitored procedural sedation is warranted for dislocations amenable to reduction in the ED.
- Traction and countertraction followed by pressure on the proximal tibia should be performed to effect reduction and decompress the popliteal vessels.
- The knee should be splinted postreduction in 20 degrees of flexion.
- Incomplete or evolving disruptions of the popliteal artery may initially produce no significant evidence of ischemia in the distal extremity and may be associated with normal pedal pulses.
- An ankle-brachial index (ABI) should be performed when feasible. A value less than 0.9 raises the possibility of damage to the popliteal artery.
- Duplex ultrasound and CT angiography have replaced catheter angiography in many institutions.

Soft-Tissue Injuries of the Knee

- Most injuries to the knee occur when the foot is firmly planted and the knee is twisted or directly struck from one side.
- Laterally originating force causes injury to the medial collateral and anterior cruciate ligaments and often the medial meniscus, while medially originating force may result in injury to the lateral collateral ligament.
- Hyperextension of the knee secondary to anteriorly originating force is most often associated with injury to the posterior cruciate.

- Injuries to the meniscus are generally the result of grinding the cartilage between the femoral condyle and tibia; this most often occurs when the foot is firmly planted and the knee flexed and externally rotated.
- The position of the knee when the injury occurred and from what direction force originated, if determinable, are extremely helpful.
- The role of the emergency physician in the evaluation of patients with knee injuries is to exclude fracture and intra-articular foreign body (e.g., avulsed cartilage), to diagnose accurately injury to the various ligaments and cartilaginous structures of the knee, and to prevent further injury by providing or recommending crutches and minimize weight bearing for a period sufficient to clarify the nature and extent of the injury.
- In patients with ligamentous injuries who are seen early before the development of effusion, passive range of motion should be full although associated with discomfort. "Locking" of the knee or the perception that the knee is mechanically prevented from moving through its normal range of motion is not expected in patients with simple ligamentous strain and should suggest intra-articular foreign body (such as radiolucent cartilage) and the need for prompt consultation before disposition.
- An effusion, which is commonly present in patients with sprains, if tense, may similarly limit full range of motion, but the sensation of mechanical interference is not present.
- In addition, patients with simple ligamentous sprain have an examination usually remarkable for tenderness at the origin or insertion of the involved ligament.
- Stress applied across the injured ligament should accentuate the patient's discomfort and is important diagnostically; laxity of the involved ligament is not expected in patients with simple sprain, and when noted, the uninjured extremity should be compared and may demonstrate a similar degree of laxity.
- To assess medial collateral integrity, the knee must be in 10 degrees of flexion; in full extension, the posterior capsule operates to stabilize the joint and may mask medial collateral injury.
- Asymmetric laxity of the joint associated with stress-related accentuation of discomfort should suggest complete ligamentous rupture, and orthopaedic consultation should then be obtained.
- Simple strains are treated initially with the application of cold for 24 to 48 hours, elevation, crutches, analgesics, and orthopaedic referral in 5 to 7 days if symptoms have not subsided; in addition, many authorities recommend the use of a nonsteroidal anti-inflammatory agent during this initial period.
- Weight bearing should be discouraged when it elicits or accentuates discomfort; this will be the case in most patients for several days.
- More significant sprains, for example, those associated with tense effusions or possible laxity, should be treated as mentioned with the addition of a knee immobilizer and strict avoidance of weight bearing.
- As in all patients, devices resulting in nonuniform compression of the lower extremity, for example, Ace? bandages, should be avoided.
- Patients with cartilaginous injuries often report that the knee "gave way," which was usually precipitated by a twisting-type or grinding-type injury.
- Patients also often report "clicking" or "popping" of the knee associated with movement; occasionally, actual mechanical locking of the joint in one position is reported as well.
- The physical examination commonly discloses an effusion with tenderness along the anterior joint line and accentuation of discomfort with movement.

- In patients with a simple or contusing injury to the cartilage, passive range of motion of the joint, unless a tense effusion is present, should be full, although associated with discomfort, and treatment should be provided as discussed with respect to simple ligamentous injuries.
- However, when mechanical locking of the joint is demonstrated, a significant avulsing or lacerating injury to the cartilage is suggested; typically, the patient resists extension, and at the limit of motion, one notes the so-called rubbery resistance associated with interposed cartilage.
- Crepitation may also be appreciated with movement of the joint in these patients. Radiologic assessment is expected to be normal, although an effusion is often noted. Orthopaedic consultation in these patients should be obtained before disposition.
- Other patients with limitation of passive motion or suspected complex meniscal injuries should similarly be discussed with the orthopaedic surgeon on call and arrangements for follow-up made.
- Very often when the history of injury is not clear, locking of the joint is not present, and localization of discomfort is not well defined, it will not be possible to absolutely differentiate injury to the meniscus or cartilage from injury to the ipsilateral ligament. In such cases, the possibility of a cartilage injury should be discussed with the patient, provide treatment as for ligamentous injuries, and recommend orthopaedic follow-up in 3 to 5 days.

Bursitis of the Knee

- A variety of bursae surround the knee, any of which may become acutely inflamed and painful.
- Blunt trauma, which may have been trivial or unrecalled, is often reported to have preceded the onset of symptoms by several days.
- Occupations that involve kneeling, climbing, or other motions that repetitively flex and extend the knee may be associated with an increased incidence of bursal inflammation.
- The prepatellar bursa (located over the patella), the infrapatellar bursa (located inferior to the patella), the anserine bursa (located medially between the tibial plateau and the pes anserine tendon), and the medial gastrocnemius bursa (located in the posterior popliteal fossa) may all become acutely inflamed; local swelling, overlying warmth, erythema, and discomfort are noted.
- Enlargement of the medial gastrocnemius bursa is commonly referred to as a Baker cyst and is more common in patients with intrinsic joint disease.
- When trauma has preceded the onset of symptoms and has involved a penetrating injury or when evidence of local cellulitis or systemic infection is present, septic bursitis must be excluded by sterile aspiration of the bursa, with cell count and differential, Gram stain, and culture and sensitivity.
- Patients with septic bursitis, of course, will require hospitalization, intravenous antibiotics to cover Gram-positive organisms (80% *Staphylococcus aureus*), and incision or aspiration and drainage.
- Gout, which may simulate acute bursitis, must also be included in the differential diagnosis in most patients.
- When infection is excluded or unlikely, treatment includes prohibition of activities or maneuvers that cause the bursa to move, the application of heat, and the institution of an oral nonsteroidal anti-inflammatory agent.
- Orthopaedic referral in 5 to 7 days is appropriate, or sooner if symptoms worsen or if fever is noted.

Osgood-Schlatter Disease

- Osgood-Schlatter disease is seen most often in adolescents, most of whom are athletic, and presumably results from a traction-type injury to the tibial tubercle at the site of insertion of the patellar tendon.
- Patients report symptoms chronically as well as acute, more severe discomfort after athletic activity.
- Point tenderness is noted over the tibial tubercle, which may be inflamed as evidenced by local swelling, erythema, and increased warmth.
- Radiologically, the proximal tibia may be normal, irregularity or prominence of the tibial tuberosity may be seen, or in some patients, an avulsion of the tuberosity may be noted.
- Cessation of sports activities is no longer recommended.
- Nonsteroidal anti-inflammatory agents are useful and should be instituted along with crutches for patients with significant symptoms. Ice may be applied initially to the area and may be helpful.
- Immobilization of the knee and surgical repair are additional options for patients with persistent symptoms; orthopaedic referral in 5 to 7 days is appropriate.

Gastrocnemius Muscle Tear and Plantaris Tendon Rupture

- These entities are considered together, because differentiation by historic or physical criteria is usually not possible and treatment is similar.
- Patients presenting with tears of the gastrocnemius muscle, which are virtually always partial, and those with plantaris tendon ruptures will report the acute onset of symptoms precipitated by physical activity of maneuvers that stress the involved muscle or tendon, respectively. This may simply involve running, jumping, pushing off at the beginning of a race, or charging the net at tennis, although often no such history is elicited. An occasional patient with an acute plantaris tendon rupture will report an audible "snap" or "pop," which, when accompanied by calf discomfort in relation to physical activity, is virtually diagnostic for this entity.
- Both groups of patients report severe calf pain that, especially in patients with gastrocnemius tears, is accentuated by plantar flexion of the foot against resistance.
- When discomfort is more distal and involves the lower posterior leg or ankle, rupture of the Achilles tendon should be considered because a very similar history may be reported.
- Physical findings in both disorders include local calf tenderness with palpation; often extensive swelling and ecchymoses; and in patients presenting somewhat less acutely, ankle swelling, warmth, and the horizontal layering of blood near the inferior calcaneous.
- These latter findings, which may include pain involving the ankle, simply occur as blood tracks distally along the fascial planes as directed by gravity.
- Rarely, when swelling and hemorrhage are extensive, local vascular compromise may occur, resulting in ischemia of the lower leg and foot; the gross appearance of the distal extremity and signs and symptoms of compartment syndrome must therefore be assessed in all patients with significant injuries involving the calf.
- Treatment for patients with plantaris tendon ruptures or partial gastrocnemius tears is symptomatic and conservative after evolving compartment syndromes and fibular fractures are excluded; fibular fractures may be associated with minimal discomfort and very subtle findings.

- The application of cold for 24 to 72 hours, elevation of the leg, immobilization, and the use of a nonsteroidal anti-inflammatory agent and analgesics are also recommended.
- Crutches should be advised for 3 to 4 days and subsequently as determined by the patient's symptoms; generally, partial weight bearing, as tolerated, is recommended to begin in 5 to 7 days.
- Orthopaedic follow-up in 5 to 7 days after the injury is appropriate.

Achilles Tendon Strain or Rupture

- Achilles tendon strains typically are seen in young adults, whereas actual tendon disruption occurs most often in men, usually between the ages of 40 and 50 years.
- Although tendon rupture may occur as a result of a direct blow to the Achilles tendon, more commonly, the tendon ruptures during a maneuver that selectively stresses it.
- A variety of histories demonstrating this fact are usually obtained, for example, charging the net at tennis, pushing a stalled car, or starting a race.
- Many patients will report the initial feeling that they were struck from behind in the area of the Achilles tendon, and many others report an audible "snap" or "pop" at the time of rupture.
- Two important points should be emphasized: (1) pain may be excruciating with partial tears or strains of the tendon and completely absent with total disruptions, and vice versa; and (2) in some patients with total tendon disruptions, plantar flexion may be present.
- Given these two points, one must be very conservative when evaluating the patient presenting with pain localized to the Achilles tendon because undiagnosed partial tears may clearly progress with activity to complete disruption.
- In the physical examination, a palpable "step-off" in the course of the tendon or a "notch" or defect along its course suggests total disruption, as does inability to plantar flex the ankle.
- One should recognize, however, that if 6 to 12 hours elapse between injury and examination, local hematoma may fill in the defect and thereby obscure any palpable step-off.
- Absence of Achilles tendon function may also be demonstrated by squeezing the gastrocnemius tendon with the patient lying face down on the stretcher with the ankles and feet extended over the edge; if plantar flexion does not occur, then injury to the Achilles tendon is highly likely.
- Immobilization through splinting is advised in patients with full and partial tears in the ED.
- In patients with complete rupture, definitive treatment is somewhat controversial (conservative therapy involving casting versus surgery).
- Orthopaedic follow-up within a week is appropriate.

Injuries to the Ankle

- The ankle is most commonly injured when inversion stress results in sprain of the anterior talofibular ligament; this structure provides the lateral ankle with stability and joins the lateral malleolus to the neck of the talus.
- Additional inverting stress results in injury to the calcaneofibular and posterior talofibular ligaments and the lateral malleolus.

- Eversion of the ankle, which is less common, results in deltoid ligament injury, and/or medial malleolar avulsion or frank fracture.
- The assessment of injury to the ankle and the provision of appropriate treatment are facilitated by viewing the ankle as a ring composed of three bones—the tibia, fibula, and talus—and their associated ligaments—the anterior and posterior talofibular and calcaneofibular ligaments laterally and the deltoid ligament medially.
- Disruption of any two of these structures, in a variety of combinations, may result in an unstable joint that must first be suspected in the ED on the basis of the examination and any radiographically demonstrated findings.
- The history is important to elicit with respect to the nature of the injury; inversion or eversion of the ankle, as previously noted, is expected to produce specific injuries or constellations of injury.
- Localized swelling, tenderness to palpation, weakness or absence of motor function as limited by discomfort, and instability of the joint with stress must all be carefully noted.
- Pedal pulses must be evaluated in all patients with significant injuries to the ankle; the Achilles tendon should be palpated and its motor function assessed.
- Radiologic assessment of the ankle includes anteroposterior, lateral, and mortise views; mortise views are anteroposterior views with approximately 20 degrees of internal rotation.
- Fractures of the lateral and medial malleolus and sliding or displacement of the talus are best observed on the anteroposterior view, whereas undisplaced fractures of the fibula and fractures of the posterior malleolus of the tibia are seen primarily on the lateral projection.
- Specific attention should be directed to the medial malleolar-talar space on the mortise view; widening of this space suggests ligament rupture.
- Similarly, transverse, avulsing, or chip fractures of the malleoli, the talus, and the calcaneous are commonly associated with ligamentous injury; such fractures when displaced should in fact be considered to be complicated by total ligamentous disruption and treated as such.
- Patients with suspected ligamentous rupture, instability as demonstrated by examination or suggested by two fractures surrounding the ankle, loss of motion not secondary to discomfort, or fractures associated with displacement should be discussed with the orthopaedic surgeon.

First-Degree Sprains
- First-degree sprains involve minor injury to the ankle and frequently present 6 to 12 hours after the injury.
- Local tenderness with palpation and mild swelling are usually noted.
- Motor function of the injured ligament is normal except as limited by discomfort.
- Ligamentous laxity is absent; pathologically minor amounts of tearing are noted to involve the ligament.
- Treatment is protective and symptomatic. Importantly, patients must be told that although injury to the ligament is minor, the time course of recovery is extremely variable. Even minor sprains of the ankle may be associated with weeks of weight-bearing discomfort—particularly if weight bearing was resumed immediately after the injury and was associated with discomfort, and treatment was delayed.
- Patients should be instructed to keep the involved ankle elevated and apply cold for 24 to 72 hours; weight bearing should be prohibited during this initial period, and

crutches or bed rest subsequently advised for patients with elicitation or accentuation of discomfort with weight bearing.
- In patients with clear first-degree sprains, partial weight bearing may be encouraged as dictated by symptoms to begin approximately 3 to 7 days after the injury and to increase thereafter as tolerated.
- An Ace™ wrap or air splint may be applied to limit local swelling and provide additional stability; a mild analgesic, preferably without aspirin, may be suggested for several days.
- Orthopaedic follow-up should be advised for 10 to 12 days if symptoms persist.

Second-Degree Sprains
- Second-degree sprains involve more significant injury to the ankle, and partial disruption of the involved ligament is identified pathologically.
- Historically, pain is present immediately after the injury, and most patients present early. Local tenderness, swelling, and hemorrhage are noted and may be impressive. There is moderate loss of function of the involved ligament, and mild laxity is often discovered.
- Radiologically, a small chip fracture of the distal malleolus is commonly noted.
- The treatment of mild second-degree sprains is as for first-degree sprains, but the duration of discomfort and disability is typically greater than for first-degree sprains.
- The importance of elevation, the application of cold for 48 to 72 hours, and the initial avoidance of weight bearing should be emphasized to the patient.
- Partial weight bearing, again as limited by symptoms, may begin in most patients by 5 to 10 days and will prevent the development of ankle stiffness.
- A more supportive dressing, such as an air splint, may be provided and will limit swelling and discomfort; analgesics may be required for 2 to 3 days.
- Crutches should be strongly recommended or provided to patients who are not able to rest in bed, and orthopaedic referral should be advised in 10 to 12 days.
- Complications include recurrent sprain related to permanent ligamentous laxity.

Third-Degree Sprains
- Third-degree sprains are diagnosed on the basis of immediate pain, loss of function of the involved ligament, and varying amounts of local swelling, edema, and hemorrhage.
- Patients benefit from a short course of casting (2 weeks).
- Orthopaedic consultation should be obtained before disposition.

Malleolus and distal fibula fractures
- Open fractures need emergent orthopaedic consultation for operative management.
- Antibiotics that cover skin flora should be administered and the patient's tetanus status assessed.
- Dislocations often complicate severe ankle fractures and should promptly be reduced (with monitored procedural sedation as needed).
- The vascular status of the foot must be assessed, especially in cases of open fractures and fracture dislocations.
- Uncomplicated ankle fractures can be splinted and closely followed up by the orthopaedist as an outpatient treatment.

Lisfranc (Tarsometatarsal) Fracture Dislocation

- This is the most common midfoot fracture and can be the result of direct trauma or, more commonly, a fall onto a plantar-flexed foot.
- This results in midfoot swelling or the inability to bear weight and sometimes paresthesias of the midfoot.
- A fracture through the base of the second metatarsal with separation between the second and first metatarsals is found on x-ray.
- Emergent orthopaedic consultation is warranted.
- Open reduction may be required for treatment.

Metatarsal Fractures

- Fracture of the proximal fifth metatarsal is the most common of the metatarsal fractures and may be treated symptomatically unless major displacement occurs, in which case open reduction and internal fixation will be required.
- Symptomatic therapy includes an initial period of cold application, elevation, prohibition of weight bearing, and a compressive dressing; in many patients, a walking cast can be applied in 2 to 5 days after local swelling has stabilized and will allow return of relatively normal activity.
- Alternatively, an orthopaedic shoe and crutches along with the local measures noted may be elected until such time because partial weight bearing can be resumed without significant discomfort; progressive ambulation is thereafter advised based on the patient's symptoms.
- Nonfifth, proximal, metatarsal fractures should be discussed with the consultant before disposition.
- Shaft fractures result from significant crushing force, and consequently, in many patients soft-tissue injuries pose a more important clinical problem than the fracture itself.
- Additionally, angulation, which frequently exists, is poorly tolerated in this location and may require correction.
- In many patients, plaster immobilization will be elected, and orthopaedic consultation is advised.

Toe Fractures

- Most toe fractures are treated symptomatically with analgesics, the application of cold for 24 to 48 hours, and elevation.
- Weight bearing should be based on the patient's symptoms.
- Fractures of toes other than the first may be treated by simply taping the fractured toe to the adjacent larger toe; this may result in increased discomfort, in which case taping should be discontinued.
- If taping is elected, a small amount of cotton may be placed between the toes to prevent maceration; this should be changed daily and the skin cleansed as usual.
- Transverse fractures involving the first toe, which may result in prolonged disability, should be referred to an orthopaedic surgeon at an interval of approximately 3 to 5 days.

Toe Dislocations

- Most metatarsophalangeal dislocations involve dorsal movement of the proximal phalanx on the metatarsal; this produces hyperextension of the involved toe, severe discomfort, and an obvious deformity.

- Lidocaine 1% or 2% without epinephrine may be infiltrated in and around the joint, followed by hyperextension, traction on the distal segment, and definitive reduction.
- Interphalangeal dislocations may be treated similarly.
- Radiographs should be obtained to screen for associated fracture.
- Joints determined to be unstable after reduction require orthopaedic consultation for possible internal fixation or casting.
- Stable reductions require only splinting for 2 to 4 weeks; orthopaedic referral within 7 to 10 days is recommended.
- A short course of analgesics, particularly in patients with metatarsophalangeal dislocations, is appropriate, as is application of cold for 24 to 48 hours, elevation, and a period of non–weight bearing as determined by the patient's symptoms.

Trauma in Pregnancy

INTRODUCTION

Every emergency room (ER) doctor or nurse knows the feeling of dread when the EMS radio announces the imminent arrival of a pregnant patient involved in a serious motor vehicle accident (MVA). Optimal care for both the woman and fetus requires the coordination of services from the prehospital providers, the ER professionals, the trauma surgeon, the obstetrician, and the neonatologist. This coordination is initiated and led by the ER practitioner. Trauma occurs in 1 out of every 12 pregnancies. The etiology of trauma in pregnancy is MVAs (55%), followed by falls (22%), assaults (22%), and burns (1%). Fetal deaths are caused by MVAs (82%), firearm injuries (6%), and falls (3%). Physical abuse occurs in 1% to 20% of pregnancies depending on the study. Trauma is the leading cause of nonobstetric deaths.

PREVENTION

- Despite case reports of uterine rupture with proper seat belt use, restrained pregnant patients likely have better outcomes after MVAs compared with unrestrained patients.
- To any EM practitioner who has witnessed the type of injuries unrestrained patients can sustain in an MVA, this makes intuitive sense.
- Current American College of Obstetricians and Gynecologists recommendations state that seat belts should be used throughout pregnancy with the lap portion placed under the uterus and across the superior iliac spines and pubic symphysis.
- The shoulder portion should be placed between the breasts.
- A pregnancy-mimicking crash test dummy demonstrated that placement of the lap belt over the uterus resulted in a three-to-four-fold increase in forces transmitted to the "fetus." Airbag deployment does not appear to increase maternal injury.

PHYSIOLOGIC CHANGES IN PREGNANCY

- Many of the normal physiologic changes in pregnancy can affect maternal injury patterns and her body's response to them.
- The uterus becomes an intra-abdominal organ after the 12th week, leaving the protective cocoon of the pelvis.
- As the uterus enlarges, it draws the bladder into the abdomen as well, increasing its potential for injury.
- Bowel is also superiorly displaced and covered by the enlarging uterus, decreasing its risk for injury, especially in penetrating trauma.
- Maternal heart rate increases by 10 to 15 beats/min, while the systolic blood pressure drops by 5 to 10 mm Hg, and diastolic blood pressure drops by 10 to 15 mm Hg.

- Maternal minute ventilation is hormonally increased leading to PCO_2 values of approximately 30 mm Hg. The kidneys compensate by lowering the serum bicarbonate to 17 to 22 mEq/L.
- In the third trimester, the enlarging uterus elevates the diaphragm by up to 4 cm, causing an enlarged cardiac shadow, and a wider mediastinum.
- Maternal blood volume changes dramatically during pregnancy. Plasma volume increases by roughly 50%, while red blood cell (RBC) mass increases by 20% to 30%. This leads to an entity known as anemia of pregnancy with hematocrit values in the low 30s.
- Uterine blood flow increases to approximately 600 mL/min, which can lead to catastrophic hemorrhage in the case of uterine injury.

PREHOSPITAL CARE

- The routine ABCs of trauma resuscitation are still followed.
- A pregnant patient's body will shift blood away from the placenta during periods of hypovolemia, so euvolemia and adequate oxygenation must be maintained. This is accomplished through two large-bore IVs, crystalloid, and supplemental oxygen.
- A situation peculiar to pregnant patients beyond 18 weeks is supine hypotension. This occurs when the gravid uterus compresses the inferior vena cava. This can be alleviated by rolling the backboard 15 degrees to the left and then securing this position with blankets. Alternatively, the uterus can be manually shifted to the left.
- If possible, the pregnant patient should be transported to a hospital that has the capability to care for the mother and to deliver and care for a distressed newborn even if the trauma seems innocuous.
- Keep in mind that placental abruption can occur after a seemingly minor trauma.

EMERGENCY DEPARTMENT CARE

- The ABCs of trauma care should be instituted for the injured pregnant patient as they are for all patients.
- Fetal mortality increases with increased maternal injury, so optimizing the mother's condition also optimizes the unborn child's chance for survival.
- During the primary survey, oxygen should be continued and crystalloid volume given to maintain euvolemia. Maternal hypovolemia threatens fetal viability.
- As in the ambulance, the backboard should be tipped to the left.
- During the secondary survey, the gestational age should be assessed. This can rapidly be accomplished via fundal height. At 12 weeks, the fundus is at the level of the pubic symphysis. By 20 weeks, the fundus is at the level of the umbilicus.
- A focused assessment with sonography in trauma (FAST) exam should also be performed as part of the secondary survey.
- Most ultrasound machines have the ability to calculate gestational age via various measurements such as biparietal diameter, and ER physicians should be familiar with this feature (Table 11-1).
- Fetuses determined to be 20 weeks' gestation and beyond should be monitored.
- The normal fetal heart rate is 120 to 160 bpm.
- Fetal tachycardia can indicate maternal or fetal hypovolemia (as occurs in placental abruption) or maternal fever.
- Fetal heart tracings should be monitored for decelerations.

Table 11-1	Maternal Anatomic Landmarks of Gestational Age

Gestational Age (Weeks)	Fundal Height
<12	Fundus not palpable
12–14	Just above pubic symphysis
22–24	Umbilicus
18–30	The distance above pubic symphysis in centimeters approximates the gestational age in weeks
36	Xiphoid process
40	Subxiphoid (fundus broadens and decreases in height)

- Decelerations in which the drop in fetal heart rate occurs early in the uterine contraction are termed early decelerations. These are benign and occur due to uterine compression of the fetal skull.
- Variable decelerations occur at varying times during uterine contractions and have a steep fall in fetal heart rate. They are of uncertain significance, but if they occur frequently, or result in prolonged fetal bradycardia, a cause should be sought.
- Late decelerations are always concerning and indicate uteroplacental insufficiency. They occur in the final stages of uterine contractions and indicate fetal distress. If they occur, an assessment of maternal volume status and oxygenation must immediately be performed, and the mother placed in the left lateral recumbent position.
- If fetal bradycardia persists, or if the late decelerations are recurrent and the fetus is 23 weeks or beyond, an emergent C-section must be performed to save the child.
- A pelvic exam should ideally be performed by an Ob/Gyn (although this is not always possible) with a sterile speculum in a nonbleeding patient, especially if a pelvic fracture is present.
- If vaginal bleeding is present, an ultrasound must be performed first to rule out placenta previa.
- Amniotic fluid presence is indicated by a vaginal pH of seven and ferning of dried vaginal secretions on a microscope slide.
- The cervix should be assessed for dilation.
- Fetal station and presentation should be determined if the cervix is dilated.
- Vaginal delivery can occur through a fractured pelvis as long as the fracture is not open, unstable, or severely displaced.
- Diagnostic imaging has revolutionized trauma care, computed tomography (CT) in particular.
- Fetal exposure to greater than 20 rad may induce adverse effects, especially within the first 8 weeks of life.
- Abdominal CT exposes the fetus to approximately 3.5 rad (Table 11-2).
- Increasing the thickness of CT slices, decreasing the number of slices, and omitting the pelvis portion of the exam are strategies to decrease fetal radiation exposure.
- Serial FAST exams along with serial abdominal exams and hemoglobin measurements can also be employed to detect intra-abdominal injury in minimally symptomatic patients.

Table 11-2	Approximate Fetal Radiation Exposure for Various Radiographic Studies Commonly Used in Trauma
Study	**Fetal Radiation in Rads**
"Trauma series": Lateral C-Spine, AP Chest, AP Pelvis	0.042
Complete C-Spine	0.002
Chest (2 view)	0.00007
Thoracic Spine	0.009
Lumbosacral Spine	0.359
Head CT	under 0.050
Chest CT	under 0.1
Abdominal CT	3.5

- Fetal-maternal hemorrhage can result in fetal and neonatal anemia secondary to hemolysis, which can ultimately lead to fetal death.
- The Kleihauer-Betke (KB) test identifies fetal red blood cells in the maternal circulation, and so can estimate the amount of fetal-maternal hemorrhage.
- All D(Rh)-negative trauma patients should receive D immune globulin.
- Among women who have symptomatic fetal-maternal hemorrhage, the mean volume of fetal blood in the maternal circulation is 15 mL.
- The 300 μg dose of D immune globulin will bind up to 30 mL of fetal red blood cells. Thus, the routine use of the KB test is useful only in the occasional D-negative patient who needs more than the standard 300 μg dose of immune globulin due to extensive fetal-maternal hemorrhage.
- D-immune globulin can be given up to 72 hours after the traumatic event.

PERIMORTEM CESAREAN DELIVERY

- The need to perform an emergency C-section on a coding mother strikes fear in the heart of every emergency practitioner, but thankfully is extremely rare.
- The entity is not well studied due to its rarity, but case series have demonstrated a viable infant salvage rate of 15%.
- Perimortem C-sections have also been documented to aid in the return of maternal pulse and blood pressure. This is perhaps due to increased blood volume in the maternal circulation after the delivery of the placenta.
- The procedure should be performed within 4 minutes of the loss of maternal pulse.
- A vertical incision is made in the midline below the umbilicus, which extends down through the uterus.
- This procedure should be performed as rapidly as possible.
- The procedure should be performed in gestations estimated to be beyond 23 weeks.

DISPOSITION

- A pregnant trauma patient who has intact membranes, has no vaginal bleeding, has been monitored for a minimum of 4 hours (if beyond 20 weeks' gestation), has

normal fetal heart tracings, and has contractions less than one every 10 minutes may be discharged.
- This decision should be made in conjunction with an Ob/Gyn.
- Patients who do not meet these criteria should be admitted for observation or transferred to a facility with the capabilities to care for the woman and her child.

PART 3

Eye, Ear, Nose, and Throat Disorders

Ear Pain

Ear pain is a common symptom in emergency medicine, particularly in the pediatric age group. A meticulous evaluation of the ear, pharynx, and general periauricular area is essential for an accurate diagnosis.

COMMON CAUSES OF EAR PAIN

- Acute suppurative otitis media*
- Acute otitis externa ("swimmer's ear")*
- Acute serous otitis media*
- Preauricular lymphadenopathy*
- Temporomandibular joint dysfunction*
- Cellulitis of the external ear*

LESS COMMON CAUSES OF EAR PAIN NOT TO BE MISSED

- Malignant otitis externa*
- Bullous myringitis*
- Acute mastoiditis*
- Foreign body in the external auditory canal

OTHER CAUSES OF EAR PAIN

- Bell palsy (idiopathic facial palsy)*
- Furunculosis of the external auditory canal*
- Herpes zoster (Ramsay Hunt Syndrome)*

*Discussed in this chapter.

- Barotrauma to the middle ear*
- Traumatic perforation of the tympanic membrane*
- Acute auricular hematoma*
- Cerumen impaction*

HISTORY

Pain followed by its disappearance in association with a bloody or purulent discharge from the auditory canal suggests acute suppurative otitis media with tympanic membrane perforation. Serous otitis media is often a cause of acute ear pain in patients with a history of a recent upper respiratory tract infection or allergies. Ear discomfort related to mastication may be caused by temporomandibular joint dysfunction or acute otitis externa. Postauricular pain developing in the setting of chronic or recurrent otitis media suggests acute mastoiditis. Recent swimming or high-altitude travel may also be noted in patients with external otitis or barotrauma, respectively. Vague pain involving the ear, often with radiation to the jaw or teeth, is sometimes reported early in patients with herpes zoster; this often occurs before the development of rash.

PHYSICAL EXAMINATION

The disappearance of the normal light reflex is noted in patients with a middle ear effusion. The tympanic membrane in patients with serous otitis media is usually amber, with or without an air-fluid level. Pain with traction on the auricle or tragus suggests an external otitic process, whereas reproduction of pain with palpation of the temporomandibular joint in the external auditory meatus suggests temporomandibular joint dysfunction. Tenderness to percussion or palpation postauricularly suggests acute mastoiditis, which requires radiologic evaluation, otolaryngologic consultation, and most often intravenous antibiotics. Erythema or vesicles involving the surrounding scalp, the pinna, or the periauricular area suggest herpes zoster, although in some patients pain may precede the development of rash.

SPECIFIC DISORDERS

Acute Suppurative Otitis Media

Acute bacterial infection involving the middle ear occurs most often in children in who high fever, pain, irritability, crying, lack of interest in nursing or eating, and pulling or brushing the affected ear are common symptoms. In some children, vomiting, usually not associated with abdominal discomfort, is prominent. Older children and adults may report varying degrees of hearing loss. Pain is intense and often described as excruciating and throbbing. After the onset of pain, a small number of patients report the sudden disappearance of pain followed by a bloody or purulent discharge from the ear canal; such a scenario suggests tympanic membrane perforation.

Findings in patients without perforation include bulging and erythema of the tympanic membrane and a disappearance of the normally present light reflex and bony landmarks of the middle ear. If perforation has occurred, blood or pus may be seen in the canal, and the site of perforation may be noted.

The organisms that commonly cause acute suppurative otitis media include pneumococci, *Haemophilus influenzae, Moraxella catarrhalis, Staphylococcus aureus,* group A streptococci, and (in infants and neonates) Enterobacteriaceae and group B streptococci.

Children

Children who are significantly ill with high fever, persistent vomiting, severe discomfort, or extreme bulging of the tympanic membrane should be considered candidates for hospitalization and intravenous antibiotics. Myringotomy or tympanocentesis is rarely needed.

Outpatient Therapy

Outpatient therapy should include fluids, antipyretics as needed, and analgesics for 3 to 5 days. Because of the intensity of discomfort, patients may require a narcotic for 2 or 3 days; we prefer acetaminophen and codeine elixir in children and codeine or an equivalent in adults. In addition, when perforation is not present, a topical analgesic, such as benzocaine (Americaine) drops, may be prescribed. A specific antibiotic should be prescribed for 10 to 14 days, the therapeutic options for which are discussed in section "Antibiotics." It is important to recommend reevaluation in 3 or 4 days if symptoms do not improve. All adults with recurrent or refractory otitis should be referred to an otolaryngologist for appropriate follow-up because a small percentage of these patients have otitis secondary to an obstructing nasopharyngeal process. Decongestants are generally not recommended and have been shown not to accelerate resolution of otitis in children.

Treatment of Perforation

The treatment of perforation secondary to acute bacterial otitis media is similar to that of suppurative otitis media; it is important to advise the patient that the ear canal should remain unobstructed. The use of ear drops is contraindicated. Perforations generally heal quite well within 3 weeks without loss of hearing; otolaryngologic follow-up should be recommended at 10 days after the initiation of therapy.

Antibiotics

The initial choice of an antibiotic in patients with suppurative otitis media remains controversial; important factors include changing bacterial resistance, complications of therapy, the convenience/practicality of the various dosing schedules, patient palatability, and cost. Based on these factors, many authorities continue to recommend initial treatment with amoxicillin; this reflects a long history of success with this agent, very low cost, reasonable palatability in children, and relatively few complications. The dose is 500 mg three times daily in adults and 80 to 90 mg/kg/day in three divided doses for 10 days in children. Because of emerging patterns of resistance in some strains of *Streptococcus pneumoniae,* some authorities have recently recommended higher doses of amoxicillin (up to 80 mg/kg/day in three divided doses). In patients with treatment failures or in communities with a high prevalence of β-lactamase–producing organisms (*H. influenzae, M. catarrhalis* species, and *S. pneumoniae*), other agents are preferred. These include azithromycin (Zithromax 10 mg/kg/day as a single dose on day 1, followed by 5 mg/kg/day given as a single dose on days 2 to 5), amoxicillin-clavulanate (Augmentin, administered as 80 to 90 mg/kg/day in three divided doses for 10 days), cefpodoxime (Vantin, administered as 10 mg/day given as a single dose for 10 days), cefuroxime axetil (Ceftin, 30 mg/kg/day divided twice daily for ten days), or ceftriaxone (Rocephin, 50 mg/kg intravenous or intramuscular daily for 3 days). In patients with penicillin allergy, we generally recommend treatment with azithromycin. In patients with **vomiting,** or when prescription or medication compliance is an issue, an acceptable treatment option is to give a single intramuscular dose of ceftriaxone, 50 mg/kg, which need not be followed with oral antibiotics.

Mastoiditis

Mastoiditis is suggested by tenderness behind the ear with percussion or palpation. Such patients should have imaging of the mastoid and should be considered candidates for hospital admission. Intravenous antibiotics and otolaryngologic consultation at the time of presentation are appropriate.

Acute Serous Otitis Media

Transudation of fluid into the middle ear may occur idiopathically or in association with upper respiratory tract viral infection, allergy, or barotrauma. An adult presenting with recurrent serous otitis media may harbor an occult nasopharyngeal neoplasm, and such patients should be referred to an otolaryngologist for evaluation. Patients report a sensation of fullness or pressure in the ear and may report vague abnormalities of balance or slight inner ear discomfort. Varying amounts of fluid can be seen in the middle ear, which often colors the tympanic membrane amber. An air-fluid level or tiny bubbles of air may be noted in the middle ear in some patients. The differentiation from acute suppurative otitis is based on the observation that the tympanic membrane is not bulging and red.

Acute Otitis Externa

Acute otitis externa ("swimmer's ear") occurs when pathogenic organisms infect the skin of the ear canal, producing often severe, local discomfort and varying degrees of swelling. Diagnosis is based on the presence of ear pain, which may radiate inferiorly toward the angle of the mandible and is accentuated by traction on the auricle or movement of the tragus. Accentuation of discomfort by these maneuvers may be an important differential point because discomfort caused by otitis media is not increased by these manipulations. Other findings include erythema and tenderness of the canal, which may appear weepy and edematous. The tympanic membrane may appear erythematous as well; however, hearing should be normal unless local swelling mechanically obstructs the canal. Local lymphadenopathy may be palpable inferiorly toward the angle of the mandible or in the pretragal area.

Fungal otitis externa is not common but should be suspected in patients with chronic symptoms, severe or prominent itching, or a cheese-like material in the canal. The usual pathogens are *Candida* and *Aspergillus* species. Fungal stains and cultures should be obtained in such patients and will be diagnostic; otolaryngologic consultation should be sought regarding specific recommendations for definitive therapy and follow-up.

Acute otitis externa occurring in the *immunocompromised host,* most often the diabetic, represents a special therapeutic problem, which is discussed in section "Malignant Otitis Externa."

Acute otitis externa occurring in other patients may generally be satisfactorily treated as follows:

- **Analgesics** should be provided for 3 or 4 days for patients with appreciable discomfort. Many patients will require a narcotic for several days because of the intensity of discomfort.
- **Local therapy** is important and may be administered as any number of topical preparations; combinations of neomycin, polymyxin, and hydrocortisone (Cortisporin Otic Suspension) or Oloxacin (Floxin Otic) are effective in most patients. An occasional patient will present with such far-advanced swelling of the walls of the canal

that the administration of topical agents by the patient may be impossible; in such cases, a small "wick" to which medication is applied may be inserted into the canal by the physician. The administration of medication is facilitated with the patient lying on the side with the affected ear up, thus allowing the agent to travel along the wick into the canal. These patients should be reevaluated in 48 hours and the wick changed or discarded. We generally recommend 3 or 4 drops four to six times per day for 10 days.

- When severe ear pain is present and associated with an obstruction of the canal to an extent that prevents the insertion of a wick, the possibility of free pus proximal to the obstruction must be considered; otolaryngologic consultation is advised before disposition in these patients to ensure drainage, wick insertion, appropriate antibiotics and analgesics, and follow-up.
- **Systemic therapy** is only necessary with high fever or preauricluar extension of the infection. An orally administered antibiotic should be used and should provide antistaphylococcal coverage. We prefer semisynthetic penicillin such as dicloxacillin tablets or elixir, cephalosporin or erythromycin. Therapy for 7 to 10 days is recommended.
- Patients should be advised to avoid getting water in the ear during the course of treatment; earplugs may be recommended for patients with recurrent infections.

Malignant Otitis Externa

The immunocompromised host, most often the diabetic subject, with acute otitis externa must be very aggressively managed, because many of these patients will have infection with *Pseudomonas aeruginosa* resistant to conventional therapy. Unless appropriate treatment is instituted, a number of serious local and systemic complications, including extensive destruction of local soft tissue and temporal bone, may develop. In all such patients, bacterial and fungal cultures should be obtained, consultation at the time of presentation requested, and admission arranged for intravenous antibiotic therapy with imipenem-cilastatin, ciprofloxacin, a third-generation antipseudomonal cephalosporin, or the combination of ticarcillin-clavulanate plus gentamicin.

Cellulitis of the External Ear

Cellulitis of the external ear is common and produces generalized erythema and pain involving the external ear. Trauma to the ear, including piercing the ears for cosmetic reasons, may be associated with such infection. Swelling is usually minimal, although discomfort may be severe in some patients.

Given the relatively poor blood supply to the external ear, many authorities recommend that patients with fever greater than 102°F should be considered candidates for several days of intravenous therapy with semisynthetic penicillin such as oxacillin. Adults without significant fever may be treated with an oral agent in high dose, such as dicloxacillin (500 mg four times daily), a cephalosporin, or erythromycin in equivalent dose. The possibility of community-acquired MRSA should be considered. An initial intravenous dose of oxacillin, 2 g in adults, may be helpful. Warm compresses to the ear, analgesics as needed, and follow-up in 48 hours are recommended. Earrings should be removed and their use proscribed for several weeks after resolution of infection.

Furunculosis of the External Auditory Canal

Furunculosis of the external auditory canal may occur spontaneously or in association with varying degrees of trauma to the canal. The diagnosis is based on demonstration of a specific furuncle or pustule in the ear canal, usually exquisitely tender, with surrounding erythema and mild swelling. Lesions perceived to be fluctuant should be gently incised and any expressed material sent for culture and sensitivity. This procedure, in many circumstances, may be more appropriately undertaken by the otolaryngologist. We generally recommend a short course of an oral antibiotic such as dicloxacillin, the application of heat three to four times per day, and follow-up in 3 or 4 days. Lesions that are not fluctuant at the time of presentation should be treated with an oral antibiotic, heat, and follow-up in 24 to 48 hours.

Preauricular Lymphadenopathy

Preauricular lymphadenopathy, if notably tender, may produce discomfort that frequently generalizes to involve the entire ear and, in some patients, the lateral face. The physician who encounters a patient with tender lymphadenopathy in the preauricular or peritragal area must carefully search the ipsilateral face, including the eye and gingiva, for evidence of infection. Frequently, a small pustule, abscess, or conjunctivitis, including herpetic keratoconjunctivitis or adenovirus infection, is noted in such patients; more commonly, acute otitis externa will be found responsible.

Herpes Zoster

Herpetic involvement of the ear is not uncommon and may present with severe pain, which is often vaguely localized to the area of the ear or jaw and *which may occur several days before the development of a rash*. If cutaneous involvement is present, the diagnosis is not difficult because erythema alone or in combination with varying stages of evolution of typical vesicles will be noted.

- **Corneal involvement** may coexist, and all patients with ocular complaints should undergo fluorescein staining of the cornea to demonstrate such involvement. If typical "ferning" or branching-type lesions are suspected or noted, immediate ophthalmologic consultation is recommended to facilitate the institution of definitive therapy. When a herpetic lesion appears on the tip of the nose (supplied by the nasociliary branch of the first division of cranial nerve V), there is a greater incidence of herpetic ocular involvement.
- **Superinfection of cutaneous lesions** is common with a number of organisms, particularly staphylococci, and when this occurs, treatment should be instituted with semisynthetic penicillin such as dicloxacillin, a cephalosporin, or erythromycin.
- Some authorities have recommended a short course of **oral steroids** (prednisone 40 mg once a day for 5 days) as a means of decreasing the incidence of postherpetic neuralgia; such therapy is said to not increase the risk of dissemination.
- **Antiviral agents** should be considered. In an immunocompromised host, consider acyclovir (Zovirax, 10–12 mg/kg intravenous every 8 hours). In a normal host, consider the following:
  - Valacyclovir (Valtrex) 1,000 mg by mouth three times daily for 7 days
  - Famciclovir (Famvir) 500 mg by mouth three times daily for 7 days
  - Acyclovir (Zovirax) 800 mg by mouth five times daily for 7 to 10 days
- Severe discomfort in affected areas is common and often requires treatment with a potent analgesic. Many patients receive additional benefit from the application

of an antibacterial ointment and a sterile dressing; such therapy may decrease the incidence of bacterial superinfection and also appears to prevent the elicitation of air current- or clothing-related dysesthesias and other discomfort. Dressings should be changed daily.

Temporomandibular Joint Dysfunction

Dysfunction of the temporomandibular joint, often secondary to malocclusion, is a relatively common problem that produces ipsilateral ear discomfort. Patients may not relate the onset or accentuation of symptoms to mastication, but such a relationship may be demonstrated by placing slight pressure on the joint with the index finger in the external auditory meatus while the patient opens and closes the mouth. Accentuation of discomfort in this manner confirms the diagnosis. Although uncommon, an occasional patient with rheumatoid arthritis will first present with temporomandibular joint involvement and discomfort.

Treatment in most patients involves reassurance, a soft diet for several days to 1 week, and the administration of aspirin or a nonsteroidal anti-inflammatory agent. Oral surgical follow-up is appropriate in most patients to exclude a surgically correctable abnormality of occlusion.

Bullous Myringitis

Approximately 10% of patients with mycoplasmal respiratory tract infection will have involvement of the tympanic membrane; other symptoms, particularly cough and sore throat, are usually present as well. Infection in this location is characterized by the presence of multiple small vesicles on the tympanic membrane and is referred to as *bullous myringitis*. Bullous myringitis may also develop secondary to viral infections of the upper respiratory tract.

Treatment includes analgesics for patients with significant discomfort and erythromycin (250–500 mg four times daily in adults, 40 mg/kg/day in children) administered for 10 days. Tetracycline is also effective against the organism but must be avoided in children younger than age 10 years and in pregnant women.

Acute Mastoiditis

Acute mastoiditis develops as a result of untreated or progressive otitis media. Patients with acute mastoiditis usually report fever, auricular and postauricular pain, hearing loss, and drainage of blood or pus or both from the canal if perforation of the tympanic membrane occurs.

Diagnosis
In cases not associated with perforation, the tympanic membrane will be inflamed and may bulge. Pain with percussion or palpation in the area just posterior to the auricle may be noted, and many patients will spontaneously report discomfort in this area. Radiologic assessment of the temporal bone will demonstrate "clouding" of the mastoid air cells and decalcification of the inner bony architecture of the mastoid; comparative views may be helpful for the nonradiologist.

Treatment
Treatment includes immediate otolaryngologic consultation, admission to the hospital, myringotomy for drainage, and intravenous antibiotics.

Barotrauma to the Middle Ear

Sudden changes in middle ear pressure, usually associated with airplane travel or diving, may produce a constellation of abnormalities involving the tympanic membrane and middle ear. Generally, the tympanic membrane is inflamed and retracted. In addition, a conductive hearing loss is noted, and air-fluid levels may be seen in the middle ear. Perforation of the eardrum and gross bleeding into the middle ear (hemotympanum) are less commonly noted but may occur secondary to pressure-related injury. In the event of a hemotympanum, the eardrum assumes a distinctly bluish color.

Mild cases may be treated with decongestants and otolaryngologic follow-up in 3 or 4 days. Severe cases should be evaluated by the otolaryngologist at the time of presentation for possible myringotomy. Perforation resulting from barotrauma requires therapy as outlined in section "Traumatic Perforation of the Tympanic Membrane". Patients with abnormalities of hearing must be followed-up to demonstrate the return of normal hearing.

Traumatic Perforation of the Tympanic Membrane

Acute traumatic perforation of the tympanic membrane may be associated with hearing loss, vertigo, tinnitus, and/or dislocation or disruption of the bony ossicles. These injuries usually occur as a result of a "slapping" -type injury to the lateral head or are related to diving injuries. Rarely, perforation may occur in association with rapid changes in middle ear pressure associated with airplane travel.

Vertigo may be prominent and is treated with meclizine, 25 mg three to four times per day, and a short course of bed rest. Patients with prominent vomiting may receive prochlorperazine either intramuscularly or by rectal suppository; severe vomiting may require hospitalization and intravenous fluids. Most patients can be treated at home and should be advised *not* to use topical ear drops and to be seen in 7 to 10 days to assess spontaneous healing. Many authorities recommend prophylactic oral antibiotics and the use of a small, sterile cotton ball, changed daily, to occlude the external meatus gently. Healing of most uncomplicated perforations is complete within 1 to 3 weeks.

Dislocation or gross disruption of the ossicles should be discussed with the otolaryngologist at the time of presentation.

Acute Hematoma of the Ear

Trauma to the external ear may result in hematoma formation; this classically involves the auricle, occurs between the cartilage and the perichondrium, and may result in permanent deformation of the external ear if left untreated.

If seen acutely, the area should be prepared and draped in the usual manner and the hematoma aspirated with a 16- or 18-gauge needle. A dressing that closely conforms to the architecture of the posterior and anterior auricle, and thereby gently but uniformly compresses the area previously occupied by the hematoma, should be constructed by the physician and *gently* applied. Sterile cotton balls or pledgets moistened with saline may be used to provide support for the convolutions of the auricle. After the ear is uniformly and comfortably supported, Kling or Webril may be circumferentially, but gently, applied. A cool compress may be applied to the area at home and the head of the bed elevated for 48 hours; reassessment in 48 to 72 hours is recommended. Patients should be advised that a repeated aspiration may be indicated if reaccumulation occurs.

Cerumen Impaction

Removal of cerumen from the auditory canal may be required to visualize the tympanic membrane in patients with possible otitis media. In addition, cerumen impaction may impair hearing or may result in mild discomfort; for these reasons, its removal may be necessary in the emergency department.

In patients with cerumen impacted firmly against the tympanic membrane, we generally prefer to avoid mechanical attempts at removal, including irrigation. In these patients, chemical agents should be prescribed, such as carbamide peroxide (Debrox), triethanolamine polypeptide oleate-condensate (Cerumenex), or half-strength hydrogen peroxide. After the daily use of any of these agents, gentle irrigation of the canal at home with warm water may be used to remove the now softened material.

In other patients, distal solid material may be easily removed with forceps or a suction catheter connected to wall suction. We have found a number 12 or 10 Frazier catheter most useful in these patients with more distal impactions. If gentle irrigation is elected, either as an initial procedure (which we have found both time consuming and not particularly successful) or after chemical treatment, a 50-mL syringe should be filled with warm water and connected to the plastic cannula of a 16- or 18-gauge Angiocath. The water jet should be directed cautiously toward the superior wall of the canal. Perforation of the tympanic membrane remains a contraindication to irrigation, and its presence therefore should be ascertained and documented prior to irrigation in all patients.

Bell Palsy

Bell palsy (idiopathic facial palsy) occurs acutely, usually over several hours, results from a presumed inflammatory reaction in or around the seventh cranial nerve near the stylomastoid foramen, and produces unilateral facial weakness involving the muscles of facial expression on the affected side. The forehead is unfurrowed, the palpebral fissure is widened, there is drooping of the corner of the mouth, and the skin folds are flattened. Upward movement of the ipsilateral eye, when the patient is asked to close the eyes, may be noted and is termed Bell phenomenon. Patients often report discomfort behind or below the ear, as well as facial numbness; however, the sensory examination of the face is normal. Hyperacusis (hypersensitivity to sounds), loss of taste on the anterior two thirds of the tongue, tinnitus, and deafness are variably noted.

Differential Diagnosis
Importantly, differentiation must be made between peripheral seventh nerve dysfunction (as discussed with respect to Bell palsy) and that caused by supranuclear interruption or more central involvement. Diagnostically, central lesions of the seventh nerve result in less involvement of the upper facial muscles, particularly the frontalis and orbicularis oculi, as a result of their bicortical (crossed and uncrossed fibers) innervation. Other neurologic signs, that is, arm or leg weakness, aphasia, or ipsilateral sixth nerve dysfunction, also suggest a more central cause. Trauma may also produce a seventh nerve deficit caused by actual interruption of the nerve as a result of direct or penetrating injury, or associated with a temporal bone fracture; urgent otolaryngologic consultation must, of course, be obtained in these patients. Otolaryngologic consultation should also be requested emergently in patients with evidence of seventh nerve dysfunction and acute or chronic suppurative otitis media, because operative repair may be necessary. Malignant involvement of the temporal bone may

also result in facial paralysis caused by seventh nerve involvement; however, in these patients, the onset of symptoms is more gradual. *Herpes zoster* similarly may involve the seventh cranial nerve (Ramsay Hunt syndrome), resulting in a facial palsy. In the great majority of these patients, at the time of presentation, an initially erythematous rash is noted to involve the lateral scalp or face and is followed by typical vesiculation. Pain in the eye, even if vague, mandates fluorescein staining of the cornea to define the typical fern-like or branching ulcer characterizing corneal involvement with this virus. If noted, urgent ophthalmologic consultation is then indicated.

Treatment

Importantly, 80% of patients with Bell palsy recover completely within 2 weeks, with partial recovery at 1 week being an important prognostic sign. Ten percent of patients will have permanent facial weakness. Treatment includes neurologic referral and ensuring that the eye is protected. Because of loss of the blink reflex and the inability to close the eye completely during sleep, the eye should be closed and a soft protective patch applied at bedtime. This ensures that the eye is covered and that drying of the cornea during sleep, with subsequent ulceration, does not occur; some authorities recommend the instillation of artificial tears at 4- to 6-hour intervals during the day and at bedtime. Prednisone, 40 to 60 mg/day for 5 days, started early in the course to be optimally effective. The use of antiviral agents remains controversial. Valacyclvir 1 gm PO TID for 7 days may be useful in severe cases.

13 Epistaxis

GENERAL CONSIDERATIONS

Because both anterior and posterior nasal bleeding may result in considerable loss of blood, the physician must first assess and correct any significant hemodynamic compromise. Careful evaluation and observation is advised for elderly or debilitated patients with significant loss of blood, particularly those living alone, or patients with complicating coagulopathies (including medication induced) and cardiovascular disorders.

The majority of nosebleeds are anterior bleeds (90%) caused by minor trauma (e.g., scratching) or desiccation in the area of Kiesselbach plexus (anterior nasal septum). Other causes include rhinitis with vigorous nose blowing, cocaine sniffing, hypertension, atherosclerosis, coagulopathies, tumors, foreign bodies, and atmospheric pressure changes. There are also uncommon causes such as the Osler-Weber-Rendu syndrome or hemorrhagic telangiectasia. Nasal fractures also cause epistaxis.

Anterior nosebleeds tend to bleed predominately from one nostril. Posterior sources tend to bleed from both nares and down the back of the throat. Patients on aspirin, NSAIDs, antiplatelet agents, and warfarin tend to require more aggressive therapy. In children, a history or family history of bleeding disorders should be sought.

The relationship between hypertension and epistaxis is unclear. There is no causal evidence between anterior epistaxis and hypertension. There may be a relationship between posterior epistaxis and elevated blood pressures. Most authorities recommend treatment of the epistaxis including adequate anesthesia of the nasal cavity and anxiolytics before treating hypertension acutely. Control of bleeding often spontaneously improves blood pressure.

INITIAL EVALUATION

The initial evaluation of the patient with epistaxis involves the differentiation of anterior from posterior bleeding. This differentiation is made on the basis of a thorough examination of the nose, which is performed with the patient sitting upright on the stretcher. For optimal visualization and treatment, the stretcher should be raised so that the patient's head is slightly below the physician's eye level. A head lamp, gown, and protective eyewear should be worn by the physician, because many patients will sneeze or cough during the evaluation. In addition, a nasal speculum, a Frazier suction catheter, and wall suction are essential to clear and visualize the point of bleeding in patients with brisk epistaxis.

ANTERIOR BLEEDING (90%)

Most instances of anterior bleeding occur as a result of self-inflicted trauma to the anterior nasal septum where small vessels (Kiesselbach plexus) may easily be disrupted.

- Many episodes resolve spontaneously, and in these patients, conservative management may be adequate. Patients should be advised to apply a cool compress to the nasal area, keep the head elevated, and avoid aspirin and exertion for 24 to 48 hours.
- When there is ongoing anterior bleeding, the patient should be urged to pinch the fleshy part of the nose firmly for 15 minutes while the examiner prepares the equipment.
  - The patient should be sitting upright on a stretcher for optimal examination and comfort. The patient should evacuate the nasal cavity gently but completely to allow visualization and instillation of vasoconstrictors. Inspection of the anterior part of the nasal septum will generally reveal either a discrete point of bleeding or shallow ulcerations or abrasions; these latter lesions are generally superficial. In either case, either pseudoephrine nasal spray should be instilled or an aqueous epinephrine (1:1,000 solution) should be applied to a cotton ball or sterile gauze that is then held against the bleeding site for 10 minutes with moderate pressure. This is most easily accomplished by bilateral alar compression. These sympathomimetic agents should be used cautiously in hypertensive or cardiac patients.
  - If a **discrete bleeding point** has been identified, the specific area may be cauterized; silver nitrate-tipped applicators are most often used. Cauterization should not be used in patients with abnormalities of hemostasis. Bilateral cauterization of the septum should also be avoided since blood flow may be significantly diminished.
  - In patients with bleeding **not confined to a discrete vessel or point**, topical epinephrine or psuedoephrine should be used and anterior nasal pack inserted. As an alternative to cauterization, Gelfoam or Surgicel can be directly applied to the bleeding area, followed by gentle pressure and light packing. A variety of nasal tampons and balloons are available and are often successful. These tampons and balloons are often easily inserted and do not require significant nasal anesthesia. Some balloons are impregnated with a procoagulant as well. If conventional anterior packing is required, cocaine, 5% to 10%, or 2% tetracaine may be applied topically to ensure anesthesia. We generally use commercially available ½- × 72-inch petrolatum-impregnated gauze. Successive folds of gauze should be layered into the nose on the side of bleeding, beginning inferiorly and continuing upward and laterally until the involved area is tamponaded. Patients should be instructed to keep the head elevated, apply a cool compress to the nasal area, and avoid aspirin, exertion, and blowing of the nose (or sneezing through the nose) for 24 to 48 hours. An appropriate oral antibiotic, such as cephalexin (Keflex), or amoxicillin-clavulanate (Augmentin) is usually prescribed to prevent sinusitis or toxic shock syndrome. The pack should be removed in approximately 48 to 72 hours, at which time the area should be inspected to ensure hemostasis. After healing, especially during the dry winter months or in the setting of an upper respiratory tract infection, many physicians recommend both humidification and the daily application of petrolatum to the mucosa of the anterior nose to prevent drying and recurrent epistaxis.
  - In the occasional patient with **persistent bleeding**, despite nasal packing, otolaryngologic consultation should be obtained. Uncontrolled hypertension and abnormalities of hemostasis should be considered in patients with recurrent or uncontrollable bleeding.

POSTERIOR BLEEDING

Direct visualization of actual bleeding sites in the posterior nose is often not possible, and because of the size of the vessels involved, bleeding may be rapid. In most patients with posterior epistaxis, anterior and posterior packing and admission for observation will be required. Significant blood loss should be treated. Early otolaryngologic referral and consultation are recommended. Patients usually do not require ICU level of care. However, the elderly and chronic alcoholics often have complicated hospital courses.

Posterior packing may be performed with any of a number of commercially available inflatable, balloon-type catheters. Epistat and Nasostat balloons are usually available and work quite well. They are typically removed in 3 to 5 days.

14 Facial Pain—Atraumatic

Facial pain occurring in the absence of trauma may be caused by a variety of disorders, many of which may be associated with referred pain, thereby making accurate localization of the source difficult. For this reason, a careful examination of the face, orbits, eyes, oral and nasal cavities, auditory canals, and temporomandibular joints is an essential aspect of the evaluation of these patients.

COMMON CAUSES OF ATRAUMATIC FACIAL PAIN

- Dental caries
- Dental or gingival abscess*
- Sinusitis
- Preorbital and orbital cellulitis*
- Facial or cutaneous abscess or infection

LESS COMMON CAUSES OF ATRAUMATIC FACIAL PAIN

- Trigeminal neuralgia (tic douloureux)*
- Parotitis*
- Salivary duct stone—parotid and submandibular
- Herpes zoster
- Acute dystonic reaction
- Temporomandibular joint syndrome*
- Temporomandibular joint dislocation*
- Malignant parotid tumors
- Lymphadenopathy (pretragal or inframandibular)
- Tetanus

HISTORY

A history of carious dentition in association with a gnawing, intolerable pain in the jaw or infraorbital region is seen in patients with gingival or dental abscesses. Pressure-like pain or aching in the area of the frontal sinuses, supraorbital ridge, or infraorbital area in association with fever, nasal congestion, postnasal discharge, or a recent upper respiratory tract infection suggests acute or chronic sinusitis. Redness, swelling, and pain around the eye are suggestive of periorbital cellulitis. The rapid onset of parotid or submandibular area swelling and pain, often occurring in association with meals, is characteristic of obstruction of the salivary duct as a result of stone. Trigeminal neuralgia produces excruciating, lancinating facial pain that occurs in unexpected paroxysms,

---

*Discussed in this chapter.

is initiated by the tactile stimulation of a "trigger point" or simply by chewing or smiling. Temporomandibular joint dysfunction produces pain related to chewing or jaw movement and is most commonly seen in women between the ages of 20 and 40 years; patients may have a history of recent injury to the jaw, recent dental work, or long-standing malocclusion. Facial paralysis associated with facial pain may be noted in patients with malignant parotid tumors. Dislocation of the temporomandibular joint causes sudden local pain and spasm and inability to close the mouth. Acute dystonic reactions to the phenothiazines and antipsychotic medications may closely simulate a number of otherwise perplexing facial and ocular presentations and must be considered. Acute suppurative parotitis usually occurs in the elderly or chronically debilitated patient and causes the rapid onset of fever, chills, and parotid swelling and pain, often involving the entire lateral face.

PHYSICAL EXAMINATION

Carious dentition, gingivitis, and gingival abscesses may be diagnosed by inspection of the oral cavity and face. Percussion tenderness over the involved tooth, swelling and erythema of the involved side of the face, and fever may be noted in patients with deep abscesses. Percussion tenderness to palpation or pain over the frontal or maxillary sinuses with decreased transillumination of these structures suggests sinusitis. Redness, tenderness, and swelling around the eye may suggest periorbital cellulitis. Pain with eye movement or exophthalmos may suggest an orbital cellulitis or abscess. Malocclusion may be noted in patients with temporomandibular joint dysfunction; tenderness on palpation of the temporomandibular joint, often best demonstrated anteriorly in the external auditory canal with the mouth open, is noted as well. Patients with temporomandibular joint dislocation present with anxiety, local pain, and inability to close the mouth. Unusual ocular, lingual, pharyngeal, or neck symptoms should suggest possible acute dystonic reactions. A swollen, tender parotid gland may be seen in patients with acute parotitis, in parotid duct obstruction secondary to stone or stricture, and in patients with malignant parotid tumors; evidence of facial paralysis should be sought in these latter patients. Palpation of the parotid duct along the inner midwall of the cheek will occasionally reveal a nodular structure consistent with a salivary duct stone. In patients with herpes zoster, typical lesions may be noted in a characteristic dermatomal pattern along the first, second, or third division of the trigeminal nerve or in the external auditory canal. It is important to remember that patients with herpes zoster may have severe pain *before* the development of any cutaneous signs. This diagnosis should always be considered when vague or otherwise undefinable facial pain syndromes are described. Simple erythema may be the first cutaneous manifestation of herpetic illness. Patients with trigeminal neuralgia have an essentially normal examination.

EMERGENCY DIAGNOSTIC TESTS

Computed tomography (CT) scanning of the sinuses will demonstrate mucosal thickening and/or air-fluid levels in patients with acute sinusitis, but the diagnosis in most instances remains a clinical one. Periorbital cellulitis is diagnosed on clinical exam. A CT scan of the orbits is required to diagnose orbital cellulitis. Soft-tissue radiographs of the cheek requested as "puff-cheek" views or CT scanning may demonstrate a calcific density in the vicinity of the parotid duct in patients with a salivary duct stone. Any purulent material expressed or noted at the duct orifice in patients with acute suppurative parotitis should be cultured.

SPECIFIC DISORDERS

Dental or Gingival Abscess

Deep dental or gingival abscesses usually develop in the setting of dental caries and are definitively treated by drainage and/or tooth extraction. Given the risk of bacteremia with manipulation of such deep lesions, antibiotics are optimally administered for 1 to 3 days before dental intervention; severe pain, however, may require that extraction be undertaken earlier. An analgesic should be given along with one of the following:

- Penicillin VK, 500 mg four times daily
- Erythromycin, 500 mg four times daily
- Clindamycin (Cleocin), 300 mg four times daily.
- Amoxicillin–clavulanic acid (Augmentin), 875/125 mg twice daily or 500/125 three times daily

Patients with severe symptoms, evidence of an extensive abscess, high fever, rigors, or other evidence of systemic infection require oral surgical consultation before disposition; hospitalization and intravenous antibiotics may be necessary. Odontogenic infection may spread into the neck causing Ludwig angina, which is discussed in Chapter 16.

Superficial gingival abscesses, which are most often noted immediately adjacent to the gum margin, may simply be incised in the usual manner, if fluctuant, and thereby definitively treated; a similar course of antibiotic therapy as discussed above, saline rinses after meals, and dental referral are also appropriate.

Preorbital and Orbital Cellulitis

Bacterial infection involving the contents of the orbit represents a major ophthalmologic emergency, and immediate consultation and referral are critical.

Clinical Presentation

Diagnosis is based upon physical exam. The periorbital area is erythematous and tender with preorbital cellulitis. With orbital extension, there is pain with extraocular movements. Ocular pain is often severe, deep, and aggravated by movement of the eye, which may be limited because of local edema. Mild degrees of proptosis may be noted. Chemosis, fever, and leukocytosis are common. Death may occur as a result of extension of infection into the cavernous sinus; diagnosis and treatment must be promptly undertaken.

Diagnostic Tests

The emergency department evaluation should include CT of the sinus and orbit, culture of any eye exudate and cultures of nose, throat, and blood. The bacteriology of orbital cellulitis is similar to that of acute sinusitis involving primarily staphylococci, pneumococci, streptococci, and *Haemophilus influenzae*.

Treatment

An otherwise healthy, well-appearing patient (>5 years of age) with preorbital cellulites may be managed as an outpatient. Orbital cellulitis requires consultation and referral, hospitalization, and early administration of appropriate intravenous antibiotics.

Trigeminal Neuralgia

Trigeminal neuralgia (tic douloureux) is an excruciatingly painful condition in which lancinating discomfort occurs in one of the three distributions of the trigeminal nerve or, less frequently, in the region of the glossopharyngeal nerve in the posterior pharyngeal wall. An acute attack may occur unpredictably or may be precipitated by stimulation of a "trigger point." Most commonly, the disease is idiopathic in origin, although occasionally it may be a presenting symptom of multiple sclerosis or a brainstem neoplasm. The initial treatment of an acute attack requires the use of a potent analgesic and neurologic follow-up in 24 to 48 hours. Long-term medical therapy with carbamazepine, baclofen, or phenytoin may provide significant and dramatic relief; patients not responding to these agents may benefit from stereotactic radiofrequency ablation of the involved nerve.

Parotitis

Acute viral parotitis develops as a result of infection with the mumps virus; suppurative or bacterial parotitis may occur spontaneously or in association with ductal obstruction secondary to stone or stricture. Bacterial infection is typically produced by staphylococci, and on palpation and "milking" of the gland and duct, purulent material may be noted to appear at the duct orifice. Treatment for patients with bacterial infection involves the culture of any expressed material, relief of obstruction by stone extrusion or surgical extirpation of a fibrotic stenotic lesion, and the administration of an antistaphylococcal antibiotic. Otolaryngologic consultation is appropriate in most patients.

Temporomandibular Joint Syndrome

Patients with the temporomandibular joint syndrome primarily complain of sharp or aching pain related to chewing or opening the mouth typically radiating to the ear. A history of recent jaw injury, dental work, or long-standing malocclusion is often obtained. Emotional stress associated with clenching the teeth or nocturnal grinding of the teeth may also be reported. Examination of the temporomandibular joint is best performed with the examiner's index fingers placed within the external auditory canals. Anterior fullness and tenderness may be noted with this maneuver, particularly with the mouth open; crepitation and limited motion may also be observed. Treatment involves the use of heat applied locally, the administration of aspirin or other anti-inflammatory agents, and limiting the diet to soft foods. The patient should be referred to an oral surgeon if symptoms persist.

Temporomandibular Joint Dislocation

Temporomandibular joint dislocation may follow trauma to the face or may occur as a result of simply opening the mouth widely with yawning, laughing, or chewing. Patients are unable to close the mouth and complain of severe discomfort and varying degrees of anxiety. Radiologic assessment of the entire mandible is indicated before attempting reduction, because condylar fractures are occasionally present and should be documented before manipulation. Bilateral dislocations often occur.

Importantly, dystonic reactions to the phenothiazines or antipsychotic medications may simulate this disorder as well as a variety of other conditions. This phenomenon should be considered in all patients with atraumatic facial pain and can usually be rapidly excluded on the basis of history. (See "Temporomandibular Joint Dislocation" in Chapter 4 for treatment of dystonic reactions and for treatment of temporomandibular joint dislocations.)

Sinusitis

See "Acute Sinusitis" in Chapter 42 for treatment of acute sinusitis.

15 Hoarseness

It is important to distinguish between acute and chronic hoarseness because therapy and prognosis differ significantly.

CAUSES OF ACUTE HOARSENESS

- Infectious laryngitis* (viral, bacterial, tuberculous, diphtheritic, fungal)
- Croup
- Epiglottitis
- Vocal cord paralysis*

CAUSES OF CHRONIC HOARSENESS

- Hypothyroidism
- Laryngeal papillomatosis*
- Laryngeal carcinoma*
- Singer's nodule*
- Vocal cord paralysis*

HISTORY

Hoarseness preceded by a sore throat or accompanied by flu-like symptoms such as cough, low-grade fever, or coryza is likely due to viral laryngitis. Epiglottitis must also be considered if the patient appears ill, has a high fever, has difficulty swallowing or is drooling, has no associated flu-like symptoms, or reports difficulty breathing. A history of chronic hoarseness must be considered suggestive of a structural or neoplastic cause, directly involving either the larynx or the recurrent laryngeal nerve. Hypothyroidism should be considered in patients with chronic hoarseness and other historical evidence of thyroid hormone deficiency.

PHYSICAL EXAMINATION

Erythema or exudate involving the pharynx suggests infectious laryngitis or epiglottitis. Unintentional weight loss, anorexia, and a smoking history suggest laryngeal carcinoma. Dry skin, fine hair, and a delay in the relaxation phase of the deep tendon reflexes should suggest hypothyroidism.

*Discussed in this chapter.

DIAGNOSTIC TESTS

A throat culture will identify patients with a bacterial cause for hoarseness, although in most patients, infection-related illnesses have a viral rather than bacterial cause. Indirect or direct laryngoscopy or a lateral soft-tissue roentgenogram of the neck usually demonstrates an edematous, enlarged epiglottis in patients with acute epiglottitis, and an elevated serum thyroid-stimulating hormone is useful in detecting the hypothyroid patient. Vocal cord polyps, squamous cell carcinoma of the pharynx or larynx, and paralysis of one or both cords may be noted by direct or indirect laryngoscopy. Apical lordotic chest radiographs and computed tomography or magnetic resonance imaging (CT or MRI) scans of the chest may be used to diagnose structural or compressive lesions involving the recurrent laryngeal nerve.

CLINICAL REMINDERS

- Do not vigorously examine the pharynx of a patient suspected of having acute epiglottitis; obtain lateral radiographs of the neck or indirect or direct laryngoscopy to identify or rule out an enlarged epiglottis.
- If clinically indicated, appropriate radiographic views of the lung apices and mediastinum should be obtained to exclude the presence of a neoplastic process compressing the recurrent laryngeal nerve in the patient with subacute or chronic hoarseness.

SPECIFIC DISORDERS

Infectious Laryngitis

Viral laryngitis is by far the most common etiology of acute hoarseness. Respiratory syncytial virus and adenovirus are the most common offending agents. Symptoms usually preceding hoarseness include coryza, fever, a watery nasal discharge, cough, and sneezing. Treatment is symptomatic and may include the use of antipyretic agents and cough suppressants. Cessation of smoking is important for the duration of the acute infection.

Diphtheria is an uncommon cause of infectious laryngitis today but should be considered in patients with an exudative pharyngitis and hoarseness because neither streptococcal nor infectious mononucleosis–related pharyngitis commonly produce an associated laryngitis. Candidal laryngitis is the most common fungal infection involving the larynx and is typically seen in patients with oral thrush or esophageal candidiasis. In children, the croup syndrome commonly includes some degree of hoarseness. Lateral neck radiographs must generally be obtained to exclude the presence of acute epiglottitis.

Laryngeal Papillomatosis

Laryngeal papillomatosis is a viral disease producing multiple, pedunculated, fleshy growths on the vocal cords. Lesions are easily excised but commonly recur. Children are at greatest risk for this disorder and recurrences are unusual after puberty.

Singer's Nodule

Persons using their voices excessively (e.g., opera singers, politicians) are prone to the development of a single, firm vocal cord nodule. If diagnosed early, nodules may regress with proper attention to reducing cord stress; however, as the nodule becomes firm, surgical excision is required.

Laryngeal Carcinoma

Smokers and alcoholics are at greatest risk for the development of laryngeal carcinoma, the lesions of which may be confined purely within the vocal cord (intrinsic) or may extend beyond the cord (extrinsic). Intrinsic laryngeal carcinoma is often heralded by a subtle development of hoarseness. After the diagnosis is made by direct laryngoscopy, a variety of therapeutic modalities may be indicated, including radiation, surgery, and chemotherapy.

Epiglottitis

See "Acute Epiglottitis" in Chapter 16.

Vocal Cord Paralysis

Mediastinal tumors and an expanding ascending aortic aneurysm are both capable of causing partial vocal cord paralysis by compression of the recurrent laryngeal nerve. Postdiphtheritic neuritis and poliomyelitis may also produce vocal cord paralysis by direct neural involvement. Operative trauma (particularly after thyroidectomy) may result in recurrent laryngeal nerve injury, which is suggested by postoperative stridor.

Hypothyroidism

See "Myxedema Coma" in Chapter 39.

16 Sore Throat

INTRODUCTION

An acutely sore throat is a common symptom in emergency medicine. The most common diagnoses are: is viral pharyngitis, strep throat or infectious mononucleosis. However, the emergency physician must remain vigilant for more serious infections such as peritonsillar abscess, retropharyngeal abscess, and acute epiglottitis. An inflamed painful throat often raises the question of viral versus bacterial infection. Most pharyngitis, regardless of the cause, resolve spontaneously. However, the standard is to treat acute group A β-hemolytic strep infections with antibiotics to minimize the risk of acute rheumatic fever. Various clinical rules in association with rapid streptococcal antigen testing successfully identify pharyngitis due to bacterial infection and can decrease the use of unnecessary antibiotics. Although the treatment for infectious mononucleosis is only symptomatic treatment, early diagnosis can be beneficial to the patient in anticipating a protracted course of the illness and the need to minimize physical activities. Peritonsillar abscess requires drainage in the emergency department. Acute epiglottitis can cause life-threatening airway obstruction and must be diagnosed. A patient with retropharyngeal abscess often requires hospitalization and drainage and should be considered in a systemically ill patient with a sore throat.

COMMON CAUSES OF SORE THROAT

- Streptococcal pharyngitis (group A, β-hemolytic)*
- Infectious mononucleosis*
- Herpangina*
- Viral pharyngitis
- Aphthous stomatitis

LESS COMMON CAUSES OF SORE THROAT NOT TO BE MISSED

- Peritonsillar abscess*
- Acute epiglottitis*
- Retropharyngeal abscess*
- Gonococcal pharyngitis
- Diphtheritic pharyngitis
- Thyroiditis
- Vincent angina
- Ludwig angina*

---

*Discussed in this chapter.

OTHER CAUSES OF SORE THROAT

- Candidiasis
- *Legionella* pharyngitis
- Mycoplasmal pharyngitis

HISTORY

Streptococcal pharyngitis ("strep" throat) is characterized by the relatively sudden onset of pain on swallowing and fever. It is important to note that acute pharyngitis associated with infectious mononucleosis or caused by gonococcus, meningococcus, *Mycoplasma*, or *Legionella* organism, although less common than streptococcal pharyngitis, is clinically indistinguishable from it. Children with streptococcal pharyngitis may present primarily with abdominal pain, and sore throat is often mild or occasionally absent. Acute epiglottitis may present dramatically with the sudden onset of high fever, severe sore throat, drooling, and dyspnea. Change or muffling of the voice, often characterized as the "hot-potato voice, " in association with severe sore throat, fever, drooling, and local neck pain or pain referred to the ear should suggest peritonsillar abscess. Fatigue, malaise, anorexia, and fever in a young adult with a sore throat should suggest infectious mononucleosis. Patients with herpangina report severe mouth, tongue, or throat pain often impairing deglutition. Patients with thyroiditis report pain and tightness of the lower throat radiating to the ears, which is often accompanied by fatigue and malaise.

PHYSICAL EXAMINATION

- Fever of 38 °C or greater associated with anterior cervical adenopathy and a pharyngotonsillar exudate are suggestive of streptococcal pharyngitis. A pharyngeal exudate, although noted in many patients with streptococcal pharyngitis, is a nonspecific finding and can be seen with gonococcal, *Haemophilus,* and diphtheritic pharyngitis, and a variety of viral syndromes including those resulting from adenovirus infection and associated with infectious mononucleosis. In many patients with streptococcal pharyngitis, simple erythema without gross exudate is noted. If the particular streptococcal strain produces erythrogenic toxin, a number of cutaneous phenomena are noted; these define the entity of scarlet fever and include a generalized, often subtle erythematous rash, circumoral pallor, a strawberry-colored tongue, and Pastia lines (accentuated flexor creases).
- "Muffling" or change in voice, often characterized as the "hot-potato voice" is noted in and should suggest peritonsillar abscess; other findings include drooling, moderate to high fever, local lymphadenopathy, and asymmetry of the pharynx manifest as swelling, fullness, or bulging of the involved soft palate and anterior pillar. In these patients, erythema and exudate are often noted to involve the pharynx generally, and the uvula may be displaced medially away from the involved side as the abscess expands. Examination of the posterior pharyngeal wall in patients with retropharyngeal abscess, most of whom will be young children, should disclose a unilateral area of erythema, swelling, and fluctuance; such patients typically (if able) report a "lump in the throat" that persists despite food intake and swallowing. Importantly, such patients may have symptoms related to or showing evidence of airway obstruction, which are typically improved by lying down.

- The oropharynx appears normal in acute epiglottitis and, especially in patients with the relatively dramatic onset of severe sore throat, high fever, and hoarseness, the absence of oropharyngeal pathology should raise one's index of suspicion that epiglottitis may be present. When the diagnosis of epiglottitis is considered, aggressive examination of the posterior pharynx is deferred (including obtaining a culture), and evaluation of the epiglottic area with a lateral neck radiograph, direct or indirect larngyoscopy should be promptly obtained. Acute upper airway obstruction induced by examination of the oropharynx in patients with acute epiglottitis is a known complication of which the physician should be aware.
- Patients with infectious mononucleosis typically also have an exudative pharyngitis; splenomegaly, prominent cervical (as well as generalized) lymphadenopathy, and palatal or uvular petechiae may be noted as well. Exquisitely painful lingual or pharyngeal ulcers or vesicles are noted in herpangina, and typical, painful, clustered vesicles on an erythematous base may be seen in patients with herpetic infections of the oral mucosa. Diphtheria produces an adherent gray membrane over the tonsils and pharynx that characteristically bleeds when rubbed with a culture swab. A shaggy, grayish membrane on the tonsils, pharynx, and gingivae with underlying granulation tissue in a patient with foul breath and cervical adenopathy should suggest Vincent angina. A tender, occasionally swollen thyroid gland is noted in patients with thyroiditis; palpation of the gland in these patients may reproduce or accentuate the patient's discomfort.

DIAGNOSTIC TESTS

Given the relatively high cost of a throat culture and the fact that a single culture in adults may have a false-negative rate as high as 30% to 40%, many clinicians elect empiric therapy and defer obtaining a culture. The rapid streptococcal antigen test has a sensitivity of more than 90%. The monospot test often allows a prompt diagnosis of infectious mononucleosis but may be negative early in the illness. A small group of patients, particularly young children, will remain **monospot or heterophile-negative** throughout their illness; in these persons, anti–Epstein-Barr virus antibody titers may be obtained and may thus confirm the diagnosis. Measurement of antithyroid and antimicrosomal antibodies aids in the diagnosis of acute thyroiditis. Lateral radiographic views of the soft tissues of the neck or direct or indirect laryngoscopy are essential in the early evaluation of the patient with suspected epiglottitis and retropharyngeal abscess; these are discussed in "Acute Epiglottitis" and "Retropharyngeal Abscess."

CLINICAL REMINDERS

- Do not neglect the examination of the oropharynx in children presenting with abdominal pain.
- Do not aggressively examine or culture the oropharynx in patients suspected of having acute epiglottitis.

SPECIFIC DISORDERS

Streptococcal Pharyngitis

Streptococcal pharyngitis is caused by group A β-hemolytic streptococci and is characterized by the rapid onset of fever and sore throat; nausea, vomiting, headache, and

Table 16-1	Treatment Regimens for Patients with Streptococcal Pharyngitis

Adults and Children Older Than 12 y
Oral penicillin V potassium, 500 mg three times daily for 10 d
Oral erythromycin, 250 mg four times daily for 10 d
Cephalexin 500 mg four times daily for ten days
Intramuscular benzathine penicillin, 1.2 million U once
Azithromycin 500 mg daily for 3 d

Infants and Children Younger Than 12 y
Oral penicillin G, 40 mg/kg/d in four divided doses for 10 d
Oral penicillin V potassium, 40 mg/kg/d in four divided doses for 10 d
Oral erythromycin ethylsuccinate, 30–50 mg/kg/d in four divided doses for 10 d
An oral cephalosporin (e.g., cephalexin oral suspension, 25–50 mg/kg/d in four divided doses for 10 d)
Intramuscular benzathine penicillin, 1,200,000 U for children >27 kg and 600,000 U for children <27 kg once

malaise may also be noted. An absence of cough is typical. In children, presenting symptoms may include abdominal pain. On examination, fever, an exudative pharyngitis/tonsillitis or simple pharyngeal erythema, and regional lymphadenopathy are found. If scarlet fever is present, circumoral pallor; a "strawberry" tongue; a generalized, erythematous rash, which ultimately develops the texture of sandpaper; and Pastia lines may be noted. Pastia lines represent the accentuation of normally present flexor creases observed most easily in the antecubital fossae. The presence of scarlet fever does not change therapy. Acceptable forms of therapy are listed in Table 16-1. If a cough, hoarseness or coryza are present, consider an alternative diagnosis.

Viral Pharyngitis

Viral pharyngitis shows erythema of the tonsils and pharynx and is often associated with rhinorrhea. Tonsillar exudate and cervical adenopathy are usually absent. Viral pharyngitis is treated with supportive care such as gargling with warm salt water, drinking warm liquids, using antipyretics and analgesics, and taking rest. Patients with severe odynophagia may be treated with dexamethasone.

Infectious Mononucleosis

Infectious mononucleosis is a disease primarily of young adults, characterized by sore throat, fatigue, anorexia, fever, and malaise. Caused by the Epstein-Barr virus, this disorder may be insidious in onset and frequently runs a course several weeks to months in length. An exudative pharyngitis or tonsillitis, palatal petechiae, cervical or diffuse lymphadenopathy, splenomegaly, hepatomegaly, and a petechial eruption may be noted on physical examination. Infrequently, pneumonitis, hepatitis, pleuritis, pericarditis, myocarditis, and meningoencephalomyelitis may develop as further complications. Pertinent laboratory data include a lymphocytosis with many atypical lymphocytes and a positive monospot test; the latter is frequently negative early in the disease, although after approximately 14 and 28 days of symptoms, 60% and

90% of patients, respectively, manifest a positive monospot test. A small group of patients, however, particularly young children, will remain monospot or heterophile negative throughout their illness but will have rising or elevated titers of anti–Epstein–Barr virus antibody. No specific therapy exists for infectious mononucleosis; however, a rapid strep test or throat culture should be obtained in all patients to rule out concomitant streptococcal infection, which should be treated if present. Corticosteroid therapy may be considered in patients with extremely severe pharyngitis, evolving airway obstruction, chronic or disabling symptoms, or profound splenomegaly. Ampicillin administered to patients with infectious mononucleosis frequently causes an extensive maculopapular rash and should be avoided. Patients should be told to avoid contact sports until the splenomegaly and risk of splenic injury resolve.

Acute Epiglottitis

The classic patient with epiglottitis is a child between the ages of 3 and 7 years in whom severe sore throat and fever develop relatively rapidly. However, the *Haemophilus influenzae* vaccine has dramatically decreased the incidence of epiglottitis in children. Most cases of epiglottitis now involve adults and have a mixed bacterial culture. Epiglottitis should be considered when the examination of the oropharynx does not reveal a source of the patient's complaints. Airway obstruction is usually more gradual in onset in adults than in children. Direct laryngoscopy is the best way to make this diagnosis. If epiglottitis is strongly considered, ENT consultation may be necessary.

- Progression to complete airway obstruction may occur quickly. Complete airway obstruction may be precipitated by manual examination or instrumentation of the mouth or pharynx; for this reason, stimulation of the oropharynx should be minimized.
- The **diagnosis** of acute epiglottitis is based on maintaining a low index of suspicion, recognizing the clinical signs, and radiologically or visually demonstrating an enlarged epiglottis.
- In severe cases that have an intact airway, "elective" intubation in the operating room by the anesthesiologist with the otolaryngologist in attendance may be the preferred manner of airway protection.
- Initial therapy includes 7 to 10 days of intravenous ceftriaxone 100 to 200 mg/kg/day in four divided doses or cefuroxime 100 to 150 mg/kg/day in three divided doses. Some authorities recommend the use of dexamethasone intravenous initially.
- **When the diagnosis is unclear,** emergency radiologic or otolaryngologic consultation should be obtained.

Peritonsillar Abscess

Suppuration involving the potential space between the capsule of the tonsil and the fascial covering of the superior constrictor muscle results in peritonsillar abscess. Infection is thought to be secondary to local extension, and most often β and anaerobic streptococci, staphylococci, or *Haemophilus* organisms are implicated.

- **History.** Typically patients present with sore throat, which may have suddenly worsened, fever, and tender cervical adenopathy. Muffling or the characteristic "hot-potato voice" and drooling are important clues in the initial encounter with the patient and should suggest the diagnosis. Neck and ipsilateral ear pain may be reported as well, and many patients are unable or refuse to open the mouth fully because this maneuver accentuates their discomfort.

- The diagnosis is made by physical examination, which discloses asymmetry, secondary to swelling, fullness, or actual bulging of the involved soft palate and anterior pillar above the tonsil. Exudate and erythema are commonly noted as well and often involve the pharynx generally. As a result of the space-occupying properties of the abscess, the uvula is often displaced away from the involved side. Actual fluctuance of the abscess is occasionally present on palpation but is more often absent or difficult to clearly appreciate.

- Recognized complications of peritonsillar abscess, all of which are related to local extension in the neck, include involvement of the retropharyngeal space and carotid sheath; the latter may result in septic thrombophlebitis of the internal jugular vein with resultant central nervous system involvement. Spontaneous drainage of the abscess may occasionally occur.

- **Treatment.** When the diagnosis of peritonsillar abscess is made, the treatment is drainage. Needle aspiration of the abscess has been shown to be an effective method that is safely conducted by emergency physicians. An 18-gauge needle should be used with a needle guard in place to prevent deep penetration if the patient should move. Successful aspiration of the abscess should result in dramatic improvement in the patient's symptoms. An initial dose of IV antibiotics may be followed by oral antibiotics with close follow-up. If aspiration of the abscess is unsuccessful or does not result in significant improvement of the symptoms, an otolaryngologist consultation should be obtained. Some patients may require IV hydration, pain medicines, and IV antibiotics.

Retropharyngeal Abscess

Retropharyngeal abscess most often affects infants and children younger than 3 years of age. Neck and throat pain, fever, difficulty swallowing, and occasionally a change in voice or cry are the presenting symptoms. In some patients, dyspnea may be a presenting symptom, and when compromise of the airway is severe, stridor may be noted. Fever is noted along with erythema, pain with palpation, swelling, and fluctuance unilaterally involving the posterior pharyngeal wall. Causative agents include streptococcal, staphylococcal, and *Haemophilus* organisms.

- A lateral roentgenogram of the neck or CT scan in addition to the physical findings previously noted are often useful to demonstrate the abscess. Particular attention should be paid to the distance between the anterior edge of C-2 and C-6 and the posterior pharyngeal and tracheal air columns, respectively. In normal adults, anterior vertebral air column distances on average are 3.4 mm at C-2 and 14 mm at C-6; however, significant variation around the mean is noted within the population. Measurements at C-2 exceeding 7 mm in children and adults, and at C-6, those exceeding 14 mm in children, or 22 mm in adults are considered to be abnormal and suspicious. An air-fluid level should also suggest the diagnosis.

- Treatment includes initial assessment and maintenance of the airway, hospital admission, immediate otolaryngologic consultation for incision and drainage, and the institution of intravenous antibiotics; a semisynthetic penicillin, such as oxacillin, 2 g intravenous every 4 hours in adults or 100 to 200 mg/kg/day intravenous in four divided doses in children, is appropriate, as discussed in "Peritonsillar Abscess." Surgery remains the definitive treatment and should be undertaken early.

Herpangina

Herpangina results from virally induced (adenovirus, coxsackie group A) ulcerations of the oropharyngeal mucosa, which may produce severe pain and occasionally limit oral intake. The physician must also consider bacterial superinfection in these patients, and when present or suspected, antibacterial treatment with penicillin or erythromycin should be instituted.

Symptomatic treatment involves reassurance and topical as well as systemic measures to control pain. Analgesics, often including narcotics, may occasionally be required and may be taken 30 minutes before meals to facilitate oral intake. Patients with a small number of erosions may benefit from the direct application of viscous lidocaine, which can be performed simply by holding a cotton-tipped applicator saturated with lidocaine against the area for 3 to 5 minutes before meals or as needed for the control of pain. In adults, more extensive involvement may require swishing or gargling a tablespoon of viscous lidocaine in the mouth for 2 to 3 minutes. If oral intake is severely limited and dehydration ensues, admission for parenteral rehydration may be required.

Common Cold

The designation "common cold" includes several syndromes resulting from infection of the upper airway with a variety of viral agents; these include the rhinovirus, herpesvirus, parainfluenza virus, coronavirus, respiratory syncytial virus, adenovirus, coxsackievirus, and echovirus. Patients present with fever, chills, myalgias, nasal stuffiness and discharge, sore throat, congestion, occasional sneezing, and a nonproductive or minimally productive cough. Children are most commonly affected, although the disease may occur at any age, and symptoms may vary widely. Presentations appear to be more common during the winter months and less common during the summer. Typically, the white blood cell count is normal or depressed with a lymphocytic predominance. Treatment includes antipyretics, antihistamines or other decongestants, nasal sprays if indicated, and a period of rest.

Ludwig Angina

Ludwig angina results from the extension of a dental abscess into the submandibular and sublingual spaces. Often, there is not a true abscess cavity but rather brawny edema. The edema pushes the tongue upward. Patients report neck pain, odynophagia, trismus, and fever. Physical exam reveals swelling, erythema, and tenderness of the anterior neck. Airway compromise may lead to stridor. Diagnosis is best made by CT scan of the neck. High-dose antibiotics (penicillin or clindamycin), surgical drainage, and intubation may be necessary. Untreated, this process can extend to the carotid sheath and mediastinum.

17 Red Eye

COMMON CAUSES OF AN ACUTELY RED EYE

- Subconjunctival hemorrhage*
- Conjunctivitis*
- Corneal abrasion (see Chapter 5)
- Corneal foreign body (see Chapter 5)
- Hordeolum (stye) and chalazion*

LESS COMMON CAUSES OF AN ACUTELY RED EYE NOT TO BE MISSED

- Acute narrow-angle glaucoma*
- Uveitis*
- Episcleritis and scleritis*
- Keratitis*
- Penetrating ocular injury (see Chapter 5)
- Corneal ulcer*

OTHER CAUSES OF AN ACUTELY RED EYE

- Traumatic iritis and hyphema (see Chapter 5)
- Ultraviolet exposure (flash burns, sunlamps, snow glare) (see Chapter 5)

DIFFERENTIAL DIAGNOSIS

The **differential diagnosis** of the acutely red eye includes subconjunctival hemorrhage, conjunctivitis, corneal abrasion and ulcer, iritis, acute narrow-angle glaucoma, uveitis, and keratitis (Table 17-1). The differential diagnosis can be refined if the physician recognizes the specific findings of conjunctival versus ciliary injection as well as the historical features that suggest a particular disorder as follows:

- Are the inflamed vessels bright red and peripheral to the limbus (conjunctival injection) or more violaceous and both emanating from and adjacent to the limbus (ciliary injection)?
- Do the affected vessels move easily with the conjunctiva when it is lightly brushed with a moistened cotton swab (conjunctival injection), or do the vessels appear deep and fixed (ciliary injection)?
- Does the patient report deep eye pain or a more superficial discomfort (conjunctivitis)?

---

*Discussed in this chapter.

Table 17-1 Differential Diagnosis of the Red Eye

	Laterality	Discharge	Adenopathy	Photophobia	Itching	Pain	Pupil	Fluorescein	Cornea
Conjunctivitis									
Bacterial	Bilateral	Purulent	None	+	−	−	wnl	None	Clear
Viral (adenoviral)	Bilateral	Watery/mucoid	Preauricular	++	−	+	wnl	P	Clear
Chlamydial	Bilateral	Watery/mucoid	Preauricular	+	−	−	wnl	P	Clear
Allergic	Bilateral	Watery	None	−	++	−	wnl	None	Clear
Iritis	Unilateral	None	None	+++	−	++	wnl	None	KP
Glaucoma									
Acute angle closure	Unilateral	Watery	None	++	−	+++	Fixed	None	E
Cornea abrasion	Unilateral	Watery	None	++	−	+++	wnl	G	E
Corneal ulcer									
Bacterial	Unilateral	Purulent	None	+++	−	+++	wnl	G	I
Viral (herpes simplex)	Unilateral	Watery	+/−	++	−	++	wnl	D	E
Scleritis	Unilateral	Watery	None	+	−	++	wnl	None	Clear
Episcleritis	Unilateral	None	None	+	−	−	wnl	None	Clear
Subconjunctival hemorrhage	Unilateral	None	None	−	−	−	wnl	None	Clear

P, punctate staining; G, geographic staining; D, dendritic staining; KP, keratic precipitates; E, edema; I, cornea infiltrate; wnl, within normal limits; +, slight; ++, moderate; +++, extreme; −, absent.

Courtesy of James J. Reidy, MD, FACS, Cornea Service, Department of Ophthalmology, SUNY at Buffalo, School of Medicine, Buffalo, New York.

- Is the visual acuity normal or reduced in the affected eye (acute glaucoma, uveitis, and keratitis)?
- Is the cornea clear or cloudy or steamy (acute glaucoma)?
- Is the pupil round and reactive, dilated and fixed (acute glaucoma), or irregular, small, and minimally reactive (acute uveitis)?
- Does the patient report any associated symptoms, such as blurred vision, colored halos surrounding lights, nausea, vomiting, abdominal pain (suggesting acute glaucoma), or severe photophobia (suggesting uveitis or keratitis)?

DIAGNOSTIC TESTS

Standard aspects of the emergency ophthalmologic examination essential for proper evaluation of the acutely red eye include inspection, determination of visual acuity, pupillary reactivity, funduscopy, tonometry, and fluorescein staining of the cornea. The last is useful for documenting corneal abrasions and herpetic keratitis and should be performed, as should tonometry, after locally anesthetizing the cornea with topical ophthalmic tetracaine.

CLINICAL REMINDERS

- Do not use topical ophthalmic steroid preparations without ophthalmologic consultation and follow-up.
- Do not use atropine-containing mydriatics when evaluating ophthalmologic symptoms, because the effect lasts for 12 to 14 days and acute narrow-angle glaucoma may be precipitated in patients with a narrow anterior chamber angle.
- Obtain consultation when ciliary injection is noted or when the cause of the patient's eye pain and redness remains undefined.

SPECIFIC DISORDERS

Subconjunctival Hemorrhage

Spontaneous rupture of a conjunctival blood vessel produces a bright red, unilateral, sharply demarcated area limited by the limbus that is totally asymptomatic, is self-limited, resolves in 1 to 3 weeks, and is not affected by treatment of any kind. Patients require only reassurance and information regarding cause (coughing, laughing, straining) and the expected time course of resolution. No specific therapy is indicated.

Conjunctivitis

Conjunctivitis may result from viral, bacterial, fungal, parasitic, allergic, ultraviolet, or chemical processes or may occur in association with systemic disease.

History

Most patients with conjunctivitis report the gradual onset of a vague, superficial discomfort associated with varying degrees of conjunctival "grittiness" or a foreign body sensation. Many patients complain of eyelid swelling or heaviness, and the former is occasionally noted on examination. A copious exudate can cause eyelid "sticking," particularly after sleep. Systemic symptoms, such as headache, nausea, vomiting, or fever are absent as are visual loss and photophobia.

Associated features may suggest a particular cause. Because it is highly contagious, multiple cases in the same household suggest infectious conjunctivitis. Many patients with allergic conjunctivitis report seasonal recurrences in association with prominent conjunctival itching, rhinorrhea, and a thin, watery ocular discharge. Fever and pharyngitis frequently occur in conjunction with conjunctival inflammation in patients with viral (particularly adenovirus) infection. Conjunctivitis in the newborn represents a special diagnostic and therapeutic problem and is discussed in "Conjunctivitis in the Newborn."

Physical Examination
On physical examination, swelling of the eyelids, edema of the conjunctiva (chemosis), and exudation may be noted. Pseudoptosis (drooping of the affected upper lid) is often noted and results from the slightly increased lid weight secondary to local edema. Chemosis of the bulbar conjunctiva is seen most often in patients with allergic reactions. Preauricular nontender lymphadenopathy may accompany viral conjunctivitis. A painful vesicular or papular eruption involving the upper or middle face and associated with a blepharoconjunctivitis strongly suggests herpes zoster. In simple conjunctivitis, peripheral conjunctival (not perilimbal) injection should be noted. These vessels are bright red and move easily with the conjunctiva when it is lightly brushed with a moistened, sterile, cotton applicator. The pupil is round and reacts well to light, which does not increase the patient's discomfort; the fundi and cornea are normal, and visual acuity is unaffected unless exudate obscures vision. Focal ulceration is not seen in patients with conjunctivitis and should suggest the need for emergency ophthalmologic consultation.

Diagnostic Tests
Diagnosis is based upon history and physical findings. Rarely, collection of material for Gram stain and culture and sensitivity is obtained in patients with severe or unusual symptoms or presentations.

Treatment
Viral Conjunctivitis
Herpetic keratoconjunctivitis is discussed in "Herpetic Keratoconjunctivitis." Other viral causes may be treated with warm compresses; many authorities suggest the use of routine antibacterial therapy as outlined in "Bacterial Conjunctivitis" to prevent bacterial superinfection. It should be noted and explained to the patient that symptoms may persist for 12 to 14 days; follow-up should be provided in approximately 3 to 4 days. Topical decongestants such as phenylephrine 1%, 1 drop twice daily, will also help to reduce symptoms. **Steroid preparations are contraindicated.**

Bacterial Conjunctivitis
Antibiotic preparations, such as sulfacetamide, erythromycin, or Polytrim, may be used and achieve a good rate of cure. Contact lenses wearers should be treated with a fluoroquinolone (Ciloxan or Ocuflox) for Pseudomonas coverage. Patients must be instructed in the use of the ointment or drops by the physician, should demonstrate an initial application, and must be advised to avoid transfer of ocular secretions to other family members if possible. Treatment should continue for 7 to 10 days, symptoms should improve within 3 to 4 days, and an ophthalmologic referral should be advised within this initial interval if improvement has not occurred. Topical decongestants such as naphazoline or phenylephrine 1%, 1 drop twice daily, will also help to reduce symptoms.

Allergic Conjunctivitis

Most authorities suggest limiting treatment in most patients to topically applied vasoconstrictors and, if symptoms are severe, oral antihistamines. We strongly advise against the use of intraocular topical steroid preparations by the emergency physician; early ophthalmologic consultation is suggested when symptoms are severe, and steroids may be administered if appropriate at that time. In some patients with particularly severe and recurrent symptoms, desensitization may be advised.

Chlamydial Conjunctivitis

Topical and systemic therapy are usually recommended. Pregnant women and children younger than 12 years should be treated with topical erythromycin ointment or sulfonamide drops, 2 to 3 four times daily for 3 to 4 weeks, and systemic erythromycin. Other adults and children older than 12 may receive topical erythromycin or tetracycline and systemic erythromycin or tetracycline (both 1 g/day in four doses) for 3 weeks. Early follow-up is essential in 3 to 4 days. Genital infection frequently coexists and should be treated in the patient and any sexual partners.

Gonococcal Conjunctivitis in the Adult

Gonococcal infection in the newborn is discussed in "Conjunctivitis in the Newborn." Adults with presumed gonococcal infection (on the basis of Gram stain) or positive cultures require immediate ophthalmologic consultation. In the patient with presumed infection, a culture planted on Thayer-Martin medium should be obtained. If there is corneal involvement, parenteral ceftriaxone (Rocephin 1–2 g/day for 5 days) should be begun.

Herpetic Keratoconjunctivitis

Ophthalmologic consultation at the time of presentation is essential for definitive therapy. **Steroid preparations are contraindicated.**

Medications for the treatment of conjunctivitis:

- Naphazoline (Naphcon) 1% solution 1 to 2 drops every 4 to 6 hours as needed
- Sulfacetamide drops (Bleph 10) 1 to 2 drops of affected eye(s) every 2 to 3 hours initially; taper by increasing time intervals as condition responds; usual duration 7 to 10 days
- Erythromycin ointment 1 cm ribbon ointment applied up to six times daily (depending on severity of infection)
- Trimethoprim/Polymyxin B (Polytrim) 1 drop in the affected eye(s) every 3 hours (maximum of six doses per day) for 7 to 10 days
    Contact lenses wearers
- Ciprofloxacin (Ciloxan) 1 to 2 drops every 2 hours while awake for 2 days and then 1 to 2 drops every 4 hours while awake for 5 days
- Ofloxacin (Ocuflox) days 1 and 2, instill 1 to 2 drops in affected eye(s) every 2 to 4 hours; days 3 to 7, instill 1 to 2 drops four times daily

Conjunctivitis in the Newborn

Conjunctivitis in the newborn is a relatively common problem and, if it occurs within the first 10 days of life, is referred to as *ophthalmia neonatorum.* Although gonococcus remains the most important causative agent to exclude, neonatal ocular prophylaxis has greatly reduced the incidence of this disease. Other infectious agents including staphylococci, streptococci, *Chlamydia,* and herpes simplex are more common, are treatable, and may present within this interval. In all patients, routine and Thayer-Martin cultures should be obtained; the cornea should then be examined under ultraviolet light after fluorescein staining to exclude herpetic infection and ophthalmologic consultation obtained.

Herpes Simplex Type 2 Keratoconjunctivitis
Herpes simplex type 2 keratoconjunctivitis may appear within the first 3 to 5 days of life, in which case fluorescein staining of the cornea will demonstrate typical dendritic, fern-like lesions characteristic of the infection. Ophthalmologic consultation and referral prior to disposition are recommended.

Acute Gonococcal Conjunctivitis
Acute gonococcal conjunctivitis appears within 5 days of birth, and findings are typically those of a severe, purulent conjunctivitis. Marked eyelid swelling and chemosis may be noted, and a predominant polymorphonuclear response is found on Gram stain. Basophilic, cytoplasmic inclusion bodies are absent, and typical, Gram-negative intracellular diplococci are commonly noted; the latter provide grounds for a clinical but tentative diagnosis. Specific confirmation should be obtained by inoculating and immediately incubating a Thayer-Martin plate. Although treatment should be instituted based on clinical grounds, culture results will confirm the diagnosis within 48 hours. Treatment requires early ophthalmologic consultation and systemic ceftriaxone 125 mg intramuscular/intravenous once.

Acute Inclusion Conjunctivitis
Acute inclusion conjunctivitis results from conjunctival contamination with *Chlamydia trachomatis,* either at birth or, subsequently, by transmission of infected genital secretions. Unless premature rupture of the membranes has occurred, chlamydial conjunctivitis is unusual before 5 days of life. Symptoms may be similar to those of acute gonococcal conjunctivitis with findings consistent with an acute, severe purulent conjunctivitis. Gram-negative intracellular diplococci are not noted on Gram stain, and basophilic, cytoplasmic inclusion bodies are demonstrable by Giemsa staining of conjunctival scrapings. Demonstration of chlamydial infection may be made by culture. Treatment includes topical erythromycin ointment or sulfonamide drops and systemic erythromycin; treatment should continue for approximately 3 weeks, and ophthalmologic consultation at presentation is recommended in all patients. Children older than 3 months can be treated with topical erythromycin or sulfacetamide ointment.

Other Bacterial Causes
Other bacterial causes are substantially more common and include staphylococci and streptococci; these infections respond promptly to topically administered antibacterial agents. The specific diagnosis depends on appropriate culture and the exclusion of herpetic, gonococcal, and chlamydial disease; therapy, however, should begin based on clinical grounds.

Acute Narrow-angle Glaucoma

Acute narrow-angle glaucoma occurs when the egress of aqueous humor from the anterior chamber of the eye is blocked, causing a rapid rise in intraocular pressure, which, if significantly elevated, may produce intraocular vascular stasis and irreversible ischemia of the retina.

Clinical Presentation
Symptoms include severe, deep, unilateral eye pain, frequently associated with headache, nausea, vomiting, and abdominal pain. An occasional patient will have only

mild nausea and minimal abdominal cramping without eye discomfort or headache. Elevated intraocular pressure produces changes in the cornea that may be perceived by the patient as reduced visual acuity, cloudy vision, or the impression of colored halos surrounding lights. The physician may note a cloudy or steamy appearance to the cornea and a reduction in acuity in the involved eye. The eye is generally inflamed with conjunctival and ciliary injection, and the pupil is generally somewhat dilated and nonreactive to light.

Diagnostic Tests
Diagnosis depends on the accurate measurement of intraocular pressure, which may be performed with a Tonopen or Schiötz tonometer. Normal intraocular pressure varies between 12 and 18 mm Hg. Pressures above this level should be considered elevated and suggestive of glaucoma.

Treatment
Treatment depends on the extent of intraocular pressure elevation and the presence or absence of visual loss. If consultation is not available and intraocular pressures exceed 40 mm Hg, treatment should be initiated immediately (see Table 17-1). Before the administration of miotics, the fundus must be completely assessed to exclude central retinal vein obstruction and retinal detachment, because the administration of miotics will make subsequent funduscopic evaluations impossible.

Treatment of acute angle glacucoma
• Topical beta blocker (Timoptic 0.5%), 1 drop
• Topical alpha agonist (Iopidine 0.5%), 1 drop
• Topical steroid (Pred Forte 1%) 1 drop every 15 minutes for 4 hours, then hourly
• Acetazolamide 500 mg IV or PO
• Mannitol 1 to 2 g/kg IV
• Recheck IOP hourly
• Topical Pilocarpine 1% to 2%, 1 drop four times daily once IOP is below 40

Uveitis

Inflammation of the uveal tract (iris, ciliary body, choroid) is termed uveitis, although inflammatory processes may involve its individual components to produce acute anterior uveitis (iritis, iridocyclitis) as a result of iris or ciliary body inflammation or chorioretinitis. The most common disorder is an acute anterior iritis, which may be idiopathic (most commonly) or caused by autoimmune disorders, trauma, or infection. Patients report the sudden or gradual onset of pain, photophobia, and blurring of vision. Exudate is absent, the cornea is clear, the pupil is small and may be irregular, perilimbal injection is noted, and fibrin and inflammatory cells present in the anterior chamber produce, by slit lamp, a characteristic "flare" reaction involving the anterior chamber. Ciliary injection suggests that immediate ophthalmologic referral is appropriate.

Keratitis

Inflammatory processes involving the cornea are termed keratitis and may result from viral, chlamydial, bacterial, drug-related, or nutritional (vitamin A deficiency) etiologies or from simple exposure and dehydration of the cornea. Herpetic keratitis and corneal ulcer are relatively common and important causes of keratitis and are briefly discussed. Varying degrees of eye pain, photophobia, and perilimbal or ciliary injection are noted; the latter indicates the need for ophthalmologic consultation and referral before disposition.

Corneal Ulcer

Corneal ulcer is easily diagnosed in the emergency department. Ciliary injection may be present, and importantly, eye pain may be absent or only mild. A gray or white opacification on the corneal surface, *frequently at the limbus,* should alert the physician to this diagnosis: it contraindicates the instillation of any antibiotic preparation until appropriate bacterial and fungal cultures are obtained (frequently by corneal scraping) and indicates the need for urgent ophthalmologic consultation. Herpes may produce a particular type of corneal ulcer that is readily diagnosed, as discussed in "Herpes Simplex Infection."

Herpes Simplex Infection

The herpes viruses remain the most common cause of **corneal ulceration** in the United States and may result from either type 1 or 2 infections. The herpes virus also produces more superficial epithelial keratitis, as well as uveitis, retinitis, conjunctivitis, and blepharitis. Children typically present with primary infection, whereas adults classically have recurrences characterized by ocular irritation, photophobia, and mild pain. Visual acuity may be reduced if the central cornea is affected; fluorescein staining of the cornea followed by examination under ultraviolet light will usually demonstrate the typical dendritic, branching, fern-like ulcer that characterizes this entity. The presence of significant corneal anesthesia is diagnostically useful. **Steroid preparations are contraindicated**; consultation and referral at the time of presentation are indicated to rapidly institute definitive antiviral therapy.

Episcleritis and Scleritis

The episclera is a thin vascular connective tissue that lies beneath the conjunctiva but superficial to the sclera. Episcleritis must be distinguished from scleritis, a potentially dangerous cause of a red eye. Episcleritis is associated with bright red episcleral discoloration and not with pain; scleritis presents with intense ocular pain, photophobia, and a deep-red or purplish discoloration.

Hordeolum (Stye) and Chalazion

Styes, which produce pain, swelling, and erythema of the involved upper or lower lid, are commonly seen in the emergency department. Typically, infection involves eyelash follicles and their associated glandular structures; surrounding erythema and swelling are often noted. True fluctuance is less commonly noted, and therefore incision and drainage are not acutely required. Ptosis may also be seen when the upper lid is involved. Warm compresses should be applied to the area four to six times per day; topical erythromycin prescribed four times per day should be adequate treatment for a stye. A chalazion presents as an acute or chronic inflammation and a reddened tender lump is present at the lid margin. Treatment is the same as for a stye with the addition of an appropriate antistaphylococcal antibiotic, such as doxycycline 100 twice per day, instituted for 7 to 14 days. Follow-up ophthalmologic evaluation should be recommended.

Although it is unusual, should incision and drainage be initially required, ophthalmologic consultation and evaluation are then appropriate. If drainage occurs spontaneously, a culture should be obtained.

Visual Disturbances

DOUBLE VISION

Double vision or diplopia is defined simply as seeing one object as two and may be monocular or binocular. The sudden onset of diplopia is a dramatic event and therefore a cause for great anxiety and concern. For this reason and because of the serious nature of many of the causes of diplopia, meticulous attention must be paid to the neuro-ophthalmologic examination.

COMMON CAUSES OF DIPLOPIA

- Acute alcohol ingestion
- Diabetic neuropathy*
- Cerebrovascular accident

LESS COMMON CAUSES OF DIPLOPIA NOT TO BE MISSED

- Orbital fracture
- Acute Wernicke encephalopathy
- Intracranial neoplasm
- Intracranial aneurysm*
- Increased intracranial pressure

OTHER CAUSES OF DIPLOPIA

- Graves ophthalmopathy
- Myasthenia gravis
- Multiple sclerosis
- Retro-orbital or periorbital hematoma or abscess
- Psychogenic causes
- Subluxation of the lens (monocular diplopia)
- Retinal detachment (monocular diplopia)
- Cataract (monocular diplopia)

HISTORY

Acute alcohol toxicity may be associated with abnormalities of accommodation, and its chronic use may precipitate Wernicke encephalopathy. A history of recent head or facial trauma in association with diplopia suggests extraocular muscle entrapment or

*Discussed in this chapter.

cranial nerve injury or compression. A personal or family history of diabetes mellitus should be investigated and may be present in patients with diplopia caused by diabetic neuropathy. However, extraocular muscle paresis may be the first clinical manifestation of their disease. Myasthenics may report neck muscle weakness, drooping eyelids, diplopia, or a change in voice. Patients with multiple sclerosis may give a history of other transient neurologic abnormalities, including transient visual loss, motor weakness, and incoordination. The sudden onset of severe headache associated with visual loss, diplopia, ptosis, neck stiffness, or change in mental status should suggest the possibility of an intracranial aneurysm or hemorrhage.

PHYSICAL EXAMINATION

Distinguishing monocular diplopia from binocular diplopia is an important initial consideration in the evaluation of patients with double vision. Monocular diplopia is usually psychogenic in origin but rarely may be associated with subluxation of the lens, cataracts, macular lesions or edema, or detachment of the retina. Each of these may be detected by a careful ophthalmologic examination. Binocular diplopia is more common than monocular diplopia and is generally caused by three general classes of disorders: metabolic, extraocular muscle, or local periorbital abnormalities.

Dysarthria, somnolence, incoordination, and the odor of alcohol on the breath all suggest recent alcohol ingestion as a cause for diplopia. Nystagmus, extraocular palsy, lower limb ataxia, and, in severe cases, coma suggest acute Wernicke encephalopathy (thiamine deficiency). An isolated sixth nerve palsy is most commonly found in diabetic neuropathy; however, the third, fourth, and fifth cranial nerves may also be involved in an asymmetric, mononeuritis multiplex pattern. In patients with diabetic neuropathy, the pupillary fibers of the third cranial nerve are "spared" pathologic change, and the pupil reacts normally to light. In contrast, in patients with mass lesions (including cerebral aneurysms) compressing the third cranial nerve externally, pupillary dilation and a sluggish or absent light response are the rule. Periorbital ecchymosis ("raccoon eyes") or edema suggests trauma-related extraocular muscle entrapment or cranial nerve contusion. Cerebrovascular accidents associated with diplopia often involve brainstem structures and findings involving other cranial nerves or the pyramidal tracts (or both) should be sought in patients in whom a stroke is suspected (i.e., patients with atrial fibrillation or elderly persons with hypertension). Weakness of the periorbital musculature, dysphonia, neck flexion weakness, and increasing weakness on repetitive muscle stimulation (i.e., repeated hand grip) are all suggestive of myasthenia gravis. Anatomically and temporally disparate associated neurologic deficits characterize multiple sclerosis. Neck stiffness accompanying headache and diplopia may be seen in patients with meningitis or intracranial aneurysm or hemorrhage.

DIAGNOSTIC TESTS

A blood alcohol level may be elevated in persons manifesting acute alcoholic toxicity. In patients with acute Wernicke encephalopathy, alcohol need not be detected in the blood, nor do patients necessarily manifest signs of alcohol toxicity. The administration of thiamine, 100 to 500 mg intravenous, serves as both a therapeutic and diagnostic maneuver in that patients with acute Wernicke encephalopathy will respond with an improvement in muscle function and a disappearance of diplopia. A random blood glucose or, if not elevated, an oral glucose tolerance test will help diagnose diabetics with neuropathy. Orbital and facial roentgenograms or computed tomography (CT) scanning are mandatory for the diagnosis of suspected orbital or facial fractures. An emergency CT scan of the head and possibly lumbar puncture are indicated in patients with diplopia and either a severe headache or abnormalities of mental status.

ABNORMALITIES OF EXTRAOCULAR MUSCLE FUNCTION

Although emergency physicians are most commonly confronted with abnormalities of extraocular muscle function caused by cranial nerve palsies, a number of other conditions affecting extraocular motor function should be noted.

Cranial Nerve Palsies

Cranial nerve palsies may involve single or multiple nerves.

Third Nerve Palsies

Third nerve palsies produce limitation of elevation, adduction, and depression of the eye; intraocular muscle involvement produces a fixed, dilated pupil with paralysis of accommodation. Diabetes is a common cause of third nerve palsy, with most patients recovering completely. Importantly, in these patients, the pupil is unaffected. Other causes are ominous and include malignant lesions, inflammatory processes such as meningitis and encephalitis, intracranial aneurysm (pain associated with pupillary involvement is particularly suggestive of aneurysm), and multiple sclerosis. Diagnostic evaluation includes neurologic consultation and CT scanning, particularly if headache is an associated symptom. Lumbar puncture or an angiogram may be required.

The Fourth Cranial Nerve

The fourth cranial nerve innervates the superior oblique muscle, which exerts vertical, horizontal, and rotatory forces on the eye, depending on its horizontal position. Patients with isolated fourth nerve paralysis present with the head tilted toward the opposite shoulder. This occurs as a compensatory maneuver to counteract the unopposed inferior oblique muscle's tendency to extort the eye. Etiologically, head injury, malignancy, and aneurysm must be considered.

Sixth Nerve Palsy

Sixth nerve palsy results in paralysis of the lateral rectus with resultant esotropia, accentuated by lateral gaze toward the involved eye. Because of the long course of the nerve, multiple causes may produce the syndrome; these include malignancy, aneurysm, inflammatory disease involving the central nervous system, heavy metal poisoning, diabetes, and middle ear infections associated with meningeal involvement producing inflammation and edema around the nerve.

Progressive External Ophthalmoplegia

Progressive external ophthalmoplegia is a bilateral myopathy affecting the extraocular muscles. This disorder may occur sporadically, or be inherited as an autosomal dominant illness, and may progress asymmetrically. In most patients, ptosis is the first clinical sign, followed by progressive paresis, with medial rectus involvement noted initially in most patients; the intraocular muscles are spared. Extraocular involvement in myasthenia gravis usually occurs before the larger muscle groups are affected, and thus ocular symptoms may be a presenting sign. Ptosis is commonly noted early along with isolated involvement of the inferior or lateral rectus muscle. The diagnosis is confirmed by electromyography or when challenged with edrophonium or neostigmine. Thyroid ophthalmoplegia in patients with exophthalmos most markedly affects elevation of the eye, probably secondary to fibrosis of the inferior rectus muscle; patients typically assume a "chin-up" head position for compensation. Fractures of the orbital floor may result in abnormalities of extraocular muscle function and may progress as edema develops.

SPECIFIC DISORDERS

Diabetic Neuropathy

Patients with diabetic neuropathy may present with a number of neurologic syndromes, the most common of which is an isolated sixth cranial nerve palsy. An isolated third nerve palsy is also occasionally noted, in which case pupillary sparing distinguishes diabetic neuropathy from a mass lesion. Diabetes mellitus may not be suspected initially in patients with abnormalities of extraocular movement, with the blood glucose and urinalysis being essentially normal. In most patients, however, an oral glucose tolerance test or measurement of 2-hour postprandial blood glucose will be abnormal, corroborating the suspected diagnosis.

Patients with diabetic cranial neuropathies complain of double vision that may be transient and may spontaneously improve.

Inability to abduct the eye or weakness of the lateral rectus muscle indicates a sixth nerve paresis; unopposed third and fourth cranial nerve action tends to produce an esotropic dysconjugate gaze. Third nerve palsies caused by diabetic neuropathy spare pupillary function; unopposed fourth and sixth nerves with a totally paretic third nerve forces the affected eye to gaze inferiorly and laterally in these patients.

Patients with diplopia caused by an isolated cranial neuropathy require a thorough neurologic evaluation to rule out other brainstem abnormalities. Once the cranial neuropathy is isolated, an essential evaluation includes measurement of fasting glucose, a urinalysis, and, if necessary, an oral glucose tolerance test. Occasionally, diabetic control improves the cranial neuropathy and diplopia.

Intracranial Aneurysm

Rupture of a saccular (berry) aneurysm into the subarachnoid space may present dramatically with severe headache, stiff neck, progressive lethargy, and coma. Aneurysms may also expand and cause mass effect on the third cranial nerve. In conscious patients, visual symptoms may include diplopia, photophobia, and visual loss, the latter secondary to optic nerve compression. CT scanning and angiography may be indicated.

LOSS OF VISION

Several major issues must be considered when evaluating the patient with acute visual loss. Involvement of one or both eyes must be determined, the presence of associated ocular pain must be identified, whether the onset of visual loss was sudden or gradual and whether return of normal vision has occurred must be determined.

COMMON CAUSES OF LOSS OF VISION

• Amaurosis fugax*
• Posterior circulation cerebrovascular accident
• Glaucoma (acute and chronic)*
• Cataract
• Vitreous hemorrhage*
• Retinal detachment*
• Migraine

LESS COMMON CAUSES OF LOSS OF VISION NOT TO BE MISSED

• Retinal artery occlusion*
• Central retinal vein occlusion*
• Uveitis

OTHER CAUSES OF LOSS OF VISION

• Optic neuritis*
• Toxic optic neuropathy
• Psychogenic causes
• Malingering

HISTORY

Sudden visual loss is seen in patients with amaurosis fugax, cerebrovascular accidents involving the posterior circulation, retinal artery or vein occlusion, acute narrow-angle glaucoma, and retinal detachment. Monocular involvement is characteristic of amaurosis fugax, retinal artery or vein occlusion, glaucoma, retinal detachment, and vitreous hemorrhage. Bilateral loss may be described in patients with posterior circulation events, hysteria, and malingering. Pain in the general vicinity of the eye or orbit usually accompanies acute narrow-angle glaucoma, uveitis, and optic neuritis. The patient's description of the details and time course of visual loss is important. Amaurosis fugax often is described as transient visual loss with "a shade coming down" over the visual field. Blurring of the visual field is noted in glaucoma, retinal vein occlusion, and optic neuritis, while loss of the peripheral field of vision, hemianopsia, or central blindness may be seen in patients with migraine. Vitreous hemorrhage and retinal detachment often produce black spots, strands, or a "film-like" perception in the visual field. Acute glaucoma often produces "steamy" or "cloudy" vision.

PHYSICAL EXAMINATION

Confirming the patient's description of involvement of one or both eyes and actually defining the presence and extent of such involvement are of primary importance in the initial assessment. Testing visual acuity will also allow for a quantitative evaluation of the severity of visual loss. Unilateral, segmental visual field deficits are noted in retinal artery branch occlusions as a result of either thromboembolism or cholesterol embolism (in amaurosis fugax). Bilateral hemianopsias or quadrantanopsias are noted in posterior circulation strokes or transient ischemic attacks. Acute iritis and acute glaucoma are often associated with increased sensitivity to light. A characteristic "ciliary flush" may be noted in acute iritis and is diagnosed on the basis of dilated perilimbal vessels. The pupil is dilated in acute narrow-angle glaucoma, whereas it is usually small and round in iritis. In both cases, the pupil may be relatively fixed in response to light.

Funduscopy is essential for the diagnosis of many of the disorders causing visual loss. Vitreous hemorrhage is readily seen on funduscopic examination, as is retinal detachment, whereas posterior synechiae may be noted in acute iritis. A pale disk with "milky" changes in the retina caused by extravascular retinal edema is noted in retinal artery occlusion; if central vision is affected, a macular red spot may be noted, and "boxcar" segmentation of vessels caused by stagnant blood may also be observed. Hollenhorst bodies (cholesterol emboli in retinal artery branches) are occasionally seen in amaurosis fugax. Blurred disk margins, distended and tortuous retinal veins, and diffuse retinal hemorrhages are noted in retinal vein occlusion. A swollen, hemorrhagic optic disk is seen in optic neuritis; if no abnormality of the optic disk is noted in a patient with a decrease in visual acuity and retrobulbar pain on movement of the globe, retrobulbar neuritis should be suspected.

DIAGNOSTIC TESTS

A thorough ophthalmologic and neurologic examination (including a slit-lamp study), visual acuity testing and measurement of intraocular pressure with a tonometer, is an essential aspect of the examination of all patients with acute visual loss.

SPECIFIC DISORDERS

Amaurosis Fugax

Transient, unilateral visual loss resulting from ischemia of the ophthalmic branch of the internal carotid artery due to cholesterol emboli is referred to as amaurosis fugax. Patients present with transient visual loss, described as a "shade coming down" over one eye, lasting a few minutes to an hour. The physical examination may demonstrate a carotid bruit and Hollenhorst bodies (cholesterol emboli) in distal retinal artery branches. Treatment is based on information provided by carotid evaluation with Doppler flow analysis, ultrasonographic examinations, and carotid angiography.

Glaucoma

Glaucoma is characterized by elevated intraocular pressure with concomitant loss of vision caused by compression of the optic nerve. Acute and chronic varieties of glaucoma exist and therapy differs.

Chronic, Open-Angle Glaucoma

In chronic, open-angle glaucoma, the trabecular meshwork in Schlemm canal remains open but has a reduced capacity to resorb aqueous outflow; in this setting, the rise in intraocular pressure is usually slow, occurring over months to years, and often not associated with acute symptoms. It is usually diagnosed by routine tonometry and is present in 2% of the population.

Acute Narrow-Angle Glaucoma

Acute narrow-angle glaucoma is a true medical emergency in which closure of the angle between the iris and the trabecular meshwork occurs suddenly, often as a result of mydriasis in a patient with a congenitally narrowed anterior chamber. Patients presenting with acute glaucoma may have no initial symptoms referable to the eye; instead, headache, malaise, nausea and vomiting, or a combination of symptoms may be reported. Other patients may report a deep pain within the eye or globe, a decrease in visual acuity associated with cloudy, smoky, or misty vision, or red or blue halos around point sources of light. On examination, the anterior chamber is variably injected, and the cornea is slightly edematous or cloudy, reducing the intensity of the red reflex. The pupil is dilated, somewhat irregular, and relatively fixed in response to light; tonometry confirms the diagnosis, demonstrating elevated intraocular pressure.

We recommend immediate ophthalmologic consultation in patients suspected of acute narrow-angle glaucoma; treatment is described in "Treatment," in Chapter 17.

Vitreous Hemorrhage

Vitreous hemorrhage is caused by retinal tears or detachment, neovascularization secondary to diabetes mellitus, or previous venous occlusion. Patients report light flashes followed by black spots, strands, floaters, or a film over the eye. Hemorrhage is diagnosed by funduscopy, and treatment includes ophthalmologic consultation and referral.

Retinal Detachment

Retinal detachment occurs either as a result of trauma to the eye or orbit or spontaneously in patients who have recently undergone cataract removal. In patients with a peripheral retinal tear or detachment, no subjective loss of vision may be noted by the patient until the macula becomes involved. Funduscopy is essential in these patients, usually after pupillary dilation, to define the presence and extent of these progressive but treatable lesions prior to macular involvement. In areas of detachment, the fundus appears gray and undulating, and the retinal vessels appear elevated and tortuous. If the macula remains attached, a true ophthalmologic emergency exists, and immediate consultation should be obtained so appropriate intervention can be undertaken.

Retinal Artery Occlusion

In an elderly patient, the sudden, painless, persistent loss of the central, superior, or inferior visual field of one eye suggests retinal artery occlusion. A pale disk and "milkiness" of the retina secondary to extravascular edema are noted on funduscopy. In patients with segmental occlusions, local retinal changes occur in the distribution of the affected artery. In central retinal artery occlusion, a macular red spot is often noted, and "boxcar" segmentation of vessels eventually develops in the setting of decreased flow.

Treatment is controversial but consists of maneuvers that may enhance perfusion of the retina. Immediate ophthalmologic consultation should be obtained because aspiration of the anterior chamber may be elected if other maneuvers are unsuccessful. Intermittent massage of the globe may occasionally dislodge an obstructing embolus; increasing systemic blood pressure with exercise may also be a useful maneuver.

Acetazolamide, 500 mg intravenous, and/or mannitol, 1.0 g/kg, may also potentially improve retinal perfusion by decreasing intraocular pressure.

Central Retinal Vein Occlusion

Central retinal vein occlusion occurs in open-angle glaucoma and a variety of hyperviscosity states, including polycythemia vera, profound leukocytosis, and the hyperglobulinemic disorders, particularly macroglobulinemia. Patients generally report that vision becomes blurred more gradually than in retinal artery occlusion and is less severely impaired. Blurred disk margins, distended, tortuous veins, and retinal hemorrhages are noted on examination. Although anticoagulation with heparin is recommended by some authorities, its use remains controversial because progression of retinal hemorrhage has occasionally been noted following its institution. The treatment of any associated or predisposing disorder (or disorders) may be of the greatest benefit.

Uveitis

See "Uveitis," in Chapter 17.

Optic Neuritis

Optic and retrobulbar neuritis are commonly associated with multiple sclerosis and typically occur in patients between the ages of 20 and 40 years. Attacks are usually self-limited, and vision usually improves over several days. Patients report loss of central visual acuity and retrobulbar pain on movement of the globe. In true optic neuritis, a swollen, hemorrhagic optic disk is noted on funduscopy, whereas in patients with retrobulbar neuritis, no such changes are apparent. The systemic administration of corticosteroids is recommended, and intracranial mass lesions should be carefully ruled out.

PART 4

Respiratory Disorders

19 Cough

The cough reflex develops in response to irritation of the tracheobronchial tree. Tracheal and bronchial mucosal dryness caused by smoke inhalation, anxiety, viral infection, acute asthma, tracheobronchial foreign body, interstitial edema as a result of congestive heart failure (CHF), and alveolar exudate associated with bacterial pneumonitis may all produce cough.

COMMON CAUSES OF COUGH

- Tobacco use
- Tracheobronchitis*
- Congestive heart failure
- Pneumonia*
- Asthma/chronic obstructive pulmonary disease

LESS COMMON CAUSES OF COUGH NOT TO BE MISSED

- Tracheobronchial foreign body
- Thoracic aortic aneurysm
- Mediastinal tumor
- Pulmonary neoplasm
- Diaphragmatic irritation

OTHER CAUSES OF COUGH

- Laryngitis
- Chemical irritants
- Interstitial fibrosis
- Anxiety

_____
*Discussed in this chapter.

HISTORY

Smokers typically report a chronic early morning cough that may or may not be productive. Patients with superimposed tracheobronchitis or pneumonia often appear systemically ill with fever, chills, and dyspnea. In such patients, a change in the amount or character of sputum or worsening dyspnea may provide the only clue suggesting an acute infectious process. Patients with CHF often note an isolated cough early in the evolution of an exacerbation and may be more prominent at night with recumbency. Cough may be the *sole* manifestation of acute asthma, especially early in an acute episode. Although a productive cough usually suggests an infectious cause, patients with CHF may produce milky or frothy sputum that occasionally is blood-tinged or pink. Intrabronchial foreign body should be suspected in all children with a persistent or unexplained cough.

PHYSICAL EXAMINATION

Basilar rales, distended neck veins, and the presence of an S_3 gallop suggest CHF. In early CHF, fine, inspiratory crackles may be heard at the bases, or the examination may be unrevealing. Focal areas of lobar consolidation (egophony, tubular breath sounds, increased fremitus) all support the diagnosis of pneumonia or a mass lesion. Although wheezing remains the hallmark of asthma or bronchospasm, isolated prolongation of the expiratory phase without wheezing may be noted early in the asthmatic episode in some patients. Foreign body entrapment in the bronchial tree may produce localized rales, wheezes, or egophony if accompanied by atelectasis and may be associated with pleuritic pain. Neurologic deficits, an aortic regurgitant murmur, or pulse deficits suggest a thoracic aortic dissection or aneurysm.

DIAGNOSTIC TESTS

Although the chest roentgenogram is the single most useful test in the evaluation of the patient with cough, it is not required in all patients. In patients who appear well and have a normal pulmonary examination, roentgenograms are usually not helpful. A chest x-ray is usually warranted with a cough associated with focal findings on examination, or if the patient appears systemically ill. Oxygenation status through pulse oximetry must be assessed in all emergency department (ED) patients with respiratory complaints. Spirometry is useful in assessing the extent of bronchospasm, even in patients without detectable wheezing.

CLINICAL REMINDERS

- Do not indiscriminately administer cough suppressants to patients with cough; attempt to determine cause.
- Administer expectorants with cough suppressants to patients with parenchymal infections; do not do so in patients with tracheobronchitis or asthmatic bronchitis, because these only serve to aggravate the primary disorder.

SPECIFIC DISORDERS

Tracheobronchitis

Tracheobronchitis is an extremely common infectious disorder of the upper respiratory tract usually caused by viruses, including the respiratory syncytial virus, the adenovirus, and the influenza viruses, as well as *Mycoplasma* or rarely pneumococcal or *Haemophilus* organisms. Cigarette smokers are particularly predisposed to developing recurrent tracheobronchitis infections, primarily because of the effect of chronic smoke inhalation on ciliary function and its tendency to produce both progressive and episodic bronchial obstruction.

- **History**. Patients with tracheobronchitis may report a dry or productive cough; yellow or green sputum (instead of clear) is said to be more suggestive of a bacterial cause. Fever, chills, and other signs of upper respiratory tract viral infection (e.g., coryza, sore throat, and myalgias) often accompany or precede the onset of cough in patients with viral tracheobronchitis.

- On physical examination, most patients appear only mildly ill, have a low-grade fever, and may be slightly dyspneic. Examination of the chest is usually unrevealing except in patients with preexisting chronic obstructive pulmonary disease.

- **Diagnostic tests**. Chest roentgenograms in patients with simple tracheobronchitis are normal. When sputum is available, examination of the Gram stain may further support a viral, *Mycoplasma*, or specific bacterial cause.

- **Treatment**. In patients with viral infections, treatment is symptomatic; to this end, cough suppressants (without expectorants) and antipyretics to alleviate the discomfort engendered by fever are recommended. In these patients, antibiotics are generally of no use; however, in persons prone to bacterial superinfection or with preexisting chronic obstructive pulmonary disease, several studies suggest a marginal benefit from the use of ampicillin, erythromycin/azithromycin, or tetracycline.

    Patients who are systemically ill, hypoxemic, or markedly dyspneic must be admitted to the hospital for additional therapy regardless of cause. These will, in general, be patients with preexisting chronic obstructive pulmonary disease. In young, otherwise healthy patients, bacterial tracheobronchitis caused by the pneumococcus or *Mycoplasma* organisms may be treated with erythromycin or azithromycin. Suspected viral tracheobronchitis in otherwise healthy patients requires only pharmacologic suppression of cough and fever and follow-up in 5 or 6 days if improvement fails to occur. Smoking should be prohibited in all patients with ongoing pulmonary infections.

Pneumonia

Diagnosis

Pneumonias may occur as a result of viral, bacterial, or atypical bacterial infection.

- **Bacterial pneumonia** often develops after an upper respiratory tract infection, and patients typically present with fever, cough productive of yellow or green sputum, and, occasionally, shaking chills, dyspnea, and pleuritic chest pain. Pneumococcus is the most common cause of bacterial pneumonia. Its classic presentation includes the abrupt onset of fever associated with a single rigor, cough with rusty sputum, and pleuritic chest pain. *Mycoplasma* is a common cause of pneumonia in the young otherwise healthy population. Streptococcal pneumonia, caused by group A organisms, is uncommon but does occur epidemically; it produces severe debility and rapidly spreads throughout the lung. Staphylococcal pneumonia may be a primary infection in infancy but most commonly follows viral infections of the upper respiratory tract, especially influenza. Community-acquired methicillin-resistant *Staphylococcus aureus* (CA-MRSA) is increasing in frequency. Patients with staphylococcal pneumonia are often extremely ill, and because the staphylococcus produces a necrotizing pneumonitis, characteristic radiologic evidence of tissue destruction (such as abscess or cysts) may be noted. *Haemophilus* pneumonia most commonly occurs in children younger than age 6 years; it is uncommon in adults, except in elderly persons with underlying chronic pulmonary disease. *Klebsiella* pneumonia also affects the debilitated patient, particularly the alcoholic. *Legionella* organisms produce an atypical pneumonia as well, which often runs a protracted, debilitating course accompanied by gastrointestinal symptoms (diarrhea), and occasional renal (acute tubular necrosis) and central nervous system involvement.

- **Viral pneumonias** are produced by the adenovirus, respiratory syncytial virus, or influenza virus. These pneumonias typically produce x-ray patterns that appear far worse than the history or physical examination would suggest. There is often a coinfection with a bacterial pathogen.
- Classically, the bacterial pneumonias produce fever, tachypnea, and tachycardia; signs of pulmonary consolidation are usually apparent on physical examination. If infection is severe, hypoxemia may be present and cyanosis may be noted.
- The **chest roentgenogram** with posteroanterior and lateral views is recommended in the evaluation of all patients suspected of harboring pneumonia. Lobar consolidation is readily demonstrated by x-ray and is suggestive of a pneumococcal or *Klebsiella* infection, the latter often producing bulging of the fissures. Streptococcal and *Haemophilus* pneumonias often produce diffuse patchy infiltrates, whereas staphylococcal pneumonias produce necrotizing changes manifest on chest roentgenogram as multiple, small, fluid-filled, consolidated cysts.
- **Examination of the sputum** is unnecessary for the outpatient management of pneumonia. Empiric therapy is adequate. Hospitalized patients and ICU patients may benefit from sputum examination if an adequate sample may be obtained and processed in a timely fashion. If tuberculosis or fungal infection is suspected or if the patient is immunocompromised, appropriate cultures and stains of these cultures should then be obtained.
- The patient's oxygenation status must be determined. Patients with chronic obstructive pulmonary disease may require arterial blood gas analysis to detect carbon dioxide retention.

Treatment

The ED care of patients with bacterial pneumonia is determined by the anticipated disposition. Outpatient, inpatient, or intensive care settings dictate different antibiotic regimens. Appropriate disposition may be determined by comorbidities, vitals signs, symptoms, patient support, and how ill the patient appears. The Patient Outcomes Research Team (PORT) prediction rules (Tables 19-1 and 19-2) may help in deciding whether an adult patient should be treated as an inpatient or outpatient. These prediction rules were formulated by the Pneumonia PORT. The rules delineate five risk classes by which mortality can be estimated. Once the decision has been made on the venue of treatment, antibiotic treatment (Table 19-3) should be initiated.

Table 19-1	Point Scoring System for Step 2 of the Prediction Rule for Assignment to Risk Classes II, III, IV, and V

Characteristic	Points Assigned[a]
Demographic factor	
Age	
Men	Age (y)
Women	Age (y) −10
Nursing home resident	+10
Coexistent illnesses[b]	
Neoplastic disease	+30
Liver disease	+20
Congestive heart failure	+10
Cerebrovascular disease	+10
Renal disease	+10
Physical-examination findings	
Altered mental status[c]	+20
Respiratory rate ≥30/min	+20
Systolic blood pressure <90 mm Hg	+20
Temperature <35 °C or ≥40 °C	+15
Pulse ≥125/min	+10
Laboratory and radiographic findings	
Arterial pH <7.35	+30
Blood urea nitrogen ≥30 mg/dL (11 mmol/L)	+20
Sodium <130 mmol/L	+20
Glucose ≥250 mg/dL (14 mmol/L)	+10
Hematocrit <30%	+10
Partial pressure of arterial oxygen <60 mm Hg[d]	+10
Pleural effusion	+10

- Young adults with pneumonia are usually sufficiently well to be treated as outpatients, provided that oxygenation is adequate and dyspnea is mild.
- Patients who appear ill, have abnormal vital signs and comorbidities, or lack adequate support may require hospital admission
- In **patients who require admission**, ED management includes supplemental oxygen, intravenous hydration, and instituting appropriate antibacterial therapy. Blood and sputum cultures should be obtained in selected patients.
- Discharged patients with pulmonary infiltrates, especially smokers older than 35 years of age, must be referred and followed-up for the resolution of all signs and symptoms; a repeat chest roentgenogram in 8 to 10 weeks is also indicated in these patients to exclude an obstructing process not previously identified or suspected.
- Critically ill patients require the intensive care unit. Blood and sputum cultures should be obtained before antibiotics. Dual antibiotic therapy should be expanded to the individual patients risk for CA-MRSA, postinfluenza pneumonia, or *Pseudomonas*. Arterial blood gas measurement may be necessary to assess

Table 19-2 Comparison of Risk-Class Specific Mortality Rates in the Derivation and Validation Cohorts[a]

| Risk Class (No. of Points)[b] | MedisGroups Derivation Cohort | | MedisGroups Validation Cohort | | Pneumonia PORT Validation Cohort | | | | | |
| | | | | | Inpatients | | Outpatients | | All Patients | |
	No. of Patients	% Who Died	No. of Patients	% Who Died	No. of Patients	% Who Died	No. of Patients	% Who Died	No. of Patients	% Who Died
I	1,372	0.4	3,034	0.1	185	0.5	587	0.0	772	0.1
II (≤70)	2,412	0.7	5,778	0.6	233	0.9	244	0.4	477	0.6
III (71–90)	2,632	2.8	6,790	2.8	254	1.2	72	0.0	326	0.9
IV (91–130)	4,697	8.5	13,104	8.2	446	9.0	40	12.5	486	9.3
V (>130)	3,086	31.1	9,333	29.2	225	27.1	1	0.0	226	27.0
Total	14,199	10.2	38,039	10.6	1343	8.0	944	0.6	2287	5.2

[a]There are no statistically significant differences in overall mortality or mortality within risk class among patients in the MedisGroups derivation, MedisGroups validation, or overall Pneumonia PORT validation cohort. The P values for the comparisons of mortality across risk classes are as follows: class I, $P = 0.22$; class II, $P = 0.67$; class III, $P = 0.12$; class IV, $P = 0.69$; and class V, $P = 0.09$.

[b]Inclusion in risk class I was determined by the absence of all predictors identified in step 1 of the prediction rule. Inclusion in risk classes II, III, IV, and V was determined by a patient's total risk score, which was computed according to the scoring system shown in Table 19-1.

Table 19-3	Treatment of Bacterial Pneumonia
	Common Infectious Agents	**Antibiotic Therapy**
Neonatal	*Escherichia coli;* group A, B, or G streptococci; *Staphylococcus aureus; Pseudomonas; Chlamydia*	Ampicillin 50 mg/kg plus gentamicin 2.5 mg/kg *intravenous* every 8 h or cefotaxime (Claforan) 50 mg/kg intravenous every 8 h. If methicillin-resistant, *Staphylococcus aureus* is suspected, vancomycin plus gentamicin (or cephotaxime)
1 mo to 4 y	Viruses, *Streptococcus pneumoniae, Haemophilus influenza, Staphylococcus aureus*	**Inpatients:** Ampicillin/Sulbactam (Unasyn) *50 mg/kg per dose intravenous every 6 hours (maximum of 2 g ampicillin per dose)* Cefuroxime (Zinacef) *50 mg/kg per dose intravenous every 8 h (maximum of 2 g per dose)* Cefotaxime (Claforan) *50 mg/kg per dose intravenous every 8 h* Consider addition of either A or B: A. *Azithromycin (Zithromax) 10 mg/kg daily* B. *or Erythromycin 5–10 mg/kg per dose every 6 h* **Outpatient:** Amoxicillin 80–100 mg/kg/d divided into two or three daily doses for 10 d Cefuroxime axetil (Ceftin) 30 mg/kg/d divided into two daily doses for 10 d Azithromycin (Zithromax) 10 mg/kg for first dose and then 5 mg/kg daily for 4 d
4–18 y	Viruses, mycoplasma, *Chlamydia pneumoniae, Streptococcus pneumoniae*	Clarithromycin (Biaxin) 7.5 mg/kg per dose twice daily for 10 d **Inpatient:** *Azithromycin (Zithromax) 10 mg/kg intravenous daily plus a or b below, or Doxycycline (Vibramycin) 2 mg/kg intravenous every 12 h plus a or b below*

(Continued)

Table 19-3	Treatment of Bacterial Pneumonia *(Continued)*

Common Infectious Agents	**Antibiotic Therapy**
	a. Ceftriazone (Rocephin) 50–75 mg/kg intravenous daily
	b. Ampicillin/Sulbactam (Unasyn) 50 mg/kg intravenous every 6 h (maximum 2 g ampicillin per dose)
	Outpatient:
	Erythromycin 10 mg/kg orally for 10 d
	Azithromycin (Zithromax) 10 mg/kg orally for first day's dose and then half of that daily for 4 d
	Clarithromycin (Biaxin) 7.5 mg/kg orally twice daily for 10 d
	Doxycycline 2 mg/kg orally twice daily for 10 d
18 y and older	Strep. Pneumoniae, mycoplasma, Chlamydia pneumoniae, H. influenzae, M. catarrhalis, enteric bacteria (coliforms), Legionella
	Inpatient:
	Cefotaxime (Clafaran) 2 g intravenous every 8 h plus a or b below or
	Ceftriaxone (Rocephin) 2 gª intravenous daily plus a or b below
	a. Erythromycin 5 mg/kg per dose intravenous every 6 h
	b. Azithromycin (Zithromax) 500 mg intravenous daily
	Outpatient:
	Azithromycin (Zithromax) 500 mg on first day and then 250 mg daily for 4 d
	Clarithromycin (Biaxin) 250–500 mg orally twice daily for 10 d
	Doxycycline (Vibramycin) 100 mg orally twice daily for 10 d
	Erythromycin 500 mg orally four times daily for 10 d

ªUse half dose in patients older than age 65.

ventilation. Lactate levels may reveal impending sepsis. Intravenous volume replacement may be necessary. Consider noninvasive positive pressure ventilation prior to intubation.

- Community-acquired aspiration pneumonias are frequently caused by one or more of the following organisms: **Bacteroides spp., Fusobacterium spp., aerobic streptococci,** and **anaerobic streptococci.** Treatment should include clindamycin, cefoxitin, amoxicillin-clavulanate, or ampicillin-sulbactam.

20 Hemoptysis

Brisk bleeding from the tracheobronchial tree is one of the more dramatic symptoms with which a patient may present to the emergency department. In all cases, it is essential to verify that blood originates from within the tracheobronchial tree and not from the gastrointestinal tract or nasopharynx. In this regard, tracheobronchial blood is usually bright red and frothy, whereas gastrointestinal blood is usually dark red or brown, acidic, and often mixed with partially digested food particles. Although vomiting usually accompanies gastrointestinal bleeding, coughing typically initiates and accompanies hemoptysis.

As in any patient with blood loss, hemodynamic stabilization is an immediate priority and should be managed as described in "Management of Hemorrhagic Shock Due to Gastrointestinal Bleeding," in Chapter 28.

COMMON CAUSES OF HEMOPTYSIS

- Bacterial pneumonitis
- Congestive heart failure (CHF)
- Bronchogenic carcinoma*

LESS COMMON CAUSES OF HEMOPTYSIS NOT TO BE MISSED

- Mitral stenosis
- Pulmonary infarction
- Pulmonary embolism
- Bronchial adenoma
- Tuberculosis*
- Acute tracheobronchitis

OTHER CAUSES OF HEMOPTYSIS

- Chronic bronchitis
- Arteriovenous malformation
- Foreign body
- Bronchiectasis
- Aspergilloma
- Goodpasture syndrome

*Discussed in this chapter.

- Wegener granulomatosis
- Strongyloidiasis
- Leptospirosis
- Trauma

HISTORY

Patients with a history of CHF may have hemoptysis developed solely on the basis of increased pulmonary venous pressure; this is particularly true in patients with mitral stenosis and associated pulmonary venous hypertension. Hemoptysis in patients with CHF is usually not massive, and patients typically produce blood-streaked or frothy pinkish red sputum. Pulmonary tuberculosis should always be considered in the differential diagnosis of hemoptysis, particularly in patients with long-standing active disease. Chronic smokers in whom hemoptysis develops should be suspected of harboring a bronchogenic carcinoma, and 50% of bronchial neoplasms are said to produce tracheobronchial bleeding at some time during their course. The bacterial pneumonias commonly produce blood-tinged sputum at some time in their course, although massive hemoptysis is unusual. Among hospitalized patients, pulmonary infarction is a more common cause of hemoptysis, and occasionally, pulmonary embolism not associated with actual infarction may produce mild tracheobronchial bleeding. If pleural pain accompanies hemoptysis, particularly in a sedentary or hypercoagulable patient, pulmonary embolism should be considered. Bronchiectasis, although a relatively uncommon disorder, is routinely accompanied by hemoptysis to such a degree that many patients are not alarmed by it.

PHYSICAL EXAMINATION

Fever and cough productive of purulent sputum suggest bacterial pneumonitis. The physical examination may confirm the presence of focal pulmonary consolidation in patients with pneumonia but is expected to be essentially unremarkable in patients with acute tracheobronchitis. Weight loss and cachexia in a smoker with hemoptysis should suggest the possibility of bronchogenic carcinoma. Cachexia, chronic cough, posttussive rales, and amphoric breath sounds at the apices are noted in patients with reactivated tuberculosis. Rales, an S_3 gallop, increased jugular venous pressure, ascites, hepatojugular reflux, hepatomegaly, and peripheral edema may be noted in patients with CHF. In particular, among patients with mitral stenosis and CHF, a loud S_1, an opening snap, and a middiastolic rumble with presystolic accentuation may be detected. Dyspnea, a pleural rub, and a swollen, tender calf or thigh may be seen in patients with pulmonary embolism secondary to deep venous thrombophlebitis of the lower extremity.

DIAGNOSTIC TESTS

A chest radiograph is essential in all patients with hemoptysis. Pulmonary infiltrates, cavitary lung lesions, CHF, radiopaque foreign bodies, bronchiectasis, apical tuberculous disease, pulmonary masses, and aspergillomas may all be detected by an adequate radiographic examination. Emergency bronchoscopy remains an essential procedure in all patients with significant hemoptysis (i.e., more than 400 mL of blood in

3 hours or 600 mL of blood in 24 hours); other management options are detailed in "Principles of Management of Hemoptysis."

In other patients, a less urgent diagnostic approach may be initiated. A complete blood count may reveal leukocytosis in patients with any of the bacterial pneumonias. Fluorescent antibody-staining techniques are more sensitive with respect to the diagnosis of tuberculous disease but are not always available. Sputum should routinely be sent for bacterial and mycobacterial culture and sensitivity, as well as for a cytologic examination for acid fast bacilli when tuberculosis is suspected.

PRINCIPLES OF MANAGEMENT OF HEMOPTYSIS

In patients with minimal hemoptysis, basic management is initially diagnostic and directed at defining and treating the underlying etiology. Hemoptysis associated with CHF or bacterial pneumonitis, for example, usually responds to appropriate therapy.

Gross, massive hemoptysis, however, is a true emergency requiring immediate attention. Massive hemoptysis is defined as tracheobronchial bleeding of more than 400 mL in the first 3 hours or more than 600 mL in the first 24 hours of observation. When the site of bleeding is known or suspected on the basis of examination, chest roentgenogram, or symptoms, the patient should first be positioned with that side down; this will minimize entry of blood into the normal lung until definitive treatment can be provided. An immediate attempt at anatomic localization of the bleeding site is essential for optimal surgical management. Although fiberoptic bronchoscopy may be used initially to localize the lung from which bleeding is occurring, most authorities believe that in patients with brisk bleeding, rigid bronchoscopy provides better access for lavaging the bronchi and thereby more accurately determining the anatomic origin of bleeding. Once the lung or lobe that contains the bleeding site has been defined, surgical resection may be indicated in patients with continued bleeding.

In patients believed not to be suitable surgical candidates, endobronchial tamponade with a balloon-tipped (Foley) catheter or embolization of the bronchial or intercostal arteries with Spongel or Gelfoam may be used. Despite optimal management, mortality in patients with massive hemoptysis still approaches 25% under the best of circumstances.

SPECIFIC DISORDERS

Bronchogenic Carcinoma

The designation *bronchogenic carcinoma* defines a group of histologic cancers involving the lung and is associated in general with a 1-year survival of 20%; tobacco smoking, asbestos exposure, and exposure to pitchblende have all been associated with an increased risk of bronchogenic carcinoma. Among the histologic subtypes, squamous cell carcinoma is the most common. It is usually centrally located and at presentation has spread beyond the thorax in more than one half of the cases. Adenocarcinoma tends to metastasize widely and is often initially localized at sites of pulmonary scarring. Oat or small cell carcinoma is routinely disseminated at the time of diagnosis, frequently presents with seizure or other neurologic phenomena, and is not generally considered a surgically treatable disease.

Clinical Presentation

All subtypes of bronchogenic carcinoma may present insidiously with progressive anorexia, cachexia, and weight loss. Chronic cough, hoarseness secondary to compression of the recurrent laryngeal nerve, hemoptysis, clubbing, and a variety of paraneoplastic disorders (most common among patients with small cell carcinoma), including Cushing syndrome, inappropriate antidiuretic hormone secretion, disseminated intravascular coagulation, and hypercalcemia (seen typically in patients with squamous cell carcinoma), may also be noted on or may precipitate the initial presentation.

Diagnostic Tests

The chest radiograph is essential for initially evaluating any patient suspected of having bronchogenic carcinoma; computed tomography scanning may be helpful in selected patients. Hilar masses or upper lobe lesions may be noted, with squamous cell carcinoma typically involving the anterior segment of the upper lobe; this is in contrast to posterior segment involvement in reactivation tuberculosis. Although cytologic examination of the sputum is important in the initial evaluation, tissue is required for histologic typing, which may be obtained by fiberoptic bronchoscopy, percutaneous needle biopsy, scalene node biopsy, or mediastinoscopy with biopsy.

Tuberculosis

Tuberculosis is caused primarily by *Mycobacterium tuberculosis,* although other mycobacterial species (*M. bovis* and atypical mycobacteria) may also produce active disease, particularly in the immunocompromised host. Primary tuberculosis is typically asymptomatic (except in the very young or immunocompromised) and leads to the production of the primary or Ghon complex (hilar adenopathy and a calcified nodule in the lung periphery) with conversion of the tuberculin skin test. In most patients, after conversion, infection enters a latent, inactive stage, although reactivation associated with debility or immunocompromise is not uncommon.

Clinical Presentation

Reactivation tuberculosis may present in a variety of ways, including tuberculous pneumonitis, pleuritis, epiglottitis, cavitary tuberculosis, osteomyelitis, "sterile" pyuria, epididymitis, or miliary tuberculosis. Furthermore, in persons who are unable to contain the initial infection, a number of primary tuberculous clinical syndromes may develop (especially in infants and young adults); these include primary tuberculous pneumonia, disseminated tuberculous infection, and, in young adults, pleuritis with pleural effusion.

Treatment

Patients suspected of having any of the various tuberculous syndromes require hospitalization for the initiation of antituberculous therapy and for isolation from the population at large. Four-drug therapy is now recommended (see Table 20-1) because of the emergence of resistant forms of tubercle bacilli. Although 2 weeks of such therapy is required to sterilize the sputum in patients with reactivated pulmonary tuberculosis, nonviable, acid-fast organisms may continue to be noted in the sputum.

Prophylaxis with isoniazid (300 mg/day for 9 months) with pyridoxine (25–50 mg/day) may be initiated in persons in whom a tubercular skin test conversion develops within 2 years of a previously negative purified protein derivative (PPD); persons with a history of untreated tuberculosis or a positive PPD and chest x-ray

Table 20-1	Initial Treatment for Active Tuberculosis with Positive Chest Radiography

Children
Isoniazid (INH) 10–15 mg/kg/d orally (up to 300 mg/d) *plus*
Rifampin (Rimactane) 10–20 mg/kg/d orally (up to 600 mg/d) *plus*
Pyrazinamide (PZA) 20–40 mg/kg/d orally (up to 2 g/d) *plus*
Ethambutol 15–25 mg/kg/d orally (up to 2.5 g/d)

Adults
Isoniazid (INH) 5 mg/kg/d orally (up to 300 mg daily) *plus*
Rifampin (Rimactane) 10 mg/kg/d orally (up to 600 mg daily) *plus*
Pyrazinamide (PZA) 15–30 mg/kg/d orally (up to 2 g/d) *plus*
Ethambutol 15–25 mg/kg/d orally (up to 1.6 g/d)

evidence of previous infection; PPD reactors younger than age 35 years; persons of any age with a positive PPD who are at high risk (e.g., diabetes, HIV); and household members and other close contact of patients with active disease with a newly reactive PPD. Exposed infants should be treated with isoniazid regardless of PPD status. The tuberculin test, however (5 tuberculin U intradermally), may not become positive in infected individuals for 6 weeks after exposure.

21 Shortness of Breath

COMMON CAUSES OF SHORTNESS OF BREATH

- Asthma*
- Pneumonia
- Bronchitis
- Croup*
- Bronchiolitis
- Hyperventilation*
- Pleuritis
- Chronic obstructive pulmonary disease*
- Congestive heart failure*
- Myocardial ischemia or infarction

LESS COMMON CAUSES OF SHORTNESS OF BREATH NOT TO BE MISSED

- Spontaneous pneumothorax
- Primary pulmonary hypertension
- Pulmonary embolism
- Cardiac tamponade
- Laryngeal or tracheal obstruction
- Superior vena cava syndrome

OTHER CAUSES OF SHORTNESS OF BREATH

- Pneumocystis carinii pneumonia
- Pleural effusion
- Interstitial lung diseases
- Endobronchial foreign bodies
- Anxiety

HISTORY

Patients who report shortness of breath in the emergency department (ED) usually experience subjective breathlessness at rest or with less exertion than in the past.
- Fever associated with dyspnea usually implies an infectious cause such as pneumonia, tracheobronchitis, or croup and bronchiolitis in children.
- Cough productive of yellow-green sputum suggests an infectious bacterial cause, whereas clear sputum is more often seen in viral infection; pink, frothy sputum may be noted in patients with congestive heart failure (CHF).

---

*Discussed in this chapter.

- A history of pedal edema, paroxysmal nocturnal dyspnea, or orthopnea suggests CHF. An associated history of hypertension, coronary artery disease, or both lends support to this diagnosis.
- Anginal discomfort accompanying dyspnea implies that either acute left ventricular dysfunction has developed in the context of ongoing myocardial ischemia or hypoxemia produced by acute CHF (pulmonary edema) has led to myocardial ischemia.
- Sudden onset of breathlessness in a patient with a history of smoking, calf swelling or tenderness, hypercoaguable state, immobilization for a prolonged period, pregnancy, or oral contraceptive use suggests pulmonary embolism (PE).
- Pleuritis of any cause may be accompanied by the sudden onset of dyspnea and pleuritic chest pain.
- Tall, thin, young men who report the sudden onset of breathlessness and pleuritic chest or back pain should be suspected to have had a spontaneous pneumothorax.
- Shortness of breath remains a common presenting symptom in patients with anxiety-related hyperventilation, although this is a diagnosis of exclusion.

PHYSICAL EXAMINATION

- Patients with severe respiratory distress from any cause use their accessory muscles of respiration and often assume a tripod position on the stretcher. Children often display nasal flaring and suprasternal and intercostal retractions. A decrease in vigilance or development of somnolence is a sign of impending respiratory failure.
- Fever may be noted in patients with breathlessness caused by an infectious cause.
- A prolonged expiratory phase and wheezing are noted in patients with bronchospasm; however, in persons with severe airway obstruction, airflow may be so limited that wheezing is absent until therapy results in increased airflow.
- Signs of lobar consolidation, including egophony, whisper pectoriloquy, and enhanced or absent breath sounds may be noted in patients with pneumonia or neoplastic disorders of the lung resulting in bronchial obstruction.
- An increased jugular venous pulse, rales, an S_3 gallop, hepatosplenomegaly, ascites, and pedal edema are all signs of CHF.
- A loud P_2 with a palpable pulmonary artery segment and a pronounced subxiphoid impulse are noted in patients with pulmonary hypertension, as are often other signs of right-sided heart failure.
- Cardiac tamponade may result in distant heart sounds, tachycardia, hypotension, and dyspnea in the setting of a relatively normal lung examination.
- Dry, "Velcro-like" rales are often noted in patients with interstitial lung disease.
- Pleural effusions produce dullness to percussion at the lung bases and may be found in the setting of CHF, pneumonia, or neoplastic disease.
- Stridor is noted in patients with obstructing lesions of the upper airway, with endotracheal or endobronchial foreign bodies, or, especially in young children, as a consequence of epiglottitis or croup.

DIAGNOSTIC TESTS

- All patients with a complaint of shortness of breath must have a complete set of vital signs including temperature and pulse oximetry.
- The chest roentgenogram may reveal an infiltrate, pulmonary vascular congestion or pneumothorax.

- In patients suspected of pneumothorax, an **upright, end-expiratory,** posterior-anterior film is most sensitive and should specifically be requested when this diagnosis is suspected.
- Radiologically, patients with CHF typically manifest cardiomegaly, often in association with bilateral alveolar infiltrates, pulmonary vascular redistribution, perihilar prominence, and peribronchial cuffing.
- A **complete blood count** (CBC) with differential may be helpful in assessing the presence of infection and may suggest a bacterial or viral etiology in some patients.
- **Brain natriuretic peptide (BNP)** is useful in identifying patients with elevated left ventricular filling pressures due to CHF. BNP is elevated early in patients with cardiac dysfunction and in symptomatic patients; a normal level should cause one to reconsider a cardiac etiology for breathlessness (Table 21-1).
- **A lateral neck radiograph** is also helpful in the differential diagnosis of stridor or upper airway obstruction. An edematous, enlarged epiglottis is noted on the lateral projection in patients with epiglottitis, while a narrowed tracheal air column is seen on the anterior-posterior (AP) projection in patients with croup. A foreign body may also be noted.
- **Direct fiberoptic larygoscopy** may reveal an enlarged, erythematous epiglottis that is diagnostic for epiglottitis or may demonstrate an obstructing foreign body.
- **Spiral chest CT or ventilation/perfusion scanning** can be used to confirm the diagnosis of PE.

Table 21-1	Median BNP Levels Among Patients in Each of the Four Heart Failure Classes[a]	
Class	**Patient Symptoms**	**BNP Level (pg/mL)**
Class I (mild)	No limitation of physical activity. Ordinary physical activity does not cause undue fatigue, palpitation, or dyspnea.	244 (±286)
Class II (mild)	Slight limitation of physical activity. Comfortable at rest, but ordinary physical activity results in fatigue, palpitation, or dyspnea.	389 (±374)
Class III (moderate)	Marked limitation of physical activity. Comfortable at rest, but less than ordinary activity causes fatigue, palpitation, or dyspnea.	640 (±447)
Class IV (severe)	Unable to perform any physical activity without discomfort. Symptoms of cardiac insufficiency at rest. If any physical activity is undertaken, discomfort is increased.	817 (±435)

[a]Data from in Maisel AS, Krishnaswamy P, Nowak RM, et al. Rapid measurement of B-type natriuretic peptide in the emergency diagnosis of heart failure. *N Engl J Med* 2002;347(3):161–167.

- **Arterial and venous blood gases** have limited utility. Pulse oximetry and clinical respiratory status should guide most management decisions. Blood gases may reveal hypoventilation and CO_2 retention. A normal or rising pCO_2 may indicate impending respiratory failure.

CLINICAL REMINDERS

- All patients with a complaint of shortness of breath must have a complete set of vital signs including temperature and pulse oximetry.
- A normal oxygenation level on pulse oximetry or ABG does not exclude pulmonary embolus.
- A chest roentgenogram is indicated in most patients with a complaint of shortness of breath. Asthmatics with a nonfocal lung exam may not require a chest roentgenogram.

SPECIFIC DISORDERS

Asthma

Clinical Presentation
History

- Patients with an acute asthmatic attack complain of shortness of breath, cough, and, occasionally, audible wheezing. Symptoms may progress over a period of minutes to hours.
- Those patients with a long history of asthma often attempt to medicate themselves with bronchodilators at home and appear in the ED when these measures fail.
- Patients may have a history of upper respiratory tract infection or may report a cough, occasionally productive, that appears to exacerbate the sensation of dyspnea and wheezing.
- In some patients with asthma, cold air or exercise often induces either cough alone as an early manifestation of bronchospasm or frank wheezing.
- Patients experiencing an acute asthmatic attack appear quite anxious and dyspneic. Respiratory rate is increased and tachycardia with an elevated blood pressure is often noted.
- In patients with severe bronchospasm, the accessory muscles of respiration are utilized, producing tracheal "tugging" and suprasternal and intercostal retractions.
- Auscultation of the chest reveals a prolonged expiratory phase with associated inspiratory and expiratory wheezes; fine basilar rales may be heard in some patients, and in others, simple prolongation of the expiratory phase in the absence of wheezing is noted.
- The heart sounds are distant as a result of air trapping and an increased thoracic diameter.
- If severe hypoxemia evolves, nail bed and perioral cyanosis may develop.

Diagnostic Tests

- Arterial blood gases should be deferred unless hypercarbia or serious hypoxemia is suspected and patients are unable to perform pulmonary function testing, particularly if symptoms are worsening despite treatment, and intubation and mechanical ventilation are being contemplated.

- If possible, all patients should have a forced expiratory volume in 1 second (FEV_1) or peak expiratory flow rate (PEFR) determined; these indices are helpful to determine attack severity and treatment strategy, the patient's response to therapy, and admission/discharge decisions (Figs. 21-1 and 21-2).
- If arterial blood gases are obtained, a low PCO_2 due to hyperventilation is expected. A normal PCO_2, suggesting significant obstruction, is worrisome. Elevation of the PCO_2 occurs only with severe attacks and may indicate impending respiratory failure.
- Patients using an oral theophylline preparation should have a baseline level obtained.
- A CBC can be obtained (preferably before systemic steroids or epinephrine administration) if pneumonia is suspected.
- A chest x-ray is necessary only to exclude pneumothorax or confirm a high clinical suspicion of pneumonia, or when patients fail to respond to therapy. An admission chest x-ray in the absence of the aforementioned indications is not indicated.

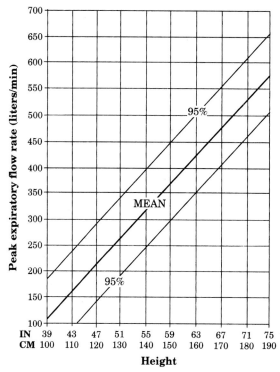

Figure 21-1. Pediatric normal peak expiratory flow (mean ± 2 SD). (Redrawn from data obtained from 382 children aged 5 to 18 years by Godfrey S, Kamburoff PL, Nairn JR. Spirometry, lung volumes and airway resistance in normal children aged 5 to 18 years. *Br J Dis Chest* 1970;64:15, reproduced with permission.)

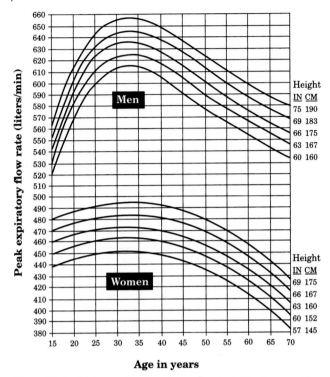

Figure 21-2. Adult normal peak expiratory flow by height, from age 15 to 70 years. (Redrawn from information in Gregg I, Nunn AJ. Peak expiratory flow in normal subjects. *Br Med J* 1973;3:282–284, with permission.)

Treatment

- In patients who appear ill, **supplemental oxygen** should be immediately administered and continuous pulse oximetry initiated. Oxygen saturation measured by pulse oximetry correlates well with hypoxemia; saturations less than 90% indicate relatively serious hypoxemia ($PaO_2 < 60$ mm Hg).
- **Inhalation of β-agonists** is the primary treatment for the patient with acute asthma. Although delivery by metered-dose inhaler (MDI) is more efficient, most patients are treated via wet nebulization. **Albuterol**, 2.5 mg, via wet nebulization repeated three times, at 20-minute intervals, is a reasonable first-line intervention.
- In patients with severe disease, administration of albuterol via continuous wet nebulization in increased doses (15 mg/h × 2 hours) with a large reservoir may be beneficial.
- After stabilization, the frequency of inhalations is reduced to hourly, or every other hour, or ever 4 hours, depending on the particular patient.
- An inhaled anticholinergic agent, such as **ipratropium**, 2.5 to 5.0 mg, is recommended. Ipratropium can be administered concurrently with albuterol and can be given at 20-minute intervals with each of the three initial inhalation treatments.

- There is evidence that albuterol and ipratropium when administered in this manner produce more bronchodilation than treatment with albuterol alone.
- Subcutaneous **terbutaline** (0.25 mg; may repeat in 20–30 minutes if needed), for those unable to comply with nebulization, produces a therapeutic response comparable to inhalation therapy with albuterol. Tachycardia often limits its use.
- The early and aggressive use of **corticosteroids** in acute asthma is recommended; commonly used initial doses are methylprednisolone, 60 to 125 mg intravenous, or prednisone, 60 mg orally. A therapeutic response can be documented within 3 hours of administration with peak effects at approximately 6 to 10 hours.
- The early use of steroids in the ED has been shown to reduce the number of patients requiring hospital admission.
- There is no evidence that parenteral administration is superior to the oral route.
- It is generally recommended that the following patients receive an initial dose of steroids in the ED: those who experience an acute attack while on, or tapering off, a steroid course; those with moderate (FEV_1/PEFR 40% to 60% of predicted) or severe (FEV_1/PEFR < 40% of predicted) attacks; and those with increasing frequent or accelerating attacks.
- Patients who appear to be dehydrated should receive intravenous fluids in the ED; routine rehydration of patients with asthma is not indicated.
- Acute episodes of asthma may be triggered by bacterial infection. When a reasonable degree of clinical suspicion exists in favor of bacterial infection, a course of antibacterial therapy is warranted.
- **Aminophylline** is not particularly helpful in the initial management of asthma in the ED, but patients who are maintained on an oral aminophylline preparation should have a baseline blood level obtained and optimized.
- Although the bronchodilatory properties of **magnesium sulfate** are well known, the role of magnesium in the treatment of acute asthma is not well defined. The use of magnesium is best reserved for severely ill patients who have not responded to other modalities and in whom intubation and mechanical ventilation appear increasingly likely. In these patients, 2 g of magnesium sulfate can be given intravenously. Side effects include nausea and vomiting, flushing, diaphoresis, weakness, hypotension, and respiratory depression; these are dose related and fortunately relatively uncommon.
- The treatment of **acute asthma in children** is similar to the treatment of adults.
- The treatment of the **pregnant patient** presenting with an acute asthmatic attack is essentially as outlined. Terbutaline, because of its inhibitory effect on uterine muscle contraction, is best avoided.

Disposition
- Patients who fail to respond to appropriate therapy should be admitted to the hospital for additional treatment and observation.
- Generally, after an initial course of inhalation therapy, patients with FEV_1 or PEFR at 70% or greater of predicted (or personal best) can be discharged from the ED provided symptoms concurrently have improved.
- Patients with an incomplete initial response to therapy (FEV_1/PEFR between 40% and 70%) should continue to receive inhalation therapy hourly along with steroids. If pulmonary function tests remain unchanged after approximately 4 hours of treatment, admission to the hospital should be strongly considered but is not mandatory; further treatment and frequent reassessments can continue, and should FEV_1/PEFR improve over this period, discharge is reasonable.
- Patients with a poor response to initial and subsequent therapy (FEV_1/PEFR < 40%) require admission and close observation.

- Typically, patients with FEV_1/PEFR less than 25% (usually associated with PCO_2 > 40 and acidosis) will require intensive care unit (ICU) admission for severe obstruction/respiratory failure; noninvasive positive pressure ventilation or intubation and mechanical ventilation will often be necessary.
- Patients who are discharged require close-interval follow-up. Patients should generally be discharged on an inhaled β-agonist, such as an albuterol inhaler, 2 puffs four times daily; Serevent, 2 puffs twice daily; or combination therapy such as Combivent (albuterol and Atrovent), 2 puffs four times daily.
- Prednisone should be prescribed on a 10-day tapering course or as 60 mg/day for 5 days after which the medication is discontinued.
- Patients whose asthma is uncontrolled by regular use of an inhaled β-agonist should also receive an inhaled steroid preparation, such as beclomethasone dipropionate, 2 to 4 puffs, twice daily or four times daily, or a combination steroid/β-agonist inhaler, such as Advair.
- All patients should be instructed to return to the ED if symptoms worsen.
- Follow-up with a primary care physician must be emphasized.

Chronic Obstructive Pulmonary Disease

Clinical Presentation
- Chronic obstructive pulmonary disease (COPD) includes both chronic emphysema and chronic bronchitis. Cigarette smoking and occupational exposures (e.g., silica) are the primary causes of COPD.
- Patients most commonly complain of increasing dyspnea. Patients may notice a change in sputum quantity or character, which may indicate an infectious cause of the exacerbation.
- Physical examination may reveal respiratory distress of varying degree, pulsus paradoxus, an increased anteroposterior thoracic diameter, bronchial breath sounds, wheezing, and clubbing.

Diagnostic Tests
- The chest roentgenogram may show bullous disease, flattened diaphragms, an increased retrosternal air space, and a small, vertical heart. An infiltrate may be visible but acute exacerbations of COPD are often not accompanied by any obvious infiltrative process.
- Arterial blood gases may show hypoxemia with hypocapnia or, if the patient has severe obstruction or has become insensitive to carbon dioxide, hypercapnia. A pH determination is quite useful in these patients in that it will reflect any acute changes in the patient's PCO_2. Recently worsening obstruction or hyperventilation will be reflected in the development of acidemia or alkalemia, respectively.
- The initial room-air PCO_2, if elevated, should alert the physician to the possibility of further carbon dioxide retention and potential respiratory failure if excessive supplemental oxygen is administered.

Treatment
- Primary treatment of decompensated COPD includes the use of supplemental oxygen, bronchodilators, and antibiotics, if indicated.
- Supplemental oxygen should be initiated promptly. COPD patients are often chronically hypoxic, and supplemental oxygen should be titrated to symptoms and not pulse oximetry levels.
- Bronchodilators are the mainstay of therapy in these patients with β_2-adrenergic agonists such as albuterol, 2.5 mg, which can be repeated three times at 20-minute

intervals. Ipratropium, 2.5 to 5.0 mg, should be given with the initial dose of albuterol, with which it exhibits synergistic bronchodilation.

- Oral or parenteral steroids should be initiated. A longer taper is beneficial for COPD patients. Prednisone 60 mg/day tapered over 9 days is a reasonable choice.
- If infection is suspected as the inciting factor (change in sputum character of quantity, increased dyspnea), an antibiotic such as Levaquin, Zithromax, or trimethoprim-sulfamethoxazole, for 7 to 10 days should be instituted.
- Noninvasive positive pressure ventilation (CPAP or BiPaP) may offer significant relief and avoid intubation in dyspneic patients. It should be considered early in the ED course.
- Progressive hypercarbia despite treatment remains an indication for intubation and assisted ventilation, particularly if associated with increasing lethargy or acidemia.

Congestive Heart Failure

Clinical Presentation

- CHF may be described in several general ways—systolic versus diastolic, dilated versus restrictive, right versus left, or low output versus high output. Specific causes of CHF may be defined in terms of each of these general categories. In the acute setting, however, therapeutic intervention is independent of the specific etiology (with certain specific exceptions, to be discussed).
- Patients with acutely worsening CHF report breathlessness, often at rest, with a history of dyspnea on exertion, paroxysmal nocturnal dyspnea, orthopnea, and/or pedal edema.
- A history of hypertension, angina, myocardial infarction, rheumatic fever or valvular heart disease, excessive alcohol use, or recent viral illness may be elicited.
- The physical examination may be quite variable but usually includes some evidence of dyspnea at rest manifested as an increased respiratory rate with or without recruitment of accessory muscles. Overt cyanosis, particularly of the lips or fingers and toes, may be noted.
- Rales are the most significant manifestation of left-sided CHF and may be auscultated only at the bases or, in patients with florid pulmonary edema, throughout the lung fields.
- If a significant degree of right-sided CHF coexists, jugular venous distention, hepatosplenomegaly, ascites, and pedal edema may be noted.
- Evidence of pleural effusion (either right sided or bilateral) may accompany rales and may significantly contribute to the sensation of breathlessness.
- An S_3 gallop may be auscultated as well but is often obscured if rales are prominent anteriorly.
- In severe pulmonary edema, patients are in extreme distress, often producing copious amounts of pink, frothy sputum. Rales are heard throughout the chest, and most patients are hypertensive at presentation.

Diagnostic Tests

- The chest roentgenogram typically reveals cardiomegaly in association with bilateral alveolar infiltrates; pulmonary vascular cephalization, perihilar prominence, and peribronchial cuffing may also be noted.
- BNP is helpful in identifying patients with elevated left ventricular filling pressures (Table 21-1). BNP levels are elevated early in patients with left ventricular dysfunction and therefore, when normal in the patient with breathlessness, should suggest that a noncardiac cause be pursued.

- The electrocardiogram (ECG) may show sinus tachycardia, evidence of left ventricular hypertrophy in patients with preexisting hypertension, or acute myocardial injury. A variety of dysrhythmias may precipitate or worsen CHF, and these should be treated as discussed in Chapter 25.

Treatment
Acute Pulmonary Edema

- Acute pulmonary edema is treated with intravenous morphine sulfate (as a pulmonary vasodilator and an antianxiety agent), intravenous furosemide (as a diuretic and a pulmonary vasodilator), supplemental oxygen, IV nitroglycerin, and elevation of the head of the bed at 90 degrees in normotensive or hypertensive patients.
- Supplemental oxygen is essential. Nasal cannula, mask, noninvasive positive pressure ventilation, or intubation may be necessary.
- Nitroglycerin (10–20 μg/min intravenous, initially; increase 10 μg/min every 3–5 minutes as needed) often results in immediate relief of symptoms.
- Morphine sulfate may be given in increments of 2 to 4 mg intravenous, which may be repeated as needed every 5 to 10 minutes.
- Furosemide, 20 to 40 mg intravenous, may be administered to patients not maintained on this agent; patients currently treated with furosemide may receive twice the daily oral dose by intravenous administration.
- Oral ACE inhibitors such as enalapril 5 mg should be initiated in the ED if the blood pressure is above 120 mm Hg and the creatinine is less than 1.5 mg/dL.
- Aspirin may be initiated if any evidence of ischemia is present.
- In patients with progressive hypoxemia despite these pharmacologic measures, noninvasive positive pressure ventilation or intubation and the institution of assisted ventilation with positive end-expiratory pressure may be required.

Hypotension and Acute Pulmonary Edema

- This scenario presents the emergency physician with a difficult management problem. Some patients with acute pulmonary edema and hypotension have modest degrees of volume depletion (pulmonary artery occlusion pressures <15 mm Hg).
- It is not unreasonable to administer a cautious fluid challenge (250 mL of normal saline over 5–10 minutes) during which time patients should be closely observed by the physician. If systolic pressure increases somewhat and/or if respiratory function remains stable, an additional 250 mL of saline can be administered.
- Patients failing to respond to a fluid bolus will require further support of blood pressure with vasopressors and positive inotropic agents. **Dopamine's** effect on the vasculature and the heart varies significantly with the dose administered; start at 5 μg/kg/min and titrate to 10 μg/kg/min. If the patient remains hypotensive, add dobutamine.
- **Dobutamine** is primarily a vasodilator, with positive inotropic effects. This agent should not be used alone in hypotensive or normotensive patients because of the risk of precipitating or worsening hypotension. Because of this agent's ability to increase cardiac output with less effect on heart rate, dobutamine is probably the agent of choice in normotensive or hypertensive patients with CHF and myocardial infarction. Dobutamine is usually started at a dose of 2 μg/kg/min and can be gradually increased to 10 μg/kg/min.

Severe Aortic Stenosis

- These patients have an absolute requirement for maximal left ventricular filling pressures given their fixed outflow obstruction and their stiffened, noncompliant left ventricular wall. Preload reduction with nitrates, a brisk diuresis, or rapid afterload reduction may theoretically depress cardiac output and thereby blood pressure. For these reasons, patients with significant aortic stenosis should be managed very conservatively. Clinically, this means permitting the patient to have bibasilar rales, thereby indicating the presence of adequate left ventricular filling pressures, generally without significantly compromising oxygenation. Small doses of diuretic and morphine sulfate may be administered to patients requiring acute intervention, albeit cautiously. Nitroglycerin should be used with extreme caution.

Diastolic Dysfunction/Mitral Stenosis

- The development of supraventricular tachycardia, particularly rapid atrial fibrillation, can be responsible for precipitating acute CHF. In these patients, diastolic filling time is reduced sufficiently to impair left ventricular filling and thereby cardiac output. In these patients, slowing the heart rate is appropriate and may be accomplished with intravenous metoprolol or Cardizem. Metopolol may be given intravenously in 5-mg increments every 5 minutes up to a total dose of 15 mg. Cardizem may be given in an initial bolus of 0.25mg/kg over 2 minutes and then as a drip of 10 to 15 mg/h. Alternatively, digoxin, 0.5 mg intravenous given over 5 to 10 minutes, may be administered initially, followed by 0.25 mg intravenous increments ever 4 hours up to a total dose of 1.5 mg in 24 hours.

Dialysis Patient

- In mild to moderately symptomatic patients, morphine sulfate and intravenous nitroglycerin (initially at 10–20 µg/min) are helpful; the nitroglycerin infusion can be increased incrementally by 10 µg/min as needed. Noninvasive positive pressure ventilation, intubation, emergency hemodialysis, or all the above may be necessary for patients critically ill or refractory to other measures.

Hyperventilation

- Hyperventilation may be a result of sepsis, metabolic acidosis, a variety of central nervous system lesions, salicylate overdose, hypoxia resulting from any cause (e.g., pneumothorax, pneumonia, pulmonary embolus), or anxiety.
- In the ED, the diagnosis of hyperventilation secondary to anxiety is common, but it must be a **diagnosis of exclusion** given the extremely serious nature of many of the other causes of shortness of breath.

Clinical Presentation

- The anxious, hyperventilating patient usually presents with a relatively acute history of dyspnea, which is often associated with distal extremity and perioral paresthesias and numbness; chest tightness; light-headedness; weakness; fainting spells or presyncope; and carpopedal spasm. Patients generally appear frightened, anxious, and occasionally hysterical.
- Increased alveolar ventilation results in a reduced PCO_2. A rapidly falling PCO_2 produces alkalosis, which in turn reduces the concentration of free ionized calcium, which produces the more striking neurologic findings in patients with hyperventilation (i.e., paresthesias, carpopedal spasm).

Treatment

- The physician should tactfully explore any possible sources of occult stress, to identify precipitants for the attack. More often, however, patients report little to explain the acute episode.

- It may be useful to explain to patients that hyperventilation may represent a response to unrecognized stress or anxiety, in much the same way that ulcer disease or high blood pressure develops in other patients. It is not unreasonable to suggest to the patient, after the attack subsides or is subsiding, that some thought be given to any as yet unidentified issue or issues that may be of concern to the patient.
- It may be useful to discuss the pathophysiology of the signs and symptoms of hyperventilation as they relate to both the rate and the depth of breathing and suggest that if these parameters can be voluntarily reduced at or near the beginning of an attack, the symptoms can resolve.
- Patients with anxiety-related hyperventilation should be told that if symptoms recur, which one would not necessarily expect them to, and if by voluntarily reducing the rate and depth of breathing one cannot terminate an attack, the patient should return to the ED.

Pulmonary Embolism

- PE is one of the most underdiagnosed, serious acute diseases confronting the emergency physician. An estimated 630,000 patients are affected each year in the United States, 11% of whom die within 1 hour of presentation.
- Pulmonary emboli typically originate from deep, venous clots in the lower extremity and iliac venous systems. Eighty percent of lower extremity DVT occurs in the deep veins of the calf and the remainder in the femoral-iliac system.

Risk Factors
- Previous DVT or PE
- Conditions associated with hypercoagulability
  - Acquired immunodeficiency syndrome (AIDS)
  - Antithrombin III deficiency
  - High-dose estrogen replacement
  - Malignancy
  - Ulcerative colitis
  - Abnormalities of fibrinogen
  - Oral contraceptive use
  - Protein C and S deficiencies
  - Systemic lupus erythematosus
- Conditions associated with venous stasis or injury
  - Congestive heart failure
  - Prolonged immobilization
  - Obesity
  - Atrial fibrillation
  - Pregnancy and the postpartum period
  - Thrombocytosis
  - Trauma
  - Varicosities
  - Indwelling venous catheters and pacemakers

Clinical Presentation
- Dyspnea (73%), pleuritic chest pain (66%), cough (37%), and hemoptysis (13%) are the most common symptoms. The classic triad of dyspnea, hemoptysis, and chest pain occurs in only 15% to 20% of patients.

- When chest pain is present, it can be pleuritic or constant and unrelated to inspiration; some patients describe pain that is identical to "classic" ischemic cardiac pain.
- The clinical severity of PE can range from asymptomatic to severe hypoxemia, shock, or sudden death.
- The physical examination is unreliable in diagnosing PE. Tachypnea (70%), rales (51%), and tachycardia (30%) are the most common signs. In any given patient, groups of physical signs have higher positive predictive value; these include DVT, diaphoresis, fever, heart rate greater than 100, cyanosis, rales, new S_3 or S_4 gallop, or murmur.

Diagnostic Tests
- All diagnostic tests for PE must be interpreted in the context of clinical probability. The modified **Wells criteria** allow the clinician to risk stratify patients into low and high risk for PE (Table 21-2). Once a pretest probability is determined, diagnostic studies can be interpreted to include or exclude pulmonary embolus or indicate further testing.
- Normal oxygenation by **pulse oximetry or arterial blood gases** does not exclude PE. Some patients with PE have an abnormal **alveolar-arterial oxygen gradient,** but this is also nonspecific.
- **D-dimer** fragment analysis by ELISA, if less than 500 ng/mL, has a high negative predictive value (>90%). When elevated, the test is nonspecific and is seen in a number of other medical conditions (trauma, malignancy, surgery, infection, cardiovascular disease) but mandates further testing for PE.
- The **ECG** may suggest evidence of right heart strain (peaking of the T wave in lead II, right bundle branch block, right-axis deviation, or an S1-Q3-T3 pattern) but more often is normal or unchanged from the patient's baseline. Sinus tachycardia and nonspecific ST-T abnormalities are the commonest abnormality.

Table 21-2	Modified Wells Criteria: Clinical Assessment for Pulmonary Embolism	
Clinical symptoms of DVT (leg swelling, pain with palpation)		3.0
Other diagnosis less likely than PE		3.0
Heart rate >100		1.5
Immobilization (≥3 d) or surgery in the previous 4 wk		1.5
Previous DVT/PE		1.5
Hemoptysis		1.0
Malignancy		1.0
Probability		**Score**
Traditional clinical probability assessment		
High		>6.0
Moderate		2.0–6.0
Low		<2.0
Simplified Clinical Probability Assessment[a]		
PE likely		>4.0
PE unlikely		≤4.0

[a]Data from van Belle A, et al. (Writing Group for the Christopher Study Investigators). *JAMA* 2006;295:172.

- Similarly, although the **chest x-ray** may be abnormal, findings are nonspecific; 30% of patients have a normal chest film, with the remainder showing a variety of abnormalities including elevation of the hemidiaphragm, atelectasis, focal infiltrates, and a pleural effusion. Hampton hump (a triangular density with its base near or resting on the diaphragm and its apex pointing toward the hilum) and Westermark sign (a dilation of pulmonary vessels proximal to and collapse of vessels distal to a presumed embolus) are uncommon but suggestive of PE, although both have been reported in other entities.
- The **ventilation-perfusion lung scan** can be helpful in making the diagnosis of PE when combined with clinical probability. Interpretations fall into essentially four categories: normal, high probability, intermediate, and low probability. A normal lung scan virtually excludes PE. A high-probability scan plus high clinical probability confirms PE. A low-probability lung scan plus low clinical probability excludes PE. All other combinations require further testing.
- **Spiral CT angiography (CTA)** is both highly sensitive and specific for larger sub-segmental, segmental clots and can effectively diagnose PE. CTA is less sensitive for smaller peripheral clots, although the true, clinical significance of these in patients without compromised cardiopulmonary reserve is not known. When there is a high clinical probability and a negative CTA, pulmonary angiography may be indicated.
- **Pulmonary angiography** remains the definitive diagnostic tool.
- An alternative diagnostic strategy is to diagnose a DVT. The demonstration of DVT via peripheral venous studies in patients suspected of PE essentially confirms the diagnosis; and no further diagnostic studies are required. Duplex ultrasound scanning remains the most useful initial study. If noninvasive venous studies are negative, contrast venography can be used to evaluate the venous system further.
- It is important to remember that positive or confirmatory studies have meaning; negative studies often do not. When the physician's degree of clinical suspicion is intermediate or high and these studies are negative or nondiagnostic, pulmonary angiography may be indicated.

Treatment
- Supportive care should include supplemental **oxygen** (which is a pulmonary vasodi-lator) and support of blood pressure with **intravenous fluids** and **vasopressors**.
- When the diagnosis of PE is strongly suspected, treatment should be initiated, unless contraindications exist, before actual confirmation of the diagnosis.
- Anticoagulant therapy is the primary therapy for PE. The goal of anticoagulation is to reduce mortality by preventing recurrent PE. Traditionally, patients have been given **unfractionated intravenous heparin** (initial bolus of 80 U/kg, followed by 18 U/kg/h as a continuous infusion). The kg-weight in obese patients is determined by using the patient's ideal body weight plus 30% of the patient's actual weight in kg in excess of ideal.
- **Enoxaparin** is thought to be equally effective as heparin, given in a dosage of 1 mg/kg every 12 hours subcutaneously.
- When unfractionated intravenous heparin is given, an activated partial thrombo-plastin time (aPTT) should be determined in 6 hours and should be at least 1.5- to 2.5-times control.
- Once daily, subcutaneous **fondaparinux** (a synthetic, antithrombotic agent) dem-onstrated efficacy and safety comparable to unfractionated intravenous heparin; this study was limited to stable patients with PE, and some patients received part of their

treatment as outpatients. Patients were treated for a minimum of 5 days and until the use of concomitantly administered vitamin K antagonists resulted in an international normalized ratio (INR) more than 2.0; patients treated with fondaparinux do not otherwise require monitoring.

- The use of **thrombolytic agents** in patients with PE should be instituted when it appears that the embolic event has overwhelmed the cardiopulmonary reserve, that is, hypotension, hypoxemia, or shock. These patients are unlikely to benefit significantly from traditional anticoagulation alone. Patients with evidence of acute right ventricular failure are also considered candidates.

- If thrombolytics are given, heparin should be discontinued (if previously started) until the PTT falls back into the therapeutic range (1.5- to 2.5-times control) and then restarted.

- Some authorities also recommend instituting thrombolytic therapy in patients with recurrent PE and those who are anticipated, based on irreversible risk factors, to have a substantially increased risk of recurrent thromboembolism and eventual cor pulmonale.

- The usual contraindications to heparin anticoagulation and thrombolytic therapy are noted below; there is no current upper age contraindication to thrombolytic therapy in this setting (Table 21-3) (the FDA has not approved the use of thrombolytic therapy in children). Intravenous heparin and oral warfarin are usually started at the conclusion of thrombolytic therapy. Common thrombolytic dosing regimens are as follows:
  - **rt-PA:** The optimal dose of rt-PA for patients with PE is unknown. The recommended dose is currently 100 mg continuously infused over a 2-hour period. In many centers, a front-loaded regimen is used, administering 15 mg as an intravenous bolus, followed by an infusion delivering 50 mg over the first hour and 35 mg over the subsequent hour. Some centers currently administer a single, large, weight-adjusted bolus of rt-PA in patients with evidence of hemodynamic instability; this is typically administered over 15 minutes with doses ranging from 0.6 mg/kg (maximum dose of 50 mg) to 1.5 mg/kg (maximum dose of 100 mg).

- **Warfarin** is typically started 24 hours after parenteral anticoagulation with heparin or Lovenox, in an initial dose of 5 to 10 mg/day; the PT is checked daily thereafter, with a goal of placing the INR between 2 and 3 or a PT 2.5- to 3.0-times control. Oral warfarin and parenteral anticoagulation should overlap by 4 days, after which parenteral therapy with heparin (or Lovenox) is discontinued, while warfarin is continued for approximately 3 months.

- **Embolectomy** is a therapeutic option for selected patients with PE. Embolectomy is used infrequently but should be considered in patients with massive PE and shock or severe, irreversible hypoxemia who are not candidates for thrombolytic therapy or have failed thrombolytic therapy.

- The treatment of **catheter-related venous thrombosis** is now routinely undertaken via the administration of thrombolytic agents directly into the catheter; typically, low doses are continuously infused and do not result in systemic anticoagulation.

- In **pregnant patients** suspected of PE, duplex ultrasound scanning of the lower extremities is the initial diagnostic modality, which if positive confirms the diagnosis. If negative, a ventilation/perfusion lung scan or CTA should be obtained. The patient will need to be counseled regarding the risks and benefits of making a diagnosis. CTA radiation exposure is directed and the abdomen can be shielded. The amount of radiation exposure with a lung scan is insignificant, with most resulting from

Table 21-3	Contraindications to Thrombolytic or Anticoagulant Therapy	
Clinical Setting	**Thrombolysis**	**Heparin**
Active major external bleeding	Absolute	Absolute
Active internal bleeding (even if minor)	Absolute	Absolute
Recent neurosurgery (past 8 wk)	Absolute	Relative
Recent hepatic or renal biopsy	Absolute	Relative
Recent ocular surgery (past 8 wk)	Absolute	Relative
Severe heparin-induced thrombocytopenia	Not contraindicated	Absolute
Recent major trauma	Relative	Relative
Recent surgery (including organ biopsy)	Relative	Not contraindicated
Recent major vessel puncture (current cannula acceptable)	Relative	Not contraindicated
Immediately postpartum	Relative	Relative
Recent past history of gastrointestinal bleeding	Relative	Relative
HTN uncontrolled at the time of thrombolysis	Relative	Relative
Long-standing diastolic HTN over 110 mm Hg	Relative	Relative
Recent prolonged cardiopulmonary resuscitation	Relative	Relative
Current pregnancy	Relative	Not contraindicated
Diabetic retinopathy with recent hemorrhage	Absolute/relative	Relative
Bacterial endocarditis	Relative	Not contraindicated
Mild heparin-associated thrombocytopenia	Not contraindicated	Relative
Central nervous system cancer	Relative	Relative

HTN, hypertension.
From Rosen P, Barkin R, Danzl DF, et al., eds. *Emergency Medicine: Concepts and Clinical Practice,* 4th ed. St. Louis, MO: Mosby; 1997: 1878,1881, with permission.

accumulation of radioisotope in the mother's bladder. This can be reduced by effecting a brisk diuresis and frequent emptying of the bladder. A high-probability scan confirms the diagnosis, whereas an indeterminate scan is of no help in excluding the diagnosis; in these patients, a CTA or pulmonary angiogram should be undertaken.

Croup

- Viral and spasmodic croup are common illnesses in children and are the commonest causes of stridor in young children.
- Viral croup, historically referred to as laryngotracheobronchitis, affects children between the ages of 1 and 3 years, with a peak age of approximately 2 years; viral

croup is more common in boys, and the illness occurs most often in the winter months.

- Patients typically come to the ED with a 2- to 3-day history of cough, fever, and rhinorrhea; worsening dyspnea and stridor typically occur at night, and many patients have a characteristic "barking" cough.
- Retractions may be noted, although patients do not appear toxic; the chest is usually clear, although transmitted upper airway stridor is heard.
- Many patients will have improved en route to the ED.
- Spasmodic croup is thought to represent airway hyperactivity, typically has no "viral" prodrome, occurs in children aged 1 to 10 years, and is not associated with fever. In other ways, the illness presents like viral croup, with a nocturnal preference, although improvement in symptoms often occurs spontaneously or with little intervention.
- The diagnosis of croup is usually made on clinical grounds.
- Radiologic confirmation of proximal narrowing of the subglottic space can be obtained by an AP radiograph of the neck; typically, a "steeple sign" is noted referring to the similar appearance of a church steeple. A lateral view should also be requested to exclude epiglottis.
- In children with mild symptoms, treatment with 2 to 4 mL of nebulized normal saline is often helpful and relieves dyspnea; other patients should be treated with supplemental oxygen and nebulized racemic epinephrine (0.5 mL in 2 mL of normal saline), which can be administered every 20 to 30 minutes as needed to a maximum of three doses in the ED. Most patients treated with racemic epinephrine will develop some degree of tachycardia; heart rates greater than 200 beats/min require that treatment be suspended.
- Many authorities recommend giving patients a "burst" or single dose of steroid (0.6 mg/kg of dexamethasone, given intramuscularly, or prednisolone, 1–2 mg/kg given orally).
- Improvement or resolution of symptoms is an indication for discharge. Outpatient treatment includes encouraging oral fluid intake, recommending humidification of inspired air, close observation of respiratory status, reassessment by a pediatrician in 12 to 24 hours, and clear instructions to return to the ED if symptoms worsen or recur.
- **Acute epiglottis** is discussed in Chapter 16 and can easily be confused with croup. In comparison, children with epiglottis are typically somewhat older (3–7 years of age), have more of a sudden onset (without the prodrome in viral croup), appear toxic with higher fever and white blood cell counts, report drooling and difficulty swallowing more often, may prefer a "sniffing" position with the head forward, less frequently manifest both stridor and the typical "barking" cough of croup, and typically present without a seasonal or time-of-day preference. The characteristic "thumb-like" appearance of the epiglottis on lateral views of the neck and the "steeple sign" characteristic of croup should be sought. When the diagnosis of epiglottis cannot clearly be excluded, otolaryngology consultation must be obtained prior to disposition.

Pneumocystis carinii Pneumonia

- *Pneumocystis carinii* causes opportunistic pneumonitis in the immunocompromised host, particularly patients with AIDS. Most patients complain of fever, dyspnea, and a nonproductive cough lasting for 2 weeks or longer.

- Typical physical findings include tachycardia and tachypnea but a relatively normal lung examination. The discordance between the paucity of findings on examination and the hypoxemia noted on blood gas analysis and bilateral dense perihilar infiltrates on chest radiograph is a hallmark of this infection.
- Diagnosis is made by histopathologic staining of material obtained at bronchoscopy.
- Trimethoprim-sulfamethoxazole, pentamidine isethionate, dapsone, and atovaquone have been used for treatment. The recurrence rate in AIDS patients is high (20%–30%).

Superior Vena Cava Syndrome

See Chapter 63.

22 Mechanical Ventilation

INDICATIONS

- Criteria for intubation and mechanical ventilation (MV) include impending respiratory failure, inadequate oxygen delivery, coma, obtundation, inability for the patient to protect the airway, or a need to urgently gather data (e.g., the need for computed tomography [CT] in an uncooperative patient).
- Poor air flow, retractions, high respiratory rates, and confusion are useful indicators of the need for MV. A blood gas showing acidosis due to retention of CO_2 or a low Pao_2 despite oxygen therapy can also help in the decision to begin MV.
- Noninvasive positive pressure ventilation (NIPPV) may be a viable option for patients with impending respiratory failure or inadequate oxygen delivery who are able to tolerate a tight-fitting mask. Patients who are agitated, confused, or unable to protect their airway are not candidates for NIPPV. Patients whose respiratory distress is due to a rapidly reversible condition (i.e., pulmonary edema or asthma) are the best candidates for NIPPV.
- In an emergent setting where a patient is not known to have a "do not resuscitate" (DNR) directive, or the applicability of a DNR directive is in question, intubation and MV should be provided with the knowledge that withdrawal of care remains an option ethically equivalent to withholding initiation of care.

SEDATION AND PARALYSIS

- NIPPV is usually well tolerated. Although the mask can be tight fitting and produce anxiety in some patients with respiratory distress, most patients are able to tolerate it without analgesia or sedation. Sedation should be used very cautiously in combination with NIPPV. Some authorities considered sedation contraindicated. A small number of patients may only be able to tolerate NIPPV with a very mild amount of anxiolytic.
- MV is uncomfortable. Sedation must be provided for patients who are awake. Neuromuscular blockade will produce the best intubating conditions. Rapid sequence activation is covered extensively in Chapter 2. Once intubated, sedation must be continued. Continuous infusion of benzodiazepines is effective. Chemical paralysis may also need to be continued. See Tables 22-1 and 22-2.

VENTILATOR SETTINGS

For an overview, refer to Table 22-3.

Table 22-1	Sedatives				
	Dose (Intravenous)				**Duration (of Induction/ Bolus) (min)**
Sedative	**Induction or Bolus (mg/kg)**	**Drip (μg/kg/min)**	**Onset (s)**	
Etomidate (Amidate)	0.2–0.4	100 × 10 min, then 10	15–45	3–12
Fentanyl (Sublimaze)[a]	5–10 (μg/kg)	2–10 (μg/kg/h)	60–90	45–60
Ketamine (Ketalar)	1.0–2.0	5–25	45–60	10–20
Lorazepam (Ativan)[b]	0.03–0.04	0.25–1.0	60–120	60–120
Midazolam (Versed)[c]	0.1–0.4	0.25–1.0	30–90	10–30
Propofol (Diprivan)	1.5–2.5	25–75	15–30	5–10

[a]Not an induction agent alone, but useful as an inductive adjunct.
[b]Not an induction agent.
[c]Drip dosing to be used in concert with opioid analgesia.

Biphasic Positive Airway Pressure

Biphasic positive airway pressure (BiPAP) provides ventilatory support via facemask. It improves oxygenation and decreases work of breathing and may obviate the need for endotracheal intubation. On inspiration, positive pressure helps to generate the tidal volume; positive end-expiratory pressure (PEEP; see later) is provided on expiration.

Table 22-2	Paralytics				
Paralytic	**Bolus (intravenous) (mg/kg)**	**Repeat[a] (mg/kg)**	**Drip (μg/kg/min)**	**Effect (min)**	**Duration (min)**
Cisatracurium (Nimbex)	0.10–0.15	0.05–0.07	1.0–2.0	5–6	25–40
Mivacurium (Mivacron)	0.15–0.20	0.08–0.15	5–10	2–3	15–30
Rocuronium (Zemuron)	0.45–0.60	0.08–0.23	5–12	1–2	25–40
Succinylcholine (Anectine)	1.0–2.0	Rare	Rare	1.0–1.5	5–10
Vecuronium (Norcuron)	0.08–0.12	0.01–0.02	1.0–2.0	5–6	25–40

[a]"Repeat" refers to intermittent doses needed for maintenance of paralysis.

Table 22-3	Initial Ventilator Settings, Adults[a,b]			
Circumstance	FiO$_2$[c]	Tidal Volume (mL/kg)	BPM	PEEP (cm H$_2$O)
Normal lung but overdose or Septic shock	0.5	10–12	10–12	5
C-spine injury Head trauma	0.5	10–12	16–20	5
Asthma	0.5	6–8	12–18	3
COPD	0.5	6–8	20–24	5
ARDS, CHF	1.0	6–8	20–24	15
Pulmonary edema Restrictive lung	0.5	6–8	18–22	5

COPD, chronic obstructive pulmonary disease; ARDS, acute respiratory distress syndrome; CHF, congestive heart failure; BPM, breaths per minute.

[a]Initial ventilator settings for the pediatric population are identical to adult settings except for breaths per minute. In children, these should be age appropriate in the normal lung (without head trauma) and modified (as in adults) for specific circumstances such as asthma or head trauma.

[b]AC (assist/control) should not be the initial mode of choice.

[c]Initial choice of FiO$_2$ can be promptly modified using pulse oximetry.

Ventilator Mode

Assist/Control (AC)

This mode provides maximal support by providing a full tidal volume when the patient triggers a breath (assist) or a full tidal volume uninitiated (control) when the triggering by the patient is at a minute rate less than the breath per minute rate selected.

Synchronized Intermittent Mandatory Ventilation (SIMV)

This allows a patient who is spontaneously breathing to trigger a breath and receive the tidal volume induced by that triggered breath. The ventilator does not assist. The ventilator does, however, note the breath and ensures a minimum minute ventilation by providing, if necessary, a preset tidal volume at a preset rate. Moreover, the ventilator coordinates and spaces the patient's native breathing effort and any ventilator breath, so that the patient does not receive breaths in rapid sequence (i.e., "stacking").

Pressure-Controlled Ventilation

AC and SIMV are volume-cycled modes, whereby a preset tidal volume is provided, and the pressure generated by the breath becomes a function of lung compliance and alveolar recruitment. In rare situations (e.g., severe bronchospasm), peak airway pressure is so high that a pneumothorax may result. Thus, a pressure-cycled mode is available that delivers only that tidal volume responsible for achieving the preset pressure. As in volume-cycled modes, the ventilator can be set to achieve a certain minute ventilation. When barotrauma is a concern, pressure ventilation may be necessary.

Minute Ventilation

This is a product of breaths per minute multiplied by the average tidal volume per minute per breath. A typical adult rate is 10 to 15 breaths/min at a tidal volume of

10 to 12 mL/kg. *Effective* tidal volume is that volume of air actually involved in oxygen and carbon dioxide exchange (tidal volume minus dead space). Dead space is determined by the tubing diameter, tubing length and compliance, and the patient's own anatomic dead space. The effective tidal volume usually runs 4 to 5 mL/kg less than the set tidal volume. Minute ventilation is adjusted by changing either the beats per minute rate or the tidal volume.

Pressure Support

Native breathing on a ventilator has been likened to breathing through a straw. The resistance of the tubing must be overcome by an increased negative inspiratory pressure, and this increases the work of breathing. In the SIMV mode, patient-triggered breaths are more work than breaths taken by unventilated persons. Pressure support addresses this problem by providing a boost to a given tidal volume when a patient has triggered his or her own breath. This, at the least, functions to overcome the resistance of the tubing.

PEEP

PEEP is used to keep alveoli inflated at the terminal phase of expiration. This support of the alveoli allows less difficult inflation of these same alveoli with the next breath. Its use can result in improved lung compliance and oxygenation, and decreased work of breathing along with decreased shunting. PEEP also results in decreased venous return, and incremental increases in PEEP to augment PaO_2 and minimize FiO_2 may result in cardiac compromise. PEEP is typically set at approximately 5 cm H_2O and should rarely exceed 15 cm H_2O in children and adults.

FiO_2

In an acute setting, 100% oxygen is reasonable. However, concentrations exceeding 50% for a lengthy period can result in oxygen toxicity: lipid peroxidation occurs, cell membranes are disrupted, and cell injury and death result. The lung and brain are the organs most susceptible to oxygen toxicity. Once the initial postintubation blood gas is obtained, the FiO_2 should be lowered to achieve a reasonable pO_2.

SPECIFIC CONSIDERATIONS

The Pediatric Patient

Endotracheal tube size may be approximated using the formula (16 + age in years) ÷ 4. (Children younger than 6 months should be considered 0 years of age.) Uncuffed endotracheal tubes should be used in children younger than age 8 and air leaks may occur.

Asthma

Bronchospasm may result in air trapping and high levels of carbon dioxide. A misguided response is either to increase the tidal volume or to increase the rate. Neither option is desirable: increasing the tidal volume risks pneumothorax because peak airway pressures are already elevated; increasing the rate simply reduces the per breath expiratory time, thus leading to even greater air trapping. "Permissive hypercapnia" refers to avoiding increased mechanical tidal volume and increased respiratory rate and allowing CO_2 levels above normal, thereby reducing the risk of pneumothorax and increased air trapping. A pH of 7.20 is the limit of tolerance because below this level, the risk of cellular dysfunction secondary to acidosis outweighs the benefits.

Acute Respiratory Distress Syndrome

Acute respiratory distress syndrome (ARDS) is caused by an excessive inflammatory response (often to infection). Its hallmark is systemically leaky capillaries, high peak airway pressures, and bilateral interstitial infiltrates on chest x-ray. The heavy interstitial burden can result in the collapse of alveoli. Here, "reversing" the normal 1:2 or 1:3 inspiratory to expiratory (I:E) ratio (i.e., changing to 1:1) allows for greater inspiratory time per breath cycle. Thus, for each breath cycle, any given alveolus sees more positive pressure and has less time to collapse. Alveoli are then fortified to withstand interstitial pressure and oxygenation is improved. Reversing the I:E ratio (inverse ratio ventilation) is a reasonable response to ARDS or similar problem, especially in a setting in which PEEP has been maximized.

TROUBLESHOOTING

Low Oxygen Saturation

Low oxygen saturation is the most common ventilator alarm. A systematic approach that considers both the equipment and the patient is warranted.

- Check the instruments. Is the pulse oximeter attached and showing a good waveform? Are there any obvious disconnections? Be sure the ventilator settings are appropriate. If ventilator malfunction is suspected, then manually ventilate the patient.
- Check the endotracheal tube. Be sure the lip line is correct and the balloon properly inflated. Check for an air leak and determine that the patient is not biting down on the tube.
- If the equipment is not the cause, then the patient must be. Aggressive suctioning is a good first step. Send an arterial blood gas. If the patient is agitated, or fighting the ventilator, consider sedation and then paralysis. Increase the FiO_2. Listen to the lungs. Are breath sounds equal? Is there evidence of a pneumothorax? Get a chest x-ray stat. Check for tracheal deviation or other evidence of a tension pneumothorax.

Air Leak

An air leak suggests a deflated cuff or misplaced tube. The tube should be repositioned or resecured and the balloon reinflated. In children, an air leak is sometimes tolerated if gas exchange is adequate.

High Peak Airway Pressure

High peak airway pressures can be ominous and suggest hemothorax, pneumothorax, worsening ARDS, worsening bronchospasm, or, perhaps, a mucus plug. A chest x-ray is needed. Suctioning often helps. Therapeutic chest percussion may clear mucous plugs.

PART 5

Cardiovascular Disorders

Chest Pain

Chest pain is one of the most common and most difficult presenting complaints in emergency medicine. Its causes are quite varied, spanning the spectrum of illness from benign costochondritis to life-threatening myocardial infarction. It is therefore important that for every patient with chest pain, the most serious possible diagnosis is at least entertained and when indicated, pursued and ruled out.

COMMON CAUSES OF CHEST PAIN

- Myocardial infarction*
- Angina pectoris*
- Pleuritis*
- Pericarditis*
- Costochondritis*
- Esophagitis*
- Pulmonary embolism and infarction
- Musculoskeletal strain

LESS COMMON CAUSES OF CHEST PAIN NOT TO BE MISSED

- Spontaneous pneumothorax*
- Spontaneous tension pneumothorax*
- Thoracic aortic dissection*
- Boerhaave syndrome

OTHER CAUSES OF CHEST PAIN

- Diffuse esophageal spasm
- Peptic ulcer disease

---

*Discussed in this chapter.

- Cholecystitis
- Herpes zoster (shingles)*

HISTORY

While the pain of pleuritis (used here to include all processes producing pleural irritation), pneumothorax, and costochondritis is often described as sharp and varying with respiration, that of myocardial infarction is usually described as dull and constant. Many patients with myocardial ischemia deny the presence of "pain," but rather insist on referring to a "discomfort," "tightness," "heaviness," or simply "pressure." Patients with esophagitis often describe a retrosternal, burning pain frequently associated with belching and often producing a bitter or acid taste in the mouth. The pain of a thoracic aortic dissection is often described as a "tearing" pain radiating toward the back.

If the patient can localize the pain to a very well-defined, discrete area, it is less likely to be due to myocardial ischemia or infarction and more likely results from processes that focally irritate or inflame the pleura or chest wall, although 15% of patients with myocardial infarction have chest wall pain with palpation. The pain of myocardial ischemia or infarction often radiates to the shoulder, arms, neck, or jaw. In fact, in some patients, the referred pain may be more severe than the chest pain accompanying it, or it may occur alone in the complete absence of any chest discomfort. Most patients with myocardial ischemic pain report discomfort generally localized to the anterior midsternal area, although patients with inferior wall ischemia may report a more epigastric location. A vertically oriented retrosternal discomfort is suggestive of esophagitis.

Pain that increases or changes with deep inspiration suggests disorders that produce pleural, pericardial, or chest wall irritation. Upper respiratory tract symptoms often precede viral pleuropericarditis and costochondritis. Fever, chills, dyspnea, and purulent sputum suggest pulmonary infection that, when involving lung segments adjacent to the pleura, may produce pleuritic discomfort. Nausea, vomiting, diaphoresis, fatigue, light-headedness, palpitations, and dyspnea often accompany the pain of myocardial ischemia or infarction. In elderly patients, women, and patients with diabetes, the pain of myocardial ischemia is often atypical in description and location (or even absent). Patients with pericarditis often note that pain worsens with recumbency and improves with sitting up; patients with acid-induced esophagitis or gastritis frequently report improvement with meals. Chest pain that is of sudden onset and is associated with varying degrees of dyspnea suggests pulmonary embolism or pneumothorax.

PHYSICAL EXAMINATION

A soft S_1 or the presence of an S_3 gallop in a patient who complains of chest pain but has no prior history of congestive heart failure suggests left ventricular dysfunction accompanying myocardial ischemia. Evidence of thrombophlebitis coupled with pleuritic discomfort should suggest pulmonary embolism. Fever, tachycardia, localized rales, dullness to percussion, decreased breath sounds, and egophony suggest pneumonia or other causes of pulmonary parenchymal consolidation. The presence of a pericardial friction rub, which may be transient, suggests pericarditis. Pleural friction rubs may also be heard in patients with pleurodynia, a pleural-based pneumonia, or pulmonary embolism. Localized chest wall tenderness at the costochondral junction suggests acute costochondritis; many patients report a subtle, subjective difference between the unaffected and affected sides with the application of pressure. A decrease in a carotid or radial pulse suggests a thoracic aortic dissection.

Typical, clustered, small vesicles on an erythematous base are noted in patients with herpes zoster (shingles). Although lesions classically occur in a radicular distribution, in some patients presenting early, only a single area of involvement may be noted. An occasional patient with severe discomfort will not manifest any rash when initially evaluated; in others presenting somewhat later, patches of simple erythema or an occasional vesicle will be noted.

EMERGENCY DIAGNOSTIC TESTS

Electrocardiogram

The electrocardiogram (**ECG**) is the single most useful diagnostic test performed in the evaluation of chest pain. It is critical to remember, however, that **when initially evaluated in the emergency department (ED), well over 50% of patients who are eventually ruled in for myocardial infarction have nondiagnostic ECGs and some have completely normal ECGs.** This test, therefore, cannot be used to independently rule out the diagnosis of myocardial ischemia in patients with otherwise compatible histories.

The ECG manifestations of **myocardial ischemia and infarction** are ST-segment depression/T-wave inversions and ST-segment elevations, respectively; a variety of cardiac and noncardiac conditions also produce these findings. These are discussed in detail in "Acute Coronary Syndrome." **Pericarditis** classically produces ECG changes that are diffuse (sometimes referred to as global) in that they involve multiple anatomically unrelated leads; these fail to correspond to any specific anatomic myocardial injury pattern, which is important diagnostically. The typical changes associated with pericarditis evolve sequentially over days to weeks and include initial PR depressions and ST-segment elevations, followed by normalization of the ST-segment and flattening of the T waves. T-wave inversions are then noted, with eventual normalization of the ECG, often requiring several weeks; Q waves are not noted. Patients with **thoracic aortic dissection** may have ECG evidence of acute myocardial infarction (AMI) as a result of concomitant (usually right) coronary artery dissection and occlusion; the inferior wall is commonly involved. **Acute myocarditis** can also produce ECG findings consistent with AMI. The ECG in patients with **pulmonary embolus** may show signs of right heart strain (peaking of the T wave in lead II, right bundle branch block, right axis deviation, or an S1-Q3-T3 pattern) but more often is normal or unchanged from the patient's baseline; sinus tachycardia and nonspecific S-T abnormalities are the most common patterns.

Serum Markers

Serum markers for AMI represent definitive evidence of myocardial necrosis. Myoglobin is the serum marker released earliest, with elevations detectable in 1 to 2 hours, but the poor specificity for a myocardial source limits its utility. Creatine kinase M and B (**CK-MB**) subunits and troponin T and I are more specific for myocardial damage and are thus superior in identifying infarction. CK-MB is detectable 3 to 6 hours after the onset of infarction, while troponin T and I detection takes slightly longer at 4 to 8 hours. For 100% sensitivity to be achieved in diagnosing myocardial infarction, an interval of up to 12 hours after the onset of pain is needed. Testing for these serum markers is available as point-of-care tests in many EDs for more rapid results.

Echocardiography

Echocardiography can visualize regional wall motion abnormalities in patients with acute injury or ischemia. A major limitation of this diagnostic modality, in addition to limited emergency availability, includes a relatively low specificity for acute infarction in that ischemia, prior infarction, and acute infarction may have similar echocardiographic appearances. A pericardial effusion, if present in patients with acute pericarditis, is usually seen with this modality.

The Chest X-Ray

The chest x-ray is helpful in diagnosing pneumothorax (an upright, posterior-anterior, expiratory film increases sensitivity) and pneumonia; some patients with pleurodynia and pulmonary infarction will have pleural-based densities as well. Pulmonary congestion may be noted as a manifestation of left ventricular dysfunction in the setting of myocardial ischemia. Mediastinal widening suggests aortic dissection, particularly if prior studies are available and demonstrate either a normal or a narrower mediastinum by comparison. The chest x-ray in patients with pulmonary embolus is usually normal; "classic" diagnostic findings, although uncommon and not 100% specific, are helpful if present and include Hampton hump (a triangular density with its base near or resting on the diaphragm and its apex pointing toward the hilum) and Westermark sign (a dilation of pulmonary vessels proximal to and collapse of vessels distal to a presumed embolus).

Arterial Blood Gases

In the past, arterial blood gases were used to help rule out the diagnosis of pulmonary embolus; because of the nonspecific nature of this particular test and the lack of sensitivity at virtually any level of PO_2, blood gases now are felt to have limited diagnostic utility.

Pulse Oximetry

Oxygen saturation as determined by pulse oximetry is not sensitive in assessing the probability of pulmonary embolus and should not be used for this purpose.

CLINICAL REMINDERS

- Admit all patients who have histories suggesting either new or changing patterns of myocardial ischemia (unstable, crescendo, or preinfarction angina) to a monitored setting or short-term observation (chest pain) unit.
- Be cautious administering sublingual nitroglycerin if the patient has significant aortic stenosis, is volume depleted, or is having an inferior infarct that includes a right ventricular infarction, since refractory hypotension may occur. Avoid nitrates completely in any patient taking one of the phosphodiesterase inhibitors used for erectile dysfunction such as sildenafil, tadalafil, or vardenafil, as severe refractory hypotension may result.
- Remember that many patients with evolving myocardial infarction have *normal* ECGs when first evaluated in the ED. Serial ECGs may be helpful in identifying an infarction in evolution.

- Remember to obtain an **end-expiratory upright** chest radiograph if pneumothorax is suspected.
- Remember that many patients with partial pneumothoraces will have bilateral breath sounds.

SPECIFIC DISORDERS

Acute Coronary Syndrome

Acute coronary syndrome (ACS) represents the spectrum of disease that encompasses any constellation of clinical symptoms compatible with myocardial ischemia, from unstable angina without evidence of infarction to AMI. AMI is generally divided into two groups: ST-elevation myocardial infarction (STEMI) and non–ST-elevation myocardial infarctions (NSTEMI). Because of its potential life-threatening consequences, myocardial infarction must be considered in all patients who present with chest pain. A system should be in place such that any patient presenting to the ED has a diagnostic ECG performed in a timely fashion given that effectiveness of treatment, as will be discussed later, is time-dependent.

History

The classic history consists of several minutes to hours of crushing substernal chest pain radiating into the neck, jaw, or arms, associated with nausea, diaphoresis, or dyspnea. Many variations of this typical presentation exist, so that the diagnosis of myocardial ischemia must be considered even when this complete constellation of symptoms is absent.

Physical Examination

On physical examination, patients may appear acutely ill, may be tachycardic, and if significant ventricular dysfunction is associated with the ongoing ischemia or infarction, may be dyspneic or hypotensive or both. Neck vein distention and pulmonary rales (or, in the extreme, frank pulmonary edema) may accompany myocardial infarction, resulting in significant hemodynamic compromise. The cardiac examination occasionally reveals a dyskinetic apex impulse, a soft S_1, and an S_3 if the patient has significant ventricular dysfunction; rarely, a pericardial friction rub may accompany an acute, transmural infarction. The murmur of mitral regurgitation can be heard in the presence of papillary muscle dysfunction or chordal rupture.

Diagnostic Tests
Electrocardiogram
The ECG, in conjunction with serologic markers for myocardial injury, is the most useful diagnostic test for the evaluation of chest pain.

It is critical to remember, however, that during initial evaluation in the ED, more than 50% of patients who are eventually considered to have ACS have nondiagnostic ECGs and a significant percentage have completely normal ECGs. In addition, the ability to exclude myocardial infarction with the serologic markers currently available depends significantly on the length of the interval between the onset of infarction and the time blood is drawn, and the absence of "stuttering" or intermittent episodes of ischemic pain and relief. In addition, serologic studies are typically negative in patients with unstable angina. These tests, therefore, can only be used to rule out the diagnosis of myocardial ischemia with an understanding of their limitations.

Typical ECG manifestations of **myocardial ischemia** are ST-segment depression and T-wave inversions, although NSTEMI can occur without these changes. A number of other conditions can also produce these findings:

- STEMI; ST-segment depression can represent reciprocal changes, and T-wave inversions can be seen late in patients with evolving STEMI.
- Left ventricular hypertrophy with strain pattern
- Digitalis effect
- Hypokalemia
- Myocarditis
- Wolff-Parkinson-White (WPW) syndrome
- Pulmonary embolus
- Some patients with acute cerebral events

ECG manifestations of **STEMI** are of course ST-segment elevations, which typically occur in two or more contiguous leads; the findings of corresponding Q waves and reciprocal ST-segment depressions are helpful in identifying patients with acute myocardial injury. One exception to this rule that acute electrocardiographically detectable infarction is only in the presence of ST elevation is a posterior wall infarction. Isolated posterior infarction produces ST-segment depression, a tall R wave, and upright T waves in leads V1 to V3 given its location relative to the chest leads. Helpful in diagnosing STEMI is the clustering of abnormalities that occurs in predictable leads, which represent specific contiguous areas of the myocardium perfused by specific vessels. The following anatomic areas correspond to changes in the following leads:

- Anterior wall: V1 to V4
- Lateral wall: I, aVL, V5, and V6
- Inferior wall: II, III, and aVF
- Right ventricular wall: V4R
- Posterior wall: V8 and V9; V1 and V2 (ST depression suggests acute infarct)

A 15-lead ECG is sometimes helpful in confirming the diagnosis of **posterior and right ventricular infarction;** after obtaining a standard 12-lead tracing, place leads V4R (the lead is placed on the right anterior chest directly opposite the standard lead V4), V8 (the lead is placed at the level of the fifth anterior intercostal space posteriorly at the left midscapular line), and V9 (the lead is placed at the level of the fifth anterior intercostal space posterior to the left parasternal border). Right ventricular infarction typically occurs in the setting of inferior infarction and produces ST-segment elevation (1 mm is considered significant) in lead V4R. Posterior infarction usually occurs in the setting of inferior or lateral wall infarction; isolated posterior infarction produces ST-segment elevation (1 mm is considered significant) in leads V8 and V9; ST-segment depression and upright T waves in leads V1 to V3 (as mentioned above), an increased (compared with old tracings) or prominent R wave in the right precordial leads, and a wide R wave (greater than 0.04 seconds) in lead V1 are additional findings.

Other conditions associated with ST elevations that may **mimic STEMI** include

- *Left bundle branch block:* Left bundle branch block, specifically, can produce findings difficult to distinguish from AMI; right bundle branch block, generally, should not. Left bundle branch block usually produces a broad, negative QS or rS in lead V1, usually 0.12 seconds or greater. In addition, poor R-wave progression or QS complexes in leads V1 to V3 or V1 to V4 are noted; ST-segment elevations and "hyperacute" T waves can also be seen in these leads; thus, the pattern resembles anterior wall infarction. In the typical pattern, neither Q waves nor S waves are noted in leads I, aVL, or V6. Although the ECG pattern of right bundle branch block can be confused with myocardial infarction (usually inferior, anteroseptal, or posterior), if one remembers the typical changes produced by right bundle branch block, this can be avoided. Typically, a broad QRS complex is noted in V1, with the characteristic rSR or qR morphology, of 0.12 seconds or greater. In general, the diagnosis of infarction should be evident in patients with right bundle branch block since characteristic ST-segment elevation cannot be attributed to the right bundle branch block alone.

- *Left ventricular aneurysm:* Patients with left ventricular aneurysms typically have a history of myocardial infarction, usually anterior; this produces persistent ST elevations in leads V1 to V6, I, and aVL; less commonly, the inferior wall is involved, producing ST elevations in leads II, III, and aVF. This pattern can easily be confused with acute myocardial injury; in the absence of a history of acute infarction or a prior ECG, the absence of reciprocal changes (ST-segment depressions) and the presence of Q waves are helpful diagnostically.

- *Pericarditis:* Pericarditis classically produces diffuse (global) ECG changes as opposed to a particular anatomic distribution.

- *Myocarditis:* Acute myocarditis can produce ST elevations consistent with AMI in virtually any distribution.

- *Early repolarization:* Benign early repolarization can produce T-wave and ST-segment changes that resemble acute myocardial injury; a prior ECG is extremely helpful in these patients. Morphologically, although the ST segment is elevated, the normal concavity (or dipping down) of the upstroke of the T wave is maintained, unlike the characteristic appearance of the T wave in patients with myocardial infarction, which most often appears to have been pulled up (convex). In benign repolarization, ST-segment elevations are usually most pronounced in leads V3 to V4; "hyperacute" T waves may also occasionally be found in these patients. Importantly, reciprocal ST-segment depressions and Q waves are not found.

- *Left ventricular hypertrophy:* Left ventricular hypertrophy can easily be confused with anteroseptal myocardial injury; Q waves and ST-segment elevations can be found in leads V1 to V2. Prominent T waves can also be noted.

- *Wolff-Parkinson-White syndrome:* Wolff-Parkinson-White syndrome results from early excitation of the ventricle via an accessory pathway; patterns resembling acute infarction can occur and are usually confused with inferior, posterior, anteroseptal, or anterolateral infarction, reflecting the variability in pathway location and thus the order of myocardial depolarization. Differentiation is assisted by remembering the ECG findings in the syndrome: short PR interval, wide QRS, and delta wave that slurs or delays the upstroke of the QRS, which is most often most apparent in lead V6. WPW can also produce QRS/T-wave discordance; this means that T waves are negative in leads in which the QRS complexes are positive. Importantly, the changes associated with the WPW syndrome may hide ST elevation in patients with infarction.

- *Hyperkalemia:* Hyperkalemia produces "hyperacute" T waves resembling acute injury.

- *Hypothermia:* The classic Osborn J wave associated with hypothermia resembles ST elevation seen in myocardial infarction.

It is important to note that although historically it has been taught that an AMI cannot be diagnosed electrocardiographically in the setting of a left bundle branch block, there are in fact electrical changes that correlate to acute infarction. These are known as Sgarbossa criteria and, if present in the setting of symptoms suggestive of ACS, are considered diagnostic of AMI.

- Sgarbossa criteria for AMI in the presence of LBBB:
  - ST elevation > or =1 mm and concordant with QRS
  - ST depression > or =1 mm in V1, V2, or V3
  - ST elevation > or =5 mm and discordant with QRS

  Diagnosis of STEMI in the setting of a right bundle branch block does not require special criteria.

Cardiac Markers

Serum markers for AMI are now rapidly available in many EDs.

- **CK-MB** subunits are generally elevated beyond normal limits within 3 to 6 hours of the onset of infarction. To approach 100% sensitivity in diagnosing myocardial infarction, an interval of up to 12 hours after the onset of pain is needed.
- Myoglobin is a small protein liberated from myocardial cells early in infarction; levels are found to be elevated within 1 to 2 hours after the onset of symptoms and peak at approximately 5 hours after myocardial injury. Myoglobin has excellent sensitivity as well as an excellent negative predictive value in acute myocardial injury, but its reduced specificity limits its utility as the sole marker for AMI. Myoglobin is also routinely elevated in patients with renal failure and with musculoskeletal injury. It is often used in conjunction with other more specific markers.
- Myocardial **troponin T and troponin I** are highly specific for the diagnosis of myocardial injury. Troponins T and I are found in the serum 4 to 8 hours after the onset of infarction, remaining elevated for 5 to 6 days. Troponin T is also elevated in approximately 50% of patients with unstable angina and, in these patients, is associated with a relatively increased incidence of proximal myocardial infarction. Troponins T and I, like CK-MB, have a high specificity for myocardial injury.

Echocardiography

Echocardiography can be useful if obtained quickly at the bedside.

The Chest X-ray

The chest x-ray is helpful in diagnosing pneumothorax and pneumonia. While not sensitive for aortic dissection, it can also suggest this diagnosis if the mediastinum is widened.

Treatment

General Approach to Treatment of Acute Coronary Syndrome

The goals of treatment of patients with myocardial infarction are to salvage myocardial cells, increase the amount of oxygen available to the myocardium, and decrease myocardial oxygen consumption. Specific therapeutic options include supplemental oxygen, nitroglycerin, analgesia, antiplatelet agents, anticoagulant therapy, and β-blockade. Ultimately, the main goal is prompt reperfusion of the myocardium experiencing vascular compromise. Options include thrombolytic therapy, percutaneous intervention via angioplasty with or without arterial stenting, or coronary artery bypass grafting (CABG). Reperfusion strategy requires a relative urgency, as "time is muscle," with the ultimate goal being to salvage ischemic myocardium and to minimize irreversible myocardial damage, and therefore to prevent the morbidity associated with ischemic cardiomyopathy and the mortality associated with pump failure and lethal dysrhythmias. The time frame is much more urgent with STEMI than with ACS/NSTEMI. The differences in treatment strategies will be discussed below.

Oxygen. Supplemental oxygen should be provided to all patients to maximize oxygen delivery to the myocardium.

Nitroglycerin. Nitrates operate to reduce preload and afterload and promote vasodilation of coronary arteries, which may enhance collateral blood flow. Patients with normal to elevated blood pressure can be given sublingual nitroglycerin (NTG, 0.4 mg); if blood pressure remains stable, this may be repeated twice at 5-minute intervals. When continued pain is noted, intravenous NTG should be started. Sublingual NTG should be administered cautiously in patients with an initially low or borderline blood pressure (<100 mm Hg systolic) and in patients with significant aortic stenosis or inferior or posterior infarctions, since hypotension may result; consider early intravenous NTG, rather than sublingual NTG, in these patients, the effect of which can rapidly be eliminated, unlike sublingual NTG. In the patient with myocardial infarction, hypotension (and its treatment if particularly low) is clearly best avoided. Intravenous NTG is usually started at 10 to 20 μg/min and can be increased incrementally by 10 μg/min q3–5 min provided the blood pressure remains stable. Antianginal effects are usually noted at doses between 50 and 80 μg/min. Avoid nitrates completely in any patient who in the last 48 hours has taken one of the phosphodiesterase inhibitors used for erectile dysfunction such as sildenafil, tadalafil, or vardenafil, as severe refractory hypotension may result.

Analgesia. In patients with continued pain following NTG therapy, small 2- to 5-mg increments of morphine can be given, which exerts both analgesic and anxiolytic effects. Hypotension is rare if doses are small and titrated; normal saline boluses (250 mL) should be given initially if blood pressure falls.

Antiplatelet Agents. Antiplatelet therapy should be provided to all patients with acute coronary ischemia, including those with myocardial infarctions; significant reductions in morbidity and mortality are produced with little risk. **Aspirin** exerts multiple beneficial effects in patients with myocardial ischemia and infarction; aspirin (162–325 mg) should be given in the ED unless allergy exists or ongoing bleeding is present. Clopidogrel can be given to those patients allergic to aspirin. Further discussion specific to other antiplatelet agents and regimens will follow in sections specific to STEMI and NSTEMI.

Anticoagulation. Anticoagulation with either unfractionated heparin or a low molecular weight heparin significantly reduces morbidity and mortality in myocardial infarction; unless contraindications exist heparin should be given. The initial loading dose for unfractionated heparin is 80 to 100 U/kg, followed by an infusion of 15 to 18 U/kg/h. In obese patients, weight is determined by determining the patient's ideal body weight plus 30% of weight in excess of ideal. The patient's aPTT should be 1.5 to 2.5 control; an aPTT should be determined 6 hours after the beginning of the infusion and 6 hours thereafter. The dose for the most commonly used low molecular weight heparin enoxaparin is 1 mg/kg every 12 hours; adjustments should be made for patients with renal dysfunction.

β-Blockers. These agents reduce oxygen demand by the myocardium. In the setting of STEMI, they should be given unless contraindications exist (see Tables 22-1 and 22-2). Their use in ACS/NSTEMI is less clear. Metoprolol, 5 mg given intravenously over 1 to 2 minutes, is appropriate; this dose may be repeated twice, with 15 mg effectively producing adequate β-blockade in most patients. Contraindications to β-blockage include reactive airway disease, chronic obstructive pulmonary disease, arteriovenous nodal block, congestive heart failure, bradycardia, and hypotension.

STEMI Treatment

Percutaneous Coronary Intervention. The key to treating a patient with STEMI is emergent revascularization. **Percutaneous coronary intervention (PCI)** by an invasive cardiologist is generally preferred over thrombolytic therapy if it is immediately available given some suggestion of superior efficacy as well as less severe bleeding complications. Patients with a contraindication to thrombolytic therapy should clearly be considered candidates for primary PCI. Ninety minutes from the time of arrival to the ED until definitive reperfusion via angioplasty ("door-to-balloon" time) is generally the current standard. Many centers that offer PCI have developed a streamlined system to minimize delays and facilitate urgent treatment once the diagnosis is made. One or more stents are often placed into the opened coronary vessel, which seem to lower the risk of restenosis and reinfarction compared with angioplasty without stenting, although a mortality benefit has not yet been shown.

Controversy exists regarding the optimal treatment of a patient who presents with STEMI to a center that does not offer PCI. For many hospitals, it is difficult to diagnose the STEMI and then proceed to coordinate a transfer of that patient to a center in which he or she can receive primary PCI all in under 90 minutes; delays can significantly jeopardize the patient's myocardium at risk. This makes thrombolytic therapy (discussed below) a first-line agent at most hospitals without this capability. The decision to transfer after thrombolytic administration depends on the institution and may or may not depend on the occurrence of reperfusion. Most patients will undergo angiography after thrombolytic treatment for STEMI, even if thrombolytic therapy is successful in establishing reperfusion, so many hospitals will initiate a transfer to a center that performs PCI either emergently or urgently within the 24 to 48 hours following reperfusion. It is reasonable to transfer to a center capable of PCI without administering thrombolytics if total "door-to-balloon time" (i.e., arrival at the door of the initial ED to PCI at the receiving hospital) is likely to be less than 90 minutes.

Adjunctive Therapy

Antiplatelet agents: Unless a contraindication exists, all patients diagnosed with STEMI who are to undergo primary PCI should receive both aspirin and a thienopyridine, the most commonly used being clopidogrel. This helps to prevent infarct-related reocclusion. Studies are ongoing to establish the optimal loading dose, with 300 to 600 mg being used currently in most protocols.

Controversy exists regarding the use of glycoprotein IIb/IIIa (GP IIb/IIIa) inhibitors prior to PCI. Many institutions have incorporated them into their ACS and STEMI treatment protocols. The timing of their use, which particular agent is used, and whether or not they are used at all will depend on local and regional protocols.

Anticoagulants: Unless a contraindication exists, all patients diagnosed with STEMI who are to undergo primary PCI should be started on an anticoagulation regimen. Either unfractionated heparin or a low molecular weight heparin is acceptable.

Oxygen, nitrates, analgesics, and β-blockers are all indicated as discussed above, again with consideration for any relative contraindications.

Studies are ongoing to determine the relative efficacy of low-dose thrombolytics, with or without GP IIb/IIIa inhibitors, combined with PCI.

Thrombolytic Therapy. Thrombolytic treatment is an alternative treatment for STEMI. As discussed above, the standard ECG evidence of STEMI manifests as 1 mm of ST elevation in two or more anatomically contiguous standard limb leads, 2 mm or more of ST elevation in two or more contiguous precordial leads, or new left bundle branch block. Patients with ACS manifested as ST depression or T-wave inversions, or those with NSTEMI, should *not* receive thrombolytic therapy.

Its efficacy is maximal if given within 3 hours after the onset of symptoms, and within this time frame, the efficacy is similar to PCI in establishing reperfusion. Patients who are treated earlier do better, and every effort should be made to facilitate rapid administration of a thrombolytic agent once eligibility criteria have been met. There is a clear benefit in patients treated within 6 hours of the onset of symptoms and a probable small benefit in patients treated within 12 hours; thrombolytic treatment should not be undertaken in patients with symptoms for more than 12 hours. A possible exception is the patient with onset and remission of symptoms during this 12-hour period, the so-called stuttering presentation; this makes determination of the onset of infarction difficult. In these patients, emergent cardiology consultation should be considered and the rewards/risks discussed in light of other factors. The beneficial effects of thrombolytics are greatest in new coronary artery occlusions and less so in occlusions of bypass grafts. Patients should be screened carefully for contraindications given the risk of hemorrhagic complications (see Table 21-3). Major bleeding occurs as a complication in 0.5% to 5% of patients receiving thrombolytics, the most concerning of which, intracranial hemorrhage, occurring in about 1% of patients.

A number of thrombolytic agents exist, all of which effect thrombolysis by converting plasminogen to plasmin. Available agents are streptokinase, an enzyme secreted by group C β-hemolytic streptococci; human recombinant tissue plasminogen activator (rt-PA or alteplase); reteplase (related to t-PA); and tenecteplase (TNK-t-PA, a genetically altered relative of t-PA). Doses in myocardial infarction are as follows:

Streptokinase: 750,000 U intravenous over 20 minutes followed by 750,000 U over 40 minutes

Alteplase; t-PA: 15-mg bolus followed by 50 mg over the next 30 minutes and 35 mg over the subsequent 60 minutes

Reteplase: 10-U bolus over 2 minutes and second 10-U bolus over 2.5 minutes, 30 minutes after the first bolus

Tenecteplase (TNK-t-PA): single weight-based bolus of 0.5 mg/kg

- **Eligibility criteria.** A table of absolute and relative contraindications is presented in Chapter 21, Table 21-3. Some specific criteria that require discussion are presented below.
  - **Age.** There is no accepted upper limit of age for excluding patients from thrombolytic therapy; the incidence of hemorrhagic stroke, however, does increase with increasing age, particularly over 75 years.
  - **Hypertension.** Patients in the ED with severe hypertension should receive treatment to reduce pain, anxiety, and blood pressure to acceptable levels; if this can be accomplished producing a systolic pressure less than 175 mm Hg, thrombolytic therapy is not contraindicated, although the risk of intracerebral hemorrhage rises with increasing systolic pressures. Patients with persistent blood pressures above 200/120 should not receive thrombolytic therapy; patients with systolic pressures persistently above 175 mm Hg should be considered candidates for PCI as an alternative.
  - **Hypotension.** The role of thrombolytic therapy in patients with hypotension is not clear; some evidence suggests a benefit from immediate thrombolytic therapy followed by PCI in patients with severe hypotension and cardiogenic shock. Cardiology and cardiothoracic surgical consultations should be obtained early in the management of these patients.

- **Retinopathy.** Active diabetic hemorrhagic retinopathy should be considered a strong, relative contraindication to thrombolytic therapy; the risk of intraocular hemorrhage and blindness is significant. Diabetic patients with minor degrees of background retinopathy should not be excluded from treatment.
- **Cardiopulmonary resuscitation (CPR).** If CPR has been prolonged (>10–15 minutes) or if as a result of CPR, evidence of traumatic injury is noted, then thrombolytic therapy should be withheld.
- **Prior stroke/TIA.** A prior hemorrhagic stroke is an absolute contraindication to thrombolytic therapy; a prior thrombotic stroke or transient ischemic attack within the last 6 months should be considered a strong relative contraindication.
- **Recent surgery/trauma.** Although this subject is controversial because of the interpretation of "recent," which has not been consistently defined in all studies, these are both relative contraindications; in patients with surgery or significant trauma within 10 days, primary PCI should be pursued rather than thrombolytic therapy.
- **Prior myocardial infarction.** This not a contraindication to treatment; patients who have received streptokinase should receive a different thrombolytic because of sensitization to streptococcal antigens.
- **Pregnancy.** Pregnancy is a relative contraindication to thrombolytic therapy.
- **Menstruation.** This is not considered a contraindication in appropriate patients, since uterine bleeding can be controlled by vaginal packing.
- **Prior CABG.** The role of thrombolytic therapy in patients presenting with myocardial infarction following CABG is controversial; many patients have been successfully treated. Some centers, because of potential resistance to thrombolytic therapy in completely occluded grafts, recommend early PCI or thrombolytic therapy followed by PCI.
- **Response to thrombolytic therapy**
  Reperfusion is suggested by any of the following three phenomena:
  - Resolution of chest pain
  - Resolution of ST-segment elevations
  - Dysrhythmias suggestive of reperfusion. An accelerated idioventricular rhythm is the most common example.

  Patients with evidence of continuing ischemia following thrombolytic therapy (continued pain or continued or increased ST elevation) should be considered candidates for emergent PCI. This requires careful observation, prompt recognition, and the capability to mobilize one's interventional cardiac team or initiate prompt transfer to a tertiary facility with PCI capability.

Hypotension and Acute Pulmonary Edema

This scenario presents the emergency physician with a difficult management problem. Initially, it is important to recognize two factors: (1) due to maximal vasoconstriction in these patients, peripheral cuff determinations of blood pressure are frequently incorrect and usually underestimated, often significantly, true arterial pressure; and (2) a relatively high percentage of patients with acute pulmonary edema and hypotension have modest degrees of volume depletion. This obviously occurs in addition to severely depressed myocardial function, which is somewhat counterintuitive; if present, it is easily remediable.

This implies that direct arterial blood pressure monitoring and objective determination of pulmonary artery occlusion pressures can be helpful. Unfortunately, in this scenario, one may not have adequate time to obtain this information; in addition, the physical examination with regard to determining left-sided filling pressures is usually not helpful. It is not unreasonable therefore to administer a cautious fluid challenge: 250 mL of normal saline over 5 to 10 minutes can be given during which time patients should be closely observed by the physician; if systolic pressure increases somewhat and/or if respiratory function remains stable, an additional 250 mL of saline can be administered.

Patients failing to respond will require further support of blood pressure with vasopressors and positive inotropic agents. **Dopamine's** effect on the vasculature and the heart varies significantly with the dose administered; at doses between 2 and 5 µg/kg/min, there is predominantly a vasodilator effect, most pronounced in the renal vasculature; at doses between 5 and 15 µg/kg/min, modest increases in myocardial contractility and heart rate are noted; at doses greater than 15 µg/kg/min, dopamine acts as a vasoconstrictive agent, resembling norepinephrine. The effects of dopamine, except when used at the lowest dosage range, in patients with acute pulmonary edema, particularly in the setting of an AMI, are not all beneficial; for this reason, dopamine is usually started at a low dose, after blood pressure has responded to α-agents, in which case the renal vasodilatory effects are helpful in maintaining renal output. **Dobutamine** is primarily a vasodilator, with positive inotropic effects. This agent should not be used alone in hypotensive patients because of the risk of precipitating or worsening hypotension; due to this agent's ability to increase cardiac output with less effect on heart rate, dobutamine is probably the agent of choice in normotensive or hypertensive patients with congestive heart failure and myocardial infarction. Dobutamine is usually started at a dose of 2 µg/kg/min and can be gradually increased to 10 to 20 µg/kg/min. **Norepinephrine** is a vasoconstrictor, which is helpful in restoring blood pressure in normovolemic patients with severe hypotension, after which low doses of dopamine or dobutamine can be added to augment renal blood flow and cardiac output. **Amrinone,** an agent that increases cyclic adenosine monophosphate in the myocardial cells, has positive inotropic effects and can be administered as a temporizing measure.

Acute Coronary Syndrome: Unstable Angina and NSTEMI

The diagnosis of **angina pectoris** implies reversible myocardial ischemia. The initial clinical presentation of patients with angina pectoris is frequently impossible to distinguish from that of patients with myocardial infarction. For this reason, any patient with chest pain that the physician suspects may be due to myocardial ischemia must be treated as having a myocardial infarction in evolution or an ACS. Only patients who have a history of chronic, stable angina pectoris and who present with chest pain representing, in all respects, a typical episode may be treated as having truly stable angina (i.e., with the administration of sublingual NTG and/or appropriate adjustment of their chronic outpatient antianginal regimen). All other patients must be considered to have at least ACS if not an evolving myocardial infarction.

The diagnosis of **unstable angina**, which is included in the spectrum of ACS, refers to anginal pain that has increased in frequency or severity compared with the patient's prior, stable anginal pattern; angina occurring at rest or the new onset or first episode of pain compatible with angina is similarly considered an unstable presentation. By definition, the diagnosis of unstable angina connotes a potentially life-threatening myocardial ischemic process that may evolve into frank infarction.

The emergency treatment of such patients with ACS is similar to that of patients with myocardial infarction, short of emergent revascularization: prompt pain relief with intravenous morphine sulfate; the administration of oxygen, aspirin, and anticoagulation; the use of nitroglycerin for pain control, additional antiplatelet agents (clopidogrel or GP IIb/IIIa inhibitors) depending on the local protocol; ECG monitoring; and prompt admission to a coronary care unit or a hospital bed with central cardiac monitoring capability. The timing of angiography and subsequent treatment (PCI, CABG, or medical management only) is ultimately the decision of the consulting cardiologist, although those patients who demonstrate elevated cardiac enzymes and are therefore categorized as NSTEMI are often treated somewhat more aggressively; that is, they create a lower threshold for urgent angiography.

Pleuritis

Pleuritis, or pleurisy, is an inflammatory process involving the pleura that has many causes, including viral pleurodynia, pleural-based pneumonia, pulmonary infarction due to pulmonary embolism, and neoplastic involvement of the pleura; pneumothorax, acute costochondritis, and intercostal muscle strain may also present with pleuritic discomfort and should also be considered.

History
Regardless of the cause, patients typically report a history of sharp, often "knifelike" pain, usually well localized to a particular region of the chest or back, that is typically increased with inspiration, cough, or sneeze.

Physical Examination
On physical examination, patients may be splinting with shallow and rapid respirations. If pleuritis is associated with a pulmonary parenchymal process such as pneumonia, signs of consolidation, including dullness to percussion, locally decreased breath sounds, and egophony may be apparent. A pleural friction rub may be heard in some patients.

Diagnostic Tests
If the chest radiograph is normal, symptoms are probably due to viral pleurodynia (Bornholm disease; coxsackie group B viral infection), early pneumonitis, or pulmonary embolism. Arterial blood gas measurements may be consistent with simple hypoventilation if splinting is severe enough to impair ventilation, or a frankly widened alveolar-arterial oxygen gradient may be noted if a pulmonary parenchymal process sufficiently impairs oxygenation.

Treatment
Treatment is directed toward the underlying cause. The diagnosis and treatment of pneumonia are discussed in "Specific Disorders," in Chapter 19, and that of pulmonary embolism in "Pulmonary Embolism." In patients with severe pleurodynia, pain relief is essential to eliminate splinting and thus prevent the development of infection and optimize ventilation. In many patients, a narcotic analgesic is required; in addition, a nonsteroidal anti-inflammatory agent such as ibuprofen or indomethacin may be helpful. If more serious diagnoses have been ruled out, outpatient treatment is appropriate.

Pericarditis

Among the causes of pericarditis (inflammation of the pericardium) are included infections (viral, tubercular, and rarely, bacterial), autoimmune disorders (systemic lupus erythematosus, rheumatoid arthritis); renal failure; and neoplastic disorders (especially adenocarcinoma of the breast and squamous cell carcinoma of the lung).

History

Patients typically relate to a history of severe, sharp, substernal chest pain made worse with inspiration, recumbency, coughing, and movement, and often relieved by sitting forward.

Physical Examination

Physical examination may reveal a friction rub, often postural, usually heard best with the patient sitting forward at end expiration. If a hemodynamically significant pericardial effusion accompanies the inflammatory process, signs of cardiac tamponade may be noted, including hypotension, tachycardia, a narrow pulse pressure, distended neck veins that do not collapse on inspiration, and faint heart sounds.

Diagnostic Tests

The earliest change on the ECG is PR-segment depression, after which J point and ST-segment elevation evolve, often globally. If a significant pericardial effusion is present, the ECG may reveal R waves of low voltage or electrical alternans. Chest radiographs may be normal or, if a large pericardial effusion is present, may demonstrate an enlarged cardiac silhouette with a "water bottle" configuration. M-mode and two-dimensional echocardiography are the diagnostic procedures of choice if a pericardial effusion is suspected; however, aside from demonstrating mild pericardial thickening and a small effusion, echocardiography in many patients with simple pericarditis is unrevealing. The diagnosis of an effusion in the presence of diastolic right ventricular collapse is diagnostic of tamponade.

Treatment

Treatment is directed at the underlying cause of the pericarditis, including antibiotics for bacterial and tuberculous infections, irradiation for carcinomatous etiologies, and hemodialysis in renal failure. When a viral infection is believed to be the cause (coxsackie virus A and B, adenovirus, echovirus 8), a nonsteroidal anti-inflammatory agent may be given (indomethacin or ibuprofen); it is important to note that if any suspicion exists that an effusion may be hemorrhagic, the use of these agents should be avoided. If hemodynamically significant tamponade exists, emergency pericardiocentesis may be lifesaving.

Costochondritis

Costochondritis is an acute, self-limited, inflammatory process involving the costosternal articulations. Patients report unilateral, pleuritic, peristernal pain, the onset of which may be perceived as gradual or sudden, is typically increased by maneuvers that produce motion of the costochondral joints, and frequently radiates along the course of the involved rib toward the side or back. A subjective sensation of breathlessness often accompanies the discomfort, and a history of a preceding upper respiratory tract infection is occasionally obtained.

Diagnosis

The diagnosis depends on the clear-cut demonstration of localized costochondral junction tenderness with palpation; elicited discomfort should be very similar to the patient's particular pain syndrome.

Treatment

Treatment involves reassurance regarding the benign nature of the disorder; discomfort usually lasts 5 to 12 days without treatment and 4 to 7 days with treatment. The use of a nonsteroidal anti-inflammatory agent such as ibuprofen or indomethacin is recommended. A narcotic analgesic may be required in some patients with severe discomfort. Some patients may find that local heat is symptomatically helpful.

Esophagitis

Esophagitis occurs as a result of the reflux of gastric acid from the stomach into the distal esophagus.

Diagnosis

Patients often give a history of epigastric or retrosternal burning radiating toward the neck; some note a bitter or acidic taste accompanying the discomfort. Symptoms are often precipitated by large meals or recumbency and are relieved by antacids or food intake. The physical examination is often unrevealing; rarely, however, subxiphoid discomfort may be noted on palpation.

It should be noted that the use of antacids as a diagnostic maneuver is ill advised. There is no evidence that relief of symptoms with antacids reliably excludes other more serious diagnoses and may in fact mislead the clinician away from the necessary pursuit of such entities.

Treatment

Treatment involves the use of antacids (30 mL 30 minutes after meals and at bedtime), the avoidance of large meals, particularly before bedtime, and elevation of the head of the bed; these latter measures simply decrease the probability of reflux. Some patients with particularly severe symptoms will respond to the addition of an H_2-receptor blocker or a proton pump inhibitor.

It is important to note that patients with the acquired immunodeficiency syndrome or those who are currently receiving immunosuppressive therapy or who have been maintained for long periods of time on broad-spectrum antibiotics may have **monilial esophagitis** or, rarely, **herpetic esophagitis.** An appropriate diagnosis in these patients requires a high degree of suspicion and confirmation by barium swallow or esophagoscopy.

Spontaneous Pneumothorax

Spontaneous pneumothorax develops when air enters the pleural space as a result of the rupture of previously asymptomatic blebs on the pleural surface.

History

This disorder most often occurs in young, healthy adults who present with a history of the sudden onset of unilateral, pleuritic, chest or back pain and varying degrees of associated dyspnea.

Physical Examination

Physical examination may be normal or may demonstrate diminished breath sounds and hyperresonance to percussion on the affected side, although breath sounds are often equal.

End-Expiratory Upright Chest Radiograph

An end-expiratory upright chest radiograph is diagnostic and demonstrates peripheral absence of pulmonary markings frequently delineated by a clearly defined pleural stripe. Nonexpiratory radiographs do not reliably demonstrate small pneumothoraces, and supine radiographs, which allow air to layer uniformly anteriorly, may also obscure the diagnosis. The perceived percent of pneumothorax based on the posteroanterior and lateral chest radiographs is often an underestimate; this is due to the inherent topologic difficulties in portraying an approximately spherical structure in two dimensions.

Treatment
Treatment depends on the size of the pneumothorax and the presence or absence of symptoms. Generally, patients with small pneumothoraces without significant discomfort or dyspnea should be managed by a simple period of observation, which is advised to ensure that the pneumothorax is stable and resolving. In patients requiring only observation, resolution of pleural air may be facilitated by breathing 100% oxygen by mask. Patients with larger pneumothoraces (i.e., more than 15%–25%) and/or significant symptoms will require chest tube insertion. Smaller pig-tailed catheters connected to a one-way valve are available as a somewhat less invasive alternative.

Spontaneous Tension Pneumothorax

A tension pneumothorax will develop in a relatively small fraction of patients with spontaneous pneumothorax. Tension pneumothorax occurs when air continues to enter the pleural space through a ball-valve or "one-way" rent in the visceral pleura; progressively increasing pleural pressures eventually compromise venous return, resulting in rapidly evolving circulatory collapse.

Diagnosis
A prompt diagnosis is mandatory and is based on unilaterally absent or decreased breath sounds, percussion hyperresonance on the affected side, and evidence of ongoing or impending circulatory compromise. Tracheal deviation away from the side of collapse is sometimes noted. Conscious patients are dyspneic and may complain of pleuritic pain.

Treatment
Patients in whom this diagnosis is suspected and who are too unstable to undergo definitive chest tube placement should be treated immediately with large-bore (14- or 16-gauge) needle aspiration of the affected side through the second intercostal space anteriorly entering along the superior margin of the third rib at the midclavicular line. As the pleural space is entered, air will rapidly escape, providing temporary treatment and confirmation of the diagnosis; chest tube insertion should then be performed promptly. If the patient is relatively stable, it is reasonable to consider proceeding right to chest tube insertion, without needle decompression, if it can be done promptly.

Acute Thoracic Aortic Dissection

Acute dissection of the aorta occurs when blood suddenly enters the aortic wall through a spontaneous intimal tear and dissects along its course. Patients (predominantly men in the fifth to seventh decades of life) give a history of the sudden onset of severe chest pain often radiating to the back; pain is frequently said to have a "ripping" or "tearing" quality. The intensity of discomfort associated with aortic dissection is typically maximal at its onset. Most patients are hypertensive when seen (unless already compromised by complications) and/or have a history of hypertension or Marfan syndrome. Other causes include atherosclerosis, cystic medial necrosis, giant cell arteritis, Ehlers-Danlos syndrome, idiopathic kyphoscoliosis, coarctation of the aorta, aortic hypoplasia, pregnancy, and relapsing polychondritis.

From the standpoint of the physical examination and patient management, it is useful to divide patients into two anatomic categories using the Stanford classification: type A dissections involve the ascending aorta; type B dissections involve only the descending aorta. This classification system is helpful in that type A dissections are generally treated surgically while type B dissections are generally treated medically.

Ascending Aortic Dissections (Type A)

In patients with ascending aortic dissections, severe chest or interscapular pain or both develop suddenly. Since these dissections originate at or near the aortic valve and sweep along the aortic arch, signs and symptoms related to the interruption of carotid blood flow are frequently present; these may be transient and include syncope, cranial nerve palsies, and hemiparesis.

Diagnosis

The absence of a carotid pulse or asymmetry of the carotid pulses is an important physical sign. In addition, a difference in the blood pressure between the right and left arm may occur. Because retrograde dissection involving the aortic valve ring develops in approximately 50% of patients with ascending aortic dissections, the development of a new aortic regurgitant murmur is especially important.

Derangements in coronary blood flow related to retrograde dissection occur in a significant number of patients, and ECG abnormalities compatible with acute myocardial injury are found in up to 45% of patients. Extension of the dissection into the pericardium may produce cardiac tamponade, the most common cause of death. Tamponade should be strongly considered when signs of right-sided heart failure and hypotension develop in patients suspected of acute dissection.

Useful diagnostic tests in the evaluation of these patients include transesophageal echocardiography, vascular magnetic resonance imaging (magnetic resonance angiography), CT angiography (generally the most widely available), and aortography. Significant widening of the upper mediastinum on posterior-anterior chest radiograph, especially if not present on prior films, is diagnostically useful, although not particularly sensitive.

Treatment

If the diagnosis of acute dissection is suspected, **medical stabilization** should be undertaken immediately while emergency imaging is arranged. Medical stabilization involves the pharmacologic control of blood pressure and the reduction of cardiac contractility. For these purposes, consider administering a β-blocker such as metoprolol (5 mg IV push q3–5 minutes, up to 15 mg) while emergency imaging is arranged. A heart rate of 60 to 80 beats/min is optimal. If constant blood pressure monitoring is available, IV nitroprusside (beginning at 0.5–1.0 µg/kg/min) should be added, the goal being to maintain the systolic pressure between 100 and 120 mm Hg. Nitroprusside should not be administered without a β-blocker having been given previously to prevent the associated reflex tachycardia. Most patients with ascending aortic dissections who are acceptable surgical candidates will require early surgical repair, and prompt thoracic surgical consultation is therefore critical. **Labetalol**, a mixed α- and β-blocker, can be used as a single agent; an initial bolus of 10 to 20 mg is given i.v., which can be increased and repeated, and followed up by a continuous infusion of 1 to 2 mg/min.

Descending Aortic Dissections (Type B)

Descending aortic dissections (type B) often begin near the origin of the left subclavian artery and then dissect distally; many patients will therefore complain of lumbar pain in addition to chest or back discomfort.

Diagnosis

Mediastinal widening on the chest radiograph is important to note because other signs and symptoms are frequently absent in these patients. For example, carotid pulses are normal and symmetric because retrograde extension from the site of origin of the dissection is rare; for the same reason, new aortic regurgitant murmurs are not noted. As for type A dissections, CT angiography, MRI/MRA, or transesophageal echocardiography is the diagnostic modality of choice.

Treatment

Medical stabilization to control blood pressure and heart rate, as discussed above for type A dissections, should be initiated immediately in these patients. Most descending thoracic aortic dissections can be managed medically, and many patients will not require surgical repair. Indications for operative repair are retrograde dissection with consequent proximal aortic involvement, continued pain despite adequate medical stabilization, and the occurrence of significant hemorrhagic (hemothorax, retroperitoneal hemorrhage) or ischemic complications (renal, spinal, lower extremity). Given the possibility of these complications, patients should be admitted to an intensive care setting with cardiothoracic and vascular surgical consultations.

24 Hypertension

INTRODUCTION

Most patients with hypertension are asymptomatic. The diagnosis is suggested in the emergency department when vital signs are routinely checked. Hypertension is defined as a systolic blood pressure (BP) greater than 140 mm Hg or a diastolic pressure greater than 90 mm Hg. A diagnosis of hypertension is established based on the average of at least two properly measured, seated BP readings on each of two or more office visits. The importance of diagnosing an individual as hypertensive rests on the observation made in multiple studies that cardiovascular and cerebrovascular mortality and morbidity correlate directly with the degree of BP elevation over time. Studies indicate that treatment of patients with even mild hypertension (i.e., diastolic pressures between 90 and 105 mm Hg) may be quite beneficial, although some experts do not agree that there is significant benefit in treating patients with borderline hypertension. Elevated BP readings in the emergency department should be repeated and addressed appropriately.

One concern with elevated BP in the emergency department is that pain or stress may transiently elevate BP. Asymptomatic patients with systolic BP greater than 140 mm Hg or diastolic BP greater than 90 mm Hg should be referred for follow-up of possible hypertension.

Most patients with hypertension will be defined as having essential hypertension in that no secondary cause is discovered after a detailed investigation. However, given that as many as 10% of patients will have a secondary cause, screening for these potential causes is important. Diseases and conditions that cause hypertension include renal disease and renal artery stenosis, primary hyperaldosteronism, Cushing syndrome, pheochromocytoma, coarctation of the aorta, estrogen use, pregnancy, medications (especially NSAIDs), various street drugs, hypercalcemia from any cause, neurologic diseases with increased intracranial pressure (ICP), acromegaly, and hypothyroidism or hyperthyroidism. Evaluation is focused on identifying cardiovascular, renal, neurologic, and ophthalmic end organ damage.

HISTORY

The patient should be questioned as to any previous history of hypertension or documented BP determinations. Symptoms of dyspnea, headaches, chest pain, or palpitations should be sought, as should any family history of hypertension. The use of birth control pills, cold preparations, nasal sprays, steroids, thyroid hormones, cocaine, or amphetamines should be identified.

PHYSICAL EXAMINATION

BP should be determined in both arms. Funduscopy should be performed to detect the presence of retinopathic changes consistent with acute or long-standing hypertension. An S_4 or signs of congestive heart failure should be noted as well. Bruits should be sought in the abdomen.

DIAGNOSTIC TESTS

Diagnostic screening tests for evidence of target organ damage in an asymptomatic patient may include urinalysis, serum creatinine level, electrocardiogram, and chest X-ray. Of these, urine dipstick is the only diagnostic ED test with evidence to support its routine use.

TREATMENT

Treatment of Patients with Newly-Discovered Asymptomatic Hypertension

Initiating treatment for asymptomatic hypertension in the ED is not necessary when patients in the ED have follow-up. Rapidly lowering BP in asymptomatic patients in the ED is unnecessary and may be harmful. Patients with persistent BP greater than 180/110 without evidence of end organ damage should be started on antihypertensive therapy in consultation with the primary physician, and close follow-up assured.

Treatment of Asymptomatic Known Hypertensive Patients with Elevated BP

Noncompliant patients should be counseled to resume their prior antihypertensive regimens with referral to their primary physician. Compliant patients may have their antihypertensive therapy stepped up, in consultation with their primary physician. Alternatively, they may be referred to their primary physician for any therapy changes.

Asymptomatic patients with markedly elevated BP without acute or progressive end organ disease may be managed on an outpatient basis. Those at higher risk of near-term complications or with existing end organ disease may be managed in consultation with their primary physician but do not require acute lowering of BP.

HYPERTENSIVE CRISES

Hypertensive Encephalopathy

Hypertensive encephalopathy consists of severe hypertension, altered mental status, and papilledema. Headache and seizures may occur. The pathophysiologic mechanism is cerebral hyperperfusion leading to loss of autoregulation with edema, hemorrhage, and coma. Brain CT may demonstrate characteristic findings in parietooccipital white matter. Treatment options include:

Labetalol	20–80 mg IV bolus every 10 min
	0.5–2.0 mg/min infusion
Nitroprusside	0.25 µg/kg/min
	Titrate upward to max 10 µg/kg/min
Nicardipine	5–15 mg/h IV
Fenoldopam	0.1–0.3 µg/kg/min IV

Accelerated Malignant Hypertension

Accelerated malignant hypertension consists of severe hypertension and retinopathy characterized by flame hemorrhages and papilledema. Headache and visual blurring occur. Mental status is normal. It is caused by decompensation of endothelial vasodilatory mechanisms. Renal insufficiency with proteinuria and hematuria occurs.

Treatment options: Same as above.

Cardiovascular Crises

Cardiovascular crises include acute coronary syndrome, acute pulmonary edema, and acute aortic dissection.

Treatment options:

1. Acute coronary syndrom (ACS): Nitroglycerin 5 to 100 µg/min IV.
2. Pulmonary edema: Nitroglycerin, plus enalaprit—1.25 to 5 mg IV (avoid in ACS) and furosemide if fluid-overloaded.
3. Aortic dissection—target systolic BP less than 120
   - Esmolol PLUS nitroprusside
     ∘ Esmolol 250 µg/kg IV bolus over 1 minute and then 50 to 100 µg/kg/min infusion.
     ∘ Must be initiated PRIOR to nitroprusside to avoid effects of possible reflex tachycardia.
     ∘ Nitroprusside 0.25 µg/kg/min; titrate to maximum 10 µg/kg/min

   OR
   - Labetalol 20 to 80 mg bolus IV every 10 minutes with 0.5 to 2.0 mg/min infusion.

Cerebrovascular Crises

Cerebrovascular crises include ischemia and hemorrhage. Loss of cerebral autoregulation is the mechanism. Allow BP to remain elevated at 220/120 in ischemic stroke to maintain cerebral perfusion. If thrombolytic therapy is indicated, control BP to less than 185/110 with

Nicardipine	5–15 mg/h IV
Labetalol	20–80 mg IV bolus
	0.5–2.0 mg/min infusion

For hemorrhagic stroke, control BP to less than 180 systolic (mean arterial pressure (MAP) <130) for patients with suspected elevated ICP. If ICP is not raised, target BP control to 160/90 (MAP 110) with

Nicardipine	5–15 mg/h IV
Labetalol	20–80 mg IV bolus
	0.5–2.0 mg/min infusion

Renovascuclar Crises

Renovascuclar crises include acute glomerulonephrites of many etiologies and renal artery stenosis. Acute renal failure occurs.

Treatment options include

Labetalol	20–80 mg bolus IV
	0.5–2.0 mg/min infusion
Nitroprusside	0.25 µg/kg/min IV
	Titrate to maximum 10 µg/kg/min

Catecholamine Crises

Catecholamine crises include drug-induced (sympathomimetics, monoamineoxidase inhibitor (MAOI) reactions), pheochromocytomas, and withdrawal syndromes (clonidine, beta-blockers, alcohol). Pheochromocytoma is treated with Phentolamine 5 to 15 mg IV. If tachycardia occurs, a beta-blocker (Esmolol) should be added.

Other catecholamine hypertensive crises may be treated with

Labetalol	20– 80 mg IV bolus
	0.5–2.0 mg/min infusion

Pregnancy Associated Hypertension

Pregnancy associated hypertension consists of preeclampsia, defined as BP greater than 140/90 (or increase >30/15 over baseline) with proteinuria and edema from 20 weeks' gestation to 2 weeks postpartum. Eclampsia is defined by the occurrence of seizures in this setting. Magnesium (2–4 g IV over 30 minutes followed by 2 g/h infusion) is indicated for seizures, with arrangements for emergent delivery. Options for treatment of hypertension include

Labetalol	20–80 mg IV bolus
	0.5–2.0 mg/min infusion
Hydralazine	5–10 mg IV every 20 min

With all hypertensive crises, patients require ICU admission. Care must be taken to avoid precipitous declines in BP with initiation of titratable antihypertensive infusions. Complications of the presenting symptom complex must be simultaneously managed appropriately. Appropriate expert consultation should be sought, including consideration to pharmacology staff if available.

25 Palpitations

INTRODUCTION

Patients who present to the emergency department reporting palpitations generally are placed into one of three pathophysiologic categories: those with tachyarrhythmias or premature contractions, those with chest wall causes, and those without discernible cause. All patients who present with palpitations must be promptly evaluated: first, for hemodynamic stability as determined by the pulse and blood pressure; and second, for the presence or absence of clinical or electrocardiographic (ECG) evidence of ventricular dysfunction or myocardial ischemia, respectively. The heart rate and rhythm may then be assessed, because these often provide the only clue to the cause of the dysrhythmia, especially if palpitations are paroxysmal and not present when the patient is subsequently evaluated. In all patients, the presence of chest pain, lightheadedness, or dyspnea in association with palpitations must be carefully investigated. An ECG is essential for all patients, and if the palpitations are paroxysmal or associated with significant symptoms, in-hospital monitoring, a 24-hour Holter monitor, and/or exercise testing may be required to unmask potential dysrhythmias.

There are two distinct classes of dysrhythmia that commonly produce palpitations: sustained tachyarrhythmias and premature depolarizations. It is interesting and remains unexplained that only some patients with these disorders sense or are troubled by palpitations. An important but benign cause for palpitations is simply forceful ventricular contractions often associated with anxiety, excitement, or exercise. Chest wall muscle contractions may also produce the symptom of palpitations and usually require no further investigation. Finally, in a significant number of patients with palpitations, there will be no discernible cause. The remainder of this chapter presents a discussion of the differential diagnosis and treatment of the dysrhythmic causes of palpitations.

SUPRAVENTRICULAR TACHYDYSRHYTHMIAS

Supraventricular tachycardias (SVTs) have rates greater than 100 beats/min, the origin of which is at or above the atrioventricular (AV) node. Various methods for classifying and diagnosing these dysrhythmias exist and must be carefully followed to ensure appropriate diagnosis and therapy. A diagnostic classification can be made on the basis of three variables readily assessable from the ECG: rate, regularity, and QRS width.

Rate

The rate of an SVT is useful in limiting the diagnostic classes to which it may belong.

Sinus Tachycardia

Sinus tachycardia may range from 100 to 180 beats/min in middle-aged or older patients but may exceed 200 beats/min in the young and very healthy.

Paroxysmal Reentrant Supraventricular Tachycardia

Paroxysmal reentrant supraventricular tachycardia (PSVT) most commonly is associated with an AV nodal reentry mechanism (60% of cases) and less so with an accessory (extranodal) bypass tract (25%). Sinus node reentry, intra-atrial reentry, and automatic atrial tachycardia compose the remainder of cases of PSVT. This dysrhythmia ranges from 150 to 220 beats/min, achieving rates as rapid as 260 beats/min in young patients and as slow as 120 beats/min in patients on quinidine or procainamide.

Nonparoxysmal AV Junctional Tachycardias

Nonparoxysmal AV junctional tachycardias range from 70 to 130 beats/min, reflect accelerated autonomic discharge in or near the bundle of His, and are often seen in association with digitalis toxicity.

Atrial Flutter

Atrial flutter ranges from 240 to 360 beats/min, with 2:1 AV conduction producing a ventricular response from 120 to 180 beats/min. Rarely, especially in young patients, 1:1 AV conduction occurs, producing ventricular rates ranging from 240 to 360 beats/min.

Atrial Fibrillation

Atrial fibrillation ranges from 100 to 160 beats/min.

Multifocal Atrial Tachycardia

Multifocal atrial tachycardia, a disorder with which atrial fibrillation is commonly confused, ranges from 100 to 160 beats/min.

Atrial Tachycardia with AV Block

Atrial tachycardia with AV block, usually associated with digitalis toxicity, commonly presents with ventricular rates ranging from 70 to 120 beats/min.

Regularity

The regularity of an SVT is useful for distinguishing between two general classes. Atrial fibrillation and multifocal atrial tachycardia are irregularly irregular, whereas all other SVTs are regular unless high-grade block develops in the AV node. For example, atrial tachycardia may be associated with 3:2 AV nodal Wenckebach block, thereby producing an irregular ventricular response.

Width

The width of the QRS complex may also be useful in determining the general site of origin of a tachydysrhythmia. **Narrow-complex tachydysrhythmias** are supraventricular (or at least high junctional) by definition. **Wide-complex tachydysrhythmias** may be supraventricular (with aberrant conduction) or ventricular. Several useful differential points may be used to distinguish SVTs with aberrancy from ventricular tachycardia (VT); these are listed in Table 25-1.

AV Bypass Tracts

The special case of AV bypass tracts as a cause for SVTs deserves further clarification. An SVT involving a bypass tract usually produces a narrow complex, given that in most cases, conduction progresses antegrade down the normal conduction pathway and retrograde up the bypass tract. Frequently, however, the bypass tract itself conducts in an antegrade fashion, producing a wide complex SVT. Patients

Table 25-1	Distinguishing VT from SVT with Aberrancy	
	VT	**SVT with Aberrancy**
QRS width	Often ≥0.14 s	Usually <0.14 s
QRS width, onset to S-trough	≥ 0.11 s	<0.11 s
Axis	Bizarre	Normal
V_1	Rs, Rsr', RsR'	rsR'
V_6	S wave present	S wave absent
Fusion beats	Present	Absent
AV dissociation	Present	Absent

with bypass tracts may present in atrial fibrillation with rapid ventricular responses (200–300 beats/min); this form of bypass conduction is most serious, because VT or ventricular fibrillation may develop. If a bypass tract is suspected because of a short PR interval or a delta wave on the ECG (Wolff-Parkinson-White [WPW] syndrome), extreme caution must be taken with the selection of therapy for tachydysrhythmias.

- WPW with *regular, narrow* complex tachycardia:
  - Adenosine—6 mg rapid IV push through a large vein followed by a 20 mL saline flush. If no conversion in 2 minutes, repeat 12 mg bolus twice.
  - Metoprolol—5 mg slow IV every 5 minutes to a total of 15 mg
- WPW with *wide* complex, *rapid atrial fibrillation*: *Note*: Calcium channel blockers are *contraindicated* because they accelerate conduction through the bypass tract, leading to rapid atrial fibrillation that may deteriorate into VT or fibrillation.
  - Amiodarone—150 mg IV over 10 minutes, followed by 1 mg/min infusion
  - Procainamide—20 mg/min IV infusion until total of 17 mg/kg. Discontinue for hypotension or widening of QRS more than 50%. Maintenance infusion 1 to 4 mg/min. Avoid procainamide in patients with impaired left ventricular function.
- WPW with rapid atrial flutter:
  - Amiodarone—If the patient is hemodynamically unstable or has evidence of myocardial ischemia or dysfunction, synchronized direct current (DC) electrical cardioversion should be immediately attempted using 50 to 100 J.

Diagnostic and Therapeutic Maneuvers
All patients should be assessed for clinical states causing tachydysrhythmias as a physiologic response, such as dehydration, hypoxemia, and fever. These primary causes of a secondary tachydysrhythmia should always be corrected prior to instituting any antidysrhythmic therapy.

Hemodynamically Stable Patient
In the **hemodynamically stable patient,** diagnostic maneuvers that may cause vagal stimulation (carotid sinus pressure, Valsalva maneuver, or cold stimulation of the face) be used to evaluate a narrow-complex tachydysrhythmia.

Carotid Sinus Pressure
Carotid sinus pressure requires that the patient has no evidence of significant carotid atherosclerosis (i.e., no bruits or previous carotid surgery) before its application. After

establishing IV access, firm digital pressure is applied to the left carotid bulb for 3 seconds with continual ECG monitoring. If significant asystole, AV block, or ventricular ectopic activity develops, digitalis toxicity should be suspected, vagal maneuvers abandoned, and appropriate treatment instituted. If left carotid sinus pressure fails to alter the SVT, the right carotid may be compressed. Some authorities believe that the right vagus nerve preferentially innervates the sinus node, whereas the left sends fibers primarily to the AV node; hence, differing response may occur to left and right carotid sinus pressure. If carotid sinus pressure alone fails, it may be effective in conjunction with other maneuvers that augment parasympathetic tone through the AV node, for example, a simultaneous Valsalva maneuver. Continual ECG monitoring must be maintained. Never compress both carotids simultaneously.

One important effect of vagal maneuvers in the patient with underlying atrial flutter is to "unmask" this dysrhythmia. When enhancement of AV block occurs as a result of carotid sinus pressure or a Valsalva maneuver, typical, regular, "sawtooth" flutter waves are often observed at a rate of approximately 300 beats/min. In these patients, elective DC cardioversion is the treatment of choice.

Pharmacologic Agents

If vagal maneuvers fail to convert the SVT or to unmask flutter, **pharmacologic agents** may be used.

- **Adenosine** is the drug of choice for initial use. Administered as a rapid bolus of 6 mg in a proximal peripheral vein, its effects occur within 15 to 30 seconds and last only a few seconds. If ineffective, 12-mg doses can be administered twice.
- **Diltiazem (Cardizem)** is effective in slowing paroxysmal atrial fibrillation and flutter. It is contraindicated when accessory or bypass tracts are suspected (short PR interval, delta waves, or rates more than 250 beats/min). Diltiazem is administered 20 mg (0.25 mg/kg) intravenously by slow push over 2 minutes and may be repeated at 25 mg (0.35 mg/kg) in 15 minutes. Initiate infusion at 5 to 10 mg/h.
- **Digoxin,** 0.5 mg, may be administered intravenously over 5 to 10 minutes, with a peak effect expected in 1 hour. This is followed by 0.25-mg doses intravenously every 2 to 4 hours up to a total of 1 to 1.25 mg. It is effective in atrial fibrillation and flutter.
- **Metroprolol,** 5 mg every 5 minutes times 3 may be administered intravenously up to 0.1 mg/kg while the ECG and blood pressure are monitored. Esmolol is given 500 µg/kg IV over 1 minute, followed by maintenance, sequential step-up infusion rates of 50, 100, 150, 200, 250, and 300 µg/kg/min, every 4 or more minutes. *Due to the myocardial depressant effects of metoprolol and diltiazem, extreme caution must be taken if they are to be used together.*

ECG Features

Table 25-2 indicates the important differential ECG features of the standard SVTs previously described; responses to vagal maneuvers and pharmacologic agents are also listed.

Hemodynamic Compromise, Chest Pain, or ECG Evidence of Ischemia

When hemodynamic compromise, chest pain, or ECG evidence of ischemia is present, electrical **cardioversion** is indicated to terminate the tachydysrhythmias. With atrial fibrillation of uncertain duration over 72 hours, 2 weeks of anticoagulation prior to cardioversion may be needed to prevent embolism from an atrial thrombus. Rate control for these cases of atrial fibrillation is preferred to cardioversion. Agents for rate control include calcium channel blockers and beta-blockers. However, if there is an accessory or bypass pathway, agents that delay impulse passage through the AV node may precipitate ventricular fibrillation and should be avoided.

Table 25-2	Electrocardiographic Features of Standard SVTs and Response to Treatment					
SVT	Atrial Rate (Beats/Min)	Ventricular Rate (Beats/Min)	Distinctive ECG Characteristics	Response to Vagal Maneuvers	Response to Verapamil	Energies Required for Cardioversion (J)
Sinus tachycardia	100–180	100–180	—	May gradually slow and then accelerate	Rarely slows	—
PSVT	150–220	150–220	May note inverted P waves in inferior leads	May abruptly terminate	May abruptly terminate	100–200
Atrial flutter	240–360	120–180	"Sawtooth" flutter waves in inferior leads and V_1 in 80%; typically 2:1 AV block	May manifest incremental block and then reaccelerate	10%–15% may convert to NSR	25–50
Atrial fibrillation	—	100–160	Irregular	Often slows	None	100–200
Multifocal atrial tachycardia	100–160	100–160	Irregular: three different P-wave morphologies with three different PR intervals	None	Usually slows	—
Atrial tachycardia with AV block (PSVT with block)	100–240	70–120	Block may vary	Block may worsen	Block may worsen	—
Nonparoxysmal AV junctional tachycardia	—	70–130	—	None	None	—

ECG, electrocardiogram; PSVT, paroxysmal reentrant supraventricular tachycardia; AV, atrioventricular; NSR, normal sinus rhythm; PAT, paroxysmal atrial tachycardia.

An awake patient should be sedated. Oxygen should be administered by nasal cannula or mask. Oxygen and CO_2 should be monitored. Twelve-lead ECG should be obtained to ensure that the patient has not spontaneously converted to normal sinus rhythm (NSR). Endotracheal intubation equipment and an external temporary pacemaker should be at hand for all patients. Blood pressure should be monitored and recorded frequently. Two key features of cardioversion are the need for appropriate QRS synchronization by the sensing mechanism and proper energy titration. The physician must be certain that the most positive deflection on the monitor sensed by the cardioversion apparatus is the QRS complex. If the QRS complex is a net-negative deflection and the T wave is positive, then the apparatus may discharge on the T wave and thereby precipitate ventricular fibrillation. Hence, if the QRS complex is not sensed properly, one may either switch chest wall electrodes or change the polarity (when possible) of the monitor tracing. Energy titration is an essential aspect of successful cardioversion.

Frequently, after synchronized cardioversion, NSR may be only briefly maintained and may be replaced by the previous rhythm or atrial fibrillation. If this occurs, additional pharmacologic intervention, as indicated by the type of tachydysrhythmia, is required before cardioversion is attempted again.

Patients on Digitalis Preparations
Patients on digitalis preparations, and particularly patients with digoxin toxicity, must be treated extremely conservatively with respect to electrical cardioversion. With digoxin toxicity, the myocardial threshold for the induction of ventricular fibrillation by electrical discharge is significantly reduced. It is recommended that in such patients, an initial 1- or 2-J synchronized discharge be applied before definitive cardioversion. The elicitation of significant ventricular ectopy (couplets, VT) or enhancement of block should suggest significant digitalis effect, and in these patients, when cardioversion is urgently required to terminate an arrhythmia associated with shock or ischemia, amiodarone or lidocaine prophylaxis should be instituted, after which the test dose of 1 to 2 J may be repeated. When this is accomplished, definitive cardioversion may proceed, although with caution. If high-grade AV block develops in response to test energies, prophylactic temporary pacing may be required before cardioversion. When complex ventricular activity is elicited despite suppressive therapy, cardioversion must be abandoned and pharmacologic conversion used.

Postcardioversion Prophylaxis

In patients successfully converted from atrial fibrillation or flutter, postcardioversion pharmacologic prophylaxis is often administered in the immediate postcardioversion period. Because long-term outpatient follow-up is required, consultation with the patient's primary physician or cardiologist is appropriate before selecting a particular agent. Postcardioversion regimens for the patients with atrial fibrillation or flutter include diltiazem or a beta-blocker. It is important to consider the common precipitating causes of such arrhythmias, including pulmonary embolism, myocardial ischemia or infarction, thyrotoxicosis, pneumonitis, and pericarditis and treat appropriately. Admission should be considered for observation, monitoring, and the exclusion of myocardial ischemic injury.

Patients successfully treated with carotid sinus pressure or electrical cardioversion for PSVT (or paroxysmal atrial tachycardia [PAT]) often require no postcardioversion prophylaxis; however, admission for observation and monitoring may be indicated when cardioversion has been required to terminate the dysrhythmia.

VENTRICULAR TACHYDYSRHYTHMIAS

VT is generally a hemodynamically unstable rhythm that often degenerates into ventricular fibrillation. Occasionally, patients manifest hemodynamically stable, sustained VT. In general, the topologic site of initiation of the tachycardia and the pattern of spread of depolarization, as well as its rate, determine how well a particular patient tolerates VT.

Most patients with VT require emergent therapy. The particular therapy (i.e., pharmacologic or electrical cardioversion) is determined by the extent of hemodynamic compromise. Patients who are hemodynamically stable may be treated pharmacologically. Correct any electrolyte abnormalities.

- Monomorphic VT
  - Amiodarone 150 mg IV over 10 minutes, followed by infusion 1 mg/min. A second 150-mg bolus may be given.
  - Lidocaine 100 mg IV slow and repeat 75 mg boluses up to 3 mg/kg, followed by infusion 1 to 4 mg/h.
  - Procainamide 17 mg/kg IV bolus at a rate of not more than 50 mg/min. Discontinue for hypotension, or widening of QRS more than 50%.
  - Magnesium 2 to 4 g IV over 5 minutes, followed by infusion 1 g/h.
- Polymorphic VT
  - Magnesium 2 to 4 g over 5 minutes. Consider overdrive pacing.

If antiarrhythmic agents fail to convert VT to NSR or if the patient is ischemic or hemodynamically unstable (i.e., hypotension, congestive heart failure, or clinical or ECG evidence of ischemia), **electrical cardioversion** should be used. DC synchronized cardioversion at 100 J is used, followed by amiodarone, procainamide, lidocaine, or magnesium to prevent recurrence.

All patients with VT should be admitted to the hospital for continuous monitoring, antiarrhythmic therapy, and an evaluation of potential cause. Myocardial infarction, cardiomyopathy, valvular heart disease, medications, and electrolyte abnormalities are common causes of VT.

The distinction between VT and SVT with aberrancy is often difficult (see Table 25-1). A therapeutic trial of adenosine may be diagnostic in hemodynamically stable patients, given that this agent has virtually no therapeutic efficacy in patients with VT. An algorithmic approach to treatment of dysrhythmias is available in standard advanced cardiac life support (ACLS) protocols.

PREMATURE DEPOLARIZATIONS

- **Premature atrial contractions** (PACs) and blocked PACs are occasionally sensed as palpitations; however, these rarely warrant treatment. If associated with ethanol, tobacco use, stimulant, or illicit drug use, avoidance of these agents should be advised and may eliminate this troublesome, but not serious, symptom.
- **Premature ventricular contractions** (PVCs) are also sensed as palpitations by many patients. They may be totally benign as well, especially in young patients without organic heart disease. PVCs that improve with exercise are generally benign. However, in patients with coronary artery disease or left ventricular dysfunction, the new development of ventricular ectopic activity or an increase in baseline activity may portend VT and therefore warrants a thorough in-hospital evaluation. Patients with abnormal ECGs or a family history of sudden cardiac death should be admitted.

Table 25-3	Grades of Ventricular Ectopy

Grade	Characteristics of Ventricular Ectopic Activity
0	None
1	Occasional (<30/h)
2	Frequent (>30/h)
3	Multiform
4a	Repetitive (couplets)
4b	Repetitive (salvos)
5	R-on-T

• Lown and his associates have devised a system that enables the physician to estimate the significance of a particular patient's ventricular ectopic activity (Table 25-3) and, therefore, the urgency of treatment. Multifocal PVCs, sustained runs of VT, and PVCs falling on or near the T wave of the preceding normal depolarization are more serious and require urgent treatment, consultation, and admission.

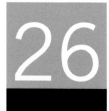

PART 6

Gastrointestinal Disorders

26 Abdominal Pain

Patients presenting to the emergency department (ED) with abdominal symptoms represent a substantial challenge to the physician. There are several critical diagnoses which cannot be missed. Several groups of patients may have atypical presentations and findings are not apparent: children, geriatric patients, the chronically debilitated, the depressed, and those patients on steroids. A conservative approach to the evaluation and disposition of these patients is recommended.

COMMON CAUSES OF ABDOMINAL PAIN

- Gastroenteritis*
- Peptic ulcer disease*
- Gastroesophageal reflux disease/erosive gastritis*
- Appendicitis*
- Biliary tract disease*
- Acute pancreatitis*
- Acute intestinal obstruction*
- Renal colic*
- Diverticulitis*
- Ectopic pregnancy*
- Ruptured ovarian cyst
- Mittelschmerz (ovarian follicular rupture)*
- Urinary tract infection*
- Premenstrual syndrome
- Pelvic inflammatory disease*
- Incarcerated hernia*
- Medications*

---

*Discussed in this chapter.

LESS COMMON CAUSES OF ABDOMINAL PAIN NOT TO BE MISSED

- Myocardial infarction or ischemia
- Pneumonitis or pleuritis*
- Enterocolitis
- Inflammatory bowel disease
- Diabetic ketoacidosis*
- Ovarian torsion*
- Streptococcal pharyngitis*
- Ischemic bowel disease*
- Acute (narrow-angle) glaucoma
- Abdominal aortic aneurysm*
- Spontaneous bacterial peritonitis*
- Testicular torsion*
- Perforated viscus
- Rectus sheath hematoma*
- Volvulus

OTHER CAUSES OF ABDOMINAL PAIN

- Mesenteric lymphadenitis
- Hepatitis or perihepatitis*
- Acute intermittent porphyria*
- Familial Mediterranean fever*
- Black widow spider bite*
- Diabetic gastroparesis
- Perforated Meckel diverticulum
- Sickle cell disease
- Intussusception*

HISTORY

To differentiate among the various causes of abdominal pain, several key features of the history must be explored in depth. These include the patient's previous medical and surgical histories; any current medications (e.g., aspirin, erythromycin); the onset, location and referral of pain; and any associated symptoms.

Onset of Pain

Abdominal pain that is maximally severe at the onset and begins abruptly—to the extent that the patient recalls the exact time of onset or the specific activity occurring when the pain began—or pain that awakens the patient from sleep must generally be regarded as serious. Conditions which may begin explosively include ureteral colic, perforated ulcer, ruptured ectopic pregnancy, ruptured corpus luteum, and, occasionally, vascular phenomena such as leaking or dissecting abdominal aortic aneurysm and mesenteric artery obstruction. Conversely, patients with acute cholecystitis, acute appendicitis, pancreatitis, and acute diverticulitis more often report the gradual onset of increasing discomfort.

Location of Pain

- In general, pain that is **initially well localized** to one area of the abdomen but then becomes generalized is suggestive of rupture or perforation of a viscus with resulting peritonitis. Immediately after rupture or perforation, many patients will report a relatively pain-free period followed by gradually increasing abdominal discomfort; this history is particularly ominous and is reported by patients with a ruptured appendix or diverticulum or perforated ulcer, as well. As pain becomes generalized, patients with evolving peritonitis have clinical evidence of peritoneal inflammation. Conversely, patients with classic appendicitis initially report vague, poorly localized, periumbilical pain, which may then localize to the right lower quadrant (RLQ) as the overlying parietal peritoneum becomes inflamed and irritated.
- Location of abdominal processes by quadrant.
  - **Right upper quadrant** (RUQ) pain is frequently reported in patients with duodenal ulcer, acute pancreatitis, cardiac ischemia, peritonitis, acute cholecystitis, retrocecal appendicitis, acute pancreatitis, acute hepatitis, acute right-sided heart failure, and right lower lobe pleuritis from any cause.
  - **Left upper quadrant** (LUQ) pain is often reported in patients with gastritis, gastric ulcer, acute pancreatitis, cardiac ischemia, peritonitis, splenic infarction or rupture, left lower lobe pneumonitis, and colonic processes involving the area of the splenic flexure (perforation, ischemia, carcinoma).
  - **Right lower quadrant** (RLQ) discomfort is frequently noted in patients with appendicitis, salpingitis, diverticulitis, mittelschmerz, ruptured ectopic pregnancy, testicular or ovarian torsion, perforated cecum, strangulated right inguinal hernia, regional enteritis, intestinal obstruction, and psoas abscess.
  - **Left lower quadrant** (LLQ) discomfort may result from any of the aforementioned conditions, with the exceptions of the pain of acute appendicitis being appreciably less common in this location and that of acute diverticulitis being more common. Patients with renal or ureteral colic may present with pain in any quadrant.
- **Diffuse abdominal pain** may be associated with peritonitis, acute pancreatitis, early appendicitis, small bowel obstruction, mesenteric thrombosis, gastroenteritis, streptococcal pharyngitis in children, and leaking abdominal aortic aneurysm. Metabolic causes of abdominal pain may also produce a diffuse picture.

Pattern of Pain Referral

The particular **pattern of pain referral** may provide valuable information. Acute cholecystitis pain may radiate laterally around the back and toward the inferior aspect of the right scapula. Acute pancreatitis most often radiates to the middle of the back. Processes that irritate the diaphragm may radiate to the ipsilateral shoulder. Mid back discomfort occurs with penetrating duodenal ulcer. Renal colic may radiate to the ipsilateral groin, testicle, or labia. In assessing patients with these patterns of pain referral, it is important to demonstrate that referral areas are not tender to palpation.

Associated Historical or Physical Features

Associated historical or physical features may provide the only clue to a diagnosis not previously considered.

- **Fever** is relatively nonspecific but may be associated with a perforated viscus, peritonitis, gangrenous bowel, cholangitis, acute salpingitis, abscess, or pneumonia.

- **Jaundice** is a relatively specific finding suggesting acute hepatitis, biliary obstruction or, in patients with high fever and rigors, acute cholangitis.
- **Polydipsia, polyphagia, polyuria, and Kussmaul respirations** suggest diabetic ketoacidosis.
- Discomfort precipitated by or fluctuating with **food intake** is often noted in acute cholecystitis or peptic ulcer disease, respectively.
- A recent **history of excessive alcohol or NSAID use** may occur with acute pancreatitis or acute gastritis.
- **Diarrhea associated with nausea, vomiting, and epigastric or poorly localized pain** occurs with acute gastroenteritis. A finding of other family members having similar symptoms further supports this diagnosis. Coryza, cough, and pharyngitis suggest a viral syndrome. With acute gastroenteritis, an episode of diarrhea may be associated with temporary relief from abdominal discomfort.
- **Diarrhea, occurring after the completion of a course of antibiotics** (typically within 2–10 days), suggests (*C. difficile*) pseudomembranous enterocolitis.
- **Severe vomiting, a history of previous abdominal surgery, and diffuse pain** suggest small bowel obstruction. Feculent or bilious vomitus occurs with mechanical obstruction. Vomiting of undigested food immediately after eating occurs with gastric outlet obstruction, which may be caused by ulcer disease or neoplasia.
- **Patients who vomit blood** after retching or after an initial episode of nonbloody vomitus may have gastroesophageal junction laceration (Mallory-Weiss tear). Hematemesis suggests bleeding lesions proximal to the mid duodenum: esophagitis, bleeding varices, gastritis, ulcer, Mallory-Weiss syndrome. Ingestion of bismuth, licorice, or beets may produce a black but non-tarlike stool negative for occult blood.
- **In women with lower pelvic discomfort,** a relatively normal appetite, and minimal or absent nausea or vomiting, a gynecologic cause should be considered. Associated vaginal discharge suggests acute salpingitis. Acute unilateral pelvic pain with an abnormal menstrual period and vaginal spotting is suggestive of ectopic pregnancy. The acute onset of unilateral pelvic pain at midmenstrual cycle (days 12–16 patients) associated with minimal gastrointestinal symptoms suggests mittelschmerz. This diagnosis should be made with caution in patients using hormonal birth control because ovulation is presumably prevented.
- **Testicular pain** associated with lower quadrant discomfort suggests torsion or ureteral colic. Because patients will not often volunteer this information, specific inquiry should be made. Examination of the genitourinary system in men should be performed in **all** cases of acute abdominal pain.
- **Rectus sheath hematoma** is a relatively uncommon diagnosis that may simulate a number of intra-abdominal processes and may also produce nausea, abdominal pain, low-grade fever, leukocytosis, referred and rebound tenderness, and local spasm. Many patients with rectus sheath hematomas have a history of anticoagulation therapy or abdominal wall trauma that may have been considered trivial.

Metabolic Conditions

A number of **metabolic conditions** may cause abdominal pain, and a high degree of suspicion must be maintained if these are to be recognized. Diabetic ketoacidosis, streptococcal pharyngitis (particularly in the child), basilar pleuritis secondary to infection, pulmonary embolus, porphyria, familial Mediterranean fever, C1 esterase inhibitor deficiency, and black widow spider bites may all produce major abdominal symptoms and signs.

Previous Abdominal Procedures

Previous abdominal procedures increase the likelihood of intestinal obstruction secondary to adhesions.

Analgesics

Improved diagnostic imaging has resulted in less reliance on serial exams. Studies suggest that narcotic analgesics can safely be given to patients while their evaluation progresses.

Antiemetics

Ondansetron (Zofran) is safe and effective.

PHYSICAL EXAMINATION

- Note the patient's **position and behavior** before initiating the formal examination. Patients with peritonitis generally will prefer to remain supine and motionless; any movement that stimulates the peritoneum, such as moving in bed, coughing, or sitting up will precipitate or worsen pain. Many patients with peritonitis will prefer to keep their hips and knees flexed in an attempt to reduce peritoneal traction-related discomfort.
- In contrast, patients with ureteral colic frequently are standing or walking around the examination room holding the affected side, unable to rest in bed.
- Patients with inflammatory processes in the area of the psoas (pancreatitis, perinephric abscess, retrocecal appendicitis, ruptured sigmoid diverticulitis) may attempt to assume positions that minimize stress on adjacent or overlying muscles. Patients with pancreatitis often prefer the "fetal" position. Patients with unilateral processes prefer a position with the ipsilateral hip and knee flexed.
- A **complete examination** includes the pharynx, chest, back (noting the presence of costovertebral angle tenderness), genitalia, pelvis, and rectum. Stool for occult blood testing should be obtained as indicated.
- **Examination of the abdomen** begins with the patient positioned supine and appropriately disrobed. Ask the patient to point with one finger to the area of maximal discomfort. It is useful to determine whether cough increases the patient's discomfort, indicating peritoneal irritation.
  - **Inspection.** The abdomen is inspected for evidence of previous surgical scars, distention associated with obstruction or ileus, and the presence of abnormal pulsations.
  - **Auscultation** should be performed to determine the presence and character of bowel sounds.
  - **Palpation** of the abdomen must be gentle to minimize anxiety and guarding. Begin palpation distant to areas of pain. Two signs suggest localized peritoneal inflammation: (1) localized abdominal pain that is worsened by palpation at a site distant and (2) elicitation of referred rebound tenderness. Voluntary or involuntary resistance to gentle palpation should be noted and the patient's area of maximal discomfort determined. **Rebound tenderness** is elicited by palpation over this site. When evidence of generalized peritoneal irritation exists, immediate surgical consultation is recommended.
- With intussusception, an abdominal mass may be palpable, often on rectal examination. Passage of mucus and blood in the stool supports the diagnosis.

- RLQ pain on **rectal examination** suggests retrocecal appendicitis.
- The **inguinal and genital regions** should be carefully examined to exclude incarcerated hernia. This diagnosis remains a commonly overlooked cause of vomiting, abdominal pain, bowel obstruction, and sepsis, particularly in the elderly or debilitated patient with a vague history.
- The **pelvic examination** evaluates the presence of endocervical discharge and whether lateral movement of the cervix intensifies the patient's discomfort. An adnexal mass should suggest ectopic pregnancy, cyst, or abscess. Bleeding may occur with ectopic pregnancy or spontaneous abortion.

DIAGNOSTIC TESTS

- **Anemia** suggests chronic or acute blood loss.
- The **white blood cell** (WBC) is neither sensitive nor specific. A low WBC count with lymphocytosis suggests viral gastroenteritis. A WBC count greater than 18,000 to 20,000/μL with a predominant polymorphonuclear leukocytosis with bands should be further evaluated. AIDS and immunosuppressed patients may fail to develop an increased number of WBCs even with serious bacterial infection.
- The **urinalysis** may demonstrate hematuria in ureteral colic, glycosuria and ketonuria in the patient with unsuspected diabetic ketoacidosis, bilirubinuria in the patient with hepatic or biliary disease, or WBCs with infectious processes.
- The **serum lipase**, when elevated twice the normal value, has greater sensitivity and specificity (both ~95%) than the serum amylase and is therefore the preferred test in pancreatitis. The **serum amylase** may be elevated in patients with acute pancreatitis as well as a variety of both extra-abdominal and intra-abdominal conditions; these include mumps, salivary duct stones, diabetic ketoacidosis, burns, renal insufficiency, a number of carcinomas, pregnancy, penetrating or perforating peptic ulcer, biliary tract disease, ruptured ectopic pregnancy, intestinal obstruction and infarction, peritonitis, and chronic liver disease.
- A serum or urinary determination of the β-**subunit of human chorionic gonadotropin (HCG)** should be obtained in all women unless post-menopausal.
- An **electrocardiogram (ECG)** should be considered in patients with upper abdominal discomfort.
- **Radiographs of the chest** may demonstrate thoracic diagnoses or free air. Abdominal films may be useful for demonstrating bowel obstruction or paralytic ileus, but have limited utility.
- **Ultrasonography** is the primary modality in the evaluation of biliary tract disease. Bedside ultrasound is indicated to evaluate the abdominal aorta in the hemodynamically unstable patient. Transvaginal or pelvic ultrasound evaluates the presence or absence of uterine or ectopic pregnancy. Ultrasound is particularly sensitive in the detection of free fluid (blood). Color Doppler ultrasound has become the procedure of choice for diagnosing ovarian and testicular torsion. Ultrasonography may also be helpful in the diagnosis of rectus sheath or abdominal wall hematoma.
- **Radionuclide imaging** is valuable in the diagnosis of acute cholecystitis if the screening ultrasound is nondiagnostic.
- **Computed tomography (CT)** is extremely sensitive and specific in diagnosing bowel obstruction, free air, appendicitis, pancreatic pseudocyst and abscess, ureteral stone, aortic aneurysm, colitis, diverticulitis, and intra-abdominal vascular pathology.

ABDOMINAL PAIN, CAUSE UNDETERMINED

Even after a thorough evaluation, a number of patients with abdominal symptoms will remain without a clear diagnosis. When potentially serious intra-abdominal processes cannot be reasonably excluded, these patients should be admitted to the hospital for continued observation and early surgical consultation. Patients who appear less ill, in whom a serious abdominal process is unlikely, and who may be reliably and continuously observed at home may be discharged with very clearly formulated and documented plans for prompt follow-up. Care should be discussed with their primary physician and plans made for a repeat evaluation in 8 to 12 hours. Patients must be instructed to return immediately if symptoms change or worsen.

SPECIFIC DISORDERS

- Although the incidence of peptic duodenal ulcer has been declining, it still remains a common disorder. In addition to acid and pepsin, infection with the Helicobacter pylori and exposure to nonsteroidal anti-inflammatory agents are the primary causative agents in ulcer formation. Peptic ulcer disease occurs in all age groups; it is the major cause of gastrointestinal bleeding in adolescents and is one of the major causes of bleeding in adults. Complications include bleeding, intractable pain, gastric outlet obstruction, and perforation.
  - **History.** Patients with duodenal ulcer disease report a gnawing mid epigastric discomfort—occasionally radiating to the back (especially if a posterior penetrating ulcer exists)—relieved by eating. Nausea with occasional vomiting may also occur. With gastric outlet obstruction (secondary to edema adjacent to a duodenal ulcer), postprandial vomiting occurs. Hematemesis may occur; however, patients with a source distal to the ligament of Treitz may present with isolated lower gastrointestinal bleeding. Melena occurs with acute or chronic bleeding. Rarely, bleeding may be so brisk that bright red blood is passed per rectum.
  - On **physical examination,** pain on palpation of the epigastrium without rebound is noted. Stool for occult blood is mandatory and often positive. Patients with gastric outlet obstruction may have abdominal distention, and a succussion splash may be noted. Free perforation produces absent bowel sounds, diffuse tenderness, rigidity, and rebound tenderness.
  - **Useful diagnostic tests** include a CBC, lipase, and *H. pylori* titers. Hypochromic microcytic anemia may be noted in patients with chronic bleeding. Lipase elevation suggests a posterior penetrating duodenal ulcer. CT or plain films should be obtained in patients with significant discomfort or physical findings to identify free air. Upper endoscopy is indicated for active bleeding.
  - The **treatment** of peptic ulcer disease is a proton pump inhibitor (PPI) (lansoprazole and omeprazole). Other agents, such as sucralfate, misoprostol, and antacids are also used. The **histamine antagonists,** which selectively block acid production by the gastric parietal cell, are less effective. **PPIs** inhibit parietal cell hydrogen ion production and release, and include omeprazole (Prilosec), 20 mg each morning before breakfast, and lansoprazole, 15 mg daily. These agents are also useful in the short-term treatment of patients with erosive esophagitis and gastroesophageal reflux. Sucralfate (Carafate), 1 g four times daily 30 minutes to 1 hour before meals, operates to provide a protective barrier from acid; bismuth subsalicylate functions in the same manner and also exhibits antibacterial activity against *Helicobacter*

pylori. Misoprostol (200 micrograms four times daily) is a prostaglandin analog that protects the mucosa in patients requiring continued therapy with the nonsteroidal anti-inflammatory agents; side effects (diarrhea and abdominal pain) are relatively common, and the drug should not be used in pregnancy. If infection with *Helicobacter pylori* is present or suspected, antibacterial therapy is indicated. A variety of antibacterial agents are effective in eliminating the organism to speed ulcer healing and reduce complications and relapse rates.

- The initial therapy is a PPI, amoxicillin 1 g and clarithromycin 500 mg, all twice daily for 7 to 14 days. Metronidazole 500 mg may be substituted for penicillin-allergic patients. There are several regimens effective for "rescue" therapy. Magnesium-containing antacids should be avoided in patients with renal impairment.
- Patients should refrain from using tobacco, alcohol, aspirin, NSAIDS, and coffee (regular and decaffeinated).
- **Complications** of duodenal ulcer, including gastric outlet obstruction, bleeding, intractable pain, or perforation require admission. In patients with **gastrointestinal bleeding**, emergent upper gastrointestinal endoscopy should be obtained for diagnosis and treatment. Blood should be obtained for CBC, clotting studies, and type and crossmatch for 2 to 4 units of packed red blood cells. Standard fluid and blood resuscitation is indicated for unstable hemodynamics. A nasogastric tube should be inserted and the return evaluated; lavage should continue until the return is clear to facilitate endoscopic evaluation. If endoscopic control of bleeding is unsuccessful, surgical consultation should be undertaken immediately; poor surgical candidates may be evaluated for selective arterial vasopressin infusion or selective arterial embolization.

- **Acute erosive gastritis** typically produces epigastric pain, nausea, vomiting, and varying degrees of gastrointestinal bleeding. It may occur as a result of, the direct, toxic effects of alcohol, aspirin, or other nonsteroidal anti-inflammatory agents. Ischemia may be causally important in the development of gastritis and may be due to physical crises (including burns, trauma, sepsis, surgery, and renal or hepatic failure). Acute massive upper gastrointestinal hemorrhage may occur.
- **Diagnosis.** Many patients with significant gastric bleeding from gastric erosions do not vomit blood. The stool should be evaluated for occult blood. If bleeding is acute, the hematocrit may be normal.
- **Treatment:**
  - Patients with **mild symptoms and no evidence of bleeding** may be discharged with carefully documented instructions to return should evidence of bleeding occur or should nausea or vomiting prevent oral intake. Treatment involves PPIs and antacid as needed. Patients should be instructed to avoid aspirin, alcohol, and other agents that may irritate the gastric mucosa. Patients with nausea are treated with ondansetron and should be advised to ingest only clear liquids for 12 to 24 hours. Patients without appreciable nausea should advance the diet as tolerated.
  - When **evidence of bleeding** is noted, hospital admission and early upper gastrointestinal endoscopy are required; treatment is as outlined. Patients should be treated with an intravenous PPI.
- **Appendicitis.** Although signs and symptoms of appendicitis may follow a fairly typical pattern, this disorder is capable of such protean manifestations that it should be considered in every patient with abdominal pain.

- In the **classic presentation,** acute appendicitis begins with epigastric or periumbilical pain, nausea, anorexia, and often one or two episodes of vomiting. Within 2 to 12 hours, pain shifts to the RLQ, where it is described as a steady ache aggravated by walking or coughing. Malaise and low-grade fever may be noted.

- On physical examination, the typical patient appears to be in mild to moderate distress with a normal temperature or low-grade fever. Periumbilical or RLQ tenderness well localized to a single point (McBurney's point) may be the only notable physical finding. When peritoneal irritation develops, referred and rebound tenderness and involuntary guarding will then be noted. Occasionally, psoas and obturator signs are present and, if so, strongly support the diagnosis. RLQ tenderness on rectal examination may be noted and, especially in patients with retrocecal appendicitis, may be more marked than abdominal tenderness.

- Moderate leukocytosis is typically noted, but the WBC may be normal. Microscopic hematuria and pyuria are occasionally noted and are due to periureteral inflammation. The test with the highest sensitivity and specificity is abdominopelvic CT. The sensitivity of CT increases from 98% to 100% with varying contrast methodologies (oral, intravenous, or colonic), making these the imaging studies of choice. The specificity is also high.

- **Variability in presentation** may be due to atypical anatomy or compromised host factors (extremes of age, chronic debility, and immunocompromised status).

- The **treatment** is emergency appendectomy, preferably within 4 to 12 hours of initial presentation. Intravenous hydration, analgesics, and antiemetics should be instituted.

- The **pregnant woman** with appendicitis presents a difficult management problem. Appendicitis occurs in approximately 1 in 1,200 pregnancies. Because the appendix is displaced cephalad and to the right by the gravid uterus, typical localization of pain to the RLQ does not occur. In at least one half of pregnant patients, the diagnosis of acute appendicitis is not made until rupture and peritonitis have evolved. Early appendectomy is indicated because delay may lead to premature labor or spontaneous abortion. Ultrasound is an appropriate initial diagnostic study. Obstetrical and surgical consultation should be obtained (CT is reasonable in the third trimester). If a definitive diagnosis is elusive, strong consideration for admission is recommended.

- Given that (1) there exists no objective means of definitively excluding appendicitis, (2) failure to diagnose or provide reasonable and documented interval follow-up care may result in significant morbidity for the patient, and (3) appendicitis is a common disease that may present in a variety of ways, a consistently conservative approach to patients suspected of appendicitis should be followed. Therefore, the threshold for confirming or excluding the diagnosis with CT should be quite low. Frequently, after discussion with the surgeon, well-documented arrangements for re-examination in 6 to 12 hours may be elected and are a reasonable option in patients who neither appear ill nor have significant abdominal findings. Patients should be instructed to return immediately to the emergency department should symptoms change or worsen.

- **Biliary tract disease.** Biliary colic, acute cholecystitis, and choledocholithiasis are the most common biliary tract conditions in patients presenting with abdominal pain.

- **Biliary colic** is a transient symptom due to passage of gallstones. Lab and ultrasound are usually normal, and pain is easily treated. If pain resolves spontaneously, ultrasound may be deferred.

- **Acute cholecystitis** occurs when a gallstone becomes impacted in the cystic duct, producing obstruction and subsequent inflammation. In these patients, if the obstruction is not relieved, gangrene, perforation, peritonitis, and local abscess may evolve.

- **History.** RUQ or epigastric pain is often precipitated by the ingestion of a large or fatty meal. Although the discomfort associated with any specific episode may gradually subside, recurrent episodes are common.
- Importantly, pain from an inflamed gallbladder often radiates to the right subscapular area. Nausea and vomiting are common.
- The **physical examination** reveals mild fever, RUQ tenderness with involuntary guarding, and mild rebound tenderness. One-fourth of patients are mildly jaundiced.
- **Diagnostic tests.** Moderate leukocytosis is often noted and mild hyperbilirubinemia (1–4 mg/dL total) may occur even in the absence of common duct obstruction. Transaminases and alkaline phosphatase are also frequently elevated. The study of choice is ultrasound with a sensitivity of 97% and a specificity of 78%. Supportive findings include stones, distention of the gallbladder, thickening of the wall, and pericholecystic fluid. Nuclear medicine scans (HIDA scans) use isotopes and which are specifically concentrated in bile (and secreted into the gallbladder) have a sensitivity and specificity of 97% and 90%, respectively. Failure to visualize the gall bladder within 1 hour of the intravenous injection of the radionuclide suggests cystic duct obstruction.
- The **treatment** of acute calculus and acalculous cholecystitis consists of hospital admission, intravenous hydration, restriction of oral intake, analgesia, antiemetics, and ampicillin/sulbactam or ciprofloxacin. Cholecystectomy may be required emergently with gangrene, sepsis, or peritonitis. Broad-spectrum antibiotic treatment is warranted. Most patients treated medically in the hospital have resolution of symptoms within several days; laparoscopic cholecystectomy is usually performed within a few days after hospitalization.

- **Choledocholithiasis** occurs in approximately 15% of patients with gallstones. This incidence increases with age, approaching 50% in elderly patients. Common duct stones usually originate in the gallbladder but may also form spontaneously in the common duct itself.
  - **History.** Frequent, recurrent attacks of severe RUQ pain persisting for hours, chills and fever, and jaundice temporally associated with RUQ pain all suggest the presence of a common bile duct stone. Charcot triad (RUQ pain, fever, and jaundice) defines the classic picture of choledocholithiasis with associated acute cholangitis.
  - The **physical examination** does not differentiate common duct stones from those in the gallbladder. Tenderness is present in the RUQ or epigastrium.
  - **Diagnostic tests.** Hyperbilirubinemia and bilirubinuria are typically noted; the serum alkaline phosphatase is also elevated. When prolonged obstruction of the common duct exists, resulting hepatocellular dysfunction may produce increases in transaminase activities. Ultrasonography is the initial diagnostic modality. Radionuclide scans, computed tomographic scans, and percutaneous transhepatic cholangiography all provide information regarding the cause, location, and extent of biliary tract obstruction, demonstrating in all cases some dilatation of intrahepatic bile ducts.
  - **Treatment.** Choledocholithiasis is treated by endoscopic retrograde cholangiopancreatography (ERCP)-based sphincterotomy and removal of stones or by cholecystectomy and choledochostomy. Given the incidence of ascending cholangitis, careful evaluation and preparation of the patient is strongly suggested unless emergency surgery is required. Antibiotic treatment should

cover Enterobacteriaceae, enterococci, and *Bacteroides* and *Clostridium* species. Antibiotic choices include ampicillin/sulbactam or metronidazole plus ciprofloxacin. Intravenous hydration, analgesia, and antiemetics are indicated.

- **Acute pancreatitis** is associated with several provocative factors including alcohol use, cholelithiasis, abdominal trauma, mumps, hyperparathyroidism, hyperlipidemias, duodenal ulcer, thiazide, clofibrate, azathioprine use, and vasculitis. Inflammation results in leakage of proteolytic enzymes into pancreatic and adjacent tissues.
  - **History.** Steady, boring, epigastric pain is typically improved on sitting forward and made worse by lying supine. The pain radiates to the back and is associated with nausea, vomiting, and occasionally severe prostration.
  - On **physical examination,** tenderness is noted primarily in the upper abdomen with occasional guarding or rebound tenderness. A paralytic ileus frequently evolves and leads to reduced or absent bowel sounds. Fever, tachycardia, pallor, and occasionally shock develop in patients with severe involvement; significant morbidity and mortality are reported in these patients. Mild jaundice may be noted but is uncommon.
  - **Diagnostic tests** typically demonstrate leukocytosis, hyperglycemia, glycosuria, proteinuria, tubular casts, and mild hyperbilirubinemia. Alkaline phosphatase activity and prothrombin time may be elevated, and the serum calcium may be decreased in association with an increase in triglycerides and lipase activity. Serum amylase is classically elevated within 6 hours of the onset of pain in 90% of patients and returns to normal levels by the third day; the serum lipase is significantly more specific in acute pancreatitis, increases more slowly, and persists for a few days longer.
  - **Complications** of acute pancreatitis include abscess, pseudocyst, chronic pancreatitis, and diabetes mellitus. Acute complications include ARDS and shock. Factors adversely affecting survival that are identifiable on admission to the hospital (Ranson criteria) include age older than 55, WBC greater than 16,000/μL, glucose greater than 200 mg/dL, serum LDH greater than 350 IU/L, AST greater than 250 IU/L, hematocrit decrease greater than 10%, increase in BUN greater than 5 mg/dL, arterial PO$_2$ less than 60 mm Hg, base deficit greater than 4 mEq/L, serum calcium less than 8.0 mg/dL, and estimated fluid sequestration greater than 6 L. Significantly increased morbidity is associated with three or more of these risk factors present on admission.
  - **Treatment** of acute pancreatitis includes restriction of oral intake and the institution of nasogastric suction in severe cases or patients with persistent vomiting, analgesics, antiemetics, and aggressive intravenous hydration. Central venous pressure monitoring may be a useful guide to intravascular volume repletion. For symptomatic hypocalcemia, calcium gluconate, 10%, 10 mL intravenously over 15 to 20 minutes is administered. Hypomagnesemia should be corrected with magnesium sulfate, 16 mEq (2 g) in 50 mL of D5W over 20 minutes. In hemorrhagic pancreatitis, the hematocrit should be maintained at approximately 30%; fresh-frozen plasma and platelets may also be required. Antibiotics are generally not indicated for uncomplicated acute pancreatitis.
  - Recurrences of acute pancreatitis are common, and morbidity remains high. Mortality is significantly higher in patients with acute hemorrhagic pancreatitis and when renal, respiratory, or cardiovascular impairment coexists.
- **Acute intestinal obstruction** occurs as a result of mechanical blockage of the intestinal lumen, which may originate either extrinsically or intrinsically, or may occur

as a result of deranged intestinal neuromuscular function resulting in decreased or absent motility.

- **Acute mechanical obstruction** may result from adhesions related to previous surgical procedures, incarcerated hernia, neoplasia, and diverticula. Obstruction that occurs as a result of deranged neuromuscular function is termed an "ileus". Paralytic or adynamic ileus, which is the most frequent type, is discussed subsequently, as is intussusception.

- Morbidity and mortality from mechanical obstruction may occur relatively suddenly as a result of intravascular volume depletion. Fluid loss occurs into the bowel wall and lumen, into the peritoneal cavity, and due to protracted vomiting. Bacteremia and sepsis may develop suddenly in patients with obstruction progressing to bowel infarction.

  ○ **History.** Pain is diffuse or poorly localized to the area of the obstruction. Pain may be mild or severe, may occur in waves associated with peristalsis, and is often described as "crampy." Frequently, pain-free intervals punctuate episodes of severe discomfort. Often, as abdominal distention increases, pain may become continuous but, in many patients, is also more tolerable. Nausea and vomiting are prominent symptoms. Very proximal obstructions may, as a result of early "reflex" vomiting, sufficiently decompress the proximal bowel so that these symptoms temporarily lessen. With less proximal obstructions, vomiting may be violent and protracted. Failure to pass flatus or feces occurs in patients with mechanical obstruction of the small intestine, but initially these functions are unaffected. Abdominal distention occurs late in the course.

  ○ In patients with colonic obstruction, early "reflex" vomiting is uncommon, and if the ileocecal valve is competent, vomiting may not occur at all. Nausea, however, is a common symptom. Failure to pass flatus or feces is common. Abdominal distention classically occurs early in the course of colonic obstruction. Pain may be deceptively mild, particularly in the elderly, and many patients present after several days of progressive constipation.

  ○ The early **physical examination** with acute intestinal obstruction may be unremarkable, particularly if examined during interperistaltic or pain-free periods. Local or generalized evidence of peritonitis or a palpable mass (except in children with intussusception) usually suggests incarcerated obstruction. Although these patients may appear deceptively well, high fever, rigors, and circulatory compromise may rapidly ensue. Varying degrees of abdominal distention may be noted. Auscultation of the abdomen in the patient with mechanical obstruction, during periods of peristalsis-induced pain, classically demonstrates bowel sounds that are high pitched, tinkling or metallic, and heard in clusters or rushes. If such patients are examined during pain-free periods, auscultatory findings are variable. In patients with paralytic ileus, in contrast, an occasional, relatively normal bowel sound is heard unassociated with increased discomfort, and this may be an important differential point. The patient with established or evolving incarceration or gangrenous obstruction typically presents with a silent abdomen. Occult or gross blood in the stool is unusual in patients with small bowel obstruction, but is frequently noted in patients with colonic obstruction because carcinoma and diverticulitis are etiologically common in these latter patients.

  ○ **Diagnostic tests.** The WBC is usually somewhat elevated, in the range of 15,000 to 18,000/μL, in patients with mechanical obstruction; however, patients seen early may have normal counts. Patients with evolving incarcerated obstruction have higher counts, often with a leftward shift; gangrenous bowel, peritonitis, and abscess should also be considered.

○ **Radiographs** should include upright posterior-anterior chest x-rays to rule out free air under the diaphragm associated with perforation of the bowel. The overall sensitivity of plain films with small bowel obstruction is marginal, varying from 40% to 80%; the specificity similarly varies from 25% to 90% and indeterminate findings are common. Diagnostic results with **CT** are much better (100% sensitivity and a specificity of 85%); CT is also excellent in identifying ischemia caused by strangulation of the bowel. These studies are also helpful in the diagnosis of acute mechanical obstruction and its differentiation from paralytic ileus.

○ **Treatment** for mechanical obstruction includes placement of a nasogastric tube with suction to decompress the proximal bowel, reestablishment of intravascular volume, restriction of oral intake, and early surgical consultation. When incarceration or gangrenous obstruction is suspected, or when evidence of peritoneal irritation or perforation is present, intravenous antibiotics and emergent surgical consultation are appropriate.

• **Paralytic ileus** is commonly seen in the ED and is due to any type of peritoneal, retroperitoneal, or intestinal insult. Paralytic ileus is an expected finding after abdominal surgery and is commonly seen in a number of medical conditions including acute severe pyelonephritis, ureteral calculi, sepsis, basilar pneumonitis, myocardial infarction, the use of drugs that decrease bowel motility, and potassium depletion.

• The differentiation of paralytic ileus from mechanical obstruction may be extremely difficult, particularly if the latter is partial or intermittent. A careful history must be taken regarding the associated factors previously noted and appropriate laboratory studies obtained. Clinically, patients with ileus, in contrast to most patients with mechanical obstruction, report a relatively steady discomfort not increased by auscultable peristalsis. Bowel sounds, which are often decreased, are typically not associated with increased pain. Vomiting is often present but is usually not protracted or severe. Most patients report nausea, and the passage of flatus and feces is absent. Abdominal distention and mild generalized abdominal tenderness are the usual findings. **Treatment** involves restriction of oral intake, administration of intravenous fluids, and nasogastric suction.

• **Intussusception.** Acute mechanical obstruction of the bowel may result when a proximal segment of intestine telescopes into the lumen of contiguous distal intestine. This occurs most often in boys between 5 and 10 months of age, most often involves the area of the ileocecal valve, and infrequently resolves spontaneously.

• Once intussusception occurs, peristaltic activity propels the invaginating segment distally, thereby placing traction on associated vascular structures, and along with evolving edema, may jeopardize blood supply to the involved segment. As the intussusception proceeds, obstruction evolves that, if undiagnosed, progresses to bowel ischemia and infarction.

○ **History.** The diagnosis of intussusception relies heavily on the history. Typically, a previously healthy child who had no symptoms on going to bed is violently awakened by severe, excruciating abdominal pain and vomiting. The hips are frequently held in flexion during paroxysms of pain. Symptoms may subside after several minutes but often recur. Blood and mucus are frequently passed in the stool at approximately 2 or 3 hours after the onset of pain and may bring the patient to the hospital, particularly if abdominal discomfort had subsided.

° **Physical examination**
  - **In patients with resolution of discomfort,** the physical examination may be remarkable only for stool positive for occult blood. These patients may be observed in the ED for several hours and, if well, may be discharged with their parents with clear instructions to return if symptoms recur. Alternatively, in-hospital observation may be elected.
    - **Patients with persisting and progressive intussusception** may appear ill, with fever, pallor, and rapidly evolving dehydration. In 90% of patients, a palpable, sausage-shaped, tender abdominal mass is palpable either abdominally or by rectal examination; blood and mucus in the stool are frequently noted.
  ° **Treatment** and diagnosis are best accomplished with a cautious barium enema or pneumatic insufflation, administered by the radiologist or surgeon. This procedure will effect reduction of the intussusception in 70% of patients, thereby avoiding surgery and general anesthesia. Surgical intervention is reserved for those patients in whom reduction by barium enema is unsuccessful.
- **Diverticulosis** of the colon increases with age and often is asymptomatic. The inflammatory complication, diverticulitis, probably affects only one fourth of patients with diverticulosis. Although diverticula may occur throughout the colon, they are most commonly found in the sigmoid. The inflammatory changes in diverticulitis range from mild cellular infiltration in the wall of the diverticular sac to extensive inflammation in the peridiverticular zone. Perforation and abscess formation may occur in a manner analogous to that of acute appendicitis.
  - **History.** Crampy lower abdominal pain is often relieved by defecation. Constipation is common, but diarrhea may also occur.
  - **Physical examination** usually reveals a moderately ill-appearing individual with low-grade fever. Tenderness with mild guarding is often noted in the lower abdomen; occult blood is found on stool analysis in 25% of patients. Massive rectal hemorrhage is infrequently seen in patients with pain; right-sided diverticula tend to bleed rather than cause severe pain or obstruction. Because diverticulitis is a lesion in which gross or microscopic perforation has occurred, clinical manifestations vary with the extent of perforation and inflammation. LLQ pain, fever, chills, ileus, and partial or complete colonic obstruction may occur.
  - **Diagnostic tests** may reveal a mild to moderate leukocytosis with an excess of polymorphonuclear leukocytes. Red and white blood cells may be seen on urinalysis. CT of the abdomen and pelvis with oral and IV contrast is the study of choice.
  - **Complications** of diverticulitis include peritonitis, abscess formation, and perforation with ensuing abdominal sepsis.
  - **Treatment** consists of antibiotic therapy, utilizing oral ciprofloxacin plus metronidazole for mild cases that may be treated as an outpatient with close follow-up. Restriction of oral intake, intravenous hydration, and early surgical evaluation are also advised. Admitted patients require IV ciprofloxacin plus metronidazole. Recurrent attacks, gross perforation, and abscess or fistulous tract formation require surgical resection.
- **Ectopic pregnancy.** (See Chapter 37, "Vaginal Bleeding," pp. 330)
- **Mittelschmerz** is unilateral adnexal pain at ovulation caused by leakage of blood or fluid at the time of follicular rupture. The sudden onset of RLQ or LLQ pain in women, occurring at mid cycle (typically days 12–16) and **unassociated** with significant gastrointestinal, genitourinary, or constitutional symptoms, suggests mittelschmerz. Vaginal bleeding or spotting should *not* be associated. A β-subunit

of HCG should be obtained to exclude ectopic pregnancy. Because regular birth control pill use is expected to prevent ovulation, and thus ovulation-related pain, the diagnosis of mittelschmerz is difficult to justify in these patients.

- Clinical presentation may show localized peritoneal irritation. Patients, although moderately uncomfortable, do not generally appear ill. Mild referred and localized rebound tenderness may be noted in the appropriate lower quadrant. A pelvic examination (with appropriate cultures) helps to exclude pelvic inflammatory disease. When right-sided discomfort is present, the exclusion of acute appendicitis may be extremely difficult, if not impossible. The duration of discomfort associated with mittelschmerz is usually less than 8 hours.
- **Diagnostic tests** are not helpful except for a pregnancy test.
- **Treatment** for mittelschmerz includes reassurance, rest, a mild analgesic, and clear instructions to return should symptoms worsen.
- In patients with right-sided discomfort in whom acute appendicitis cannot be excluded, appropriate diagnostic evaluation should be obtained.

- **Urinary tract infection**
  - **Acute cystitis**
    - **Diagnosis.** Dysuria, pelvic pressure, and urinary frequency and urgency are common. Systemic symptoms, such as high fever, rigors, or prostration, are absent, and the physical examination is unremarkable except for mild pelvic discomfort with palpation. Dipstick of a midstream, clean-voided specimen of urine will demonstrate pyuria, positive leukocyte esterase, and varying degrees of hematuria. Hemorrhagic cystitis is manifest by grossly bloody urine. Urine C & S is unnecessary in the nonpregnant, sexually active woman unless recurrent or complicated. Sexually transmitted infections should be ruled out.
    - **Treatment** includes oral hydration and completion of the entire course of antibiotics. Dysuria, frequency, and urgency will benefit from phenazopyridine (Pyridium), 200 mg three times daily for 2 days. Phenazopyridine should not be used during pregnancy. Treatment options include 3 to 5 days of 1 double-strength tablet of trimethoprim-sulfamethoxazole twice daily. Alternatively, a course of ampicillin, 250 mg four times daily or nitrofurantoin, 50 to 100 mg four times daily with food may be considered. Ciprofloxacin may be used for complicated cystitis.
  - **Acute pyelonephritis** involves the renal parenchyma and is frequently associated with bacteremia. It presents with back pain, high fever, rigors, nausea, and vomiting. Some patients report symptoms suggestive of recent cystitis.
    - **Diagnosis** is based on the patient's history, clinical presentation, unilateral or bilateral percussion tenderness over the involved kidney (or kidneys), and pyuria.
    - With suspected pyelonephritis, a clean-voided midstream or catheter-obtained specimen of urine should be collected and urinalysis, and culture and sensitivity of urine or blood obtained.
    - **Treatment.** Those who appear ill or are elderly, whose vomiting limits oral intake, in whom bacteremia is suspected, and who have high fever should be admitted. Admitted patients require intravenous fluid, intravenous antibiotics, analgesics, antiemetics, and antipyretics. Shock requires aggressive sepsis management. Initial therapy choices are ceftriaxone, ciprofloxacin, or ampicillin 2 g intravenously every 4 to 6 hours.
    - Acute, uncomplicated pyelonephritis can be treated as outpatients with ciprofloxacin 500 mg twice daily for 10 to 14 days. **Repeat urine culture** is advised

5 days after therapy. Follow-up in 3 to 4 days is indicated should improvement fail to occur or other symptoms develop.

- ○ **Recurrent episodes** of pyelonephritis in women and *initial* episodes in men require nonemergent urologic evaluation to exclude anatomic abnormalities.

- **Acute urethral syndrome** is found in 30% to 40% of women who present with clinical cystitis but who fail to demonstrate significant bacterial growth when urine is appropriately collected. Urinalysis frequently shows pyuria but no microorganisms nor casts. Infection with *Chlamydia trachomatis* or *Ureaplasma urealyticum* may be the cause.

- Acute urethral syndrome is a self-limited illness. Treatment with phenazopyridine (Pyridium), 200 mg three times daily, and azithromycin 1 g orally as a single dose, or a short course of doxycycline, 100 mg twice daily may be considered.

- **Pelvic inflammatory disease** (See chapter 33, p. 293)

- **Abdominal aortic aneurysm** is clinically significant at a diameter of 4 cm.

  - **Diagnosis.** Leaking AAA causes middle or lower abdominal pain radiating to the back or back pain alone. Hypertension, ischemic lower extremities, and renal artery emboli or obstruction may also be important initial manifestations.

  - Physical findings include a palpable, pulsatile, midabdominal mass. Aneurysmal dilation of the abdominal aorta may be noted on an abdominal radiograph, particularly the cross-table lateral view, due to calcification in the wall of the aneurysm. Abdominal ultrasonography and CT are useful diagnostic procedures in defining the aneurysm in stable patients.

  - **Aneurysmal rupture** occurs when diameters exceed 6 cm (~50% rupture by 1 year) and is a true surgical emergency. Patients report severe abdominal or back pain and present with or develop shock. Patients presenting with shock require emergency operative intervention; extensive diagnostic testing should be avoided, as should prolonged efforts to normalize blood pressure. Large-bore intravenous access should be established, crystalloid infused, blood (usually 7–10 U packed red blood cells) made available, and the surgical team mobilized. In stable patients with normal blood pressure, both ultrasound and CT are useful, although each has specific limitations. Ultrasound can be obtained quickly, often at the bedside, but has low sensitivity for retroperitoneal blood. When a high level of clinical suspicion exists, many surgeons will proceed to surgery when an aneurysm is demonstrated by ultrasound. CT, although more time consuming than ultrasound, provides considerable additional information, including rapid confirmation of rupture or leak, size and extent of the aneurysm, and information regarding other diagnostic possibilities. Despite optimal emergency care and prompt operative intervention, once rupture ensues mortality approaches 50%.

- **Ischemic bowel disease** may produce chronic or acute symptoms depending on the rapidity with which occlusive lesions progress in the mesenteric arterial bed and on the number of vessels involved. **Chronic intestinal ischemia** generally results from atherosclerotic occlusive lesions at or close to the origin of the celiac, superior mesenteric or inferior mesenteric arteries, producing a marked reduction in intestinal blood flow under conditions of acute demand (i.e., postprandially). **Acute intestinal ischemia** is produced by embolic occlusion of visceral branches of the abdominal aorta or by thrombosis of one or more visceral arteries or may occur as a result of nonocclusive, mesenteric vascular insufficiency in patients with decompensated heart failure.

  - **Diagnosis.** Patients with "abdominal angina" complain of epigastric or periumbilical postprandial pain lasting from 1 to 3 hours. To avoid discomfort, patients do not eat and consequently often lose weight. Acute mesenteric ischemia produces the acute onset of steady, crampy epigastric or periumbilical abdominal pain lasting for several hours, often associated with prostration. Physical examination may be unrevealing in both chronic and acute intestinal ischemia, with patients commonly presenting with symptoms that are discordant (i.e., far in excess) of physical findings. Occasionally, a bruit may be auscultated. Absent bowel sounds in a patient complaining of severe pain with minimal physical findings should suggest the diagnosis. In patients with **infarction,** peritoneal irritation evolves, often associated with stool positive for occult blood. Laboratory tests are unrevealing in chronic intestinal ischemia but may reveal a marked leukocytosis and elevated lactate levels with acidosis with acute mesenteric ischemia.

- **Treatment.** Emergency angiography with plans for surgery to bypass the obstructed vessel (or vessels) or resection of infarcted bowel is essential for immediate management. Volume resuscitation and correction of metabolic abnormalities should be instituted while surgical consultation is obtained.

- **Spontaneous bacterial peritonitis** (SBP) develops in cirrhotic patients with ascites. No source for the introduction of the bacteria into the peritoneal cavity may be apparent. Organisms involved are primarily Gram-negative enteric organisms, but *Streptococcus* spp., *Klebsiella,* and *Streptococcus pneumoniae* can be involved. The mortality rate for SBP is high.
  - The **history** reveals diffuse abdominal pain, fever, chills, and hypotension. Onset of SBP may correspond with worsening hepatic encephalopathy.
  - The **physical findings** of SBP range from no abdominal tenderness to severe tenderness with peritonitis.
  - **Diagnostic tests** include a CBC, electrolytes, BUN/Cr, and liver function studies but do not pinpoint SBP. The test of greatest diagnostic significance is analysis of aspirated peritoneal fluid obtained by paracentesis. Typically, there will be more than 300 WBCs/mL, of which more than 250 will be polymorphonuclear leukocytes (PMNs), and a decreased protein content, usually less than 1 g/dL. Ascitic fluid should be both aerobically and anaerobically cultured.
  - **Treatment** recommendations are IV ceftriaxone +/– vancomycin or oral ciprofloxacin for the stable outpatient.

27 Constipation and Diarrhea

CONSTIPATION

Although frequently a functional problem, constipation may be caused by a variety of treatable organic processes. Any new change in bowel habits should be evaluated for organic causes.

COMMON CAUSES OF CONSTIPATION

- Irritable bowel syndrome*
- Diabetes
- Diverticulitis
- Anorectal disorders (hemorrhoids, anal fissure, fistula or stricture, perianal abscess)*
- Drug ingestion (opiates, anticholinergics, barium sulfate, iron supplements, calcium channel blockers, parasympatholytics, phosphate-containing antacids)

LESS COMMON CAUSES OF CONSTIPATION NOT TO BE MISSED

- Hypothyroidism
- Hypercalcemia
- Rectal carcinoma
- Scleroderma
- Hypokalemia
- Hernia
- Sigmoid volvulus
- Bowel obstruction

OTHER CAUSES OF CONSTIPATION

- Hirschsprung disease
- Prolonged inactivity or immobilization
- Chagas disease
- Myotonic dystrophy

HISTORY

Chronic constipation alternating with episodes of diarrhea suggests **irritable bowel syndrome. Anal fissure, perianal abscess, anal fistula, and external hemorrhoids** often cause intense pain with defecation, thereby producing constipation through

---

*Discussed in this chapter.

avoidance. Narrow-caliber stools, with or without blood coating, suggest a **rectal fissure, stricture,** or **rectal carcinoma.** Dysphagia, Raynaud phenomenon, and characteristic skin changes suggest **scleroderma.** Profound constipation is seen in the rare, congenitally acquired **aganglionic colon** of Hirschsprung disease. Constipation associated with megacolon occurring in patients from Central and South America is often caused by **Chagas disease.** Vomiting and abdominal pain accompanying constipation are frequently noted in patients with **bowel obstruction.**

PHYSICAL EXAMINATION

Lower quadrant abdominal pain often accompanied by occult blood in the stool suggests **diverticulitis** or **colorectal carcinoma** (although colorectal carcinoma is usually painless early in its course). **Anorectal pathology** (i.e., anal fissure, external or internal hemorrhoids, perianal abscess) will be noted on examination. **Hypothyroidism** (obesity, dry skin, coarse hair, and delayed reflexes) may be accompanied by constipation. A mass lesion on digital rectal examination suggests **rectal carcinoma. Inguinal hernias** and colonic volvulus produce constipation by partial (or complete) bowel obstruction.

DIAGNOSTIC TESTS

Analysis of the stool for gross or occult blood provides information about some of the nonfunctional causes of constipation including diverticulitis and rectal carcinoma. Anoscopy may demonstrate internal hemorrhoids or fissures. The abdominal roentgenogram often demonstrates excessive colonic stool.

SPECIFIC DISORDERS

Irritable Bowel Syndrome

Irritable bowel syndrome (IBS) consists of abnormal intestinal motility, manifest by an increase in slow-wave activity in the colon. Three clinical variants of the disease are recognized: chronic constipation with abdominal pain (IBS-C), chronic intermittent diarrhea without pain (IBS-D) and alternating constipation, and diarrhea usually without pain. Patients with the first two varieties are more commonly seen in the emergency department (ED).

History
- IBS affects young or middle-aged adults with a 2:1 female-to-male ratio. Diarrhea occurs intermittently for months or years, with or without intermittent constipation and crampy lower abdominal pain, usually somewhat relieved by passing flatus or stool.

Physical Examination
- **Physical examination** may reveal these a somewhat distended abdomen during episodes of pain. Between episodes of pain, a tender sigmoid filled with feces may be palpated. No definitive tests are available to diagnose IBS; its diagnosis rests entirely on the clinical history and the exclusion of other pathology including celiac disease (gluten intolerance).

Treatment
- **Treatment** includes encouraging the patient to adapt to the symptoms in a way that minimizes impact on lifestyle. Pharmacologic therapy may be helpful in predominant constipation by an increasing dietary bulk. Bloating and cramping

may be relieved with antispasmodic or anticholinergic agents (hyoscyamine or dicyclomine); a mild sedative or a trial of low-dose tricyclic antidepressant therapy may be beneficial. Current specific therapy for IBS-C is lubiprostone (Amitiza), which promotes fluid secretion into the intestinal lumen. IBS-D treatment includes rifaximin (Xifaxan), which inhibits intestinal bacteria, and alosetron (Lotronex), which is a 5-HT$_3$ receptor antagonist.

Anorectal Disorders

- **Hemorrhoids** are varicosities of the hemorrhoidal venous plexus. External hemorrhoids involve only the inferior venous plexus and lie below the anorectal line. Those cephalad to the dentate line are internal hemorrhoids.
  - **External hemorrhoids** cause pain and bleeding, worsened by defecation. A tender perianal mass is noted on examination.
    - **Conservative treatment** consists of sitz baths, systemic and local analgesics, stool softeners and avoidance of straining at stool. A topical cream or suppository containing both anesthetic and anti-inflammatory properties, such as Anusol-HC, should be used twice daily.
    - **Surgical treatment.** Thrombosed hemorrhoids require incision and clot removal. This may be performed in the ED with local anesthesia. With the patient in the lateral decubitus position, the area is prepared and draped and incised to an extent sufficient to allow the removal of the clot. Minor bleeding frequently occurs and may persist for 1 to 3 days. A dry, sterile dressing should be applied and patients should be instructed to start warm sitz baths three to four times daily for 5 to 7 days along with surgical follow-up.
    - **Caution** is advised to avoid mistaking a nonthrombosed or incompletely thrombosed hemorrhoid for a fully thrombosed hemorrhoid. Nonthrombosed or incompletely thrombosed hemorrhoids are generally pink or erythematous and fluctuant, whereas fully thrombosed hemorrhoids, which may safely be incised and evacuated, are purple or black in color and hard or nonfluctuant; both lesions may be extremely tender. Recognizing these differences is essential because the incision of a partially thrombosed hemorrhoid may precipitate significant hemorrhage.
  - **Internal hemorrhoids** frequently produce a prolapsing anal mass and significant rectal bleeding. Prolapse typically occurs during defecation early in the course of the disease, but eventually permanent prolapse may develop. Anal irritation and intense pruritus often develop in the setting of a mucoid anal discharge. Bleeding is usually intermittent and is rarely massive except in patients with portal hypertension or abnormalities of hemostasis. Hospitalization and surgical excision are recommended when bleeding is significant, when symptoms are severe or disabling, or when conservative treatment has been ineffective.
- **Anal fissures** are linear disruptions of the anal epithelium. The treatment of simple acute fissures is based on maintaining regular, soft bowel movements and the use of sitz baths three to four times per day. Chronic fissures may require surgical excision if conservative measures fail to produce healing and control pain.
- **Perianal abscess.** A perianal abscess is often the acute stage of an anal fistula. When fluctuance is present, incision and drainage is the treatment of choice. When nonfluctuant, warm sitz baths three to four times daily, appropriate antibiotic if systemic evidence of infection is present, and surgical follow-up in 24 to 48 hours are recommended.
- **Anal fistula.** Most anal fistulas are preceded by an anal abscess and arise in an anal crypt. If an anal fistula opens into the rectum above the pectinate line, inflammatory

bowel disease, tuberculosis, lymphogranuloma venereum, rectal cancer, or a foreign body should be considered. Local pruritus, tenderness, and pain worsened by defecation are reported, and recurrent abscesses may develop. Surgical incision or excision under general anesthesia may be required for definitive therapy.

- **Anorectal stricture.** Surgery or trauma to the rectum that denudes the epithelium of the anal canal may result in a rectal stricture. Lymphogranuloma venereum and granuloma inguinale may also lead to stricture formation, as may gonococcal infection. Pain on defecation, constipation, and stools of narrow caliber are the commonest symptoms. Surgical correction may be necessary for patients with severe, chronic stenoses.

TREATMENT

Treatment of constipation involves treatment of any organic causes. Symptomatic treatment includes increasing the patient's intake of fiber and the use of laxatives, stimulant cathartics or stool softeners. Laxatives (docusate sodium, 50 to 200 mg orally daily, or docusate calcium, 240 mg orally daily, each with mineral oil, 15 to 45 mL orally (or per rectum) every 6 to 8 hours) are usually effective. Stimulant cathartics (cascara, 5 mL orally daily and bisacodyl, 10–15 mg orally at bedtime) or the 10-mg rectal suppository are also effective. Cathartics containing nonabsorbable salts (such as milk of magnesia, 15–30 mL orally every 8–12 hours or magnesium citrate, 200 mL orally) cause water to be osmotically retained in the colon and are also effective (not to be used in patients with renal failure). Phosphosoda, 1.5 oz with 500 mL of water orally is given twice within an 8-hour interval; it is contraindicated in patients with renal failure. Enemas are also effective; sodium biphosphate (Fleet) enemas are a common initial choice and can be given per rectum once or twice (also avoid in patients with renal failure). Tap water enemas (1 L) are also used, with oil-based preparations usually reserved for patients failing other forms of therapy.

DIARRHEA

Cases of acute diarrheal illnesses include viruses, invasive bacteria, toxin-producing bacteria, protozoa, drugs, neoplastic processes, autoimmune disorders, and functional abnormalities.

COMMON CAUSES OF DIARRHEA

- Viral gastroenteritis (especially Norwalk virus)*
- Bacterial gastroenteritis*
- Staphylococcal toxin
- Invasive *Escherichia coli*
- Enterotoxigenic *E. coli*
- *Salmonella* sp. (salmonellosis)
- *Campylobacter jejuni*
- Shigella*
- *Vibrio cholerae**
- *Vibrio parahaemolyticus**
- Drugs (antibiotics, cholinergics, magnesium-containing antacids [Maalox, Mylanta, Riopan])
- Diverticulitis
- Irritable bowel syndrome

LESS COMMON CAUSES OF DIARRHEA NOT TO BE MISSED

- Protozoal gastroenteritis
- Amebiasis (*Entamoeba histolytica*)
- Giardiasis (*Giardia lamblia*)
- *Yersinia enterocolitica*
- Inflammatory bowel disease (especially Crohn disease)
- Pseudomembranous enterocolitis (*Clostridium difficile*)*
- Villous adenoma
- Fecal impaction*

OTHER CAUSES OF DIARRHEA

- Traveler's diarrhea*
- Bacterial overgrowth syndromes
- Pancreatic insufficiency
- Bile salt enteropathy
- *Clostridium perfringens*
- *Bacillus cereus*
- Cathartic abuse
- Carcinoid
- Lactase deficiency with lactose intolerance
- Hyperthyroidism
- AIDS-related diarrhea

HISTORY

- The **time interval** between the ingestion of a presumptively contaminated substance and the development of symptoms is often very helpful in assessing cause. Diarrhea developing within 6 to 12 hours after a meal is most likely caused by ingestion of a preformed toxin, such as **staphylococcal exotoxin,** and is frequently preceded by severe vomiting. The ingestion of food contaminated with *Salmonella* **sp.** may be associated with a symptom-free interval of up to 2 days. Similarly, the ingestion of **coliform organisms producing enterotoxin** or associated with invasion of the bowel wall may not produce symptoms for 1 to 3 days after the ingestion. To substantiate a food-borne cause, it is useful to determine whether any of the patient's close associates or family members have similar symptoms.
- The **gross appearance** of the stool is also helpful in suggesting a cause. Frankly bloody diarrhea is often seen in patients with *Shigella* **or** *Campylobacter* **infections,** whereas bulky, foul-smelling stool is suggestive of **pancreatic insufficiency.** The so-called rice-water stool is seen in **typhoid fever,** and gross pus is occasionally noted in the stool of patients with **inflammatory bowel disease. Cholera, toxigenic** *E. coli* **enteritis, diarrheogenic pancreatic tumors,** and **bile salt enteropathy** all produce a secretory diarrhea that, by history, examination and laboratory analysis, is quite watery and dilute.
- A history of recent travel suggests **traveler's diarrhea;** the specific cause of this disorder remains unclear. It is usually self-limited, and patients fully recover 2 to 3 weeks after returning home. A history of recent antibiotic use should always suggest

pseudomembranous enterocolitis, a diarrheal illness produced by a necrolytic toxin synthesized by *C. difficile.* Diarrhea secondary to **diverticulitis** may be accompanied by tenesmus, rectal urgency, fever, and left lower quadrant discomfort. Diarrhea persisting for weeks or months is usually either functional or may be associated with several less common illnesses, including **carcinoid, bile salt enteropathy, pancreatic insufficiency,** the **bacterial overgrowth syndromes,** or **hyperthyroidism;** it is rarely infectious. In addition, the **habitual use of cathartics** should be considered, which often produces a rather perplexing, prolonged history of diarrhea.

PHYSICAL EXAMINATION

- Fever may be noted in the more severe bacterial illnesses, especially **salmonellosis, Campylobacter infections and shigellosis; ulcerative colitis** and **Crohn disease** are also often accompanied by fever during their acute exacerbations. In elderly patients, **fecal impaction** may be noted on physical examination, around which small amounts of liquid stool may be expelled, producing the symptomatic report of diarrhea. Perirectal fissures are suggestive of **Crohn disease.**

DIAGNOSTIC TESTS

- Stool exam for **fecal leukocytes** and for the presence of **occult blood** is essential. Fecal leukocytes are present in the invasive bacterial diarrheal illnesses, including salmonellosis, shigellosis and *C. jejuni* infections, whereas viral gastroenteritis usually does not produce a fecal leukocytosis. Occult or frank blood may be observed in the stool of patients with shigellosis and *C. jejuni* infections. The diagnosis of pseudomembranous enterocolitis is made by identifying *C. difficile* toxin in the stool.
- Osmotic diarrhea includes lactase deficiency, the use of magnesium-containing cathartics, and unabsorbed carbohydrates associated with the malabsorption states.
- A **complete blood count** (CBC) may suggest invasive bacterial infection. **BUN and electrolytes** help determine the extent to which the patient has lost fluid, sodium, potassium and bicarbonate.
- **Stool cultures** should be obtained when salmonellosis, shigellosis, or *Campylobacter* infections are suspected. A fresh specimen of stool should be analyzed for the presence of ova and parasites in patients in whom amebiasis or giardiasis is suspected.

CLINICAL REMINDERS

- Vigorously replenish fluid and electrolyte losses in patients with secretory and osmotic diarrheal illnesses; this is especially essential in infants and children.
- Analyze stool specimens for the presence of occult blood and fecal leukocytes.
- Culture stool specimens in suspected bacterial illness.
- Patients with suspected infectious diarrhea should be treated with ciprofloxacin 500 mg twice daily for 3 days and loperamide.

SPECIFIC DISORDERS

Viral Gastroenteritis

Viral gastroenteritis is the most common cause of infectious diarrhea. Echoviruses, reoviruses (especially Norwalk virus), and adenoviruses are common.

History
- The patient may report upper respiratory tract symptoms in addition to diarrhea, abdominal cramping or discomfort, headache, fever, and generalized malaise. Typically, crampy abdominal discomfort is somewhat improved after an episode of diarrhea.

Physical Examination
- On **physical examination,** hyperactive bowel sounds and mild lower abdominal tenderness are noted.

Diagnostic Tests
- Stool examination reveals no pus or blood. The CBC is usually within normal limits. A lymphocytic predominance is common.

Treatment
- **Treatment** includes fluid replacement, either orally or parenterally. Outpatient therapy includes restriction of caffeine, lactose, and dairy products, encouraging clear liquid intake for several hours and advancing the diet as tolerated. Diarrhea typically subsides within 3 to 5 days. If vomiting coexists and is severe, admission for fluid replacement is warranted, especially in the very young and elderly.

Bacterial Gastroenteritis

Bacteria produce gastrointestinal symptoms, either by the elaboration of a toxin that stimulates the secretion of water into the intestinal lumen or by actual invasion of the intestinal mucosa.

- ***Escherichia coli*** may cause diarrhea by either of the aforementioned mechanisms. In patients with enterotoxic coliform diarrhea, the syndrome is usually mild and self-limited; the invasive coliform diarrheal illnesses, however, are somewhat more protracted and associated with fever, crampy abdominal pain, profuse diarrhea, and, occasionally, frankly bloody stools. These two forms of coliform diarrhea may be differentiated by Gram or Wright stain of the stool; numerous polymorphonuclear leukocytes and erythrocytes are seen in patients with invasive infections. **Traveler's diarrhea** is typically self-limited but may be debilitating; it is experienced primarily by travelers to developing countries, caused by infectious agents transmitted through food and water. The most common causative agent is **enterotoxigenic *E. coli.*** Illness lasts 3 to 5 days and is not associated with excessive fluid losses. The severity of symptoms can be reduced with bismuth subsalicylate (Pepto-Bismol), 60 mL four times daily. Antimotility drugs and ciprofloxacin, 500 mg orally twice daily for 3 days, reduce severity and duration of illness. Avoiding ingestion of contaminated food and water remains the most effective prophylactic measure.
  - Stool C & S should be obtained in children, those with bloody diarrhea, systemic illness or immunocompromised state. Other treatment is fluid supplementation and, occasionally, antispasmodic agents.
- *Salmonella enteritidis* causes diarrhea 24 to 36 hours after ingestion of contaminated food or water. There is relatively sudden onset of headache, nausea, vomiting, fever, and diarrhea lasting 2 to 4 days. Some serotypes may cause a more severe illness lasting up to 3 weeks without therapy, occasionally accompanied by bacteremia. Physical examination is nonspecific, but the stool examination reveals many polymorphonuclear leukocytes. Stool culture is important for an accurate diagnosis. In mild cases, adequate salt and water repletion are effective. Loperamide and 3 days of ciprofloxacin are indicated. Patients with severe illness or documented bacteremia

require hospitalization for intravenous hydration and ciprofloxacin (400 mg intravenous every 12 hours) or trimethoprim-sulfamethoxazole (1 double-strength tablet twice daily for 2 weeks).

- *Shigella* may cause severe diarrhea, particularly in infants and elderly patients. Stools may be bloody and patients may appear quite ill with rapidly progressive dehydration. The stool contains abundant polymorphonuclear leukocytes and erythrocytes, and a stool culture is mandatory. Therapy involves volume and salt repletion as well as treatment with ciprofloxacin, 500 mg orally every 12 hours, or trimethoprim-sulfamethoxazole, 1 double-strength tablet twice daily for 2 weeks.

- **Staphylococcal exotoxin** causes nausea, vomiting, and diarrhea 2 to 6 hours after ingestion of inadequately cooked or improperly refrigerated food. It lasts 24 hours, and foods containing mayonnaise or creams are usually implicated. The physical examination is nonspecific and stool cultures are unrevealing. Fluid repletion is the mainstay of therapy.

- *Campylobacter jejuni* causes bloody stool; crampy, periumbilical abdominal pain; fever; chills; and headache. The physical examination is nonspecific; stool contains many polymorphonuclear leukocytes and erythrocytes. Stool culture is mandatory for appropriate diagnosis. Therapy involves salt and water repletion, ciprofloxacin, 500 mg orally every 12 hours, or erythromycin ethylsuccinate (EES) 50 mg/kg/day orally divided four times daily.

- *Vibrio cholerae* is uncommon in advanced Western nations. It causes a profusely secretory diarrhea requiring vigorous salt and water repletion. The disease usually runs a 5- to 7-day course. Trimethoprim-sulfamethoxazole (Bactrim) twice daily is effective.

- Ingestion of raw seafood may cause *V. parahaemolyticus* diarrhea. It occurs 6 to 48 hours later with crampy abdominal pain. The physical examination is nonspecific, and a stool culture will reveal the pathogen. Therapy requires repletion of salt and water and doxycycline.

Protozoal Gastroenteritis

The most common causes in the United States are *E. histolytica* and *G. lamblia.* Amebiasis either can produce an intermittent diarrheal syndrome or can occasionally lead to a severe, fulminating illness with an initial presentation similar to that of inflammatory bowel disease. Giardiasis typically produces a more chronic diarrheal illness that is associated with epigastric distress secondary to duodenal infestation with parasites. The travel history is important in both of these conditions; amebiasis is seen in patients who have traveled to the tropics, whereas giardiasis is worldwide in contaminated surface water.

Physical Examination
- The **physical examination** may show periumbilical tenderness with amebiasis and mild epigastric tenderness with giardiasis. Amebiasis frequently produces occult blood in the stool.

Diagnostic Tests
- **Diagnostic tests** include an analysis of freshly obtained stool for ova and parasites. Serology may show giardia antigen in stool.

Treatment
- Once the diagnosis of amebiasis is established, the patient should be treated with metronidazole, 750 mg three times daily for 10 days (or 500 mg intravenous every 8 hours for 5–10 days), followed by paromomycin, 500 orally three times daily for 7 days, or iodoquinol, 650 mg twice daily for 3 weeks. Asymptomatic

carriers should be treated with iodoquinol, 650 mg orally three times daily for 3 weeks. Giardiasis may be treated with metronidazole, 250 mg three times daily for 5 days; tinidazole, 2 g as a single dose; quinacrine hydrochloride, 100 mg three times daily after meals for 7 days; or furazolidone, 100 mg orally three times daily for 7 to 10 days for children.

Pseudomembranous Enterocolitis

Pseudomembranous enterocolitis (antibiotic-associated enterocolitis) is caused by a necrolytic toxin elaborated by *C. difficile,* an organism that commonly inhabits the bowel. Typically, this illness develops subsequent to or concurrent with exposure to antibiotics, which alter the normal ecologic balance of the bowel flora, permitting *C. difficile* to proliferate. Every antibiotic has been implicated, although vancomycin and aminoglycosides rarely.

Diagnosis
- Diarrhea in these patients is typically profuse and watery but may be frankly bloody in approximately 5% of cases. Colonoscopy shows the characteristic multiple, discrete yellowish plaques that on biopsy reveal the features of a pseudomembrane. The diagnosis is made by identifying *C. difficile* toxin in the stool.

Treatment
- **Treatment** involves the use of oral metronidazole, 250 to 500 mg orally three times daily for 7 to 14 days or oral vancomycin, 125 mg four times daily for 7 to 10 days. Antidiarrheal agents should be avoided.

Inflammatory Bowel Disease

- Both **ulcerative colitis** and **Crohn disease** produce bloody diarrhea and diffuse abdominal pain. Extracolonic manifestations of inflammatory bowel disease include uveitis, dermatitis, erythema nodosum, pyoderma gangrenosum, pericholangitis, spondyloarthritis, sclerosing cholangitis, and peripheral arthritis. Extraintestinal manifestations should suggest an inflammatory bowel disease. Perirectal fistulas are commonly seen in Crohn disease. Examination of the stool reveals both erythrocytes and polymorphonuclear leukocytes. Stool culture is negative for enteropathogenic bacteria. Fresh stool specimens should be examined for ova and parasites. Rectal involvement is 100% in ulcerative colitis. Diagnosis is made by biopsy.
- **Toxic megacolon** is the most serious complication of ulcerative colitis; it occurs much less commonly in Crohn disease. Megacolon develops due to a decrease in neuromuscular tone in the bowel wall. The use of hypomotility agents has been reported to precipitate this complication. Abdominal roentgenogram shows colonic dilation with a diameter greater than 6 cm and air in the wall of the colon ("pneumotosis coli"). Risk of bowel perforation is extremely high, and for this reason, toxic megacolon should be considered a true medical emergency. Perforation is associated with a mortality of greater than 30%. In patients with severe, fulminant ulcerative colitis or toxic megacolon, anticholinergic and opioid drugs should be avoided because they can precipitate or aggravate toxic megacolon.
- **Treatment** includes repletion of intravenous fluids and electrolytes, initiation of broad spectrum intravenous antibiotic coverage and parenteral glucocorticoids. An initial steroid regimen of hydrocortisone, 300 mg/day (or an equivalent dose of methylprednisolone [48 mg/day]) or prednisolone (60 mg/day) is recommended. Patients with ulcerative colitis, if not previously treated with steroids, should receive ACTH (120 U/day) in place of hydrocortisone. Patients with ulcerative

colitis are at risk for the development of toxic megacolon. If suspected, a surgical consultation should be obtained and complete bowel rest started. If signs of toxic megacolon increase despite therapy, or fail to improve, emergent surgery may be required.

- Mild to moderate flares of inflammatory bowel disease are treated with glucocorticoids in ulcerative colitis and with sulfasalazine (Azulfidine, 3–4 g/day), in Crohn disease; steroids are used less frequently in Crohn, except for severe symptoms. Sulfasalazine is useful for maintaining remissions in ulcerative colitis; the role of maintenance therapy in Crohn disease is less clear, although success has been reported with the immunosuppressive agents (6-mercaptopurine and azathioprine).

- The usefulness of sulfasalazine is often limited due to side effects (anorexia, diarrhea, vomiting, headache, abdominal pain, and allergic complications). Newer agents, which are derivatives of 5-aminosalicylic acid, are efficacious and associated with far fewer complications. These agents (mesalamine, olsalazine, and balsalazide) are available in oral and topical (by enema) preparations. The topical preparations are useful in patients with distal colonic involvement, including proctitis. Topical steroid preparations are also useful.

- Diarrhea in Crohn disease usually responds to diphenoxylate (Lomotil), 5 to 20 mg/day or loperamide (Imodium), 4 to 16 mg/day.

28 Gastrointestinal Bleeding

COMMON CAUSES OF HEMATEMESIS

- Peptic ulcer disease
- Gastritis
- Esophagitis
- Mallory-Weiss tear*
- Esophageal varices*

LESS COMMON CAUSES OF HEMATEMESIS NOT TO BE MISSED

- Artifactual causes
- Aortoenteric fistula*
- Occult blood ingestion
- Malignancy

COMMON CAUSES OF RECTAL BLEEDING OR MELENA

- Hemorrhoidal bleeding*
- Colorectal carcinoma*
- Diverticulosis
- Any cause of brisk upper tract bleeding
- Inflammatory bowel disease
- Infectious diarrhea

LESS COMMON CAUSES OF RECTAL BLEEDING OR MELENA NOT TO BE MISSED

- Angiodysplasia of the colon
- Meckel diverticulum
- Osler-Weber-Rendu syndrome

HISTORY

Epigastric or right upper quadrant discomfort, often described as "gnawing" or "burning," may be reported in patients with **peptic ulceration** involving either the stomach and distal esophagus or the duodenum. The history may reveal that discomfort

---

*Discussed in this chapter.

is relieved with food or antacid intake and that it often recurs several hours after eating. Recent or chronic ingestion of **steroids, aspirin, or other nonsteroidal anti-inflammatory agents,** or antithrombotic and antiplatelet therapy may predispose to gastrointestinal bleeding. Lower quadrant discomfort may be present in patients with **diverticulitis, inflammatory bowel disease,** and infectious diarrhea.

A variety of substances, including licorice, beets, spinach, chard, charcoal, coal, dirt, lead, iron, bismuth (Pepto-Bismol), and sulfobromophthalein, may sufficiently discolor either the gastric contents or stool to produce alarm; these artifactual causes may be established by history and actual blood loss excluded by a negative stool guaiac determination.

Hematemesis beginning after an initial bout of retching is often caused by the development of a Mallory-Weiss mucosal laceration. In Laennec cirrhosis, one half of patients presenting with hematemesis are bleeding from a nonvariceal source.

A history of narrowing of the caliber of stools and weight loss is suggestive of colorectal carcinoma. Perianal pain or pruritus is commonly reported in patients with hemorrhoids. A family history of gastrointestinal bleeding suggests the Osler-Weber-Rendu syndrome.

PHYSICAL EXAMINATION

- Abdominal tenderness is noted in peptic ulcer, diverticulitis, inflammatory bowel disease, colorectal carcinoma, and infectious diarrhea.
- Signs of **hyperestrogenism** secondary to chronic liver disease, including gynecomastia and testicular atrophy, support the diagnosis of significant liver damage, which may be associated with portal hypertension and esophageal varices.
- External hemorrhoids are seen on **inspection of the rectum;** internal hemorrhoids, which are much more likely to produce significant hemorrhage, are best documented by anoscopy or proctosigmoidoscopy. Because 60% to 70% of all colorectal cancers arise in the rectosigmoid, digital rectal examination may detect such lesions.

DIAGNOSTIC TESTS

Stable patients presenting with hematemesis require passage of a nasogastric tube and a rectal examination for the analysis of occult or gross blood. Admission should be considered in all patients with evidence of upper tract bleeding. Blood should be obtained for typing and cross-matching, determination of hematocrit and clotting parameters, and other routine admission studies. A negative nasogastric aspirate for occult blood does not exclude an upper tract source. In approximately 25% of patients with duodenal bleeding, a competent pyloric sphincter prevents reflux of blood into the stomach resulting in negative NG aspirates for blood.

The hematocrit is useful for corroborating chronic or subacute gastrointestinal hemorrhage but is normal in patients seen early in the course of bleeding. Eight hours is required to permit complete equilibration between the extravascular and intravascular compartments; in the setting of acute hemorrhage, the hematocrit is an insensitive indicator of the extent and subsequent rate of blood loss. A platelet count and prothrombin time (PT) and partial thromboplastin time (PTT) should be measured and, if abnormal, corrected with platelet transfusions or fresh frozen plasma (FFP), respectively. Antithrombotic or antiplatelet medications are reversed with FFP or platelet transfusions, respectively.

Consultation for urgent colonoscopy should be obtained for active lower tract bleeding. If bleeding is massive, adequate visualization of the bleeding site is often impossible and mesenteric arteriography is the diagnostic procedure of choice. It should be arranged promptly after initial stabilization. The rate of spontaneous resolution of lower tract bleeding is high, although approximately 25% of patients rebleed. Although hemorrhoidal bleeding is relatively common, with significant lower tract bleeding, this must be a diagnosis of exclusion.

CLINICAL REMINDERS

- Clinical status may require aggressive resuscitation with crystalloid and blood products.
- Do not assume that lower tract bleeding is hemorrhoidal unless a bleeding hemorrhoid is visualized.
- Obtain early gastroenterologic and surgical consultation in all patients with gastrointestinal bleeding.

MANAGEMENT OF HEMORRHAGIC SHOCK DUE TO GASTROINTESTINAL BLEEDING

Rapid initial response to hemorrhagic shock due to gastrointestinal bleeding includes the establishment of a functional airway, if required, correction of hypoxemia, insertion of a nasogastric tube and Foley catheter; beginning continuous monitoring of blood pressure, pulse oximetry, and cardiac rhythm; and insertion of two large-bore short-length, peripheral intravenous catheters. Administer 2-L bolus of normal saline in adults and two 20 mL/kg in children. If necessary, un–cross-matched blood may be transfused. HCT should be maintained at approximately 30% to 35% and the central venous pressure at 8 to 12 cm H_2O.

Multiple, closely spaced transfusions of packed red blood cells may lead to clinically significant hypocalcemia as well as abnormalities of hemostasis. Hypocalcemia results from chelation of intravascular calcium by the citrate preservative and occurs with packed red blood cells at transfusion rates greater than 100 mL/h. Calcium chloride, 0.2 g (2 mL of a 10% calcium chloride solution), may be given slowly through a separate intravenous line. A relative depletion of clotting factors, simply as a function of dilution, may evolve in multiply transfused patients if fresh frozen plasma is not administered concomitantly. Administer 1 U of fresh frozen plasma for every 4 U of packed red blood cells.

MANAGEMENT OF UPPER TRACT BLEEDING

Gentle lavage with room-temperature saline is useful both for slowing upper tract hemorrhage and monitoring the rate of blood loss. For upper gastrointestinal (UGI) bleeds, fiberoptic endoscopy is the diagnostic study of choice and should be employed early. Begin Protonix 80 mg IV bolus and subsequent infusion or octreotide for suspected variceal bleeding.

When bleeding is so brisk that it exceeds one's ability to sustain or normalize blood pressure, emergency surgical consultation must be obtained.

If bleeding is so rapid that that the mucosa cannot be adequately visualized on endoscopy, abdominal angiography may establish a diagnosis and provide additional therapeutic options, for example, selective vasopressin infusion or embolization.

MANAGEMENT OF LOWER TRACT BLEEDING

After hemodynamic stabilization, patients with persistent, life-threatening, lower gastrointestinal tract bleeding require emergency diagnostic angiography to determine the anatomic site and rate of bleeding. When hemodynamic stabilization is not possible because of massive bleeding, operative intervention is emergently required. In patients with less significant bleeding, colonoscopy may also be used to identify bleeding sites. Early surgical consultation is recommended.

SPECIFIC DISORDERS

Esophageal Varices

History
- Esophageal and esophagogastric varices develop in the setting of portal hypertension and may be the source of exsanguinating hemorrhage. Because bleeding occurs directly into the esophagus, copious hematemesis develops. Many patients have a history of previous UGI hemorrhage, alcohol abuse, hepatitis, or chronic liver disease.

Physical Examination
- The **physical examination** usually demonstrates signs of chronic liver disease and portal hypertension. Palmar erythema, spider angiomata, gynecomastia, testicular atrophy, caput medusae, splenomegaly, jaundice, peripheral edema, and ascites may be present.

Treatment
- **Treatment** should be directed at maintaining hemodynamic stability, replenishing blood and clotting factors, and arresting hemorrhage. Octreotide should be administered by infusion (50–100 μg bolus, followed by an infusion at 25–50 μg/h); this agent reduces portal pressures with limited side effects. The role of peripheral vasopressin (0.3 U/min intravenous, followed by increments of 0.3 U/min every 30 minutes until bleeding ceases, side effects develop, or the maximal dose of 0.9 U/ min is achieved) is less clear; this is primarily caused by the precipitation of serious side effects (myocardial ischemia, ventricular arrhythmias, mesenteric ischemia, and cutaneous ischemic necrosis). ECG monitoring is recommended during vasopressin infusion to detect myocardial ischemia. In patients with coronary artery disease, vasopressin must be used with great caution. Additional therapeutic interventions are endoscopic variceal ligation or banding and endoscopic sclerosis or sclerotherapy. A variety of surgical procedures (transjugular intrahepatic portosystemic shunts and portacaval or distal splenorenal shunts) can be considered if bleeding continues despite ligation or sclerotherapy or if bleeding remains uncontrolled.

Mallory-Weiss Tears

Mallory-Weiss tears are mucosal lacerations occurring at the gastroesophageal junction, usually following an initial episode of vomiting nonbloody material or retching.

Diagnosis
- Patients present with painless hematemesis. Dietary or alcohol indiscretion is commonly reported.

Treatment
- Although bleeding may be significant, treatment is generally conservative, using antacids and PPIs, providing aggressive replacement of blood to a hematocrit of 35%, and correcting abnormalities of hemostasis. Often bleeding spontaneously abates and surgical intervention is rarely required.

Hemorrhoidal Bleeding
See Chapter 27.

Colorectal Carcinoma
Colorectal carcinoma most often affects people aged 50 to 70 years.

History
- Right-sided colon cancers are frequently sessile or polypoid and may reach palpable size before producing symptoms of obstruction; this is attributed to the liquid nature of the fecal stream in the ascending colon. Because left-sided cancers often grow more circumferentially, constipation or a change in stool caliber is the presenting symptom. Most colorectal cancers bleed at some time but this is usually occult. Right-sided cancers are the exception to this rule and may bleed massively. Diarrhea, abdominal pain, tenesmus, anorexia, and weight loss may be presenting symptoms.

Physical Examination
- The **physical examination** may reveal a palpable abdominal mass if the cancer involves the right colon or a mass palpable by rectal examination. Stool may contain occult blood.

Treatment
- No emergency treatment is required for suspected colorectal carcinoma unless significant rectal bleeding, pain, or signs of obstruction or perforation are present. In other patients, a careful evaluation regarding staging is essential, and consultation should be obtained before disposition.

Aortoenteric Fistula
Aortoenteric fistula is an uncommon cause of upper GI bleeding, but one that is suggested by a history of previous aortic/aortic graft surgery. The fistula is typically between the aorta and the duodenum but can occur anywhere in the bowel. Bleeding can occur months or years after a procedure. Identification of the "warning or herald" bleed (which occurs at a variable period before major bleeding) is essential if mortality is to be avoided. Although a CT scan or endoscopic procedure can confirm the cause of bleeding, when the diagnosis is suspected based on history and examination, emergent surgical remediation should proceed before confirmation.

29 Hiccups (Singultus)

Hiccups are usually a benign and transient phenomenon that most often occurs idiopathically, although included in the differential diagnosis are a variety of disorders. Continuous symptoms lasting greater than 48 hours often have an organic cause.

COMMON CAUSES OF HICCUPS

- Idiopathic
- Excess alcohol
- Excessive smoking
- Eating large boluses of food with inadequate liquid
- Air swallowing
- Anxiety
- Esophagitis
- Uremia
- Cyclical diaphragmatic spasm (after laughing, crying, coughing)

LESS COMMON CAUSES OF HICCUPS NOT TO BE MISSED

- Acute myocardial infarction
- Mediastinal or peridiaphragmatic irritative processes
- Gastric irritation or distention
- Foreign body in the ear canal irritating the tympanic membrane
- Pancreatitis
- Pneumonia
- Subphrenic abscess
- Cholecystitis
- Perforated intra-abdominal viscus with subdiaphragmatic free air
- Phrenic nerve tumors

TREATMENT

After the important causes of hiccups are considered, a variety of treatments are available. Most of the simple, well-known "home remedies" probably act by simply diverting the patient's attention. Medical measures that are occasionally effective include nasopharyngeal stimulation with a soft rubber catheter; mild sedation; gargling and swallowing viscous lidocaine, chlorpromazine (Thorazine), antacids, antispasmodics, Reglan; and, for patients with rare intractable hiccups, bilateral phrenectomy.

In persistent cases refractory to other measures, chlorpromazine (Thorazine), 25 to 50 mg intravenous, or haloperidol, 2 to 10 mg intramuscular, will often terminate the episode.

30 Jaundice

INTRODUCTION

Jaundice, a yellow discoloration of the skin, sclerae, and mucous membranes, has been recognized for centuries as a sign of liver disease. Bilirubin, the pigmented product of heme metabolism, accumulates in the body primarily as a result of its affinity for elastin, imparting a yellow color to these tissues. Although hyperbilirubinemia is present when the total serum concentration of bilirubin exceeds 1.2 mg/dL, clinically jaundice is not recognizable in most patients until the total bilirubin concentration exceeds 3 mg/dL.

The etiology of hyperbilirubinemia may be prehepatic, hepatic, or posthepatic in origin. Prehepatic hyperbilirubinemia results from excess intravascular liberation (i.e., hemolysis); hepatic hyperbilirubinemia is caused by hepatocyte dysfunction (i.e., faulty uptake, metabolism, or excretion of bilirubin); posthepatic hyperbilirubinemia occurs when the removal of bilirubin from the biliary system is impaired (i.e., by common bile duct obstruction or intrahepatic cholestatic obstruction).

COMMON CAUSES OF JAUNDICE

- Cholecystitis
- Hemolysis
- Hepatitis (e.g., infectious, drug induced, alcohol related)*
- Hepatic cirrhosis (e.g., Laennec, primary biliary)
- Carcinoma (primary or metastatic liver)
- Pancreatic carcinoma
- Common bile duct obstruction (usually secondary to gallstones)

LESS COMMON CAUSES OF JAUNDICE NOT TO BE MISSED

- Cholangitis
- Chronic heart failure
- Spirochetal infections (syphilis, leptospirosis)

OTHER CAUSES OF JAUNDICE

- Sarcoidosis
- Prolonged fasting
- Gilbert disease

---

*Discussed in this chapter.

- Crigler-Najjar syndrome
- Dubin-Johnson syndrome
- Rotor syndrome
- Recurrent jaundice of pregnancy
- Neonatal hyperbilirubinemia
- Infectious mononucleosis

HISTORY

Symptoms of hyperbilirubinemia are nonspecific and include pruritus, malaise, a loss of "taste," and anorexia. Dark urine and light- or clay-colored stools are noted in disorders that cause hepatic and posthepatic jaundice. A history of close or intimate exposure to other persons with jaundice or infectious hepatitis, ingestion of shellfish, or use of contaminated needles suggests **infectious hepatitis** as a cause. A history of exposure to **drugs or toxins** known to be associated with toxic hepatitis suggests these agents as potential causes. A history of excessive, regular **alcohol** use raises the possibility that the patient's jaundice may be secondary either to progressive Laennec cirrhosis or alcoholic hepatitis. Colicky right upper quadrant (RUQ) pain suggests **acute biliary obstruction** secondary to a stone or compression of the common duct. Cholangitis, which may follow common duct obstruction due to stone, should be considered in patients with high fever, rigors, abdominal pain, and fluctuating jaundice. Painless jaundice and a history of weight loss suggest carcinoma of the pancreas or chronic alcoholism.

PHYSICAL EXAMINATION

Splenomegaly may be noted in patients with intravascular hemolysis (e.g., **sickle cell anemia**) and in hepatic disorders producing portal hypertension (**cirrhotic disorders**). Estrogenization secondary to chronic acquired hepatic disease (e.g., **Laennec cirrhosis**) may produce gynecomastia, testicular atrophy, and sparse axillary and pubic hair. RUQ discomfort on palpation suggests **hepatitis, cholecystitis,** or **extrahepatic biliary obstruction.** A painless, palpable gallbladder (Courvoisier sign) with jaundice suggests **carcinoma of the head of the pancreas.** Needle tracks should suggest intravenous drug abuse and associated acquired **infectious hepatitis.**

DIAGNOSTIC TESTS

A predominant **unconjugated** hyperbilirubinemia is noted in all prehepatic disorders, some drug-induced hepatic diseases, Gilbert disease, and the Crigler-Najjar syndrome. A predominant **conjugated** hyperbilirubinemia is observed in all posthepatic disorders, most drug-related hepatitic disorders, Dubin-Johnson and Rotor syndromes, and all other intrahepatic causes of hyperbilirubinemia.

An elevated serum AST and serum ALT suggest hepatocellular dysfunction, whereas a markedly elevated alkaline phosphatase suggests extrahepatic obstruction or intrahepatic cholestasis. An elevation of gamma-glutamyltranspeptidase or 5'-nucleotidase further confirms these two mechanisms of jaundice, respectively. The determination of hepatitis A antibody is specific for diagnosis of acute hepatitis A, and acute hepatitis B may be diagnosed by the presence of hepatitis B surface antigen (HB$_s$Ag) or "e" antigen (HB$_e$Ag). On occasion, levels of HB$_s$Ag are too low to be detected during acute infection, circumstances under which the diagnosis can be made by detecting the presence of IgM anti-HB$_c$ (or antibody against core, "c," antigen). Chronic active or chronic persistent hepatitis causes persistent viremia manifested as hepatitis B surface antigenemia; its presence may confound the diagnosis of an acute hepatitic process in these patients. Prolongation of the prothrombin time, an indication of depressed hepatic synthetic function, portends a poor prognosis in the patient with acute infectious hepatitis.

In patients presenting with jaundice, it is imperative to distinguish obstruction from other etiologies. This is especially true when abdominal pain, fever, or evidence of systemic infection prevails. This may reliably be accomplished in 85% of patients with ultrasonography, computed tomography (CT) scans of the abdomen, or radionuclide imaging. Intrahepatic bile duct dilation may be demonstrated by the first two of these techniques and is diagnostic of biliary obstruction. Radionuclide imaging of the biliary tree with hepatobiliary iminodiacetic acid (HIDA) and diisopropyl iminodiacetic acid (DISIDA) is accurate even in patients with extreme hyperbilirubinemia. When the gallbladder is not visualized with these agents, the diagnosis of cholecystitis is confirmed. In addition, failure of the agent to reach the duodenum is noted in patients with biliary obstruction.

Ultrasonography and CT scans of the abdomen are useful to estimate liver and spleen size, exclude hepatic metastases, and evaluate the pancreas for mass lesions.

Another useful diagnostic technique is endoscopic retrograde cholangiopancreatography obtained by gastroenterologic consultation.

SPECIFIC DISORDERS

Viral Hepatitis

Distinct viral agents cause acute infectious hepatitis: hepatitis A (HAV), B (HBV), C (HCV), D (HDV), E (HEV), and G.

- **Hepatitis A** occurs sporadically in an epidemic form. Transmission of the hepatitis A virus (HAV) usually occurs through the fecal-oral route; outbreaks can occur with contamination of food and/or drinking water. Although transmission by sexual contact and contaminated needles is reported, it is uncommon. Shellfish have also been implicated. The incubation period ranges from 2 to 6 weeks. No known carrier state exists in hepatitis A, and morbidity and mortality are quite low.
  - Patients present with anorexia, nausea, vomiting, malaise, flu-like symptoms, and an aversion to tobacco among smokers. The physical examination may be remarkable for fever, jaundice, and an enlarged, tender liver. Hepatocellular enzyme elevations dominate the laboratory studies with hyperbilirubinemia and a less marked elevation of alkaline phosphatase activity. Hepatitis A infection is established by demonstrating seroconversion for hepatitis A.
  - Hepatitis A is diagnosed by finding anti-HAV antibody (IgM); anti-HAV IgG antibody is present in patients recovering from the illness or after vaccination.
- **Hepatitis B** is caused by the hepatitis B virus (HBV) and transmitted by inoculation of infected blood or blood products as well as by oral and/or sexual contact. Mother-to-infant transmission is also reported. High-risk groups include homosexuals, intravenous drug abusers, hemodialysis staff, dentists, and other medical professionals. Approximately 1% to 5% of infected individuals become chronic carriers, thereby providing a substantial reservoir of infection. The incubation period for hepatitis B ranges from 6 weeks to 6 months.

- Symptoms of hepatitis B infection are similar to those of hepatitis A but are more insidious. The spectrum of illness is quite variable, ranging from asymptomatic infection to fulminant, lethal hepatitis. Prodromal symptoms include malaise, anorexia, nausea, vomiting, myalgias, arthralgias, and fever. Dark urine and light, clay-colored stools are often reported as prodromal symptoms are subsiding. RUQ or epigastric discomfort often develops. Jaundice evolves after 1 week of prodromal symptoms; a small number of patients never develop clinical jaundice.
- **Physical examination** reveals icterus, lymphadenopathy, liver tenderness, and hepatomegaly in approximately one half of patients.
- **Diagnostic tests.** Hepatocellular enzyme elevations are common. A "cholangiolitic" variety of hepatitis B infection exists with a significant elevation of alkaline phosphatase activity.
- Serologic analysis is useful to document the state of disease activity, to identify carriers, and to define infectivity. $HB_s Ag$ is the antigen routinely measured in serum. Its presence is the first manifestation of hepatitis B infection, occurring before biochemical evidence of liver disease and persisting throughout the clinical illness. Disappearance of $HB_s Ag$ occurs when the virus is eliminated. The development of antibody against $HB_s Ag$ (anti-HB_s) is associated with recovery from clinical illness and noninfectivity (this is also seen after vaccination). Persistence of $HB_s Ag$ without significant anti-HB_s antibody evolution is associated with the development of chronic active or persistent hepatitis. Core antibody (anti-HB_c) develops soon after $HB_s Ag$ is detected and appears simultaneously with the onset of clinical illness. Patients who are anti-HB_c–positive and $HB_s Ag$-negative are considered infective. $HB_e Ag$ is found only in $HB_s Ag$-positive sera, appears during the incubation period soon after the appearance of $HB_s Ag$, and accompanies $HB_s Ag$ antigenemia. $HB_e Ag$ is a sensitive index of viral infectivity. Transmissibility of hepatitis B is increased in the presence of $HB_e Ag$ and impaired once antibody to $HB_e Ag$ develops (usually by the fourth week of illness).
- **Hepatitis C.** Hepatitis C virus (HCV) is usually subclinical and is responsible for most cases of transfusion-related viral hepatitis (75%–90%). Transmission also occurs via contaminated needles. HCV may also be transmitted sexually and from mother to infant, although at a rate lower than HBV; 80% of infected individuals develop chronic hepatitis. HCV is diagnosed by antibody to HCV via enzyme-linked immunosorbent assay (ELISA). ELISA assay may not be positive until 8 weeks after the onset of clinical illness. ELISA is not used to screen for disease in asymptomatic individuals. The incubation period for HCV is generally 7 to 8 weeks, ranging from 2 to 20 weeks. A carrier state occurs in a small percent of infected individuals.
- The **treatment** of patients with acute viral hepatitis consists of bed rest, avoidance of substances potentially damaging to the liver (alcohol, acetaminophen), and close follow-up. Most patients can be managed as outpatients. Persistent nausea and vomiting may require rehydration in the hospital. If hepatic function becomes markedly impaired, protein intake should be reduced until liver injury improves. The prognosis for most patients with infectious hepatitis is good, clinical recovery occurring by 15 weeks. A small percent of patients will develop severe and progressive hepatic failure; ICU admission, aggressive supportive measures, and early consideration of transplantation are recommended. Hepatitis B and C infection cause chronic hepatitis (active or persistent) in 5% to 10% of patients and requires close follow-up.

Prophylaxis

Hepatitis A
Pre-exposure

Hepatitis A vaccine should be administered to individuals traveling to endemic areas; other individuals who should receive the vaccine are intravenous drug users, patients with abnormalities of hemostasis requiring blood products, homosexual men, and persons with chronic liver disease. For travelers, the vaccine is given 4 weeks before departure; if an unexpected departure to an endemic areas is urgently required, immunoglobulin (Ig), 0.02 mL/kg should be given intramuscularly along with the first dose of vaccine (at different anatomic sites).

Postexposure

Immunoglobulin (Ig) given intramuscularly in a dose equal to 0.02 mL/kg is useful for the prevention of hepatitis A in persons with close or intimate exposure to confirmed infectious individuals of their serum (for example, needle sharing), sexual contact, or household contact. Ig can be administered up to 2 weeks after exposure but should be given as soon as possible. Hepatitis A vaccine should be administered at the same time to unvaccinated individuals (at a different anatomic site). Should a case of hepatitis A infection occur in a **day-care center**, Ig should then be given to all unvaccinated children and unvaccinated staff. For hepatitis A cases occurring in two or more households of individuals attending any center (children or staff), Ig should be administered to prevent other cases. In both settings, vaccine should be given at the same time as Ig (at different anatomic sites). Hepatitis A occurring in an individual **handling or preparing food** requires that staff and customers receive Ig (and vaccine) if treatment can be provided within 2 weeks of exposure. Contact with local public health officials is recommended.

Hepatitis B
Pre-exposure

- **Hepatitis B vaccine** has been shown to be effective in pre-exposure prophylaxis of individuals at high risk (injections at 0, 1, and 6 months) and in postexposure prophylaxis. In the latter group, the vaccine may be given with hepatitis B Immunoglobulin.

Immunoglobulin

- Immunoglobulin has been shown to be protective if given within 10 days of exposure to hepatitis B virus. This is recommended only for persons with clear exposure to HB_sAg-contaminated material or for individuals with intimate contact with patients known or determined to be specifically positive for HB_sAg. When possible exposure is reported, often as a result of needle puncture or sexual contact, efforts should be made, if possible, to determine whether HB_sAg positivity exists in the contact. HB_sAb should also be measured in the exposed individual. If the contact is determined to be HB_sAg-positive, transmission of infection to the patient is possible. The exposed person's antibody status dictates prophylactic therapy with hepatitis B immunoglobulin. Persons with exposure to HB_sAg and who are HB_sAb-negative should receive prophylactic therapy as soon as possible with hepatitis B immunoglobulin, 0.06 mL/kg intramuscularly, with the same dose repeated at 28 days. Those who are HB_s Ab-positive are immune and require *no* prophylactic therapy.

Drug-Related Hepatitis

A wide variety of drugs and toxins may cause hepatic injury. The diagnosis of such injury is often difficult, because drug-induced liver disease can produce both hepatocellular as well as obstructive enzyme profiles.

Treatment consists of promptly discontinuing the suspected drug or toxic agent.

Direct Hepatotoxicity
Drugs in this group produce dose-related injury in all patients.
• Acetaminophen
• Ethanol (chronic)
• Carbon tetrachloride
• Tetracycline

Viral Hepatitis–like Injury
These drugs produce idiosyncratic reactions.
• Chloramphenicol
• Halothane
• Isoniazid
• Phenylbutazone
• Streptomycin

Cholestatic Pattern of Injury
Whereas methyltestosterone, mestranol, and norethandrolone directly reduce bile secretion without producing signs of inflammation on biopsy, other agents produce a true periportal inflammatory response leading to a cholestatic reaction.
• Chlorothiazide
• Chlorpropamide
• Erythromycin estolate (in adults)
• Prochlorperazine

Chronic Active Hepatitis–like Injury
These agents produce a syndrome clinically and histologically indistinguishable from chronic active viral hepatitis.
• Acetaminophen
• Aspirin
• Chlorpromazine
• Halothane
• Isoniazid
• Methyldopa
• Nitrofurantoin

Nausea and Vomiting

Nausea and vomiting result from a wide variety of diverse causes. Nausea appears to be produced by stimulation of the central nervous system chemoreceptor trigger zone, which may be activated by a wide variety of drugs and endogenous stimuli. Vomiting is induced by stimulation of the vomiting center in the medulla, which receives input from the gastrointestinal tract, the cerebral cortex, the vestibular apparatus, and the chemoreceptor trigger zone. Complications of vomiting include dehydration, fluid and electrolyte disturbances (including metabolic alkalosis, hypokalemia, and hyponatremia), aspiration of vomitus, gastroesophageal mucosal laceration (Mallory-Weiss syndrome), and postemesis rupture of the esophagus (Boerhaave syndrome).

CAUSES OF NAUSEA AND VOMITING COMMONLY ASSOCIATED WITH ABDOMINAL PAIN

- Gastroenteritis
- Anxiety
- Mechanical obstruction of the gastrointestinal tract
- Biliary tract disease
- Food poisoning
- Alcoholic gastritis
- Renal colic
- Pancreatitis
- Peptic ulcer disease
- Drugs (narcotics, nonsteroidal anti-inflammatory agents, antibiotics)

CAUSES OF NAUSEA AND VOMITING NOT ASSOCIATED WITH ABDOMINAL PAIN

- Pregnancy
- Labyrinthine disorders
- Uremia
- Migraine headache
- Drugs (narcotics, nonsteroidal, anti-inflammatory agents)

LESS COMMON CAUSES OF NAUSEA AND VOMITING NOT TO BE MISSED

- Myocardial ischemia or infarction
- Cerebrovascular accident
- Concussion or postconcussive syndrome

- Testicular or ovarian torsion
- Hypertensive encephalopathy
- Increased intracranial pressure
- Alcoholic ketoacidosis
- Diabetic ketoacidosis
- Glaucoma
- Functional (bulimia)
- Diabetic gastroparesis
- Pyelonephritis

OTHER CAUSES OF NAUSEA AND VOMITING

- Systemic infections
- Radiation sickness
- High-altitude illness

HISTORY

Vomiting must occasionally be distinguished from regurgitation, especially in infants, which is the expulsion of food in the absence of nausea or contraction of the abdominal or diaphragmatic musculature. Regurgitation of gastric contents is typically noted with gastroesophageal sphincter incompetence.

It is important to separate patients who have nausea and vomiting associated with abdominal pain from those without pain. Causes of abdominal pain with nausea and vomiting range from the obvious (mechanical obstruction of the small bowel) to the less apparent (myocardial infarction or diabetic ketoacidosis). Nausea and vomiting associated with diarrhea, low-grade fever, myalgias, and crampy abdominal pain that improves on defecation suggest viral gastroenteritis; constant or severe pain should suggest more serious diagnoses.

A variety of drugs may produce these symptoms, the most common being the nonsteroidal anti-inflammatory agents (including aspirin), as well as erythromycin, digoxin toxicity, and steroids.

The temporal relationship of nausea and vomiting to eating may be useful diagnostically. Early morning nausea and vomiting are noted in pregnancy (especially the first trimester) and in uremia. Gastritis secondary to alcohol use often leads to epigastric discomfort and early morning "dry heaves." Gastritis and gallbladder disease produce vomiting soon after eating. Nausea and vomiting developing 4 to 6 hours or more after eating and often involving the expulsion of large volumes of undigested food suggest gastric retention (diabetic or idiopathic gastroparesis, or gastric outlet obstruction). Vertigo is commonly reported in association with the labyrinthine etiologies of nausea; symptoms are typically increased by head movement.

PHYSICAL EXAMINATION

Abdominal tenderness may suggest a specific cause, such as cholecystitis, intestinal obstruction, peptic ulcer disease, or pancreatitis. Patients whose history suggests mechanical obstruction (previous abdominal operation, progressive discomfort, vomiting large amounts several hours after meals, or a history of chronic duodenal ulcer disease) may have only minimal abdominal findings on examination. If the gastric outlet is obstructed, a succussion splash may be noted. Biliary tract disease may produce jaundice and colicky right upper quadrant discomfort, whereas pancreatitis is usually associated with midepigastric pain radiating directly through to the back. Early morning nausea and vomiting of pregnancy (so-called morning sickness) may be the only sign of early pregnancy. Nausea and vomiting of labyrinthine disorders (Ménière syndrome, benign positional vertigo, vestibular neuronitis) are usually positional. Uremia may produce progressive nausea and vomiting. Acute inferior myocardial infarction is often accompanied by isolated nausea and vomiting as a result of vagal or diaphragmatic "irritation," especially in diabetics. Vomiting due to cerebrovascular accident results from either increased intracranial pressure secondary to hemorrhage or direct brainstem involvement.

DIAGNOSTIC TESTS

Vomitus may provide clues to the cause. A feculent odor to the emesis demonstrates that bacterial action has occurred and suggests that intestinal obstruction or a gastrocolic fistula may be present. Bile is often noted whenever vomiting has been excessive or prolonged; therefore, it signifies no specific disorder except when present in large quantities, in which case an obstructive lesion below the ampulla of Vater is suggested. Blood or "coffee ground" emesis suggests an esophageal, gastric, or duodenal hemorrhagic process.

A complete blood count may suggest either subacute or chronic blood loss if anemia is present; leukocytosis may be noted in patients with acute (infectious) gastroenteritis, biliary tract disease, renal colic or pyelonephritis, or pancreatitis. The serum lipase may be elevated in pancreatitis. Elevated alkaline phosphatase and total and direct bilirubin are noted in obstructing biliary tract disorders. A serum β of human chorionic gonadotropin will diagnose pregnancy. Morning sickness rarely persists beyond the first trimester, and if it does, a hydatidiform mole or a multiple pregnancy may be present. An electrocardiogram should be obtained if myocardial infarction is suspected. An elevated blood urea nitrogen and creatinine define azotemia and may explain nausea and vomiting as part of the uremic syndrome. Patients with a renal stone will have nausea or vomiting and pain.

TREATMENT

There are three aspects of the treatment of nausea and vomiting: (1) treatment of any identifiable underlying causes; (2) replacement of blood and fluid losses as indicated by physical examination, by associated vital signs and postural changes, and by abnormal laboratory values; and (3) symptomatic treatment of the nausea and vomiting with antiemetics. At times, nasogastric suction is necessary.

Antiemetics work in one or more of the following fashions: (1) by depressing the vomiting center, (2) by depressing the chemoreceptor trigger zone in the area postrema, (3) by limiting impulses from the vestibular apparatus to the chemoreceptor trigger zone, and (4) by limiting impulses from the peripheral receptors in the gut to the vomiting center. Many antiemetics have unknown mechanisms of action. In pregnancy, a safe antiemetic is ondansetron (Zofran).

The most efficacious antiemetic with the fewest adverse effects is ondansetron (Zofran). This agent has replaced most other antiemetics due to its efficacy and lack of adverse effects. Prochlorperazine (Compazine), 5 to 10 mg intravenous or 25 mg per rectum (useful in headache), promethazine (Phenergan—useful particularly for motion-related disorders or vertigo), 25 mg intramuscular or intravenous, and metoclopramide (Reglan), 10 mg intravenous or PO, are effective, but with more side effects. Oral agents include meclizine (Antivert—also used in motion-related disorders or vertigo), 25 mg orally every 6 hours, and trimethobenzamide (Tigan), 250 mg orally three times daily as required.

PART 7

Genitourinary and Pregnancy-Related Disorders

32 Hematuria

Blood in the urine may be either microscopic or macroscopic, the latter generally causing patients to come to the emergency department. In patients who present with "blood in the urine," artifactual causes must be considered and excluded. These include hemoglobinuria, myoglobinuria, beet ingestion, and the use of phenolphthalein-containing laxatives. Although significant blood loss is unusual except in patients with bleeding secondary to trauma or anticoagulation, as in any patient with blood loss, hemodynamic stability should be evaluated early and corrected as needed.

COMMON CAUSES OF HEMATURIA

- Hemorrhagic cystitis
- Nephrolithiasis
- Pyelonephritis
- Acute prostatitis
- Urethral stricture

LESS COMMON CAUSES OF HEMATURIA NOT TO BE MISSED

- Genitourinary malignancy
- Papillary necrosis
- Renal infarction
- Genitourinary tuberculosis
- Glomerulonephritis
- Urethral foreign body
- Excessive coagulation therapy
- Traumatic urethritis

HISTORY

- The artifactual causes of hematuria are excluded by history.
- Fever, chills, suprapubic or flank pain, dysuria, frequency, and urgency suggest urinary tract infection with associated hematuria.
- Severe flank pain, often radiating to the lower quadrant or groin, associated with restlessness, diaphoresis, nausea, and vomiting should suggest nephrolithiasis. A personal or family history of renal calculi may be noted in addition.
- Fever, suprapubic or perineal pain, and referred testicular pain suggest acute prostatitis.
- Renal emboli with infarction should be considered in all patients with flank pain, atrial fibrillation, and hematuria.
- When hematuria occurs in the context of therapeutic anticoagulation, a structural abnormality occurring at some location in the genitourinary tract is likely.
- Urethral foreign bodies should be considered in all children with hematuria.
- Gross, painless hematuria in the patient with sickle cell trait should suggest papillary necrosis. Other causes of papillary necrosis, including diabetes mellitus and analgesic nephropathy, although usually not associated with gross hematuria, should be considered as well.
- Gross hematuria may be reported in men with traumatic urethritis; this entity is self-limited, results from intercourse-related trauma to the urethra, and typically presents 2 to 12 hours after coitus.

PHYSICAL EXAMINATION

- Costovertebral angle tenderness with percussion is noted in patients with pyelonephritis, whereas suprapubic tenderness may be noted in patients with cystitis, both of which may be accompanied by fever.
- Patients with renal colic similarly may have percussion tenderness over the involved kidney and tenderness with palpation over the involved ureter on abdominal examination.
- Prostatic tenderness and bogginess are noted on rectal examination in patients with acute prostatitis.

DIAGNOSTIC TESTS

- The urinalysis is the most important test in the evaluation of the patient with hematuria.
- Even in patients who present with gross hematuria, erythrocytes must be identified microscopically.
- The ingestion of beets or phenolphthalein-containing oral laxatives, myoglobinuria and hemoglobinuria all produce red urine without erythrocytes.
- In glomerulonephritic hematuria, red cell casts may be noted on urinalysis.
- In selected patients with potentially more serious causes of hematuria, a complete blood count, chemistry panel, prothrombin time, and partial thromboplastin time should be obtained to assess the presence of chronic blood loss and exclude coagulopathy.
- In patients without clear genitourinary infection, a renal and bladder ultrasound or abdominal and pelvis CT should be obtained to identify any structural abnormali-

ties of the kidney, renal pelvis, ureter, or bladder, as well as the presence of calculi. In suspected cases of ureterolithiasis, the CT should be performed without contrast.

- Referral for a cystoscopy is necessary in persons in whom imaging does not provide a definitive diagnosis; biopsy of any suspicious lesions will be undertaken by the urologist at the time of study.
- Urinary cytology is also an important element in the evaluation of patients with hematuria of unknown cause.

SELECTED DISORDERS

Acute Prostatitis

- Acute prostatitis most commonly affects men between the ages of 20 and 40 years.
- Patients present with fever, chills, dysuria, increased urinary frequency and urgency, and suprapubic or perineal pain, which may be referred to the testes.
- Initial or terminal hematuria or hematospermia or both may be noted by the patient.
- Acute urinary retention may occur if the acute inflammatory process produces sufficient periurethral prostatic edema.
- Many patients give a history of gonococcal or nonspecific urethritis.
- On physical examination, suprapubic and epididymal tenderness and a tender, boggy prostate gland may be noted.
- Occasionally, a well-defined or localized area of discrete swelling, tenderness, and fluctuance may be noted and suggests a prostatic abscess.
- Erythrocytes and leukocytes may be noted on microscopic examination of the urine.
- Because cystitis frequently coexists, a urine culture may be useful in identifying the causative organism; prostatic massage to obtain a specimen should be avoided because of the possibility of inducing epididymal seeding or generalized bacteremia.
- In patients with equivocal findings, the Stamey three-glass test is useful in differentiating the site of hematuria or pyuria. It is performed by asking the patient to void and collect separately the first 10 mL, the midstream, and the last few drops of urine into each of three labeled containers. Anterior urethral disorders produce the largest number of cells in the first container, whereas prostatic, bladder neck, or posterior urethral disorders produce the greatest number of cells in the last container.
- A similar number of cells in all containers usually indicates disease above the bladder neck.
- Although chlamydial, coliform, enterococcal, *Klebsiella,* and gonococcal organisms may produce acute prostatitis, in many patients no bacterial pathogen is identified by culture.
- *Cryptococcus neoformans* may be the causative agent in human immunodeficiency virus (HIV)-infected men.
- Patients with evidence of bacteremia (high fever, rigors, markedly elevated white cell count) or urinary obstruction require admission and intravenous antibiotic therapy; gentamicin (1 mg/kg every 8 hours) or tobramycin (1 mg/kg every 8 hours) plus ampicillin (2 g every 6 hours) is an appropriate initial regimen in such patients.
- Alternatively, intravenous ciprofloxacin or ofloxacin may be used.
- Patients not requiring hospitalization may be treated according to age. If younger than age 35 years, when the primary organisms are *Neisseria gonorrhoeae* and *Chlamydia trachomatis,* patients may be treated with one of the two following regimens:

- Ceftriaxone 250 mg intramuscular once plus doxycycline 100 mg orally for 10 days
- Ofloxacin 400 mg orally once followed by 300 mg twice daily for 10 days
- If older than age 35 years, when the primary organism is Enterobacteriaceae, treatment is with one of the following three regimens:
- Ciprofloxacin 500 mg orally twice daily for 14 to 28 days
- Ofloxacin 200 mg orally twice daily for 14 to 28 days
- TMP/SMX DS 1 tablet orally twice daily for 14 to 28 days

Traumatic Urethritis

- A benign, self-limited entity resulting from an abrading injury to the distal urethra associated with sexual intercourse or masturbation.
- Frequently, initial hematuria or a bloody penile discharge is the presenting complaint.
- Treatment includes reassurance and avoidance of sexual activity for several days.

33 Sexually Acquired Disorders

GONOCOCCAL INFECTION

- *Neisseria gonorrhoeae* is the causative organism.
- Uncomplicated infections are limited to the transitional and columnar epithelium of the anterior urethra.
- The gonococcus may also infect other sites (pharynx, cervix, rectum, or conjunctiva) or extend locally, producing epididymitis, prostatitis, or pelvic inflammatory disease (PID).
- Regardless of the initial site of infection, unless treated, an asymptomatic carrier state may evolve and provide a source for endemic transmission of the organism.
- For unclear reasons, disseminated gonococcal infection (DGI) may occur in some individuals, producing septicemia, arthritis, dermatitis, endocarditis, perihepatitis, or meningitis.
- Symptoms of urethritis usually occur within 2 to 5 days of exposure, although delays of more than 9 days are occasionally reported.
- Dysuria and penile discharge are the usual symptoms in men, whereas women report dysuria, vaginal discharge, and lower abdominal pain.
- The discharge, when present, is usually creamy yellow, gray, or white and often copious.
- In men, aside from urethral discharge, occurring either spontaneously or exuded on "milking" the urethra, the physical examination is otherwise normal.
- Women may demonstrate a chronic cervicitis, vaginitis, or inflammation of Bartholin and the periurethral Skene glands.
- In men, Gram stain reveals leukocytes with intracellular Gram-negative diplococci, the presence of which is considered evidence for a presumptive diagnosis of gonorrhea; specific therapy should be initiated after a urethral or cervical culture is obtained.
- In women, Gram stain is not diagnostically helpful, because the test has a 50% false-negative rate and a 5% false-positive rate.
- The culture, which is plated directly on Thayer-Martin medium, is essential both to establish the diagnosis and, in patients presenting with recurrent symptoms after appropriate therapy, to document the existence of a resistant or penicillinase-producing strain.
- Cultures should be taken with calcium alginate swabs, because rayon and cotton inhibit growth of the organism.
- Nucleic acid amplification tests (NAATs) that amplify DNA sequences of *N. gonorrhoeae* have supplanted culture in many clinical settings due to their ease of use.
- It is also important to note that up to 45% of patients infected with the gonococcus may concomitantly be infected with one of the agents causing nonspecific urethritis

(NSU), especially *Chlamydia*, and this should be considered in the treatment strategy.

- Importantly, in selected patients with suspected gonorrhea, pharyngeal and rectal cultures should also be obtained in addition to urethral or cervical/vaginal cultures; this optimizes the likelihood of culturing the organism and determining its sensitivity.
- A serologic test for syphilis (RPR) and HIV should be obtained in all patients as well.
- Treatment regimens for patients with uncomplicated gonococcal urethritis/cervicitis/pharyngitis/rectum (two-drug therapy is necessary to treat both gonococcus and chlamydia).
- Fluoroquinolones are no longer recommended for first-line treatment unless there is documented sensitivity by culture to this drug class.
- Use one antibiotic listed as "A" and one listed as "B" for men and nonpregnant women, and one "A" plus one "C" for pregnant women:
  - A. Cefixime 400 mg orally once
  - A. Ceftriaxone 125 mg intramuscularly once
  - A. Spectinomycin 2 g intramuscularly once (for patients allergic to the aforementioned antibiotics)

PLUS
  - B. Azithromycin 1 g orally once
  - B. Doxycycline 100 mg orally twice daily for 7 days
  - B. Erythromycin 500 mg orally four times daily for 7 days

OR
  - C. Erythromycin 500 mg orally four times daily for 7 days
  - C. Amoxicillin 500 mg orally three times daily for 7 days
  - C. Azithromycin 1 g orally in a single dose

Note the following:
- If spectinomycin is used for proctitis, use 4 g intramuscularly.
- Ceftriaxone or spectinomycin alone do not treat chlamydial infection or incubating syphilis; an RPR should therefore be repeated in approximately 4 weeks after treatment to exclude the former, and a re-examination in 5 to 7 days is advised.
- Spectinomycin is not effective as treatment for pharyngeal gonorrhea; use ceftriaxone 125 mg IM.
- The pregnant patient should *not* receive tetracycline, doxycycline, or a quinolone.
- Patients presenting with clinical gonococcal infection after appropriate treatment should have cultures taken from all potential sites of infection and treatment with ceftriaxone or spectinomycin instituted.
- Follow-up cultures should be advised 4 to 7 days after the completion of therapy.
- All sexual partners exposed to the patient should be examined, cultured, and treated prophylactically; sexual activity should be prohibited for 5 to 7 days.
- DGI should be treated with parenteral ceftriaxone, cefotaxime, ceftizoxime, or spectinomycin for at least 24 hours after clinical improvement and then switched to oral cefixime for at least 7 days of total treatment.
- Gonococcal conjunctivitis in adults can be a severe, sight-threatening condition. Patients demonstrate copious purulent discharge. Most patients should be admitted. Treatment is with parenteral ceftriaxone.
- Neonatal conjunctivitis is often gonococcal, requires hospitalization, and is also treated with ceftriaxone (25–50 mg/kg up to 125 mg IM or IV).

POSTGONOCOCCAL URETHRITIS

- Patients who present with persistent or recurrent symptoms or signs of urethritis after recent appropriate therapy for gonococcal urethritis are said to have postgonococcal urethritis; all such patients should be reexamined and recultured.
- In the evaluation of these patients, it must first be appreciated that approximately 40% of patients with gonococcal urethritis have coexistent chlamydial or ureaplasmal infection, the course of which is unaffected by treatment with penicillin, spectinomycin, or a cephalosporin, such as ceftriaxone.
- Failure to treat these patients with tetracycline or doxycycline, therefore, or to provide simultaneous treatment for the patient's sexual partner(s), typically results in persistent or recurrent symptoms.
- In such patients, one must always consider simple reinfection as a result of interval exposure to a new contact.

NONSPECIFIC URETHRITIS

- NSU is caused by *Chlamydia trachomatis* or *Ureaplasma urealyticum,* although in approximately 20% of patients, the cause remains obscure.
- Patients may report dysuria, penile discharge, or burning; however, asymptomatic cases are common in both men and women.
- The discharge when present is scant and mucoid, and typically, only leukocytes are noted on Gram stain.
- The causative agents of NSU are fastidious and cannot be grown on routine culture media.
- NAATs have become a widespread method to diagnose *Chlamydia.*
- Treatment regimens include 100 mg of doxycycline twice daily for at least 7 days, azithromycin, 1 g orally, in a single dose, *or* 500 mg of erythromycin four times daily for at least 7 days.
- All sexual partners of patients with NSU should be examined and treated with one of these regimens plus coverage for Gonococcus and serologic testing for syphilis and HIV as outlined above.
- Persistent or recurrent NSU is usually caused by failure to treat the sexual partner (or partners); however, less common causes of recurrent urethritis should also be considered.

PELVIC INFLAMMATORY DISEASE

- PID is a syndrome resulting from infection of the reproductive organs and their supporting structures; involvement may be unilateral or bilateral.
- Most commonly, acute salpingitis, secondary to bacterial infection with *N. gonorrhoeae, C. trachomatis,* or other indigenous pelvic organisms, including streptococci and a variety of anaerobes, is present.
- Severe lower quadrant cramping or aching, usually bilateral, with fever, menometrorrhagia, leukorrhea, and adnexal tenderness is noted in most patients.
- Profound tenderness associated with lateral motion of the cervix should suggest the diagnosis.
- It is important to note that PID is an important differential diagnosis in any woman presenting with abdominal pain.

- Although the white blood cell count is typically elevated and Gram-negative intracellular organisms may be noted on Gram stain of endocervical or vaginal smears, the diagnosis of PID should be based on the patient's history and physical findings.
- Patients with severe illness (high fever, chills, a "toxic" appearance, peritoneal signs, pregnancy, suspected pelvic abscess, failure to respond after 72 hours with outpatient therapy, need for laparoscopy for diagnosis), those who are immuno-deficient (human immunodeficiency virus [HIV] infection with low CD4 counts) or are on immunosuppressive therapy, or those who are unlikely to comply with outpatient therapy require hospital admission for hydration and antibiotic therapy.
- Adolescents with PID have a potential for developing infertility, and some authors recommend inpatient treatment for these patients.
- Organisms commonly involved in PID include gonococcus, *Chlamydia*, *Mycoplasma hominis*, Enterobacteriaceae, and anaerobes.
- Outpatient regimens include ceftriaxone 250 mg intramuscularly once plus 14 days of doxycycline 100 mg orally twice daily, or cefoxitin 2 g intramuscularly once with 1 g orally of probenecid and doxycycline 100 mg orally twice a day.
- Inpatient therapy can be started with either cefoxitin 2 g intravenous every 6 hours (or cefotetan 2 g IV every 12 hours), plus doxycycline (100 mg IV or oral) every 12 hours, or clindamycin 900 intravenous every 8 hours plus gentamicin 2 mg/kg intravenous initially, then 1.5 mg/kg every 8 hours.
- Adequate analgesia should be provided to patients as needed along with instructions for gynecologic follow-up if outpatient therapy is chosen.

HERPES GENITALIS

- Infection of the lower genital tract by the herpes simplex type 2 virus is a sexually acquired disease of increasing importance and morbidity.
- Initial exposure, with an incubation period from 3 to 12 days, results in primary infection, which, in most patients, is followed by recurrent outbreaks.
- The primary infection is characterized by severe pain, tender inguinal adenopathy, and fever.
- Symptoms are often disabling, particularly in women, who may experience difficulty with walking or urination.
- In men, in addition to painful penile lesions, urethritis, dysuria, and penile discharge may also be noted.
- In women, vulvovaginitis is severe and associated with widespread erosions, vesicles, and edema; a profuse, malodorous vaginal discharge may also be noted along with tender, inguinal adenopathy.
- Anorectal herpes is characterized by the typical cutaneous lesions as well as painful rectal and perirectal erosions and ulcerations.
- After primary infection, the virus remains latent in sensory ganglia; recurrent outbreaks, which may occur spontaneously or in association with a number of precipitants, include emotional stress, genital trauma, the menses, fever, and systemic infection.
- Recurrent episodes are less severe than the primary infection and are associated with the typical lesion (multiple, small, clustered vesicles overlying a small area of confluent erythema).
- Vesicles are initially clear, but subsequently become cloudy, with healing by 10 days; yellow crusting of older lesions indicates bacterial superinfection.

- Lymphadenopathy is usually also noted.
- Microscopic examination of scrapings from the base of vesicular lesions may reveal the characteristic multinucleated giant cells and acidophilic inclusion bodies.
- Viral cultures of the lesions may demonstrate the organism, and antibody titers against the virus increase in most patients.
- The use of acyclovir in the treatment of herpes simplex genital infections can be summarized as follows: intravenous acyclovir (5 mg/kg intravenous every 8 hours) should probably be reserved for patients with potentially life-threatening illnesses, such as herpes encephalitis and disseminated herpes.
- Oral acyclovir (400 mg three times per day for 7–10 days) promotes resolution of primary infections if started early (within 2 days of onset); such treatment has no effect on subsequent outbreaks.
- It has also been shown that patient-initiated administration of oral acyclovir within 48 hours of symptoms (given as 800 mg twice daily or 200 mg five times per day) may shorten healing times and reduce symptoms in patients with recurrent episodes.
- Patients with frequent outbreaks (more than six per year) may benefit from continuous or prophylactic administration of acyclovir (200 mg two to five times per day); such therapy may prevent outbreaks or may reduce their frequency while the medication is being administered.
- Valacyclovir has demonstrated equal efficacy with acyclovir for primary, episodic, and suppressive therapy with less frequent dosing.
- Other supportive treatment measures include providing adequate analgesia; some patients with primary infection will require a narcotic analgesic.
- Patients may also benefit symptomatically from a sitz bath; women with severe discomfort associated with urination may be able to void in the tub or after the application of a local anesthetic.

SYPHILIS

- Syphilis is caused by the spirochete *Treponema pallidum*, an organism that may infect any organ system in the body, resulting in protean manifestations; sexual contact is the usual means of transmission.
- The natural history may be divided into the early stage (primary syphilis), the secondary stage (dissemination), and the late stages.
- The primary stage of syphilis is characterized by the chancre, a painless, usually single ulcer occurring on the shaft or glans of the penis or the labia; painless inguinal adenopathy is also noted at this time.
- The chancre usually appears within 21 days of exposure and heals spontaneously (without treatment) in 3 to 4 weeks.
- Asymptomatic dissemination of *T. pallidum* occurs within the first few days after exposure.
- The secondary lesions of syphilis usually occur 6 to 12 weeks after the appearance of the chancre.
- Generalized fatigue, fever, malaise, diffuse lymphadenopathy, and symmetric, discrete, pink-tan macules appearing first on the chest and abdomen are the typical findings in secondary syphilis.
- In time, the lesions become hyperkeratotic, and the palms and soles may become involved.

- Large, soft, moist papules may appear in the perianal and vulvar areas and on mucosal surfaces; these are referred to as condyloma lata.
- "Moth-eaten" alopecia may also be noted on the scalp.
- The lesions of secondary syphilis are abundant in spirochetes so that appropriate care must be taken during the examination.
- A symptom-free latent stage of the illness ensues with resolution of the secondary rash after 3 to 4 weeks.
- Many years later, the late or tertiary stage of the illness may develop, at which time benign (gummatous) lesions of the skin, bones, and viscera evolve.
- Cardiovascular and central nervous system complications become manifested, including aortitis, general paresis of the insane, paralytic dementia, tabes dorsalis, and Charcot joints.
- Dark-field microscopic examination of scrapings from the base of the chancre may reveal the spirochete.
- The laboratory tests of greatest importance in diagnosing syphilis include the commonly used nontreponemal antigen test (RPR) and the specific fluorescent antitreponemal antibody absorption test or FTA-ABS.
- The RPR becomes positive 4 to 6 weeks after the onset of infection or 1 to 3 weeks after the appearance of the chancre.
- The RPR tests serum reactivity that is present in patients with syphilis to a cardioli-pin-cholesterol-lecithin antigen.
- It is almost uniformly positive in patients with secondary syphilis and may become negative in the latent and late stages of the illness.
- Because the FTA-ABS is a specific test, it is routinely used to distinguish a false-positive RPR (occurring in 10% of patients) from a true-positive RPR.
- In addition, the FTA-ABS is positive in most patients with primary syphilis, in virtually all patients with secondary syphilis, and in most patients with late syphilis; the test remains positive even after successful therapy.
- Primary, secondary, or latent syphilis with a duration of less than 1 year should be treated with 2.4 MU of penicillin G benzathine intramuscular as a single dose (50,000 U/kg intramuscular as a single dose in children up to a maximum dose of 2.4 MU) or, if the patient is penicillin allergic, doxycycline, 100 mg orally twice daily for 14 days, or tetracycline 500 mg four times daily orally for 14 days.
- Latent syphilis with a duration of more than 1 year, late syphilis, or syphilis in HIV-positive patients should be treated with 2.4 MU of penicillin G benzathine intramuscular weekly for 3 consecutive weeks or doxycycline, 100 mg orally twice daily for 4 weeks.
- Patients treated for early syphilis may develop the Jarisch-Herxheimer reaction, an acute febrile reaction manifested by myalgias and headache. The Jarisch-Herxheimer reaction generally occurs within 24 hours of treatment. The reaction can induce early labor in pregnant women, but this possibility should not delay therapy. There is no known way to prevent the Jarisch-Herxheimer reaction, but antipyretics may relieve the symptoms of the reaction.
- Sexual contacts must be examined and treated as needed in all cases.

VAGINITIS

Trichomonas vaginalis

- Infection produces a thin, frothy, slightly green or yellow vaginal discharge and local pruritus; the causative organism is easily visualized on a saline or wet preparation of the discharge.

- The slide is prepared by mixing a drop of the discharge with a drop of saline, covered with a coverslip, which is then viewed at 100 to 400 magnification with the condenser down; motile 10- by 20-μm organisms are noted in 80% of culture-positive patients.
- Treatment must include the patient as well as any sexual partner(s) and is accomplished with a single 2-g dose of metronidazole, and patients should be cautioned against the use of alcohol when this agent is administered (to avoid a disulfiram-like effect).
- This regimen is also permissible in pregnancy.
- An alternative treatment is metronidazole, 500 mg twice daily for 7 days.

Candidiasis

- Candidiasis is not considered to be a sexually acquired disorder, but it may be exacerbated by or reintroduced through sexual contact.
- Diabetics with poor glucose control, patients receiving antibiotics for bacterial infections, pregnant patients, and women taking birth control pills are more susceptible to candidal infections.
- Vaginal candidiasis produces a "cheesy" vaginal discharge that is associated with severe itching and burning in the perineum.
- Erythematous, "raw"-appearing vaginal and labial tissues are noted on examination, and a microscopic analysis of the vaginal discharge with 10% potassium hydroxide (KOH) demonstrates the organism.
- Fluconazole 150 mg orally in a single dose is a highly effective treatment but is not recommended during pregnancy.
- Topical treatment with one of the imidazole compounds is also effective; these are available in a variety of preparations, including clotrimazole vaginal suppositories 100 mg intravaginally at bedtime for 7 days, clotrimazole 1% vaginal cream one applicator intravaginally at bedtime for 7 days, miconazole vaginal suppositories 200 mg intravaginally at bedtime for 3 days and butoconazole 2% cream, one applicator intravaginally at bedtime in a single dose. Miconazole is felt to be safe in pregnancy.
- Patients should also be advised to wear cotton underwear, which will help eliminate moisture, and to avoid tight-fitting clothing such as pantyhose or jeans.

Gardnerella Vaginalis

- *Gardnerella vaginalis* causes bacterial vaginosis and produces a thin, slightly watery vaginal discharge with accompanying dysuria.
- The discharge has "clue cells"; *G. vaginalis* adherent to sloughed epithelial cells is seen upon microscopy.
- A characteristic fishy odor is noted when KOH is applied to a slide, and a pH greater than 4.5.
- Vaginal infection with this agent may be treated with metronidazole 500 mg orally twice daily for 7 days, or clindamycin, 300 mg orally twice daily for 7 days, or clindamycin cream 2% one applicator intravaginally at bedtime for 7 days.
- Patients given metronidazole should be instructed to avoid alcohol.

PEDICULOSIS PUBIS

- Lice may infest the pubic areas and typically produce extreme pruritus.
- As the lice feed, their products of digestion are injected into the skin and result in intense pruritus.

- Pyoderma, itching, and mild inflammation of the pubic area or tender local or inguinal adenopathy without another clear-cut explanation should suggest pediculosis.
- Adult lice, nits, or both should be searched for, as should linear scratch marks.
- Treatment is with permethrin 1% cream applied to affected areas and rinsed off after 10 minutes.
- Although one application is usually sufficient, a second application should be recommended in 7 to 10 days if living organisms are noted or eggs (nits) are observed directly at the hair-skin junction.
- Patients should be instructed to expect several days of persistent pruritus, which does not necessarily imply a treatment failure.
- Similarly, dead organisms may also be noted for several days, and nits may be found attached to the hair shaft at some distance from the hair-skin junction, neither of which implies active infection.
- If nits are noted along the hair shaft, they may be removed with a fine-tooth comb or forceps.
- Eyelash involvement should be treated by thickly applying petrolatum twice daily for 7 days, followed by manual removal of nits. Oral ivermectin was reported effective in a case series.
- Close friends, family members, and sexual contacts should be screened for involvement and the last prophylactically treated.

SCABIES

- Caused by the mite *Sarcoptes scabiei*, scabies is usually acquired through close or sexual contact and produces a severe pruritus that is presumably caused by an acquired sensitivity to the organism.
- The characteristic burrow is an S-shaped ridge or dotted line, frequently ending in a vesicle.
- Lesions are typically located in the interdigital web spaces of the hands, the wrists, antecubital fossae, nipples, umbilicus, genitalia, and gluteal cleft.
- The diagnosis is suggested by the characteristic lesions and their particular pattern of distribution and confirmed by recovering the mite from the burrow after scraping the superficial dermis from the lesion using a sterile needle or number 15 scalpel blade after mineral oil is applied to the skin.
- The organism, which has a characteristic appearance, can then be observed microscopically under low power.
- Treatment consists of topical permethrin 5% cream which is applied to the entire body from the neck down at bedtime and removed by shower or bath 8 to 14 hours later; special attention should be paid to the interdigital webs, axillae, breasts, buttocks, perianal region, and genitalia.
- The fingernails should also be trimmed and these areas treated.
- One treatment is usually adequate.
- Ivermectin is an oral treatment alternative.
- Clothing and bed linens should be changed and washed concurrent with treatment.
- Patients should be told that persistent pruritus should be expected for several days and does not necessarily suggest treatment failure; reapplication at 7 days is occasionally necessary.
- Family and household contacts should be screened and, if symptomatic, should receive simultaneous treatment, as should all sexual contacts.

CONDYLOMATA ACUMINATA (GENITAL WARTS)

- Papillomas of the perianal or genital skin that are sexually transmitted, autoinoculable, and probably caused by a papillomavirus.
- They may be distinguished from the condyloma lata of syphilis by their more fleshy and pedunculated appearance.
- Treatment consists of the cautious application of 25% podophyllin, taking care to avoid contact with normal skin; the drug should be washed off 6 hours after application.
- Patient-applied agents include podofilox, 0.5% solution or gel, or imiquimod, 5% cream.
- Laser, cryotherapy, and surgical excision are alternative therapies often applied to refractory cases.
- Despite meticulous application, lesions tend to recur, and all patients should be referred for follow-up and additional care.

GRANULOMA INGUINALE

- Rare in the United States, it is caused by *Klebsiella granulomatis*, an intracellular Gram-negative organism that affects the anogenital areas.
- Donovan bodies contained in intracytoplasmic cysts are noted in cells obtained from tissue scrapings and are seen in most patients.
- The incubation period is from 8 to 12 weeks, and a beefy red, friable, shallow, sharply demarcated ulcer is produced that is typically painless; inguinal adenopathy may also develop.
- Lesions spread contiguously.
- Treatment includes doxycycline 100 mg orally twice a day for 21 days and ciprofloxacin 750 mg orally twice a day for 21 days.

CHANCROID

- *Haemophilus ducreyi* causes chancroid, which infects the genital or anal area with an incubation period of 1 to 5 days.
- Like syphilis and herpes, chancroid is a cofactor for HIV transmission.
- At the site of inoculation, the initial lesion is a small macule, which rapidly becomes a vesicopustule; the latter breaks down to form a painful soft ulcer with ragged or irregular edges, a necrotic base, and surrounding erythema.
- Painful inguinal adenopathy is also noted, which is usually unilateral and consists of multiple, tender matted nodes that may soften and spontaneously rupture.
- Treatment consists of ceftriaxone, 250 mg intramuscularly once.
- Alternatives include ciprofloxacin, 500 mg orally twice daily for 3 days or azithromycin, 1 g, given orally in a single dose.
- Note that syphilis must be excluded in all patients as 10% of chancroid patients are co-infected.

LYMPHOGRANULOMA VENEREUM

- *Chlamydia trachomatis* produces lymphogranuloma venereum with an incubation of 5 to 21 days after genital contact.

- This is a rare entity in the United States.
- The initial vesicular or ulcerative lesion often goes unnoticed, with inguinal buboes appearing 1 to 4 weeks after exposure; inguinal lesions are usually bilateral and have a tendency to fuse and develop draining sinuses.
- Because local lymph drainage in women leads to the perirectal glands, early manifestations may include proctitis with tenesmus and a bloody purulent rectal discharge.
- These symptoms are often seen in homosexual men as well and lead to perianal fistula formation.
- The diagnosis is made by clinical suspicion and NAATs that confirm the presence of *C. trachomatis* in lesion swabs or bubo aspirate.
- Doxycycline, 100 mg orally for 21 days, is the treatment of choice (except in pregnancy); alternatives include erythromycin, 500 mg orally four times daily for 21 days.

34 HIV Disease and AIDS

HUMAN IMMUNODEFICIENCY VIRUS

- Human immunodeficiency virus (HIV) is a cytopathic retrovirus that kills the cells it infects.
- It targets the T-helper (CD4) lymphocytes and depletes them.
- This depletion creates a profound defect in cellular immunity, leaving the infected individual susceptible to opportunistic pathogens and tumors.
- The natural history of HIV infection is divided into stages based on CD4 cell counts and clinical manifestations.
- The average CD4 count in the peripheral blood of healthy individuals is 800 to 1,000/mm^3, but most laboratories use a normal range of 450 to 1,400/mm^3.
- The first stage is the acute retroviral syndrome, which usually occurs 2 to 4 weeks after an exposure.
- It has a clinical presentation similar to infectious mononucleosis. Common features are fever, adenopathy, hepatosplenomegaly, sore throat, myalgias, and leukopenia with atypical lymphocytes.
- A high-grade viremia with a transient decrease in CD4 cell count is also present.
- This is followed by a spontaneous recovery in 1 to 3 weeks.
- Stage two involves a seroconversion, which usually occurs 1 to 3 months after viral transmission.
- During this phase, there is an interplay of the cytotoxic T-cell response (responsible for the destruction of HIV-infected CD4 cells), humeral immunity, and cytokine release that reduces the viral load and returns the CD4 cell count to levels near, but not equal to, those that predated infection.
- The third stage is an asymptomatic infection in which the CD4 count may be greater than or equal to 500 to 200/mm^3.
- The patient may have no symptoms or may have a generalized lymphadenopathy, but in this stage has developed a gradual decrease in CD4 counts.
- The average decline is 30 to 60/mm^3/y for 5 to 8 years, followed by an accelerated decline over the 2 years preceding an opportunistic and/or acquired immunodeficiency syndrome (AIDS)-defining infection.
- However, the rate of decline in CD4 counts and the rate of progression to full-blown AIDS are variable.
- The fourth stage involves an early symptomatic HIV infection in which the CD4 count is 100 to 300/mm^3.
- Those with CD4 counts greater than 200/mm^3 are susceptible to the same pathogens that infect immunocompetent hosts, while those with CD4 counts less than 200/ mm^3 are vulnerable to major complications such as bacterial pneumonia, vaginal candidiasis, thrush, oral hairy leukoplakia, shingles, idiopathic thrombocytopenic purpura, and pulmonary tuberculosis.

Table 34-1	Positive HIV Serology with Any of the Following

Candidiasis, esophageal, or pulmonary
Cervical cancer
Coccidioidomycosis
Cryptosporidiosis with diarrhea >1 mo
Cytomegalovirus
Histoplasmosis
Kaposi sarcoma
Lymphoma
Mycobacterium avium infection
Mycobacterium kansasii infection
Mycobacterium tuberculosis infection
Pneumocystis carinii pneumonia
Pneumonia, recurrent bacterial
Progressive multifocal leukoencephalopathy
Salmonellosis, recurrent
Toxoplasmosis

- The fifth stage involves a late symptomatic infection in which the CD4 count is less than $200/mm^3$.
- This phase is characterized by a low CD4 cell count and/or the AIDS-defining illnesses (see Table 34-1) and represents the transition from HIV infection to the development of the AIDS.

EPIDEMIOLOGY

- Worldwide more than 33.4 million people are HIV-positive, and in 2006, there were more than 1.1 million individuals living with HIV in the United States.
- Approximately 56,000 new cases are diagnosed each year in the United States.
- With improvements in antiretroviral therapy, the mortality and morbidity from AIDS are decreasing faster than the incidence of AIDS.
- Highly active antiretroviral therapy (HAART) allows people to live longer and healthier lives with HIV, a terminal disease, but it does not prevent HIV infection.
- Prevention of HIV disease remains crucial in stopping this epidemic.
- Initially, the majority of US cases occurred in homosexual men, but today, the rate of HIV infection within the heterosexual community exceeds that seen in most homosexual communities.
- Minorities and socioeconomically disadvantaged groups continue to have a disproportionate number of cases and spread of HIV infection.
- The proportion of women infected with HIV is increasing, especially among women of reproductive age.
- Women currently comprise 22% of adult AIDS cases in the United States.
- Behavior or risks associated with a greater likelihood of acquiring HIV include male homosexuality or bisexuality, intravenous drug abuse, prostitution, heterosexual exposure to a partner at risk, a large number of sexual partners, a history of receiving blood products before 1985, and being born to an HIV-infected mother.

TRANSMISSION

- The HIV virus is concentrated in cells, which makes cellular fluids more infectious than acellular fluids.
- Highly cellular fluids include blood, semen, pleuroperitoneal fluids, cerebrospinal fluid (CSF), amniotic fluid, breast milk, and vaginal secretions.
- Urine, sweat, saliva, and tears do not transmit HIV.
- The greater the viral load, the more infectious; thus, exposure to body fluids during periods of high viremia as seen in seroconversion and advanced disease carry the greatest risk of transmission.
- HIV is most frequently transmitted through unprotected sexual intercourse, and that risk increases in the presence of mucosal disruption seen with sexually transmitted diseases, especially chancroid.
- High-risk sexual behaviors include anal intercourse and intercourse during menses.
- Transmission during oral intercourse with ejaculation has been reported.
- Parenteral transmission occurs with needle sharing among intravenous drug abusers, via blood transfusion with HIV-infected blood without detectable antibodies (risk 1 in 40,000–250,000), or transfer of the virus by a HIV contaminated needle-stick (risk 0.3%–0.4% per exposure).
- Vertical transmission from an HIV-infected mother to her infant occurs in 13% to 39% of deliveries.
- Breast-feeding also poses a risk of transmission up to 29% and is discouraged in women with HIV.
- The risk of HIV seroconversion after a needle-stick injury when the source patient has known HIV disease is 0.3% to 0.4%.
- However, that risk is influenced by the depth of penetration, gauge of the needle, amount of blood injected, and the viral load of the source patient.
- The likelihood of mucocutaneous transmission of HIV is less than 0.09% and is influenced by the cellularity and viral load of splashed fluid, and the fluid's contact time.
- Early prophylaxis after HIV exposure may reduce the risk of HIV seroconversion by as much as 81% and should be recommended or offered to all high-risk parenteral exposures (see Tables 34-2 and 34-3).
- Chemoprophylaxis is effective, but not absolute.
- The current recommendations from the CDC for HIV postexposure prophylaxis (PEP) is a 4-week regimen of two drugs (zidovudine [ZDV] and lamivudine [3TC]; 3TC and stavudine [d4T]; or didanosine [ddI] and d4T) for most HIV exposures and an expanded regimen that includes the addition of a third drug for HIV exposures of increased risk for transmission (see Tables 34-2 through 34-4).
- When the source person's virus is known or suspected to be resistant to one or more of the drugs considered for the PEP regimen, the selection of drugs to which the source person's virus is unlikely to be resistant is recommended. This means when selecting a PEP regimen, choose at least two antiviral drugs that the source patient is not taking and add a third drug if needed to ensure two new drugs.
- When there is a delayed exposure report, unknown source person, pregnancy in the exposed person, resistance of the source virus to antiretroviral agents, or toxicity of the PEP regimen, then consultation with local experts or the National Clinicians' Post-Exposure Prophylaxis Hotline is advised (see Table 34-5).

Table 34-2	Recommended HIV Postexposure for Percutaneous Injuries				
	Infection Status of Source				
Exposure Type	**HIV-Positive Class 1**[a]	**HIV-Positive Class 2**[a]	**Source or Unknown HIV Status**[b]	**Unknown Source**[c]	**HIV-Negative**
Less severe	Recommend basic two-drug PEP.	Recommend expanded three-drug PEP.	Generally, no PEP warranted; however, consider basic two-drug PEP[d] for source with HIV risk factors.[e]	Generally, no PEP warranted; however, consider basic two-drug PEP[d] in settings where exposure to HIV-infected persons is likely.	No PEP warranted.
More severe[f]	Recommended expanded three-drug PEP.	Recommend expanded three-drug PEP.	Generally, no PEP warranted; however, consider basic two-drug PEP[d] for source with HIV risk factors.[e]	Generally, no PEP warranted; however, consider basic two-drug PEP[d] in settings where exposure to HIV-infected person is likely.	No PEP warranted.

[a] HIV-positive, Class 1, asymptomatic HIV infection or known low viral load (e.g., <1,500 RNA copies/mL); HIV-positive, Class 2, symptomatic HIV infection, AIDS, acute seroconversion, or known high viral load. If drug resistance is a concern, obtain expert consultation. Initiation of postexposure prophylaxis (PEP) should not be delayed pending expert consultation, and, because expert consultation alone cannot substitute for face-to-face counseling, resources should be available to provide immediate evaluation and follow-up care for all exposures.

[b] Source of unknown HIV status (e.g., deceased source person with no samples available for HIV testing).

[c] Unknown source (e.g., solid needle and superficial injury).

[d] The designation "consider PEP" indicates that PEP is optional and should be based on an individualized decision between the exposed person and the treating clinician.

[e] If PEP is offered and taken and the source is later determined to be HIV-negative, PEP should be discontinued.

[f] More severe (e.g., large-bore hollow needle, deep puncture, visible blood on device, or needle used in patient's artery or vein).

Table 34-3   Recommended HIV Postexposure Prophylaxis for Mucous Membranes and Nonintact Skin[a] Exposures

Exposure Type	HIV-Positive Class 1[b]	HIV-Positive Class 2[b]	Infection Status of Source Source or Unknown HIV Status[c]	Unknown Source[d]	HIV-Negative
Small volume[e]	Consider basic two-drug PEP.[f]	Recommend basic two-drug PEP.	Generally, no PEP warranted; however, consider basic two-drug PEP[f] for source with HIV risk factors.[f]	Generally, no PEP warranted; however, consider basic two-drug PEP[f] in settings where exposure to HIV-infected persons is likely.	No PEP warranted.
Large volume[h]	Recommended basic two-drug PEP.	Recommend expanded three-drug PEP.	Generally, no PEP warranted; however, consider basic two-drug PEP[f] for source with HIV risk factors.[g]	Generally, no PEP warranted; however, consider basic two-drug PEP[f] in settings where exposure to HIV-infected person is likely.	No PEP warranted.

[a]For skin exposures, follow-up is indicated only if there is evidence of compromised skin integrity (e.g., dermatitis, abrasion, or open wound).

[b]HIV-positive, Class 1: asymptomatic HIV infection or known low viral load (e.g., <1,500 RNA copies/mL). HIV-positive, Class 2: symptomatic HIV infection, AIDS, acute seroconversion, or known high viral load. If drug resistance is a concern, obtain expert consultation. Initiation of postexposure prophylaxis (PEP) should not be delayed pending expert consultation, and, because expert consultation alone cannot substitute for face-to-face counseling, resources should be available to provide immediate evaluation and follow-up care for all exposures.

[c]Source of unknown HIV status (e.g., deceased source person with no samples available for HIV testing).

[d]Unknown source (e.g., splash from inappropriately disposed blood).

[e]Small volume (i.e., a few drops).

[f]The designation, "consider PEP," indicates that PEP is optional and should be based on an individualized decision between the exposed person and the treating clinician.

[g]If PEP is offered and taken and the source is later determined to be HIV-negative, PEP should be discontinued.

[h]Large volume (i.e., major blood splash).

Table 34-4	PEP Treatment Regimens

Basic Regimen

Zidovudine (Retrovir; ZDV) + Lamivudine (Epivir; 3TC); available as Combivir
ZDV: 600 mg/d, in two or three divided doses, and
3TC: 150 mg orally twice daily
Combivir: 1 tablet twice daily

Alternate Basic Regimen

Lamivudine (Epivir; 3TC) + Stavudine (Zerit; d4T)
3TC: 150 mg orally twice daily, and
d4T: 40 mg orally twice daily (30 mg orally twice daily if body weight is
<60 kg)

Expanded Regimen

Basic regimen plus one of the following:
Lopinavir/Ritonavir (Kaletra; LPV/RTV)
LPV/RTV: 3 capsules twice daily with food

Table 34-5	Situations for Which Expert[a] Consultation for HIV PEP is Advised

Delayed (later than 24–36 h) exposure

Unknown source (e.g., needle in sharps disposal container or laundry). Decide use of PEP on a case-by-case basis. Consider the severity of the exposure and the epidemiologic likelihood of HIV exposure. Do not test needles or other sharp instruments for HIV.

Known or suspected pregnancy in the exposed person does not preclude the use of optimal PEP regimens. Do not deny PEP solely on the basis of pregnancy.

Resistance of the source virus to antiretroviral agents. Influence of drug resistance on transmission risk is unknown. Selection of drugs to which the source person's virus is unlikely to be resistant is recommended, if the source person's virus is known or suspected to be resistant to ≥1 of the drugs considered for the PEP regimen resistance. Testing of the source person's virus at the time of the exposure is not recommended.

Toxicity of the initial PEP regimen. Adverse symptoms such as nausea and diarrhea are common with PEP symptoms and often can be managed without changing the PEP regimen by prescribing antimotility and/or antiemetic agents. Modification of dose intervals (i.e., administering a lower dose of drug more frequently throughout the day, as recommended by the manufacturer), in other situations, might help alleviate symptoms.

[a] Local experts and/or the National Clinicians' Post-Exposure Prophylaxis Hotline (PEPline) (1-888-448-4911).

National Clinicians' Post-Exposure Prophylaxis Hotline
- Phone: **1-888-448-4911** or Web site: **http://www.ucsf.edu/hivcntr**
- Both the source patient and the exposed individual should be tested for hepatitis B and C, syphilis, and HIV antibody.

HIV TESTING

- The enzyme-linked immunosorbent assay (ELISA) detects HIV antibodies.
- ELISA is currently the best screening test available for HIV, with sensitivities and specificities of more than 98.5% and 99%.
- ELISA can be false-negative in the first 6 weeks of HIV infection.
- There are false-positives, and all positive ELISA test results should be repeated.
- If the second ELISA is positive, it must be confirmed by Western blot to establish HIV infection.
- The sensitivities and specificities of Western blot approach 100%.
- Rapid HIV tests can be performed on saliva, blood, or plasma and are being used by more and more ED's nationally.
- Rapid assays can take as little as 5 minutes to provide results.
- Positive tests must be confirmed by Western blot.
- Polymerase chain reaction tests are used to determine the quantitative viral load and are extremely sensitive.
- They are being used to assess the magnitude of HIV replication and its associated rate of CD4 T-cell destruction, whereas the CD4 counts indicate the extent of HIV-induced damage already done.
- Viral load is also used to monitor the development of resistance to antiretroviral therapies and/or treatment failures.
- Resistance is assumed when a compliant patient's viral load begins to increase, whereas treatment failures are generally defined as a plasma viral load more than 400/mL after 4 to 6 months of continuous therapy.

CLINICAL MANIFESTATIONS AND MANAGEMENT OF AIDS-ASSOCIATED DISEASE

- As the CD4 cell count decreases, the HIV-infected individual becomes immunocompromised and susceptible to opportunistic infections and tumors (see Tables 34-6 and 34-7).

MALIGNANCIES

- Kaposi sarcoma (KS) is the most common cancer associated with HIV and may present during any phase of HIV disease.
- Typical lesions are raised, red to purple nodules or papules.
- KS is usually widely disseminated with mucous membrane involvement.
- Diagnosis is made by punch biopsy, and treatment is recommended as long as it does not cause a further immune suppression.
- Non-Hodgkin lymphoma (NHL) typically occurs late in the course of HIV infection at CD4 cell counts less than 200/mm^3.
- The clinical course of systemic NHL is more rapid in the AIDS patient and may present as a rapidly growing mass, fever, night sweats, or weight loss.

Table 34-6	Correlation of CD4 Cell Count and Opportunistic Infection	
CD4 Count	**Organism**	**Presentation**
<500	*S. pneumoniae*	Pneumonia
	H. influenzae	Pneumonia
	M. tuberculosis	Pulmonary TB
	Candida	Oropharyngeal and vaginal candidiasis
	Herpes simplex	Orogenital herpes
	Herpes Zoster	Shingles
	Epstein-Barr virus	Oral leukoplakia
<200	*P. carinii*	PCP pneumonia
	Cryptosporidium	Chronic diarrhea
<100	*Toxoplasma gondii*	Encephalitis
	Microsporidia	Diarrhea
	Candida	Esophagitis
	Cryptococcus neoformans	Meningitis
	M. tuberculosis	Extrapulmonary tuberculosis
	Herpes simplex	Disseminated herpes
	Herpes zoster	Disseminated zoster
	Epstein-Barr virus	CNS lymphoma
<50	*Mycobacterium avium* complex (MAC)	Disseminated MAC
	Cytomegalovirus	Retinitis, gastrointestinal disease, encephalitis

- CNS lymphoma may present with focal neurologic deficits, headache, altered mental status, or seizures.
- On a head CT with contrast, it may be confused with CNS toxoplasmosis because both appear as ring enhancing lesions.
- Currently, antibiotic therapy directed at toxoplasmosis is recommended to establish a tentative diagnosis.
- Only those patients who do not show improvement with a trial of antibiotics should be considered for a brain biopsy to confirm the diagnosis.
- Treatment of CNS lymphoma is not curative, but radiation therapy and steroids may be palliative.
- Anogenital malignancies are more common as a result of coincidental HPV infection; therefore, periodic rectal and pelvic examinations with Papanicolaou smears are warranted to identify early cervical and squamous cell carcinomas.

PULMONARY INFECTIONS

- In early or intermediate HIV disease, there is an increased incidence of bacterial pneumonia, especially those caused by encapsulated pathogens such as *Streptococcus pneumoniae* and *Haemophilus influenzae*.
- As the CD4 cell count drops below 200, a variety of opportunistic infections begin to appear.

Table 34-7	Treatment and Prophylaxis for HIV-Related Opportunistic Infections	
Opportunistic Infection	**Preferred Treatment**	**Alternative Treatment**
Pneumocystis Carinii (PCP)		
Acute infection	Trimethoprim (15 mg/kg/d) + sulfamethoxazole (75 mg/kg/d) po or IV q8h for 21 d TMP/SMX DS 2 tabs po q8h for 21 d.	Pentamidine 4 mg/kg/d IV for 21 d
		Clindamycin 600 mg q8h IV + Primaquine 30 mg po qd for 21 d
	For PaO_2 <70 mm Hg, A-a gradient >35, or an O_2 saturation <90% on room air. Add prednisone 40 mg po bid tapered over 3 wk.	
Prophylaxis	TMP/SMZ DS 1 tab po three times per week or one single-strength tab (400/800 mg) po qd. Dapsone 100 mg po qd.	Pentamidine aerosol 300 mg once monthly. (Dapsone 200 mg po qd + Pyrimethamine 75 mg po + Folinic acid 25 mg po) All once per week.
Toxoplasma Encephalitis		
Acute infection	(Pyrimethamine 20 mg po loading dose and then 75–100 mg po qd + folinic acid 10–15 mg po qd + sulfadiazine 1–1.5 g po q6h) for 6–8 wk or until CT evidence of Toxoplasmosis has resolved. Continue folinic acid for 1 wk after stopping pyrimethamine. All acute infections must be followed by suppressive therapy.	Pyrimethamine 200 mg po loading dose and then 75–100 mg po qd + Folinic acid 10–15 mg po qd with one of the following: Clindamycin (600 mg po/ IV q6h for 6–8 wk) or Azithromycin (1.5 g po qd) or Dapsone 100 mg po qd. Follow treatment with suppressive therapy.

(Continued)

Table 34-7   Treatment and Prophylaxis for HIV-Related Opportunistic Infections *(Continued)*

Opportunistic Infection	Preferred Treatment	Alternative Treatment
Prophylaxis	TMP/SMZ-DS 1 tab po qd	Dapsone 50 mg po qd + pyrimethamine 50 mg po q week + folinic acid 25 mg po q week. Atovaquone 1,500 mg po qd.
Suppressive therapy	Sulfadiazine 2–4 g/d ÷ qid + pyrimethamine 25–50 mg po qd + folinic acid 10 mg po qd	Clindamycin 300–450 mg po q6–8h + pyrimethamine 25–50 mg po qd + folinic 10–25 mg po qd. Atovaquone 750 mg po q6–12h.
Candida		
Thrush, vaginitis, and esophagitis	Fluconazole 200 mg po first dose then 100 mg po qd for 7–14 d. Itraconazole oral solution (200 mg po qd or 100 mg po bid) for 14 d. Caspotungin 50 mg IV qd	Nystatin 500,000 U swish and swallow qid or 500,000 U 2 tabs tid for 14 d. Amphotericin B 0.3–0.5 mg/kg IV qd. For vaginitis may also use Intravaginal miconazole suppository (100 mg) or (2%) cream for 7 d. Clotrimazole cream or troches for 7 d Fluconazole 400 mg po qd for 6–10 wk
Cryptococcal Meningitis		
Acute infection	Amphotericin B 0.7–1.0 mg/kg/d IV + Flucytosine 25 mg/kg/d po q6h for 2 wk Amphotericin B 0.7–1.0 mg/kg/d IV for 2 wks or until afebrile and headache and vomiting gone. Then stop Amphotericin B and start Fluconazole 400 mg po qd for 8–10 wk. Then start maintenance or suppression therapy.	Fluconazole 400 mg po qd + Flucytosine 37.5 mg/kg po q6h for 10 wk
Suppressive therapy	Fluconazole 200 mg po qd	Amphotericin B1 mg/kg IV for 1 wk. Itraconazole 200 mg po bid.

Histoplasmosis

Acute infection — Amphotericin B 0.5–1.0 mg/kg/d IV for 7 d followed by 0.8 mg/kg qod to total dose of 10–15 mg/kg and then start suppressive therapy. Use Liposomal Amphotericin if increased risk for nephrotoxicity: 3 mg/kg/d IV for 14 d followed by suppressive therapy. — Itraconazole 400 mg po qd for 12 wk (Not recommended to treat meningitis.)

Suppressive therapy — Itraconazole 200 mg po bid

Coccidioidomycosis

Acute infection — Fluconazole 400–800 mg po qd — Amphotericin B 0.6–1.0 mg/kg/d for 7 d IV and then 0.8 mg/kg IV qod for a total dose of 2.5 g or more followed by: Fluconazole (400 mg po qd) or Itraconazole (200 mg po/IV bid) for 3–12 mo.

Mycobacterium Tuberculosis — **Consult Infectious Disease Expert**

Acute infection — Multidrug therapy with combination of INH (isoniazid), RIF (rifampin), PZA (pyrazinamide), ETB (ethambutol), RFB (rifabutin), and SM (streptomycin). — RIF 600 mg + PZA 15–20 mg/kg/d for 2 mo or RIF 600 mg po qd for 4 mo

Previously Referred to us "Prophylaxis"

Latent infection — INH 5 mg/kg/d po + pyridoxine 25 mg po qd for 9 mo (maximum does INH is 300 mg in adult)

M. avium **Complex**

Acute infection — Clarithromycin (500 mg po bid) or Azithromycin (600 mg po qd) + ETB 15–25 mg/kg/d + RFB 300 mg po qd — Clarithromycin or Azithromycin + ETB And RFB with one of the following: Cipro 750 mg po bid Ofloxacin 400 mg po bid Amikacin 7.5–15 mg/kg qd IV

(Continued)

Table 34-7 Treatment and Prophylaxis for HIV-Related Opportunistic Infections *(Continued)*

Opportunistic Infection	Preferred Treatment	Alternative Treatment
Prophylaxis	Clarithromycin 500 mg po bid Azithromycin 1,200 mg po weekly	RFB 300 mg po qd Azithromycin 1,200 mg po weekly + RFB 300 mg po qd
Herpes Simplex		
Initial treatment	Acyclovir 200 mg po five times per day for 10 d. Valacyclovir 1,000 mg po bid for 7–10 d. Famciclovir 250 mg po bid for 7–10 d.	Famciclovir 250 mg po bid for 7–10 d
Severe/refractory	Acyclovir 400 mg po five times per day for 14–21 d. Acyclovir 5 mg/kg IV over 1 h q8h for 7 d. Famciclovir 500 mg po bid for 7 d.	Foscarnet IV: HSV recurrence common when IV stopped; thus suppressive therapy with po Famciclovir needed in Acyclovir resistant HSV. Valacyclovir 1,000 mg po bid for 7–10 d.
Herpes Simplex		
Chronic suppression	Acyclovir 400 mg po bid qd Famciclovir 250 mg po bid qd	
Herpes Zoster		
Immunocompromised	Acyclovir 800 mg po five times per day for 7 d	Acyclovir IV: more than one dermatome involved, Trigeminal nerve involved or disseminated. Foscarnet 40 mg/kg IV q8.
Cytomegalovirus		
Retinitis	Foscarnet 90 mg/kg IV q12h for 14–21 d. Ganciclovir (5 mg/kg IV bid) for 14–21 d. Valganciclovir 900 mg po bid for 21 d with food.	

po, orally; q, every; h, hour; qd, every day; qid, four times daily; tid, three times daily; bid, twice daily; IV, intravenous.

- The most common of these pulmonary infections is *Pneumocystis (jirovecii) carinii* pneumonia (PCP).
- PCP is the most common life-threatening opportunistic infection in patients with HIV disease.
- PCP is frequently associated with prodromal symptoms of fever, fatigue, and weight loss before the onset of dyspnea and nonproductive cough.
- The chest radiograph commonly shows diffuse bilateral interstitial infiltrates but may demonstrate alveolar infiltrates and pleural effusions or may appear normal.
- Diagnosis is made by induced sputum examination with immunofluoresent staining.
- Treatment of PCP is trimethoprim-sulfamethoxazole (TMP-SMZ) orally or intravenous for 3 weeks.
- For those allergic to TMP-SMZ, dapsone and pentamidine are alternate therapies.
- In addition, steroids (40 mg orally, twice daily with a tapered course over 3 weeks) should be added to the treatment regimen of any individual with a PaO_2 less than 70 mm Hg, an A-a gradient more than 35 on room air, or an oxygen saturation less than 90% on room air.
- *Coccidioides immitis* may be encountered by HIV-positive individuals in the deserts of the Southwest.
- It typically presents with slowly progressive respiratory and constitutional symptoms.
- *Histoplasmosis encapsulatum* is endemic to the Ohio and Mississippi River valleys and is found in soil contaminated by bat or bird droppings.
- Patients infected with histoplasmosis present with fever and pneumonia.
- Diagnosis is made by culture or by the histologic appearance of the organism in blood or infected tissues.
- *Mycobacterium tuberculosis* infections have increased with the spread of HIV.
- HIV-infected patients are more susceptible to both reactivation and primary infection.
- The chest radiograph may show apical infiltrates and cavitary lesions.
- A PPD may be negative despite infection because of anergy produced by the HIV destruction of cell-mediated immunity.
- The diagnosis is made by sputum stains for AFB with confirmatory cultures.
- Treatment guidelines in HIV-infected and immunocompetent hosts are the same.
- Suspected cases of TB should be treated with a four-drug regimen of isoniazid, rifampin, pyrazinamide, and ethambutol.
- All HIV patients with a PPD more than 5 mm in diameter and a negative chest x-ray should receive 12 months of isoniazid plus pyridoxine as prophylaxis.

NEUROLOGIC COMPLICATIONS

- *Toxoplasma gondii* is a protozoan infection acquired by the ingestion of undercooked meat or substances contaminated with cat feces.
- The primary infection generally passes without notice in childhood.
- The toxoplasmosis seen in AIDS is caused by the reactivation of *T. gondii* cysts.
- It is the most common cause of focal encephalitis among AIDS patients and may present as a focal neurologic deficit, fever, headache, altered mental status, and seizures.

- Diagnosis is made by contrast enhanced head CT, which demonstrates a ring enhancing lesion(s) which may be indistinguishable from CNS lymphoma.
- The presence of antibodies to *T. gondii* in the CSF is helpful, whereas the presence of serum antibodies is not.
- When a head CT is suggestive of toxoplasmosis, appropriate treatment should be instituted and, if this fails, other diagnoses (lymphoma, abscess) should be considered.
- *Cryptococcus neoformans* is the most common cause of meningitis among HIV-infected individuals.
- It is an encapsulated yeast with low virulence and does not appear in HIV-infected hosts until the CD4 cell count is less than 100/mm^3.
- Cryptococcal meningitis presents with headache, fever, meningismus, and photophobia.
- Lumbar puncture reveals an elevated opening pressure greater than 200 mm Hg in 70% of patients.
- CSF analysis shows leukocyte counts of 0 to 700/mm^3, protein elevation (55%), a low glucose (24%), positive India ink stains (75%), and detectable cryptococcal antigens (95%).
- The definitive diagnosis is confirmed by culture of *C. neoformans* from the CSF.
- AIDS dementia is a progressive process caused by HIV infection and manifests with impairment of recent memory as well as progressive deterioration of cognitive, motor, and behavioral function.
- CT/MRI shows cerebral atrophy, ventricular enlargement, subcortical gray matter lesions, and white matter changes.
- CSF may show a mild pleocytosis. There is no clearly effective treatment.
- Peripheral neuropathies are common in HIV and in addition may be caused by one of the reverse transcriptase inhibitors (ddI, ddC, and d4T).

GASTROINTESTINAL COMPLICATIONS

- The most common gastrointestinal (GI) complication seen with HIV disease is diarrhea.
- HIV itself may cause diarrhea (AIDS enteropathy), as may a host of opportunistic infections and tumors.
- In addition, many antiretroviral medications (nelfinavir, ritonavir, amprenavir, lopinavir, indinavir, and didanosine) are associated with diarrhea, and antibiotic use may lead to *Clostridium difficile* colitis.
- For these reasons, the differential diagnosis of diarrhea in the HIV/AIDS patient presents a diagnostic and therapeutic challenge.
- Treatment is symptomatic with repletion of fluid losses and antimotility agents and appropriate stool studies (ova, parasites, bacterial culture, acid fast stain, trichrome stain, *C. difficile* enterotoxin, etc.).
- Esophagitis with odynophagia and dysphagia may be caused by *Candida albicans* or *Candida krausei*, herpes simplex virus, or cytomegalovirus.
- Endoscopy, fungal stains, viral cultures, or even biopsy may be needed to make the diagnosis.
- Oral hairy leukoplakia and *Candida albicans* may be present in the oropharynx.
- Oral hairy leukoplakia has thick, painless, white lesions that cannot be removed with scraping, whereas oral candidiasis has lacy white plaques that are easily scraped off.

- Treatment of oral candidiasis has traditionally been with clotrimazole troches 10 mg orally five times per day or nystatin suspension 400,000 to 600,000 U four times a day. Oral fluconazole is replacing topical therapy and is given as a 200-mg loading dose followed by 100 to 200 mg daily for 7 to 10 days.
- Painful oral lesions may be caused by herpes simplex virus or mycobacterium avium complex.

CUTANEOUS COMPLICATIONS

- Most patients with HIV/AIDS demonstrate cutaneous pathology at some point in their disease.
- Acute HIV infection leads to a diffuse macular or maculopapular eruption that occurs 2 to 3 days after the onset of flu-like symptoms.
- Varicella-zoster eruptions that involve multiple dermatomes are commonly seen in AIDS patients. Consider admitting any patient with systemic involvement, ophthalmologic involvement, or extensive dermatomal zoster. Intravenous acyclovir is the treatment.
- Uncomplicated dermatomal zoster, in patients with CD4 counts more than 200, may be treated with oral acyclovir, famciclovir, or valacyclovir.
- The primary and secondary courses of syphilis are unchanged in HIV, but treatment failure after penicillin therapy is more common in AIDS.
- Norwegian scabies (crusted scabies) is a severe form of scabies that occurs in AIDS patients and consists of a severe infestation of the skin involving thousands of mites that eventually causes scales to form. The entire skin can be involved eventually.
- Pruritic papular eruption is a condition associated with HIV that causes a papular eruption that is symmetric and occurs on the extensor surfaces of the arms, the trunk, and the face with palmer and plantar sparing. Its etiology is unknown.
- Morbilliform and urticarial rashes are common side effects of HIV medications and are more prevalent in the patient with a low CD4 count.

OPHTHALMOLOGIC COMPLICATIONS

- Cytomegalovirus retinitis produces a severe necrotic vasculitis and retinitis that usually occurs when the CD4 cell count is less than $50/mm^3$.
- The diagnosis is based on retinal findings such as fluffy, white perivascular lesions; hemorrhages; and exudates.
- If untreated, it rapidly causes blindness.
- The treatment is foscarnet or ganciclovir.

HIV THERAPY

- Reverse transcriptase inhibitors include zidovudine (AZT), didanosine (ddI), zalcitabine (ddC), stavudine (d4t), and lamivudine (3TC) and must be given on a long-term basis.
- Common side effects are nausea, diarrhea, fatigue, sleep disturbances, pigment changes, anemia, neutropenia, peripheral neuropathy, and pancreatitis.
- Protease inhibitors are a newer class drugs, and each has a unique side effect profile.
- Saquinavir is the best-tolerated protease inhibitor and is associated with headache and GI upset.

- Indinavir is partially excreted in the urine, and its administration may increase the incidence of renal calculi and renal colic.
- Nelfinavir is commonly associated with diarrhea.
- Ritonavir is the most poorly tolerated, with associated GI upset, fatigue, rash, fatigue, malaise, altered taste sensation, and perioral paraesthesias.
- The long-term safety of protease inhibitor therapy is unclear.
- The principles of HAART in HIV infection can be simplified as follows. First, anti-retroviral therapy should be started early. Second, assume that mutations and associated drug resistance are present from the start (therefore, to successfully inhibit viral replication of each HIV variant, combination therapy with two nonnucleoside reverse transcriptase inhibitors plus an HIV protease inhibitor must be started simultaneously). Third, the treatment goal is to completely suppress viral replication and, finally, to restore immune constitution.
- Treatment is lifelong and requires compliance for success.
- Resistance to an antiretroviral therapy is assumed when the viral load begins to climb in a compliant patient.
- Treatment of HIV-infected mothers should follow the same treatment guidelines as established for nonpregnant individuals.
- Antiretroviral therapy in an HIV-positive mother reduces the mother-to-child transmission rate from 30% to less than 1%.

35 Sexual Assault

PATIENT'S IMMEDIATE EMOTIONAL NEEDS

- Rape represents a profound, true emotional crisis for virtually all patients.
- It should be made clear at the beginning of the patient encounter that he or she is no longer in danger of harm. Patients should first be placed in a quiet, comfortable, private room, where a member of the staff should remain with the patient at all times.
- Although details of the incident should not be explored at this time, the patient should be comforted and allowed to express any feelings he or she feels are appropriate.
- Before the physical examination, the patient should be discouraged from changing clothes, washing, urinating, or defecating; oral intake should be prohibited when oral penetration may have occurred.
- Although serious physical injury may occur, in most patients, emotional or psychological damage is initially and ultimately more disabling and must be thoroughly addressed.
- It is the responsibility of the emergency provider to consider these initial psychological needs and to make clearly available appropriate counseling services.
- It is strongly recommended that the appropriate counseling service, whether it be a designated nurse responsible for rape counseling or a member of the psychiatry or social service department skilled in the initial care of such patients, comes to the emergency department and establish contact with the patient before discharge.
- This contact will not only allow an initial assessment of the patient but also make clear the availability of psychological assistance if it becomes necessary over the next 24 to 48 hours.
- Aside from acute care, a psychological referral at an appropriate interval as suggested by the consultant should be strongly advised.

CONSENT AND THE CHAIN OF EVIDENCE

- Consent must be obtained from the patient for each part of the evaluation process.
- Some patients will not wish to prosecute and, on this basis, will wish to forego the formal collection of evidence substantiating the allegation of rape; this is clearly the right of the individual and in no way alters other care.
- Patients should, however, be encouraged to allow a complete formal evaluation for the collection of evidence, because they may change their minds and then wish to proceed with prosecution; this clearly will be made difficult or impossible without the initial substantiation of rape through the proper collection of evidence.
- Again, the evaluation and treatment, medically and psychologically, of patients who elect to forego the forensic evidence gathering are unchanged in all other respects.
- The "chain of evidence" refers to the orderly and recorded transferal of information and evidence from the person obtaining it to its ultimate destination in the crime laboratory or court.

- The transmittal form is designed to make clear the person or agency responsible at any given time for the collected material.
- Each time information or collected material is transferred to another person or institution, its custody must be formally recognized and signed for.
- Separate transferal forms should be generated for each group of collected specimens.
- Each collected specimen must be labeled with the date and time of collection, the patient's name and hospital number, the origin of the particular specimen, and the name of the individual who collected the specimen.
- Failure to document formally and in writing the transferal of information or evidence with each passage and to identify or label collected information correctly and completely may result in the rejection of such material by the court.

HISTORY

- In some jurisdictions, a specially trained nurse conducts the history and physical examination, whereas in other jurisdictions, the physician is responsible for the pertinent medical evaluation; details related to the actual incident are more appropriately obtained by police officers with an appropriate member of the staff available at all times to provide emotional support to the patient.
- Medically pertinent facts should be investigated sequentially.
- These are as follows:
  - The date, time, and location of the incident
  - Whether force or the threat of force was used to coerce or intimidate, whether drugs or alcohol were used, or whether the patient was unconscious or intellectually abnormal in any way before or during the incident
  - What specific type of assault the patient believes to have occurred?
  - Was there oral, anal, and/or vaginal penetration?
  - Was such penetration attempted and with what specifically?
  - Did ejaculation occur and, if so, then where?
  - Was a condom used?
  - When was the patient's last voluntary intercourse?
  - A negative history of previous intercourse should specifically be noted.
  - What specific type of birth control is used by the patient?
  - Note whether there has been compliance with contraception over the previous 30 days.
  - Have periods been regular, particularly the last two or three?
  - Was there any evidence of pregnancy or pelvic infection present before the incident?
  - Has the patient changed clothing, douched, showered, bathed, eaten, or brushed teeth subsequent to the episode?
  - Does the patient have any medical problems or drug allergies?
  - What, if any, regular medicines were prescribed and when were they last taken?
  - Have any other drugs or alcohol been taken voluntarily before or after the incident?

PHYSICAL EXAMINATION AND COLLECTION OF EVIDENCE

The physical examination, which must be undertaken gently and tactfully, should address three primary issues:
- Is there physical or significant emotional injury to the patient or other medical or surgical problems that require emergency treatment? If so, these obviously are initial priorities.

- Is or was the patient intellectually capable of consenting to voluntary intercourse? Minor children, as defined by most state laws, are unable to provide consent; penetration of the penis into the genitalia in such patients is referred to as statutory rape. Persons with abnormalities of mental status that are the result of mental retardation, mental illness, lack of normal psychosexual development, or the voluntary or coerced ingestion of drugs or alcohol are also generally considered unable to consent to voluntary intercourse. When mental retardation, mental illness, or other abnormalities of mental status are noted and are thought significant with respect to the issue of consent, formal psychiatric consultation should be undertaken before discharge from the emergency room. After written permission is obtained, specimens of blood and urine may be obtained for determination of toxic substances.

- Is there physical evidence of force, and is there physical evidence that substantiates the alleged assault? The patient should be discouraged from urinating, defecating, or washing before the examination; similarly, oral intake should be restricted if oral penetration has occurred. Before the patient disrobes, a photograph of the patient, if written permission has been granted, may be taken. The necessary instruments and specimen containers should be assembled before undertaking the examination; a "kit" containing the proper permission forms, the emergency department protocol for rape victims, and the necessary instruments and specimen containers should be present in all emergency departments. If not, such kits are commercially available and are recommended for the orderly and proper collection and identification of information and specimens.

- The patient should be asked to undress and to place each garment individually into a separate labeled paper bag, stapled closed at multiple sites, and the proper protocol for the chain of evidence initiated by the individual collecting or obtaining the specimen. Members of the emergency department staff should refrain from touching the patient's clothing because cross-contamination of blood group antigens present in perspiration or foreign genetic material may interfere with the subsequent analysis of similar antigens contained in semen or blood deposited on the patient's clothing by the alleged rapist.

- The patient should be examined for any evidence of trauma; this may include bites, scratches, bruises, areas of ecchymoses, lacerations, and fractures, etc. These should carefully and precisely be described and, if possible, a diagram or photograph obtained. Important areas include the wrists and ankles, breasts, and perineal area.

- Any semen identified on the patient should be collected with a moistened, cotton-tipped applicator, placed in a dry sterile collection tube, and evaluated in the laboratory for acid phosphatase activity. Identification of semen may be aided by ultraviolet illumination; however, it must be remembered that urine as well as a variety of other substances may also fluoresce. Pubic hair that appears to contain semen should be clipped, labeled, retained, and submitted as described. The patient's pubic hair should then be combed and any foreign material, particularly hair, that may have originated from the assailant be labeled as "pubic hair combings" and retained. A sample of the patient's pubic hair should be obtained by clipping and similarly retained separately. Scrapings from under the nails should be collected and retained, because they may reveal tissue from the assailant if the assailant was scratched during the attack.

- The pelvic examination should note any evidence of external or internal trauma. It is important that the entirety of the vaginal mucosa be visualized to exclude occult laceration. This is particularly true in patients with evidence of vaginal laceration or vaginal bleeding in whom a source is not otherwise identified. Water should be the only lubricant used during the examination because other substances may interfere with the determination of acid phosphatase. The posterior fornix should be inspected after insertion of the speculum for the presence of any secretions. If present, these should be aspirated and placed in a properly labeled sterile container and submitted according to the chain of evidence protocol for determination of sperm, acid phosphatase, and blood group antigens; this material may then be cultured in Thayer-Martin medium or via PCR probe to exclude gonococcal infection. In patients without such secretions, materials must be collected from the vagina for analysis. A cotton-tipped applicator may be used to swab the vaginal wall; material obtained is smeared onto two slides that are then examined for the presence of sperm and determination of acid phosphatase activity. A wet mount using nonbacteriostatic normal saline may be made for analysis for the presence of motile sperm. Additionally, in patients without available secretions, the vaginal wall may be irrigated with 10 to 20 mL of normal saline, which is then aspirated from the posterior fornix and analyzed for the presence of acid phosphatase, sperm, blood group antigens, and culture if not already obtained. It is important that the laboratory assessment for motile sperm be undertaken immediately after the specimen is obtained and labeled. At some hospitals, examiners who are trained in its use may examine the patient with a colposcope for signs of genital trauma not generally seen by the eye alone.

- If the patient reports rectal penetration, the rectum must be inspected for evidence of injury. Samples should be obtained, labeled, and submitted. The rectum may similarly be irrigated with 10 to 20 mL of saline and studies obtained as outlined.
- If oral penetration is reported, the oral cavity must be inspected for evidence of trauma; to substantiate penetration, swabbing from between the teeth should be submitted for sperm and acid phosphatase activity.
- Blood should be obtained from the patient for typing (to assist with blood group analysis), RPR, and quantitative determination of the serum β-subunit of human chorionic gonadotropin (HCG).

SPECIFIC PROBLEMS

Prevention of Pregnancy

- Women who have been raped should have a quantitative determination of the serum β-subunit of HCG obtained as soon as possible; no treatment to prevent pregnancy should be administered until a pregnancy existing before the rape is clearly excluded by β-HCG testing. Patients presenting within 24 to 48 hours of the alleged incident with a positive urine HCG were pregnant before the rape and should not receive any medication contraindicated in pregnancy. After the HCG has been returned and is negative, treatment to prevent pregnancy may be elected if pregnancy is possible based on the patient's menstrual history, and the patient wishes termination of possible pregnancy and so indicates formally in writing on the permission or consent form.
- A number of medical regimens to prevent pregnancy are available and are effective if given within 72 hours of intercourse. All protocols may be complicated by nausea and vomiting. Plan B® (levonorgesterel), a recently approved drug for the secondary prevention of pregnancy, may be started within 72 hours of intercourse.

Prevention of Infection

- The victim of rape is considered to be a venereal disease contact. Although the incidence of gonorrhea, *Chlamydia,* syphilis, hepatitis B, and the human immunodefi-

ciency virus (HIV) is relatively low in victims of rape, prophylactic treatment may have significant psychological as well as medical benefits.
- Of the potential venereal diseases, gonorrhea is the most commonly acquired.
- The Centers for Disease Control and Prevention (CDC) recommends an empiric antimicrobial regimen that covers *Chlamydia,* gonorrhea, *Trichomonas,* and bacterial vaginosis.
  - Cultures or PCR testing for gonorrhea and *Chlamydia* from involved areas should be obtained before treatment, along with serum for RPR (VDRL) determination; the latter would be expected to be negative unless preexisting exposure has occurred.
  - Prophylactic treatment for gonorrhea, *Chlamydia*, *Trichomonas*, and bacterial vaginosis may be undertaken as follows (CDC recommendation):
  - Ceftriaxone 125 mg intramuscularly in a single dose plus metronidazole (for trichomoniasis) 2 g orally in a single dose plus azithromycin 1 g orally in a single dose or doxycycline 100 mg orally twice daily for 7 days
- The CDC also recommends postexposure hepatitis B vaccination if not already done (without hepatitis B immunoglobulin) at the time of initial examination. Follow-up doses of the vaccine should be given at 6 weeks and 4 months after the first dose.
- Postexposure HIV prophylaxis (PEP) is controversial since the rate of conversion is so low. However, the patient should be counseled about the risks and benefits of the drug regimen and allowed to make his or her own decision. Refer to the CDC website (CDC.gov) for current medication recommendations.

FOLLOW-UP

- Psychological and medical follow-up for victims of sexual assault is often inadequate.
- Each patient will require information from the physician regarding the possibility of pregnancy, the possibility of infection, and whether any permanent psychological, physical, or sexual abnormalities are likely. Frequently, these issues become unclear soon after leaving the emergency department despite a thorough discussion.
- For this reason, it is prudent that the person who will psychologically support the patient longitudinally should come to the emergency department before discharge to establish contact and thereby make available a means for the patient to obtain information and reassurance.
- All patients should additionally receive an appropriate gynecologic referral, and interval follow-up should be suggested; patients should have medical follow-up at 2 and 6 weeks. Patients should be reevaluated for pregnancy and sexually transmitted diseases at the 2-week follow-up.
- Because the drug regimen to treat sexually transmitted diseases as listed is not optimal for treating syphilis, a follow-up serologic test for syphilis should be obtained at 6 weeks.
- It should also be made clear to the patient that he or she may return to the emergency department at any time if needed.

36 Testicular, Scrotal, and Inguinal Pain or Swelling

COMMON CAUSES OF TESTICULAR AND SCROTAL PAIN OR SWELLING

- Acute orchitis
- Acute epididymitis
- Testicular torsion
- Inguinal hernia
- Hydrocele
- Varicocele
- Spermatocele

COMMON CAUSES OF INGUINAL PAIN OR SWELLING

- Inguinal hernia
- Inguinal adenopathy
- Muscle strain

HISTORY

- The development of a "bulge" or swelling in the groin or scrotum after heavy lifting or exercise suggests an inguinal hernia.
- When this history is associated with nausea, vomiting, and a change in bowel habits or abdominal pain, bowel incarceration is suggested.
- Tender inguinal swelling that develops gradually may represent a soft-tissue abscess or inguinal adenopathy secondary to lower extremity or venereal infection; a history of recent sexual exposure or urethral discharge may be elicited in the latter.
- A diffusely swollen, tender testis associated with fever and signs of systemic illness suggests testicular ischemia, infarction, or orchitis.
- The sudden onset of testicular pain in a young man or child suggests testicular torsion, a true urologic emergency.
- Inguinal area discomfort after exercise or exertion made worse by movement or elevation of the leg against resistance suggests muscle strain.

PHYSICAL EXAMINATION

- Local abscess or inguinal lymphadenopathy in the setting of lower extremity infection or a urethral discharge poses no great diagnostic difficulty.
- Fever is commonly noted in patients with orchitis or epididymitis.
- Inguinal hernia may contain bowel loops; therefore, on auscultation, bowel sounds may be noted.

- Direct and indirect inguinal hernias may be readily palpated in the upright patient and may be reducible with recumbency or Trendelenburg position and slight pressure; if they are not, however, or if significant tenderness is present, incarceration must be ruled out.
- A hydrocele or spermatocele may be transilluminated, whereas an inflamed epididymis, a torsed testicle, or a hernia generally cannot be.
- Varicoceles are most commonly seen on the left because the venous drainage of the left testicle occurs into the left renal vein.
- Examination of the lower extremity, particularly the toes, may demonstrate an infectious process responsible for inguinal adenopathy.
- Swelling, retraction, and severe discomfort are important signs of testicular torsion.
- Testicular elevation in patients with orchitis (Prehn sign) often causes some improvement in pain and may therefore be a useful, although absolutely not a definitive, diagnostic maneuver.
- Enhancement of inguinal area discomfort associated with movement of the extremity against resistance is found in patients with musculoligamentous injuries; to elicit such discomfort, internal or external rotation of the leg against resistance is often helpful.

DIAGNOSTIC TESTS

- The white blood count is normal or mildly elevated in orchitis or epididymitis but may be significantly elevated in patients with incarcerated hernia.
- An abdominal CT will prove the diagnosis in patients with a possible incarcerated obstructing inguinal hernia.
- Color Doppler ultrasound is now considered the diagnostic procedure of choice in patients suspected of torsion; also potentially seen by ultrasound are an edematous epididymis, a varicocele, or a spermatocele.
- A urinalysis and urethral swab should also be obtained in the patient with suspected epididymitis.

CLINICAL REMINDERS

- Obtain an emergency Doppler ultrasound, or immediate urologic consultation in patients in whom testicular torsion is suspected.
- Attempt to reduce inguinal hernias whenever possible. Use procedural sedation if necessary.

SPECIFIC DISORDERS

Inguinal Hernia

- An indirect hernia consists of a protrusion of the abdominal contents through the internal inguinal ring into a congenital peritoneal diverticulum.
- This diverticulum is the unobliterated processus vaginalis that accompanies the descent of the testis in men and ovarian fixation in women.
- These hernias are nine times more prevalent in men than women and occur most commonly during the first year of life and between 10 and 30 years of age.
- Indirect inguinal hernias are demonstrated by examining the patient in the standing position.

- Invagination of the scrotal skin with the index finger placed well within the external inguinal ring while the patient coughs forces the hernia against or past the examining finger and is diagnostic.
- Indirect inguinal hernias are often bilateral.
- Surgical repair remains the only satisfactory treatment and should be advised based on the patient's symptoms and lifestyle.
- The recurrence rate is approximately 1% to 5%.
- Symptoms of direct inguinal hernia are similar to those of indirect hernia; however, a globular bulge in the vicinity of the external inguinal ring is often noted.
- Direct hernias often reduce immediately on recumbency and are rare in women.
- Treatment is also ultimately surgical via laparoscopic or open techniques employing mesh.
- Incarceration of a hernia is suggested by irreducibility and is often associated with severe local pain, tenderness, fever, and signs of intestinal obstruction.
- Emergency surgical consultation is essential in these patients.

Acute Epididymitis

- Acute epididymitis may be caused by a variety of organisms, including *Chlamydia* and gonococci, or may occur in association with prostatitis.
- Symptoms include marked pain and swelling of the epididymis and, very frequently, the testis as well.
- Pain is generally of a gradual onset, and fever is commonly observed.
- Physical examination reveals a swollen, tender scrotal mass located below, behind, and often lateral to the testicle.
- Pyuria may be present on urinalysis.
- Doppler studies often show increased flow.
- Treatment consists of adequate analgesia, cold compresses, and scrotal support.
- For men younger than 35 years of age who commonly have sexually transmitted organisms as a cause, give ceftriaxone 250 mg intramuscular once followed by doxycycline 100 mg orally twice daily for 10 days.
- Anal insertive homosexual men or men older than age 35 should be treated for Enterobacteriaceae with ciprofloxacin 500 mg orally twice daily for 10 days, or ofloxacin 300 mg orally twice daily, for 10 days.
- Importantly, the physician should consider testicular torsion in all patients with suspected epididymitis.

Acute Orchitis

- Testicular torsion must once again be entertained in the differential diagnosis.
- Acute orchitis may be caused by a variety of viral or bacterial agents, the most common of which is the mumps virus (70% of cases), or may be secondary to an associated epididymitis.
- Eighty percent of cases of mumps orchitis occur in boys under the age of 10.
- In patients with viral orchitis, antibiotics are of no use; care is supportive (ice, analgesia, scrotal support).
- Bacterial orchitis usually spreads from an associated epididymitis, or in men with prostatic hypertrophy.
- Age-based treatment and differential diagnosis of suspected bacterial orchitis are similar to those of acute epididymitis.

Testicular Torsion

- Testicular torsion occurs unilaterally and may follow or be precipitated by exercise or may occur spontaneously.
- This leads to the abrupt cessation of blood flow and testicular ischemia and infarction, which is likely to be irreversible after 12 hours.
- Peripubertal men are most commonly (but not exclusively) affected, in whom the subacute or sudden onset of testicular or lower quadrant abdominal pain is reported.
- Patients with a history of having had torsion in the past with orchiopexy can redevelop torsion months to years later because some urologists use absorbable suture when performing an orchiopexy.
- Torsion is common in patients with an undescended testis in whom a painful, inguinal mass is noted.
- An affected descended testis is swollen, retracted, and tender. Patients presenting very early may have minimal physical findings.
- An emergency color Doppler ultrasound is essential for the noninvasive evaluation of patients with suspected torsion; decreased or absent perfusion is noted on the affected side and is diagnostic.
- Immediate surgical exploration by urologist and detorsion with bilateral orchiopexy are then undertaken.
- An effort at detorsion is usually undertaken by the emergency practitioner after the diagnosis is confirmed and if urologic consultation is delayed. This is a temporizing maneuver.
- In most patients (2/3), the testis torses or turns medially (the anterior aspect of the testis has turned medially).
- After parenteral analgesia, it is reasonable to attempt to detorse the testis by turning the anterior portion of the testis laterally (in a direction on the right or left as if opening a book, the right side going counterclockwise and the left clockwise as one looks at the patient in a lithotomy position). If "lengthening" or relaxation of the testicle occurs, then detorsion may have been successful. Conversely, if "shortening" of the cord appears to occur (the testicle ascends somewhat), then torsion probably occurred laterally initially, and an attempt to turn the testis medially is warranted.
- When urologic subspecialty consultation or imaging capabilities are not available, emergent transfer is appropriate.

Hydrocele

- Hydrocele consists of a collection of clear yellow fluid within the tunica or process vaginalis; it may develop rapidly, secondary to local injury, epididymitis, or orchitis.
- Hydrocele produces swelling in the inguinal area or within the scrotum.
- Although hydrocele is typically painless (unless accompanied by epididymitis or orchitis), patients may complain of its size or weight.
- The mass typically transilluminates.
- Treatment by the urologist with aspiration or surgery is indicated if the hydrocele is tense, impairs testicular circulation, or is otherwise symptomatic.

Varicocele

- Varicoceles are common in young men and consist of a dilated, venous pampiniform plexus.

- The left testis is more commonly affected because of a higher incidence of incompetent venous valves on the left, which permit engorgement of the ipsilateral plexus.
- The patient may report pain or a bulky mass.
- Treatment is not necessary unless the varicocele is unusually large or infertility is present.
- The sudden onset or increase in the size of a varicocele in a middle age or older man should suggest the possibility of tumor invasion of the renal vein, because the left testis drains directly into the left renal vein.

Spermatocele

- Spermatocele is a painless cystic mass containing sperm whose genesis is from the head of the epididymis most often.
- Spermatoceles are typically less than 1 cm in diameter but occasionally become quite large and may be mistaken for hydroceles.
- Treatment is conservative unless the spermatocele becomes symptomatic.

37 Vaginal Bleeding

INTRODUCTION

In the United States, menstruation usually begins between the ages of 10 and 15 and may be irregular for several years. For most women, cycles become regular in the late teens, and as menopause approaches, cycles once again become irregular. This natural history of menstrual cycle fluctuation must be kept in mind when evaluating patients with vaginal bleeding. For the emergency physician, vaginal bleeding that produces hemodynamic compromise or is associated with pregnancy is of the greatest concern. In these cases, a urinary HCG should be obtained if the patient is of reproductive age. Pregnancy must not be ruled out solely on the basis of the patient's sexual or menstrual history; this is particularly true in the adolescent and in the perimenopausal woman.

- In children younger than 10 years of age presenting with vaginal bleeding, a number of age-specific diagnoses must be considered:
  - Precocious sexual development
  - Genital malignancy
  - Vaginal candidiasis
  - Occult "straddle-type" injuries
  - Sexual assault
  - Vaginal foreign body
  - Occult birth control pill ingestion
  - Pregnancy
- In patients older than 35 years of age, anatomic causes of vaginal bleeding are common and include endometrial and cervical polyps and a variety of gynecologic malignancies.
- Because structural abnormalities are common in this age group, it is important that bleeding should not be designated simply as "perimenopausal" without a thorough pelvic examination as well as other appropriate studies.
- Pregnancy must always be excluded.
- In patients of reproductive age, vaginal bleeding is most often related to normal menses or to an anovulatory cycle; the latter is common near the menarche or menopause or can be related to a number of other phenomena, such as stress or rapid change in weight.
- The emergency practitioner should remember the importance of Rh sensitization in Rh-negative women delivering Rh-positive infants; this is preventable by administering $Rh_0(D)$ immune globulin (300 μg) after delivery.
- $Rh_0(D)$ immune globulin should also be administered to Rh-negative women after abortion, miscarriage, amniocentesis, and severe antepartum hemorrhage.

COMMON CAUSES OF VAGINAL BLEEDING

- Menstruation
- Oral contraceptive use

- Anovulatory cycle
- Spontaneous abortion
- Ectopic pregnancy
- Intrauterine pregnancy
- Intrauterine contraceptive device
- Persistent corpus luteum

LESS COMMON CAUSES OF VAGINAL BLEEDING NOT TO BE MISSED

- Gynecologic malignancy
- Vaginal or cervical injury
- Vaginal foreign body
- Gestational trophoblastic disease
- Abruptio placenta
- Placenta previa
- Vasa praevia
- Uterine rupture

HISTORY

- The age of the patient is very helpful in suggesting a number of possible causes of vaginal bleeding.
- Precocious sexual development, pregnancy, malignancy, candidal vaginitis, occult "straddle-type" injuries or sexual assault, occult birth control pill ingestion, and vaginal foreign body should be considered in children younger than 10 years of age.
- In patients older than 35 years of age, endometrial and cervical carcinoma and polyps, pregnancy, vaginal or cervical trauma related to coitus, perimenopausal bleeding, and pelvic inflammatory disease must be considered.
- In all patients of child-bearing age, pregnancy (intrauterine and ectopic), infection, spontaneous abortion, and coital trauma are common causes of bleeding.
- In patients with an intrauterine contraceptive device, menorrhagia with midline, crampy abdominal pain is often reported.
- A history of recent sexual exposure, fever, vaginal discharge, and pain with intercourse all suggest pelvic inflammatory disease.
- A history of vaginal spotting, often after a normal, missed, or slightly abnormal menstrual period, when associated with lower quadrant pain should suggest ectopic pregnancy; rapidly evolving evidence of circulatory compromise completes the clinical picture.

PHYSICAL EXAMINATION

- Vaginal or cervical laceration or injury will be apparent on pelvic examination, as will the presence of a foreign body; a foul-smelling vaginal odor may be noted in patients with a long-standing foreign body.
- A blue vaginal or cervical discoloration, softening of the cervicouterine junction, breast enlargement, and nipple tenderness suggest pregnancy, either intrauterine or ectopic.

- Fetal tissue in the vagina or cervical os is sometimes noted in patients with incomplete abortion, whereas vaginal bleeding or ruptured membranes in a patient in the first or second trimester associated with a dilated cervix without extruding tissue suggests that abortion is imminent.
- Third-trimester, bright red painless bleeding suggests placenta previa, whereas painful bleeding with uterine tenderness or tetany suggests abruption.
- Patients who present with painless third-trimester bleeding should not have a pelvic examination until ultrasound has excluded or documented the position of placenta previa.
- Patients with ectopic pregnancy may also present with abdominal pain and a palpable adnexal mass or fullness, although subtle presentations with relatively painless vaginal spotting are common.
- In patients with pelvic inflammatory disease, fever, lower pelvic pain with abdominal palpation, mild to moderate rebound tenderness, a purulent discharge from the cervix, and profound discomfort when the cervix is laterally displaced are often noted.

DIAGNOSTIC TESTS

- The hematocrit may be used to assess the significance of bleeding if intravascular equilibration has been achieved.
- Because most patients tend to overestimate the extent of blood loss, a pad count per hour is useful as an estimate of the severity of bleeding.
- The urine or serum β-subunit of HCG is one of the most important studies to perform in the patient with vaginal bleeding; the urine or serum HCG may become positive as early as the third to fifth day after conception.
- If ectopic pregnancy is a diagnostic possibility, a quantitative determination of the serum HCG should be obtained.
- Hydatidiform mole and choriocarcinoma may produce false-positive results, whereas early ectopic pregnancy, intrauterine fetal demise, and a missed abortion may produce false-negative results.
- A blood type and screen should be obtained to determine the patient's Rh status and subsequent need for $Rh_0(D)$ immune globulin.
- Abdominal and pelvic ultrasonography is useful in defining the presence of both intrauterine and ectopic pregnancies and should be performed in all stable patients suspected of having an ectopic pregnancy.
- This can rapidly be performed at the bedside in the hypotensive or tachycardic female patient with abdominal pain to determine the presence of free fluid suggesting a ruptured ectopic pregnancy.
- Ultrasound is also necessary to evaluate for placenta previa in the patient with vaginal bleeding in the third trimester.

CLINICAL REMINDERS

- Perform a pelvic examination on all patients unless, based on painless, third-trimester, bright red bleeding, placenta previa is suspected.
- Obtain a urine or serum HCG to determine pregnancy, and when ectopic pregnancy is a consideration, obtain a quantitative serum HCG.
- Request emergency Ob/Gyn consultation in patients with third-trimester bleeding.

- Remember to administer $Rh_0(D)$ immune globulin to Rh-negative women after abortion, miscarriage, trauma, antepartum hemorrhage, and delivery of an Rh-positive infant.

SPECIFIC DISORDERS

Ectopic Pregnancy

- An ectopic pregnancy should be suspected when a woman who is or may be pregnant presents with abdominal pain or vaginal bleeding.
- Pregnancies in which the zygote becomes implanted in extrauterine locations are said to be ectopic.
- Ectopic pregnancy occurs in approximately 0.5% to 1.0% of all pregnancies, and 98% of these implant in the fallopian tube.
- Shock, which occurs in approximately 10% of patients, results from local rupture and hemorrhage.
- Most patients report a missed period or a most recent period that, in some frequently subtle way, was unusual.
- Patients may report symptoms suggestive of pregnancy: breast tenderness, morning nausea, or easy fatigability.
- A history of right or left lower quadrant pain, often of abrupt onset and associated with vaginal bleeding or spotting, is usually obtained and should suggest the diagnosis.
- The pain is generally mild and is poorly localized.
- Some patients present with syncope or shock.
- Shock, syncope, or left shoulder pain suggests rupture with free blood in the peritoneum.
- Ectopic pregnancies are more common in women who use IUDs, have had pelvic inflammatory disease, have had tubal ligations, have had a previous ectopic pregnancy, have had lower abdominal and gynecologic surgery, and have used fertility drugs.
- On physical examination, patients with brisk intraperitoneal or vaginal bleeding may be hypotensive and diaphoretic; postural changes in blood pressure or pulse rate may suggest significant acute blood loss.
- If intraperitoneal bleeding has occurred, the classic signs of peritonitis will be noted; however, these signs generally are absent in patients bleeding into the uterine cavity.
- Pelvic examination may demonstrate varying degrees of vaginal bleeding, mild to moderate discomfort on lateral movement of the cervix, and an adnexal mass or bulging of the cul-de-sac in approximately 50% of patients.
- A quantitative serum HCG should be obtained in all patients with suspected ectopic pregnancies.
- Current pregnancy tests are highly sensitive and can be positive at 4 days after implantation (hCG levels of 15–50 mIU/mL).
- Emergency pelvic ultrasonography should be obtained in all stable patients to guide the gynecologist regarding treatment.
- Normally, intrauterine pregnancies can be detected by abdominal ultrasound when the quantitative HCG is 6,500 mIU/mL and by vaginal ultrasound when it is 1,000 to 2,000 mIU/mL.
- Shock should be managed in the usual fashion.

- Patients presenting with shock, postural hypotension, or brisk vaginal bleeding should be typed and cross-matched for Rh determination and transfusion.
- Large-bore intravenous access should be established, repletion of intravascular volume instituted with Ringer lactate solution or normal saline, and emergency gynecologic consultation obtained.
- Patients who are Rh negative should receive 50 to 300 μg of anti-D immunoglobulin (RhoGAM) intramuscularly, unless the father is known to be Rh negative.
- Under certain circumstances, the gynecologist may elect medical treatment (methotrexate), typically for patients with mild symptoms, no evidence of rupture or fetal cardiac activity by ultrasound, stable vital signs, a β-hCG less than 10,000 mIU/mL, and a tubal mass less than 4 cm.
- Medical therapy is unsuccessful approximately 10% of the time.
- Patients returning to the emergency department after medical treatment and who report increased abdominal or pelvic discomfort, or other evidence of intraperitoneal bleeding, require reevaluation of the ectopic pregnancy and assessment of the presence and extent of intraperitoneal bleeding.
- A surgical approach may be needed in these patients, and a gynecologist should be consulted early.

Spontaneous Abortion

Threatened Abortion
- Threatened abortion is usually associated with mild to moderate lower pelvic cramping and is by definition not associated with the passage of fetal tissue.
- The cervical os is closed, the uterus is appropriately enlarged for the length of gestation, and the cervix and adnexa are nontender.
- Treatment is conservative and expectant, including reassurance, bed rest, abstinence from vaginal intercourse, and gynecologic consultation before disposition.

Inevitable or Imminent Abortion
- Inevitable or imminent abortion is diagnosed on the basis of a dilated or effaced cervix or fetal membranes noted or palpated in the os.
- Ultrasound can determine the completeness of the abortion and help guide the need for dilation and curettage (D&C).
- Treatment is often expectant.
- Consultation with the gynecologist should be obtained in the ED.

Incomplete Abortion
- Incomplete abortion occurs when the fetus in incompletely expelled from the uterus.
- It occurs more often after 12 weeks.
- It is confirmed by ultrasound.
- Treatment is via D&C, and thus gynecologic consultation in the ED is warranted.

Complete Abortion
- Complete abortion occurs when all of the products of conception are passed and documented to be complete by pathologic examination.
- It occurs most often prior to 12 weeks.
- In most patients, the cervical os will be closed, bleeding is minimal, and the uterus is normal in size.
- Ultrasound can confirm the absence of intrauterine fetal parts.

- Occasionally ultrasound is equivocal, and D&C will need to be performed to confirm that the abortion is complete.
- These patients need close gynecologic follow-up.

Missed Abortion

- Missed abortion occurs when intrauterine fetal death goes unrecognized; patients present several days to weeks later with vaginal spotting or frank bleeding.
- On examination, the cervix is closed, and the uterus, which may or may not be tender to palpation, is smaller than expected for gestational age.
- It is important to note that the HCG may or may not be positive; a pelvic ultrasound provides definitive evidence for missed spontaneous abortion and should be obtained in all patients.
- Sepsis or disseminated intravascular coagulation may occur in these patients.
- Treatment is D&C or dilation and extraction depending on the gestational age of the fetus.

Septic Abortion

- Septic abortion is characterized by abdominal pain, fever, rigors, and sanguinopurulent vaginal discharge.
- Physical exam may demonstrate a boggy, tender uterus with purulent discharge from a dilated cervical os.
- Patients may progress to peritonitis and severe sepsis.
- It is caused by a variety of aerobic and anaerobic Gram-positive and negative organisms.
- Treatment is with broad spectrum antibiotics and emergent D&C.

Persistent Corpus Luteum

- Patients whose early pregnancy is complicated by the presence of a persistent and enlarging corpus luteum or corpus luteum cyst typically report one or two missed periods, followed by the acute onset of unilateral cramping pain in the lower pelvis in association with spotting or frank vaginal bleeding.
- The physical examination may reveal asymmetry of the cul-de-sac or a palpable adnexal mass that is frequently tender.
- An ovarian or peritubal mass will be noted on ultrasonographic examination, and depending on the gestational age at presentation, an intrauterine pregnancy may be noted as well.
- The urine or serum HCG is positive in most patients.
- If rupture occurs, circulatory compromise may be the presenting symptom or may develop, in which case operative intervention will be required.
- Given the lack of specificity of the signs, symptoms, and laboratory evaluation, unless an intrauterine pregnancy is dearly demonstrated by ultrasonography, it may be difficult or impossible to differentiate this entity from ectopic pregnancy.

Placenta Previa

- Implantation of the zygote most often occurs in the upper uterus.
- Even when lower uterine implantation results, upward placental migration occurs during pregnancy in most patients.
- In 1% of patients, however, the zygote implants and the placenta develop near the cervical os.
- During the third trimester, as the contour of the lower uterus changes, the placenta may separate from the uterine wall; this typically produces brisk, bright red, painless vaginal bleeding.

- Because manipulation of the uterus may result in further separation of the placenta, pelvic examinations are deferred.
- In unstable patients (those in labor, with fetal distress, or with significant bleeding), intravenous access is established, fluid resuscitation instituted, preoperative bloods obtained, 2 to 4 U of packed red cells made available, and emergency obstetric consultation obtained.
- In stable patients, an emergency ultrasound will establish the diagnosis or exclude it.
- As discussed, RhoGAM (300 μg, intramuscular) administration, to prevent Rh sensitization in Rh-negative patients, should be considered, unless the father is known to be Rh negative as well.

Abruptio Placentae

- Abruption occurs when a normally implanted placenta separates prematurely from the uterine wall.
- Uterine pain, tenderness to palpation, and varying degrees of vaginal bleeding and uterine spasm are noted.
- Hemodynamic compromise, fetal distress, and disseminated intravascular coagulation are found in severe abruption; the definitive treatment is delivery, most often by cesarean section.
- As discussed, RhoGAM (300 μg, intramuscularly) administration, to prevent Rh sensitization in Rh-negative patients, should be considered, unless the father is known to be Rh negative.

38 Childbirth and Emergency Delivery

NORMAL DELIVERY

When an obstetrician is unavailable or when delivery is precipitous, the emergency physician may be required to perform a routine vaginal delivery. When delivery is not imminent, all attempts should be made to obtain obstetric assistance. All expecting mothers presenting to the ED in possible labor should have an IV established, and uterine contraction and fetal monitoring initiated.

Examination
- Maternal blood pressure, heart rate, respiratory rate, and temperature are noted.
- Elevated maternal blood pressure may indicate preeclampsia.
- Elevated maternal temperature may indicate chorioamnionitis.
- Fetal heart rate and maternal uterine contractions are evaluated.
- The normal, baseline (measured between uterine contractions) fetal heart rate, which is most easily assessed by Doppler analysis or palpation of the umbilical cord if prolapsed, varies from 120 to 160 beats/min.
- Tachycardia (rates more than 160) may be associated with early fetal hypoxia, maternal fever, hyperthyroidism, and the administration of atropine or sympathomimetic agents to the mother.
- Baseline rates 100 to 120 beats/min represent mild bradycardia; rates less than 100 beats/min are referred to as marked bradycardia.
- Bradycardia is noted in patients with fetal hypoxia and when placental transfer of β-blocking or local anesthetic agents occurs.
- Changes in fetal heart rate in relation to uterine contractions may provide additional and important information regarding fetal oxygenation.
- Early decelerations are defined when slowing of the fetal heart rate and uterine contractions begin together and are thereafter similar in extent; early decelerations are thought to be caused by transient increases in intracranial pressure from head compression, although early fetal hypoxia may be manifest in this manner as well.
- Late decelerations in fetal heart rate occur well after a uterine contraction is established and persist after the contraction is over; this pattern represents fetal hypoxia from any cause.
- Variable decelerations occur randomly without relation to uterine contractions and commonly represent fetal hypoxia caused by umbilical cord compression.
- When fetal hypoxia is diagnosed or suspected, immediate measures to improve oxygenation (administering O_2 to the mother, changing her position, and administering a fluid bolus) are indicated, along with emergent obstetric evaluation for cesarean section.
- An ultrasound, if available, can aid in the determination of a breech presentation and identify the presence of twins.

- A sterile speculum should next be employed to assess for rupture of membranes (suggested by pooling of fluid in the vagina that is nitrazine-positive (turns blue) and exhibits a ferning pattern when dried (for 10 minutes) and examined by microscope.
- The presence of meconium-stained amniotic fluid should be noted and preparations made for the potential need to intubate the child for the purposes of deep suctioning if he or she exhibits respiratory distress after delivery.
- The presence and amount of vaginal bleeding should be noted.
- If significant maternal bleeding has occurred, a manual exam is deferred until placenta previa has been ruled out by US.
- Cervical dilation should be assessed with a sterile-gloved hand and ranges from 0 to 10 cm.
- Next cervical effacement is assessed and ranges from 0% effacement (cervix is 3–4 cm in length) to 100% effacement (the cervix is completely thinned).
- Finally, fetal station is assessed at 1-cm intervals relative to the ischial spines. When the child's head is 5 cm above the ischial spine, it is a –5 station. When the child's head is at the ischial spine, it is at 0 station. When the child's head is at the perineum (crowning), it is a +5 station.

Preparation

- Under all circumstances, oral intake should be prohibited, and if time permits, intravenous access should be established and blood obtained for a complete blood count and routine typing.
- A "delivery kit" is available in most emergency rooms and will be helpful.
- The vulva and perineum should be prepared and draped in the usual fashion.
- Sterile gloves should be worn by the physician.

Episiotomy

- When the vulva is tightly stretched around the infant's head forming a circle of tissue (crowning), an episiotomy may be performed.
- This procedure should be undertaken no sooner than when crowning occurs and only when stretching of the perineum and tearing of tissue are believed to be imminent.
- Episiotomy is often not required in multiparous women.
- When necessary, this procedure may be accomplished by making a midline or posterolateral perineal incision with scissors to such an extent that relaxation of the perineal musculature is achieved.
- Caution must be exercised to guard against extending the incision too far posteriorly toward the rectum.

Delivery of the Infant

- Delivery of the head is assisted by exerting upward and posterior pressure, with the draped hand, on the area of the rectum.
- Once the infant's head is delivered, the physician should pass a finger around the infant's neck to ensure that the umbilical cord does not encircle the neck; if it does, fetal hypoxia caused by cord compression, avulsion of the placenta, or uterine invagination as the delivery progresses may result.
- A cord encircling the infant's neck should be slipped over the head as soon as noted; if this is not readily possible, the cord should be clamped in two places and cut.
- After delivery of the head, foreign material should be aspirated from the nose and mouth with a bulb syringe.

- Ordinarily, as soon as the head is delivered, turning will occur spontaneously in such a way that the infant is positioned with the shoulders in the mother's sagittal plane.
- If turning does not occur spontaneously, the shoulders should be rotated manually, thereby facilitating movement of the most anterior shoulder under the symphysis pubis and its subsequent delivery.
- This maneuver is initiated by applying firm but gentle downward traction on the infant's head while grasping the head between the hands.
- Downward traction will engage the anterior or uppermost shoulder beneath the symphysis pubis, and further downward traction will deliver the shoulder, after which upward movement of the infant's head toward the symphysis will result in delivery of the posterior shoulder.
- Completion of the delivery usually occurs soon thereafter.
- After delivery, the infant's oropharynx should be gently aspirated to remove any foreign material.
- Within the first moments of extrauterine life, most newborns will quickly begin spontaneous respirations.
- Keeping the child warm, postdelivery suctioning of the oropharynx and nasal passages with a bulb syringe, and gentle toweling are generally all that are required to initiate respirations.
- After delivery of the infant, the umbilical cord should be clamped in two places, the most proximal of which should be placed 1 inch from the infant's abdomen.
- After dividing the cord between clamps, a specimen of cord blood should be obtained for a blood gas, and blood type and Rh screen.
- The child is then placed on the mother's abdomen and covered, provided respiration and color are normal.
- Apgar scores, as described in Table 38-1, are recorded 1 and 5 minutes after delivery.

Delivery of the Placenta

- In most patients, delivery of the placenta will occur spontaneously approximately 10 minutes after delivery of the infant.
- This event is often preceded by increased vaginal bleeding.
- Simultaneously, the uterus becomes firm, and as the placenta descends, the umbilical cord lengthens.
- Early cord clamping, mild traction on the cord, and oxytocin (20 U/L at 10 mL/min intravenous) have been shown to reduce the incidence of uterine postpartum hemorrhage.

Table 38-1	Apgar Scoring		
	Score		
Sign	**0**	**1**	**2**
Color	Blue, pale	Blue extremities	Completely pink
Heart (pulse)	Absent	<100	>100
Reflex irritability	None	Grimace	Cough; sneeze
Muscle tone	Limp	Some extremity flexion	Active motion
Respirations	Absent	Slow; irregular	Good; crying

- Uterine massage through the anterior abdominal wall will also assist in arresting hemorrhage.
- Once complete delivery of the placenta occurs, the cervix and vagina must be carefully inspected for the presence of lacerations.

Rho(D) Immune Globulin

- Although the Rh status of the mother and child is not always known in the emergency department, the physician should remember the importance of Rh immunization in Rh-negative women delivering Rh-positive infants.
- In this setting, the administration of Rho(D) immune globulin to the mother (300 μg) after delivery is critical.
- The emergency physician must also remember to administer Rho(D) immune globulin to Rh-negative women after abortion, miscarriage, antepartum hemorrhage, and trauma.

MALPRESENTATIONS

- Abnormalities of presentation may be classified as face, brow, breech, hand or arm alone, or compound.
- Prolapse of the umbilical cord may complicate a normal cephalic delivery or, more commonly, occurs in the context of one of the malpresentations noted.
- Compound presentations occur when a limb, which may be either the upper or the lower extremity, is prolapsed during a cephalic or breech delivery; this is differentiated from a hand, arm, or leg presentation occurring alone.
- Breech presentation simply means that although the fetus is positioned along the correct axis, the head is high in the uterus, and the buttocks, knees, or feet will be the presenting part when delivery begins. Isolated hand or arm presentations imply that the fetus is positioned transversely (a transverse lie), a malposition frequently complicated by umbilical cord prolapse.
- When prolapse of the umbilical cord is noted or suspected (by a steep fetal bradycardia), immediately place a hand into the vagina and support the presenting part, so that as much pressure as possible is taken off of the cord.
- This should be done until the Ob/Gyn is available to take the patient for an emergent cesarean section.
- If immediate cesarean section is not possible, a Foley catheter should be placed and at least 500 mL of saline should be instilled. This aids in elevating the fetal presenting part and reducing pressure on the prolapsed cord.
- In all patients with malpresentations, immediate obstetric consultation should be obtained and fetal oxygenation assessed by determination of fetal heart tracing.

PERIMORTUM CESAREAN SECTION

- When an expectant mother is in cardiac arrest and the fetus is at least 24-weeks-old, an emergent cesarean section must be accomplished by the emergency physician.
- Series have shown that children can survive neurologically intact from this procedure, but the best outcomes are in children delivered within 5 minutes of maternal cardiac arrest.
- Often maternal survival is enhanced after the cesarean section due to the removal of the burden of placental blood flow upon the maternal circulation.

- CPR should continue during the procedure, and ideally, a second individual with knowledge of neonatal resuscitation will be present to tend to the neonate while maternal resuscitation continues.
- A midline incision should be utilized, and the incision extended to the child with care not to lacerate the child.
- If the mother is expected to survive, antibiotics should be administered and her wounds carefully closed in a multilayer fashion.

PART 8

Neurologic Disorders

39 Coma, Seizures, and Other Disorders of Consciousness

Patients who present to the emergency department (ED) with a history of transient loss of consciousness or impaired consciousness require a thorough and systematic evaluation by the physician. It is important to obtain as much history as possible from family, friends, and other observers. A history of trauma; previous illness; medication, alcohol, or drug use; or psychiatric illness is important to elicit to guide appropriate additional studies and therapy.

COMMON CAUSES OF IMPAIRED CONSCIOUSNESS

- Head trauma
- Intracerebral hemorrhage
- Thromboembolic cerebrovascular disease
- Seizure disorder*
- Hypoglycemia*
- Alcohol or drug intoxication
- Diabetic ketoacidosis*
- Hyperosmolar hyperglycemic nonketotic coma*
- Syncope (see Chapter 40)
- Orthostatic hypotension
- Lactic acidosis*

OTHER CAUSES OF IMPAIRED CONSCIOUSNESS NOT TO BE MISSED

- Subarachnoid hemorrhage
- Meningitis
- Encephalitis
- Wernicke encephalopathy

---

*Discussed in this chapter.

- Hypertensive encephalopathy
- Intracranial neoplasm
- Uremic encephalopathy
- Hepatic encephalopathy
- Hyponatremia
- Myxedema*
- Hypocalcemia
- Hypercalcemia
- Dehydration
- Carbon monoxide inhalation
- Chronic obstructive pulmonary disease with acute decompensation
- Hyperthermia
- Hypothermia
- Hyperthyroidism (thyroid storm)*

HISTORY

- The use of medications, alcohol, or illicit drugs or a history of trauma, which may have been remote or trivial, is an important differential feature to ascertain early in the evaluation of all patients with an alteration in mental status.
- The presence of palpitations, chest or abdominal pain, headache, fever, or neck stiffness should specifically be investigated.
- A history of diabetes mellitus, hypothyroidism, hypoparathyroidism or hyper-parathyroidism, liver disease, hypertension, renal failure, or chronic obstructive pulmonary disease is important to determine.
- Changes in mental status or loss of consciousness associated with standing or on arising from sitting or recumbency suggest postural hypotension.

PHYSICAL EXAMINATION

- A complete set of vital signs including an oral or rectal **temperature** should be obtained in all patients; **postural vital signs** should also be obtained when a history of syncope is present. **Pulse oximetry** must be measured.
- Signs of trauma, the stigmata of liver disease, needle tracks, and infectious or embolic phenomena should be sought in the examination of the skin.
- Examination of the **head** may reveal "raccoon's eyes," suggesting an orbital or basilar skull fracture; Battle sign, suggesting a mastoid fracture; or nasal or aural bleeding, suggesting a basilar skull fracture.
- **Examination of the eyes** is a crucial aspect of the neurologic examination of the comatose patient. The position of the eyes with respect to the head and to one another should be ascertained. **Conjugate displacement** of the eyes occurs toward the side of a destructive cortical mass lesion, away from the side of an irritable (epileptiform) cortical focus, and away from the side of a pontine lesion. **Dysconjugate eye positions** virtually always suggest a brainstem abnormality. Pupils that are **midposition** (3–5 mm diameter) and nonreactive to light are found in patients with midbrain damage. Conversely, if the pupils react to light, the midbrain is intact. **A unilaterally dilated, unreactive pupil** implies third nerve compression secondary to temporal lobe herniation. **Small, reactive pupils** with a dysconjugate gaze directed toward the nose suggest a pontine lesion.
- **Funduscopy** should also be performed and may reveal papilledema, suggestive of increased intracranial pressure, or a subhyaloid hemorrhage, occasionally noted in patients with ruptured intracranial aneurysms.

- Both subarachnoid hemorrhage and meningitis may produce **neck stiffness**.
- Fetor hepaticus, the fruity smell of ketoacidosis, alcohol, or acetaldehyde on the breath may be noted.
- **Posturing** is helpful in discerning the cause of coma. Decorticate posturing consists of flexion and adduction of the arms and extension of the legs and suggests a deep hemispheric process. Decerebrate posturing consists of extension, adduction, and internal rotation of the arms and extension of the legs; this posturing localizes the lesion to the upper brainstem.
- Spontaneous **seizure activity** is also important to note; diffuse, generalized tonic-clonic movements suggest a grand mal seizure, whereas lip smacking and other automatisms indicate a temporal lobe focus. Focal seizures or generalized seizures that begin with a discrete focus suggest a local structural lesion.
- In patients with coma, the **respiratory pattern** is useful in localizing lesions. **Cheyne-Stokes respirations,** characterized by periods of hyperventilation tapering to periods of apnea, suggest bilateral deep hemispheric disease or basal ganglia dysfunction and may be seen as well in congestive heart failure, uremia, or hypertensive encephalopathy. **Central neurogenic hyperventilation** refers to continued, regular, rapid respirations that have no specific localizing significance but are said to increase in regularity with increasing depth of coma. A prolonged inspiratory phase followed by expiratory apnea defines **apneustic breathing,** which implies lower pontine damage. **Ataxic breathing** suggests a lesion in the medullary respiratory center and is best described as a chaotic, random respiratory pattern.
- **Motor responses** must also be observed during the neurologic examination of the comatose patient, both spontaneous and induced by painful stimuli. Focal seizures may be of localizing value, whereas generalized seizures are not. Myoclonic jerks and asterixis should be noted and imply metabolic encephalopathy. Localized absence of movement may be caused by a structural lesion or may be a manifestation of the postictal state (Todd paralysis). Higher level motor movements, such as yawning or withdrawal from painful stimuli, imply that the corticospinal tracts are intact.

DIAGNOSTIC TESTS

- Measurement of sodium, BUN, creatinine, glucose, calcium, magnesium, and blood ammonia, a toxic screen; computed tomography (CT) or magnetic resonance imaging (MRI) studies of the head; an electrocardiogram (ECG); and lumbar puncture may all provide useful information.
- The selection and sequential performance of each of these tests must be judicious and guided by both history and physical examination. If meningitis or encephalitis is suspected, a lumbar puncture is indicated.

TREATMENT

- The physician's immediate therapeutic responses to comatose patients should include standard airway maintenance and ventilation, intravenous catheter placement, and, after drawing blood for the appropriate studies, the intravenous administration of one ampule of 50% D/W, 100 mg of thiamine, and 0.8 to 2.0 mg of naloxone. Comatose and semicomatose patients who cannot protect their airways will need endotracheal intubation and ventilator support. Care should be taken not to overhydrate the patient with suspected brain edema. In patients with malignant hypertension, intravenous labetalol or continuous infusion nitroprusside should be administered as described in Chapter 24. In patients with suspected bacterial meningitis, antibiotics should be administered as early as possible.

- Most patients with unexplained abnormalities of mental status require admission. In addition, patients with syncope that is not clearly benign (i.e., vasovagal syncope in a young person, intoxication, rapidly resolving insulin-induced hypoglycemia) must be admitted to the hospital or an observation unit for monitoring and further evaluation. Importantly, patients with hypoglycemia secondary to treatment with one of the oral sulfonylurea agents (tolazamide, acetohexamide, and especially chlorpropamide) may require admission because of the long half-life of these agents and the consequent need for continuous intravenous glucose therapy.

CLINICAL REMINDERS

- Consider postural vital signs, a pregnancy test, an ECG, a complete blood count, and stool for occult blood analysis in patients who present with a history of syncope; observation and monitoring may be appropriate (see Chapter 40).
- Administer thiamine to patients in coma before the administration of glucose to prevent the precipitation of acute Wernicke encephalopathy.
- Administer antibiotics to all patients with suspected bacterial meningitis as soon after lumbar puncture as possible. If the lumbar puncture will be delayed or if it is unobtainable for any reason, antibiotics should then be given before obtaining cerebrospinal fluid.
- Do not overhydrate patients with suspected brain edema.
- Hyperventilate to a PCO_2 of 25 to 30 mm Hg, and administer mannitol (1.0–1.5 g/kg over 20–30 minutes) to patients with increased intracranial pressure. Dexamethasone (10 mg followed by 4–6 mg every 6 hours) should be administered early.

SPECIFIC DISORDERS

Seizure Disorder

Diagnosis

- Seizures may be classified as generalized or partial (focal). Generalized seizures include tonic-clonic (grand mal), absence (petit mal), and febrile seizures. Partial seizures may be either simple (focal seizures) or complex (focal with alteration in mental status).
- Patients may present to the ED during a seizure or postictally. Because most grand mal seizures last no more than 5 or 10 minutes, patients are usually postictal on arrival.
- Confusion, evidence of fecal or urinary incontinence, postictal paralysis, and perioral injury are commonly noted and suggest a recent tonic-clonic seizure.
- Most patients presenting to the ED with a seizure have a prior history of seizures. Medication noncompliance and alcohol or benzodiazepine withdrawal are common causes of recurrent seizures.
- Head trauma is the leading cause of seizures in all age groups.
- In the absence of head trauma, in infants and children up to age 5, fever is the likeliest cause of a first seizure. From ages 5 to 30, idiopathic convulsive disorders predominate, whereas from ages 30 to 60, intracranial malignancy and AIDS-related intracranial processes become increasingly more common. Beyond age 60, cerebrovascular disease represents the greatest single cause of seizures, including both acute embolic and thrombotic events.

- A first-time seizure in pregnant women in the third trimester or postpartum period may represent eclampsia.
- The physical examination must be directed toward uncovering any underlying disease processes, including neoplasia or infarct of the central nervous system, evidence of head trauma, metabolic derangements (e.g., hypocalcemia, hypoglycemia, or hypomagnesemia), or drug abuse.
- The neck should be examined for evidence of rigidity and the anterior neck should be specifically examined for signs of previous surgery, suggesting possible hypocalcemia related to thyroid or parathyroid disease.
- In particular, the neurologic examination should be directed at defining lateralizing or focal signs. A Todd or postictal paralysis, although suggesting a focus, may be noted in patients with generalized epilepsy for 24 to 48 hours after the seizure. In this case, the usefulness of neurologically defined focal findings is minimal; beyond 48 hours, however, any focality noted on examination likely has a structural counterpart.

Diagnostic Tests

- Testing in all patients having a first seizure should include a measurement of serum electrolytes, calcium, BUN, and glucose. All women of childbearing age should have a pregnancy test. A noncontrast CT of the brain should be completed in the ED or arranged for as an outpatient in the near future. Toxicology screening and ECG should be considered on a case by case basis. If CNS infection is suspected, a lumbar puncture should be performed after elevated intracranial pressure (related to focal mass effect) has been excluded. A CT scan of the head should be obtained immediately and before lumbar puncture in all patients with suspected focal processes, continued abnormal mental status, and elevated intracranial pressure.
  - Patients with recurrent seizures should have anticonvulsant medication levels measured.

Generalized Seizures

- An initial and immediate loss of consciousness and extensive autonomic phenomena are common clinical features. Motor activity may be either absent (akinetic) or convulsive (tonic-clonic or grand mal). Frequently, this seizure pattern is preceded by a preictal phase consisting of bilateral, generalized myoclonic jerks, usually occurring in flexion and lasting several seconds. Autonomic changes begin in the preictal phase, are maximal toward the end of the tonic phase, and decrease during the clonic phase; these consist of tachycardia, hypertension, bladder distention, piloerection, glandular hypersecretion, mydriasis, and apnea. Tonic contractions, in flexion then extension, herald the ictal phase. Tonic rigidity lasts from 10 to 20 seconds and evolves through a vibratory tonus while progressing into clonus. Tonic tremors slow in frequency but increase in amplitude until distinct clonic activity, manifested by alternating muscular relaxation and violent flexor contractions, appears. Clonus usually lasts for approximately 30 seconds, during which time the relaxation cycles progressively increase in duration until the seizure terminates with a final flexor jerk. Intraoral injury is common during the clonic phase, while urinary and fecal incontinence typically occur in the immediate postictal period.

Febrile Convulsions

- Febrile convulsions typically manifest as generalized tonic-clonic seizures. These constitute the most common childhood neurologic problem and affect 2% to 5% of all children younger than 5 years of age. In general, a febrile seizure may be defined as a convulsive episode in a child between the ages of 6 months and 5 years in whom other causes have been excluded. Most febrile seizures are generalized from the outset and subside within 10 to 20 minutes. Episodes usually develop 2 to 6 hours after the onset of fever and are most commonly noted in children with upper respiratory tract infection, otitis media, pharyngitis, roseola infantum, or *Shigella* gastroenteritis. Fifty percent of patients report a family history of febrile seizures. Two percent of children with febrile seizures will develop idiopathic epilepsy while up to 33% will have a recurrence associated with fever.

- The physician must bear in mind that the diagnosis of febrile seizure is one of exclusion; other causes, such as trauma and meningoencephalitis, must be ruled out before concluding that the convulsion was due only to fever. A first seizure in a febrile child in whom a central nervous system infection cannot be excluded remains an indication for lumbar puncture and a period of observation. Typically, these are children less than 1 year of age. Meningitis can often be excluded in older children based upon clinical appearance after the seizure and postictal period.

- After the airway, breathing, and circulation have been evaluated and secured and the diagnosis of febrile seizure has been made, promptly reducing fever with antipyretics and sponging with tepid water as needed is essential for the prevention of short-term recurrences. Occasionally, treatment with intravenous lorazepam (0.05 to 0.1 mg/kg intravenous) or diazepam (0.1–0.25 mg/kg intravenous given at 1 mg/min up to 10 mg) may be required to terminate the seizure.

Alcohol Withdrawal

- Alcohol withdrawal is a common cause of secondary tonic-clonic seizures. The occurrence of an alcohol withdrawal seizure clearly reflects physiologic dependence, which may develop after as few as 2 to 3 weeks of daily, heavy alcohol intake. Alcohol withdrawal seizures occur as a distinct clinical syndrome and typically begin 6 to 48 hours after the termination of a period of sustained heavy alcohol consumption; 95% occur within the first 12 hours after cessation of alcohol. Treatment consists of aggressive intravenous benzodiazepines. Lorazepam (Ativan) 2 mg intravenously followed by 6 hours of observation is a common practice. Importantly, patients must be evaluated for other causes of seizure, including electrolyte abnormalities (especially hypokalemia, hypocalcemia, and hypomagnesemia), head trauma, and meningoencephalitis.

Partial Seizures

- Partial seizures are distinguished by their initial focal manifestations and may, when simple, include sensory, autonomic, or motor manifestations. They are usually brief, begin and end abruptly, and involve little or no alteration of consciousness. However, generalization may occur and lead to an impairment of consciousness. If alteration of consciousness occurs at the onset of seizure activity, the seizure is referred to as complex; complex partial seizures involve extensive areas of the cortex and are often expressed as psychic symptoms consisting of changes in affect, automatisms, confusion, disturbed ideation, hallucinations, and memory loss. These seizures usually last longer than simple partial seizures and have a more gradual onset and termination. An aura usually precedes the onset of complex partial seizures and varies from a variety of vague somatic sensations to elaborate dreams. Typical autonomic changes are described in this form of epilepsy and are often followed by automatisms, such as lip smacking and chewing or sucking movements. The entire seizure lasts for several minutes and usually stops with only momentary postictal confusion and amnesia for peri-ictal events. Psychomotor seizures also commonly terminate with secondary generalization.

Treatment

- In most patients presenting with seizure, emergency intervention is rarely required. Continuous tonic-clonic seizures require emergency intervention only if protracted or if the patient develops significant acidosis or hypoxia.

Table 39-1	Prophylactic Therapy of Tonic-Clonic (Grand Mal) Seizures		
Choice	Drug	Dosage	Therapeutic Range
1	Phenytoin (Dilantin)	5 mg/kg/d	7.5–20 mg/L
2	Phenobarbital (Phenobarbital)	3–5 mg/kg/d	15–40 mg/L
3	Carbamazepine (Tegretol)	7–15 mg/kg/d	4–12 µg/mL

- All patients should be given oxygen and placed flat in the lateral decubitus position with the head down. An oral airway should be inserted unless it induces gagging or vomiting or is traumatic; in which case, if ventilation is adequate, it may be removed. Restraints must be avoided. Side rails should be up and padded appropriately with blankets or pillows, and if possible the physician should remain in attendance during the seizure. Pulse oximetry should be monitored to detect evolving hypoxia. Fingerstick glucose should be obtained.
- The pharmacologic treatment modalities available for the **chronic prophylaxis** of the various common seizure disorders are listed in Tables 39-1 through 39-4. Note that although phenytoin is listed as the first choice in all but petit mal seizures, many authorities currently recommend carbamazepine as the initial prophylactic drug of choice in other seizures because of its reduced incidence of side effects. Carbamazepine is less effective for short-term treatment, and for this reason, phenytoin remains the first-line choice in the ED setting. To prevent recurrent seizures, phenytoin may be administered orally or intravenously in doses of up to 1 g in adults (or 10–15 mg/kg), in 50 mL of **normal saline** (because precipitation occurs in dextrose solutions) at a rate not to exceed 50 mg/min. Cardiac monitoring should accompany intravenous administration. An alterantive, Fosphenytoin is a prodrug of phenytoin and is administered in PE (phenytoin equivalent) units (15–20 PE/kg) at a faster rate (100–150 PE/min) and unlike phenytoin may be given IM.

Table 39-2	Prophylactic Therapy of Absence (Petit Mal) Seizures	
Choice	Drug	Dosage
1	Ethosuximide (Zarontin)	20 mg/kg/d
2	Valproate (Depakene or Depakote)	15–60 mg/kg/d
3	Clonazepam (Klonopin)	Adults: 0.5–6.5 mg orally three times daily Children younger than 10 y: 0.01–0.03 mg/kg/d orally in three divided doses up to 0.1–0.2 mg/kg/d orally in three divided doses
4	Paramethadione (Paradione)	20–40 mg/kg/d
5	Methsuximide (Celontin)	300–1,200 mg/d in adults and children older than 10 y

Table 39-3	Prophylactic Therapy of Focal (Epilepsia Partialis Continua) Seizures	
Choice	**Drug**	**Dosage**
1	Phenytoin (Dilantin)	5 mg/kg/d
2	Phenobarbital (Phenobarbital)	1–5 mg/kg/d
3	Felbamate (Felbatol)	Adults and children older than 14 y: 1.2 g/d orally in three to four divided doses
		Children 2–14 y: 15 mg/kg/d orally in three to four divided doses

- **Status epilepticus** is generally accepted as a seizure that persists for more than 30 minutes or two or more seizures without a lucid interval. Among epileptic patients, the incidence is reported to range from 1% to 10%. Status epilepticus can occur at any age and may be produced by any of the causes of seizures in general. Status epilepticus is a serious medical disorder with a 10% acute mortality. In experimental studies, neuronal damage has been observed in animals in whom sustained seizure activity was maintained; this occurred despite muscle paralysis, controlled ventilation, maintenance of normal body temperature, and normal hemodynamics. It has therefore been theorized that neuronal cellular injury results from a severe and prolonged derangement in intracellular energy metabolism.

- Although the treatment of status epilepticus is somewhat controversial, most authorities would agree with the approach outlined in Table 39-5. All patients should be given oxygen and placed in the prone position with the head down. An oral airway should be inserted unless it induces gagging or vomiting, in which case, if ventilation is adequate, it may be removed. Restraints should be avoided; however, side rails should be up and appropriately padded. The adequacy of oxygenation must be serially assessed with continuous pulse oximetry.

- Despite the fact that the longer acting agents, such as phenytoin and phenobarbital, remain commonly used drugs for the prophylactic treatment of many seizure disorders, their use alone in status epilepticus should be tempered by their relatively long onset of action (20–60 minutes) and safe infusion time (10–30 minutes). For this reason, **intravenous diazepam and lorazepam** are most useful as first-line agents. Diazepam should be administered to adults in 5- to 10-mg increments intravenous and to children as 0.1 to 0.25 mg/kg, given intravenously at a rate no faster than 1 mg/min to a maximum dose of 10 to 15 mg, titrating to control seizure activity and

Table 39-4	Prophylactic Therapy of Partial Complex (Temporal Lobe Epilepsy) Seizures	
Choice	**Drug**	**Dosage**
1	Phenytoin (Dilantin)	5 mg/kg/d
2	Carbamazepine (Tegretol)	7–15 mg/kg/d

Table 39-5 Treatment of Status Epilepticus

Agent	Dosage
Children	
50% D/W	1–2 mL/kg by rapid intravenous administration
Lorazepam	0.1 mg/kg intravenous given over 2–5 min, repeat prn 10–15 min, not to exceed 4 mg/dose
Fospheytoin	15–20 PE/kg not to exceed 150 mg/min
Or	
Phenytoin	18–20 mg/kg intravenous not to exceed 50 mg/min
Repeat lorazepam or consider Midazolam drip 0.1–0.4 mg/kg/h	
Propofol (with mechanical ventilation)	2 mg/kg IV load followed by 0.1–0.2 mg/kg/min drip
General anesthesia	—
Adults	
Thiamine	100 mg intravenous given rapidly
50% D/W	One ampule by rapid intravenous administration
Lorazepam	0.1 mg/kg intravenous given over 2–5 min, repeat prn 10–15 min, not to exceed 4 mg/dose
Fospheytoin	15–20 PE/kg not to exceed 150 mg/min
Or	
Phenytoin	18–20 mg/kg intravenous not to exceed 50 mg/min
Repeat lorazepam or consider Midazolam drip 0.1–0.4 mg/kg/h	
Propofol (with mechanical ventilation)	2 mg/kg IV load followed by 0.1–0.2 mg/kg/min drip
Phenobarbital	15–20 mg/kg IV followed by 100 mg/min infusion
General anesthesia	—

the degree of respiratory depression. Lorazepam, 0.1 mg/kg intravenous at 2 mg/min, may be substituted for diazepam and has the advantages of a longer duration of action and less respiratory depression. Simultaneously, given the relatively short half-life of diazepam, a longer acting agent such as phenytoin or phenobarbital should be coadministered as described in Table 39-5. A fingerstick glucose should be monitored and supplemental glucose may be needed due to the increased metabolic demands.

- If these standard measures fail to control status epilepticus or if hypoxia or significant acidosis evolves, endotracheal intubation should be performed after the administration of additional diazepam, lorazepam, and a neuromuscular blocking agent (see Chapter 2).

Alterations in Mental Status Due to Diabetes

- Coma in the diabetic patient may be related to a variety of causes not directly associated with diabetes (e.g., cerebrovascular accidents, meningitis, subdural hematoma). However, more common causes include hypoglycemic and hyperglycemic coma (ketoacidotic and hyperosmolar nonketotic forms) and lactic acidosis secondary to dehydration. A careful physical examination and specific laboratory studies are essential to differentiate these causes of coma in the diabetic. Patients with hypoglycemic coma are generally hypothermic and breathe normally, whereas diabetics with metabolic acidosis breathe rapidly and deeply (Kussmaul respirations) in an effort to compensate for the acidosis. A laboratory determination of blood glucose, serum ketones, and an arterial or venous pH will confirm the diagnosis.

Hypoglycemia

- Symptoms caused by hypoglycemia result from both epinephrine excess (sweating, tremor, tachycardia, and anxiety) and central nervous system (CNS) dysfunction (confusion, headache, abnormal behavior, seizure, and coma). Hypoglycemia is classified as either postprandial or fasting; fasting causes are divided into those caused by overuse of glucose (insulinoma, exogenous insulin, or oral hypoglycemic agent administration) and underproduction of glucose (hypopituitarism; adrenal insufficiency; severe hepatitis; cirrhosis; drugs including alcohol, propranolol, and salicylates; and possibly during severe malnutrition and late pregnancy).
- The **most common presentation** involves the insulin-dependent diabetic patient who becomes hypoglycemic in association with increased insulin doses, reduced caloric intake, or increased caloric expenditure. The onset of renal failure in the diabetic may also be heralded by clustering of hypoglycemic episodes (as renal clearance of insulin falls).
- The **treatment** of significant hypoglycemia, after blood is obtained for analysis, involves the rapid, intravenous administration of 50 mL of 50% D/W. This should completely eliminate symptoms caused by hypoglycemia, usually over 1 to 2 minutes.
- An uncomplicated reaction in the insulin-dependent diabetic patient can be managed as described, and generally admission is not required; generous caloric intake is encouraged (which includes protein in the meals) for 24 hours along with instructions to see a private physician in this interval for possible alterations in future insulin dose or schedule.
- Patients with hypoglycemia due to oral sulfonylurea agent therapy may require hospital admission and therapy with continuous, intravenous 5% to 10% D/W; this recommendation reflects the prolonged serum half-life of many of these agents and therefore the high probability of recurrent hypoglycemia.

Diabetic Ketoacidosis

- **Diagnosis.** Coma secondary to diabetic ketoacidosis (DKA) is typically preceded by 1 or more days of fatigue, nausea, vomiting, polyuria, and polydipsia, after which stupor and coma evolve. Physical evidence of dehydration, hypotension, tachycardia, Kussmaul respirations, and the "fruity" odor of acetone are noted on examination. Glycosuria, ketonuria, hyperglycemia, ketonemia, an increased anion gap, acidemia, and variable serum potassium are found on initial presentation in most patients. Leukocytosis and hyperamylasemia are often noted as well.

- The **pathophysiologic events** leading to DKA include insulin lack and hyperglucagonemia. Increased hepatic gluconeogenesis in the setting of decreased peripheral tissue uptake of glucose results in hyperglycemia and a resultant osmotic diuresis, often with rapidly evolving salt and water depletion. Insulin lack and glucagon excess further accelerate adipose tissue breakdown and enhance hepatic ketogenesis; acetoacetate and β-hydroxybutyrate are thereby produced; the latter typically presents in markedly greater concentration than the former and, importantly, is not detected by the standard nitroprusside Acetest. This fact has particular importance as treatment proceeds and is further discussed.

- **Treatment** involves meticulous attention to electrolyte and fluid balance during salt and water repletion and insulin therapy. During the first 2 to 3 hours of therapy, determination of serum potassium, blood sugar, and pH at approximately 30-minute intervals is recommended, after which, if stabilization has occurred, measurements may be obtained hourly. Treatment must be focused on four issues: the administration of insulin, the repletion of fluid and electrolyte losses (including potassium and phosphate), the correction of acidosis, and the diagnosis and treatment of any precipitating conditions.

  - Appropriate and aggressive repletion of **fluid and electrolytes** remain a mainstay of effective therapy for DKA. Most patients have an enormous fluid deficit, often approximating 5 to 10 L; the rate of fluid replacement and the specific solute used are determined by the patient's clinical presentation. Patients who are initially hypotensive require aggressive treatment with normal saline, often receiving 1 to 2 L in the first hour; central venous pressure measurements may be useful in guiding fluid replacement in selected patients. After normalization of blood pressure, half-normal saline should be used to replete additional free water and electrolyte losses.

  - **Low-dose continuous-infusion insulin** regimens, all of which use regular insulin, are the currently favored manner of providing insulin. In all patients, an intravenous loading dose of 0.1 U/kg of regular insulin should be rapidly administered, after which a continuous infusion should be initiated at 0.1 U/kg/h of regular insulin through a separate, dedicated, intravenous line and infusion pump. A dedicated, separate line and an infusion pump are strongly recommended to provide accurate titration of the insulin dose. If the plasma glucose fails to decrease by 10% in the first hour of treatment, the loading dose of regular insulin should be repeated.

  - If the **serum potassium** is normal at presentation or when a serum level of 4.0 is attained during therapy, supplemental intravenous potassium should be administered, because even with apparently normal serum potassium levels, patients with DKA are typically severely depleted of total body potassium; this fact is often not reflected in the initial serum level because of the extracellular shift in serum potassium engendered by concurrent acidosis. Potassium replacement may be given initially as rapidly as 20 to 25 mEq/h, with the average deficit being approximately

200 mEq. This may be administered as potassium phosphate, because 40 to 50 mmol is the average deficit of the phosphate anion. A stock solution of 15 mL of potassium phosphate is available and provides a total of 66 mEq of potassium and 45 mmol of phosphate. Five milliliters of this solution may be placed in 1 L of solution and when infused at 200 mL/h will replace phosphate at the optimum rate of 3 mmol/h. Additional potassium (20–40 mEq/L) may be added to the liter in the form of potassium chloride, thereby increasing its delivery to 20 to 25 mEq/h.

- **Acidosis** is best treated with insulin and repletion of salt and water and bicarbonate is rarely indicated. The use of bicarbonate has been associated with cerebral edema in children.
- The treatment of DKA is often complicated by the **correction of hyperglycemia before the elimination of ketoacidosis.** Clearly, in this setting, further therapy with insulin, which is absolutely required, will result in marked hypoglycemia unless measures are taken to prevent it. It is most often advised that when the serum glucose decreases to approximately 300 mg/dL, an infusion of 5% dextrose in one half normal saline be instituted and continued until such time as acidosis is corrected and the patient is able to eat normally and be converted to a subcutaneous insulin regimen.
- Another potential pitfall in the treatment of patients with DKA involves the failure to recognize that the standard nitroprusside or Acetest test used for the determination of serum ketones primarily measures acetoacetate, the concentration of which may actually increase during the resolution of ketoacidosis. This occurs because β-hydroxybutyrate, which is not detected by the test, is converted to acetoacetate during therapy. Therefore, an apparent increase in serum ketones during the course of treatment must not be interpreted as treatment failure.
- **Precipitating factors** of DKA are not always easily identifiable; infection is the major factor, but increased ambient temperature, stress, and poor compliance with one's insulin regimen are all recognized precipitants.
- **Morbidity and mortality.** With better central pressure monitoring and careful attention to the finer points of metabolic correction, the mortality rate of DKA has declined dramatically over the years to approximately 2% per episode. Elderly patients presenting in profound coma and those with serious other concurrent illnesses experience the highest mortality.

Hyperglycemic Hyperosmolar Nonketotic Coma

- The second most common form of hyperglycemic coma is hyperosmolar hyperglycemic state (HHS) formally known as hyperglycemic hyperosmolar nonketotic coma (HHNK), which is characterized by profound hyperglycemia, hyperosmolarity, and severe dehydration in the absence of significant ketosis. It is especially common in middle-aged or elderly patients with mild or occult diabetes, and, again, a common precipitating cause, such as infection or recent surgery, is often noted. A relative, rather than absolute, insulin deficiency is usually present, which reduces glucose use by muscle, fat, and liver while inducing hyperglucagonemia and increasing hepatic glucose output. Ketosis fails to occur in these patients, probably because of the presence of some insulin activity, only a small amount of which is necessary to inhibit ketogenesis.

Diagnosis

- The onset of HHS may be insidious, occurring over a period of days or weeks, during which time progressive polyuria, polydipsia, and dehydration develop. Lethargy and confusion ultimately ensue, progressing to seizures and coma. The physical examination confirms profound dehydration in a lethargic or comatose patient without Kussmaul respirations. Severe hyperglycemia is the rule, with blood glucose values typically ranging from 800 to 2,400 mg/dL. In mild cases when dehydration is less severe, excess urinary sodium losses and dilutional hyponatremia protect against extreme hyperosmolality. With progressive dehydration, however, osmolalities of 330 to 440 mOsm/L may be noted. Osmolalities of more than 350 are generally seen. Ketonemia and acidosis are usually absent, but if dehydration is severe enough to limit tissue perfusion, lactic acidosis may develop. The serum osmolality, normally ranging from 280 to 300 mOsm/L, may be estimated using the following equation: **serum osmolality = 2(Na) + (glucose)/18 + (BUN)/2.8.** An osmolar gap should not be present with HHS.

Treatment
- Fluid replacement is the mainstay of therapy in patients with HHS. If profound hypotension is present, the initial resuscitation effort should employ saline; in other cases, half-normal saline is preferred because all patients are more severely deprived of water than of salt. As much as 4 to 6 L of fluid may be required in the first 6 to 8 hours. Insulin therapy may also be required with regular insulin, 0.1 U/kg intravenous loading dose followed by 0.1 U/kg/h by intravenous infusion. **It is important to note** that patients with HHS are generally **very sensitive to the action of insulin** when compared with patients who have DKA. For this reason, many authorities recommend using only an initial loading dose of regular insulin without a continuous infusion and repeating the loading dose every 4 to 6 hours as needed. This approach is generally adequate, because rehydration alone in these patients who have some circulating insulin improves glucose use and clearance.

Mortality
- With the best therapy, the **mortality** of HHS exceeds that of DKA, remaining at 10% to 20%. The increased age of these patients and their often more serious concurrent illnesses contribute to the higher mortality associated with this disorder.

Lactic Acidosis

- An accumulation of excess lactate in the blood produces lactic acidosis. This by-product of glucose metabolism is principally produced by erythrocytes, skeletal muscle, skin, and brain. The liver and to a minor extent the kidney contribute to the removal of lactate. Thus, overproduction from tissue hypoxia, deficient removal associated with hepatic failure, or both in patients with shock may produce an excess accumulation of lactate. Lactic acidosis is common in all seriously ill patients with septic, cardiogenic, or hypovolemic shock; severe respiratory or hepatic failure; bowel infarction; or excessive ethanol intake.

Diagnosis
- Because lactic acidosis most often develops secondary to tissue hypoxia or vascular collapse, the primary clinical presentation varies depending on the inciting catastrophic illness. Clinically, the major features of lactic acidosis are marked hyperventilation and changes in mental status, which include stupor and coma. Profound acidosis and acidemia are typically noted in the laboratory analysis with minimal or absent ketonemia and ketonuria. Lactic acidosis is one of the main causes of a high anion gap metabolic acidosis and, in the absence of appreciable azotemia, ketonemia, aspirin, methanol, or paraldehyde ingestion, should be seriously considered in the differential diagnosis of such an acidosis. Normal plasma lactate typically ranges from 0.1 to 1.8 nmol/L; in lactic acidosis, the plasma lactate may increase to 30.

Treatment
- Treatment of the primary precipitating disorder is the mainstay of therapy. Shock should be treated with aggressive fluid resuscitation. In addition, sepsis should be treated with early broad-spectrum antibiotics. Bicarbonate therapy should be reserved for resistant, critically ill patients in consultation with a nephrologist.

Mortality
- Despite optimal therapy, the mortality rate of spontaneous lactic acidosis remains high.

Myxedema Coma
- Myxedema coma should be considered in the differential diagnosis of all patients presenting with stupor or coma. In the United States, hypothyroidism most commonly follows surgical or radioiodine ablative treatment of the thyroid for Graves disease or as a result of chronic or Hashimoto thyroiditis. Less commonly, autoimmune-mediated, drug-mediated, and pituitary or hypothalamic causes are responsible for progressive failure of the thyroid. Half of cases occur after age 60 and present more frequently in women.

Diagnosis
The diagnosis of myxedema coma rests on a high degree of suspicion and a clear recognition of the usual or expected signs of hypothyroidism.
- Classic findings in patients with hypothyroidism include cool, dry skin that has a doughy feel; coarse, often sparse hair; periorbital swelling or puffiness; nonpitting edema of the lower extremities (myxedema); glossomegaly; "hung-up" reflexes (the relaxation phase of the deep tendon reflexes is delayed or prolonged); and often, but not always, an enlarged thyroid. In patients with myxedema coma, the mental status may be described as stuporous or comatose. In addition, hypothermia, which is said to be a cardinal sign, is consistently noted. Hypotension, bradycardia, distant heart sounds, and clinically obvious hypoventilation are additional findings in many patients.
- **Laboratory findings** include hyponatremia and elevation of the serum creatine kinase, AST, and lactic dehydrogenase enzymes. Measurement of arterial blood gases may confirm hypoventilation, and frequently both a respiratory and a lactic acidosis are present. The ECG may demonstrate bradycardia associated with generally reduced QRS amplitude and flattening or inversion of T waves. The chest roentgenogram often demonstrates cardiomegaly, which may be caused by dilation or pericardial effusion.
- **Precipitating factors** should be investigated and include exposure to cold temperatures, ingestion of central nervous system depressants, trauma, and any variety of infectious illnesses.
- The **diagnosis of myxedema coma is clinical;** treatment must be instituted before laboratory confirmation of hypothyroidism. Blood must be initially obtained for the rapid determination and exclusion of the other causes of stupor and coma. Rapidly reversible causes must be treated or excluded as soon as possible. Thyroid function studies, including thyroid-stimulating hormone (TSH), free T_4, and a serum cortisol, should be obtained.

Treatment
- Administer levothyroxine (T_4) intravenous in a loading dose equal to 300 to 500 µg, followed by 50 µg/day intravenous.
- Give dexamethasone in a dose equal to 6 mg intravenous push initially, followed by 4 mg intravenous every 6 hours, *even* in patients who are not frankly hypoadrenal;

the coadministration of steroid is appropriate, because treatment with thyroxine alone to these patients may precipitate an acute state of cortisol deficiency. This occurs because of the ability of thyroxine to enhance steroid catabolism and utilization.

- Institute assisted ventilation if respiratory failure or compromise is present based on arterial blood gases.
- Gradual rewarming with blankets is advised when hypothermia is present; more aggressive rewarming is usually not needed and may be contraindicated.
- Treat hypoglycemia in the usual manner with 50 ml of intravenous 50% D/W; a continuous infusion of 5% glucose in normal saline may be required to maintain a normal serum glucose.
- Pay careful attention to water balance and electrolyte status; minimize free water administration because water retention may occur.
- Rapidly exclude or treat other causes of an abnormal mental status (e.g., hypoglycemia, meningitis, overdose, acute thiamine deficiency).
- Initially withhold all central nervous system depressants and reduce dosage of most other medications until thyroid status is normalized.
- Consider any precipitating events.

Thyrotoxic Crisis (Thyroid Storm)

- Most patients who present with thyrotoxic crisis either have not had hyperthyroidism diagnosed or have been inadequately treated for hyperthyroidism. Under these circumstances, a variety of precipitating events, including acute medical or surgical illnesses, may then initiate thyrotoxic crisis.
- The **initial diagnosis** of thyrotoxic crisis is **a clinical one.** The usual signs and symptoms of hyperthyroidism, including fever; tachycardia; tremor; goiter; diarrhea; increased pulse pressure; warm, moist skin; lid lag; exophthalmos; chemosis; and a variety of mental status abnormalities, may be noted. In patients with thyrotoxic crisis, however, these findings are often exaggerated. Temperature, often reaching 106°F; tachycardia, often atrial fibrillation; and dramatic aberrations in mental status characterize the clinical picture. Vomiting and diarrhea may be profound and, in association with extreme diaphoresis, may produce severe dehydration and electrolyte abnormalities. Coma and delirium have also been described. Thyrotoxic crisis may induce a state of relative adrenal insufficiency, which must be considered in the treatment strategy.
- Routine blood studies and serum triiodothyronine (T_3), T_4, T_3 resin uptake, TSH, and serum cortisol should be obtained in all patients.
- **Treatment** should be directed at both supportive measures and definitive interventions.
- **Supportive measures** include repletion of intravascular volume and electrolytes, the administration of supplemental B-complex vitamins and glucose intravenously, a cooling blanket for patients with severe hyperthermia, intensive care monitoring for several days, and pressor support for maintenance of blood pressure as needed.
- **Definitive interventions** include blockade of hormone synthesis using propylthiouracil, 100 mg orally every 2 hours or by nasogastric tube; inhibition of hormone release using potassium iodide, 30 drops/day in four divided doses orally or by nasogastric tube, or sodium iodide, 1 to 2 g in 1 L of normal saline/day; inhibition of the peripheral sympathomimetic effects of thyroid hormone with propranolol, 2 mg intravenous over 15 to 30 minutes followed by 20 to 40 mg orally every 6 hours; and treatment of presumptive cortisol deficiency with dexamethasone, 4 to 6 mg intravenous every 6 hours (dexamethasone also inhibits hormone release from the thyroid gland and the peripheral conversion of T_4 to T_3).

Stroke and Syncope

INTRODUCTION

- Thrombotic and embolic infarctions of the brain are major causes of human morbidity and mortality. Eighty-five percent of strokes are ischemic, whereas the remaining fifteen percent are hemorrhagic. The 1-month mortality for stroke varies with etiology: 15% for ischemic stroke, 50% for subarachnoid hemorrhage (SAH), and 80% or greater with intracerebral hemorrhage (ICH). Concurrent cardiovascular disease, pulmonary complications, and recurrent stroke may complicate patient recovery. Fully 25% to 40% of patients will have a repeat stroke within 5 years of their initial insult.

- The World Health Organization (WHO) defines stroke as the sudden onset of a neurologic deficit accompanied by a focal dysfunction and symptoms lasting more than 24 hours, which is not caused by a traumatic vascular problem. Transient ischemic attacks (TIAs) are focal neurological events resolving completely within 24 hours. A reversible ischemic neurologic deficit (RIND) is defined as a focal neurological event that resolves within 3 days to 3 weeks. A variety of conditions may mimic stroke, including complex migraine with hemiparesis, postictal paralysis (Todd paralysis), hypoglycemia, cerebral tumors, cerebral infections or encephalitis, subdural hematoma, multiple sclerosis, and malignant hypertension. Misdiagnosis is more common in younger patients or those who present with complex or atypical symptoms.

- Risk factors for stroke include systolic and diastolic hypertension; advancing age; cardiovascular factors including atrial fibrillation, ischemic disease, cardiomyopathy, and mechanical valves; diabetes; smoking; nonwhite racial background; male sex; and heavy alcohol use. TIAs are strong predictors of risk, with 12% of those with TIAs going on to experience a significant stroke within 12 months. Most strokes, however, are not preceded by a TIA.

CLINICAL FEATURES

- Stroke usually involves the development of a focal neurologic deficit, the nature of which can help localize the vascular territory affected. Transient loss of consciousness is not generally a feature of stroke. Seizures may also occur as a feature of stroke caused by focal cerebral irritation. Headache may result from a hemorrhagic stroke or SAH. Other features may include vomiting or coma.

- Careful clinical evaluation may localize the infarct in many cases. The neurologic deficits in stroke relate to the area of the brain damaged because of interrupted perfusion from specific supply vessels. Angiographically, 62% of thrombotic stroke patients have stenosis or occlusion of the internal carotid artery, 10% have occlusion or stenosis of the middle cerebral artery, and 15% have vertebrobasilar artery occlusion or stenosis.

Cerebral Infarction
Thrombotic Infarction
- Cerebral occlusions result in well-described, sudden, focal neurologic deficits, usually without vomiting, headache, or obtundation unless a large portion of the cerebrum is involved. Deficits caused by cerebral arterial thrombosis usually develop over minutes to hours and may often develop overnight. Patients at risk for thrombotic cerebral infarction may also have generalized atherosclerotic disease or hypercoagulable states caused by malignancy, thrombocytosis, and hyperosmolar states.

Embolic Infarction
- Cerebral embolic infarction occurs suddenly without warning and may occur at any time of the day or night. The neurologic deficit develops within seconds. Common sources of emboli include atrial thrombi in patients with chronic or paroxysmal atrial fibrillation, valvular vegetations, and myocardial infarction with mural thrombi and in patients with extracranial vascular disease who have ulcerated plaques in the carotid system. The acute phase of embolic stroke may present with focal or diffuse seizures corresponding to the area of the infarcted brain; loss of consciousness is unusual except in complete carotid occlusions with cerebral edema. Patients who have had a cerebral embolism caused by a cardiac source should be rapidly anticoagulated with heparin after cerebral imaging has ruled out acute hemorrhage.

Transient Ischemic Attacks
- TIAs present as focal neurologic deficits lasting less than 24 hours; in most cases, resolution is seen within 15 to 60 minutes. The causes of TIAs include fibrin/platelet emboli, vasospasm, arterial hypertension, hypercoagulable disorders, and polycythemia. Management is controversial, and is discussed in "Transient Ischemic Attacks" under "Evaluation and Management of Specific Stroke Syndromes."
- A series of TIAs occurring over days or weeks before ED presentation (crescendo TIAs) requires urgent evaluation and probably anticoagulation with heparin after normal cerebral imaging.
- Transient focal neurological deficits may also be caused by seizures (Todd paralysis), complex migraine headaches, and closed head injuries; however, history and physical examination of the patient should aid in the differentiation of these conditions from TIAs.

Intracranial Hemorrhage
- Hemorrhagic stroke, SAH, and intracranial hemorrhage (ICH) may occur during stress or exertion. Precipitating events may include sexual intercourse, labor and delivery, and Valsalva maneuver. Alcohol appears to contribute to an increase in ICH and SAH. Focal deficits rapidly evolve and may be associated with confusion, coma, or immediate mortality.
- Severe headache of sudden onset (the "worst ever") is a cardinal symptom of a subarachnoid hemorrhage and may be accompanied by nuchal rigidity. Arteriovenous malformations (AVMs) may bleed into the subarachnoid space with lateralizing findings if cerebral parenchyma is involved. Spontaneous SAH is usually caused by rupture of a saccular aneurysm. Apart from focal seizures, lateralizing deficits are usually absent with SAH.
- ICH will present with well-demarcated focal deficits because of intraparenchymal damage. Intracranial hemorrhage is often a complication of long-standing hypertension, amyloid angiopathy, or anticoagulation therapy. Common sites include the thalamus, putamen, cerebellum, and brainstem (in decreasing order of incidence).

Table 40-1	Ischemic and Infarction Syndromes in Acute Stroke

Vascular Territory	Clinical Syndromes
Internal carotid artery	Hemiparesis and aphasia in dominant hemisphere
Anterior watershed	Hemiparesis greater in leg with sensory loss
Posterior watershed	Hemianopia
Middle cerebral artery watershed	Hemiparesis, hemisensory loss, aphasia in dominant hemisphere
Deep anterior cerebral artery	Movement disorders
Lacunar infarction	Pure motor or sensory loss
Middle cerebral artery	
Superior division	Contralateral face, arm, or leg sensory and motor deficit; ipsilateral head and eye deviation, Broca aphasia
Inferior division	Homonymous hemianopia, Wernicke aphasia, coma, quadriplegia
Basilar and/or vertebral artery	Nystagmus, vertigo, ipsilateral limb ataxia, ipsilateral Horner syndrome

Cerebellar hemorrhage is a critical diagnosis to make, because it may be amenable to neurosurgical intervention. Onset usually occurs during activity. Hemorrhagic infarction should be considered in patients who are anticoagulated, who have an unexplained headache history, or who have sustained craniocerebral trauma.

Ischemia and Infarction Syndromes

Table 40-1 lists common areas of cerebrovascular ischemia and infarction with their sequelae.

Internal Carotid Artery Lesions

• Carotid artery disease may present with a carotid bruit in asymptomatic individuals. Patients with symptomatic carotid disease may present with TIA, which is characteristically short-lived. Clinical symptoms of internal carotid (ICA) occlusion vary with extent of collateral blood flow but generally reflect ischemia in the middle cerebral artery (MCA) territory with contralateral hemiparesis and aphasia (if the dominant hemisphere is involved).

Watershed Infarcts

• Watershed infarcts involve the extreme reaches of collateral circulation supplied by the larger intracranial arteries. These are vulnerable areas of circulation, especially during periods of relative hypotension. These infarcts present with hemiparesis, hemisensory loss, or even aphasia if the dominant hemisphere is involved.

Middle Cerebral Artery

• The MCA supplies most of the convex surface of the brain and a significant portion of "deep" brain tissue, including the basal ganglia, putamen, caudate nucleus, and portions of the internal capsule. Occlusion of the MCA is responsible for most stroke syndromes, with embolism from the ICA or heart to the MCA being the most common cause. Occlusion of the upper MCA produces a large infarct characterized by contralateral hemiplegia, deviation of the eyes toward the side of the infarct, global aphasia (in the dominant hemisphere), hemianopia, hemianesthesia, and hemineglect. The hemiparesis affects the upper body more than the lower body and leg. Loss of consciousness may occur after MCA infarct, often at 36 hours or more after the insult, and is caused by peri-infarct edema, elevated intracranial pressure, or cerebral herniation.

- Hand dominance of the patient allows the clinician to infer hemispheric dominance. Infarcts of the dominant hemisphere will cause damage to areas of the brain responsible for speech. Broca aphasia (motor aphasia) is caused by infarction to the insular cortex from MCA occlusion and results in hesitant and broken speech caused by dyspraxia between the oropharyngeal muscles and respiratory elements responsible for smooth phonation. Wernicke aphasia (sensory aphasia) occurs after infarction to the posterior temporal and lateral temporo-occipital regions caused by lower MCA occlusion. The language disturbance is seen in the acute infarct phase and is recognized by speech containing few recognizable words.

Posterior Cerebral Artery

- The posterior cerebral artery (PCA) generally originates from the vertebrobasilar (VB) system and supplies clinically significant areas in the occipital lobe and thalamus. Occlusion lesions manifest as a homonymous visual field defect with macular sparing; oculomotor palsies or intranuclear ophthalmoplegias may also be seen. Thalamic infarcts may result in sensory losses of pain, temperature, and touch on the affected side of the body.

Vertebrobasilar (VB) Arteries

- The vascular anatomy of the VB system is complex and leads to a variety of clinical syndromes. Brief occlusion of a VB artery by a fibrin-platelet embolus (TIA), vasospasm, hypotension, or a fixed stenotic lesion may result in some or all of the following neurologic symptoms: perioral numbness, dizziness or vertigo, diplopia, dysarthria, hemiparesis, ataxia, vomiting, or impaired hearing. VB infarction is generally caused by occlusion of the basilar artery, which supplies the pons, midbrain, and a portion of the cerebellum. Clinical manifestations include coma, abnormal breathing patterns, quadriplegia with decerebrate posturing, and bilateral sensory loss. Occlusion of a vertebral artery results in lateral medullary infarction (Wallenberg syndrome), which is clinically manifested as vertigo, headache, facial pain, disequilibrium, nausea, vomiting, and an ipsilateral Horner syndrome.

Lacunar Infarctions

- Whereas large-vessel occlusions typically have predictable symptomatology, lesions of small penetrating branch arterioles have a separate set of symptoms. Lacunar ("island") infarcts are common and involve the deep central regions of the brain, particularly the basal ganglia, thalamus, and pons. Lesions are characterized by a lack of visual disturbance, aphasia, or impaired consciousness. Pure motor hemiparesis or pure sensory loss of the face, arm, or leg is a common result of lacunar infarction. Other lacunar syndromes include ataxia/leg hemiparesis or a dysarthria/clumsy hand clinical presentation. Lacunar infarctions have a good prognosis, with a lower overall mortality than MCA infarctions. Predisposing causes to lacunar infarction include atherosclerotic disease, amyloid angiopathy, and nonneurologic causes such as pneumonia and coronary events.

EMERGENCY MANAGEMENT OF ACUTE STROKE

• Management of acute stroke includes appropriate imaging techniques, involvement of a multidisciplinary "stroke team," and emergency department (ED) assessment of treatment options including blood pressure–lowering agents, antiplatelet therapy, and potential anticoagulation or antithrombolytic therapy.

Initial Evaluation

• ED evaluation of an acute stroke must begin with airway and circulatory stabilization, rather than focusing on the neurologic disability. Supplemental oxygen should be provided via mask or nasal cannula to keep oxygen saturation above 95%. Airway patency may require use of a nasal airway, or, in those with a Glasgow Coma Score of 8 or less, intubation and mechanical ventilation. Venous access should be secured; appropriate intravenous fluids include normal saline or Ringer lactate solution given at 100 mL/h or less. Initial physical examination and history should include a careful neurologic and cardiovascular examination, screening for other diseases that may mimic acute stroke such as seizure disorders, hypoglycemia, complex migraine, dysrhythmias, or syncope. The patient should be assigned a score from the National Institute of Health Stroke Scoring system (NIHSS) found in Table 40-2.

Table 40-2	NIH Stroke Scale	
Item	**Name**	**Response**
1A	Level of consciousness	0 = Alert
		2 = Not alert
		3 = Unresponsive
1B	Level of questions	0 = Answers both correctly
		1 = Answers only one correctly
		2 = Answers neither correctly
1C	Level of commands	0 = Performs both tasks correctly
		1 = Performs one task correctly
		2 = Performs neither task
2	Best gaze	0 = Normal gaze
		1 = Partial gaze palsy
		2 = Total gaze palsy
3	Visual fields	0 = No visual loss
		1 = Partial hemianopsia
		2 = Complete hemianopsia (one eye)
		3 = Bilateral hemianopsia
4	Facial palsy	0 = Normal
		1 = Minor paralysis
		2 = Partial paralysis
		3 = Complete paralysis
5	Motor: arm	0 = No drift
	a. Left	1 = Drift before 10 s
	b. Right	2 = Falls before 10 s
		3 = No effort against gravity
		4 = No movement

Item	Name	Response
Table 40-2	**NIH Stroke Scale** *(Continued)*	
6	Motor: leg a. Left b. Right	0 = No drift 1 = Drift before 5 s 2 = Falls before 5 s 3 = No effort against gravity 4 = No movement
7	Ataxia	0 = Absent 1 = One limb 2 = Two limbs
8	Sensory	0 = Normal 1 = Mild loss 2 = Severe loss
9	Language	0 = Normal 1 = Mild aphasia 2 = Severe aphasia 3 = Mute or global aphasia
10	Dysarthria	0 = Normal 1 = Mild 2 = Severe
11	Extinction/inattention	0 = Normal 1 = Mild 2 = Severe
12	Distal motor a. Left arm b. Right arm	0 = Normal 1 = Some extension after 5 s 2 = No extension after 5 s

The time of symptom onset should be carefully ascertained for consideration of thrombolytic therapy, which has a discrete therapeutic window. Acute stroke events that are present when a patient wakes up should be assumed to have taken place when the patient went to sleep for thrombolytic timing purposes.

- Initial laboratory investigation includes urgent ECG, complete blood count (CBC), electrolytes, blood sugar, BUN, creatinine, and a clotting profile to include international normalized ration (INR) and partial thromboplastin time (PTT).
- Vital signs should be monitored every 15 minutes. Hypotension (systolic blood pressure less than 100 mm Hg) may require fluid support; if the patient has cardiovascular shock, vasopressors may be required. Hypertension requires careful consideration before intervention is contemplated (see "Blood Pressure Considerations"). Increased blood pressure in the cerebral circulation has a purpose, serving to perfuse the brain and possibly tamponade bleeding areas.
- A noncontrast CT scan of the head is mandatory to rule out hemorrhage or mass lesion. This CT should be obtained and interpreted within 30 minutes. If the NIHSS is greater than 10, and there is a significant neurological deficit, consideration should be given to CT perfusion scanning in centers capable of this study.
- A CT perfusion scan involves rapid intravenous contrast injection followed by multiple scans of the brain at the level of the basal ganglia. The perfusion scan will give

an indication of those areas of the brain that are and are not perfused and may serve to guide further intervention.

- Newer imaging techniques include rapid diffusion-weighted magnetic resonance imaging (MRI); however, this modality may not be available in all centers.

EVALUATION AND MANAGEMENT OF SPECIFIC STROKE SYNDROMES

Transient Ischemic Attacks

- Evaluation of the patient should localize the insult to the anterior or posterior circulation and help determine whether the patient is in a high-risk category. Localization of the lesion is based on the symptomatology discussed earlier. Seventy-five percent of patients will have resolution of symptoms within 30 minutes or less. Patients who have symptoms and present 1 hour after onset have only a 15% chance of recovery by 24 hours.
- Physical examination should include attention to carotid artery bruits, which, in the presence of TIA, signify significant carotid artery stenosis. The presence of atrial fibrillation is also a potential source for cardiac emboli.
- Investigative workup includes EKG, CBC, electrolytes, BUN/creatinine, PTT/INR, and blood sugar. Nonenhanced CT scanning of the brain is also mandatory to rule out ICH or mass lesions.
- TIAs are harbingers of further stroke. Patients are triaged to a higher risk category if they have experienced multiple TIAs within the preceding 2 weeks, if the neurological deficit was severe or appeared in a crescendo-like manner, if the TIA was caused by a cardioembolic event, or if the patient has significant medical co-morbid conditions (advanced age, decompensated cardiac disease, uncontrolled diabetes, significant infection).
- High-risk patients require admission for further workup, including echocardiography and Doppler ultrasound of the carotid circulation. Patients with an unremarkable head CT in whom a cardioembolic source is suspected should be anticoagulated with heparin (15–17 U/kg/h without an initial bolus dose) to maintain a PTT 1.5- to 2.0-times normal, followed by Coumadin.
- Younger, healthier patients with no evidence of a cardioembolic cause of their TIA are considered at lower risk and may be discharged home on ASA 81 to 1,300 mg/daily with close follow-up by the primary physician or neurologist. In those unable to tolerate ASA, clopidogrel 75 mg daily is an alternate but a more expensive choice.
- For patients presenting with TIA who are already on ASA or Coumadin, adding clopidogrel 75 mg daily may provide additional benefits but is not without controversy. Management of these patients is best performed in consultation with the primary care physician or the consultant neurologist.

Acute Stroke

- Initial ED evaluation and management includes a focused history, physical examination, NIHSS value, documentation of time of onset of symptoms, and stabilization of airway, breathing, and circulation.
- Basic laboratory investigations should include CBC, electrolytes, blood sugar, BUN/creatinine, PTT/INR, serum cardiac markers, and an ECG. A stat noncontrast CT of the brain should be performed and interpreted within 30 minutes of the

patient's presentation to the ED. A chest radiograph should also be ordered. If an on-call neurologist or stroke team is available, they should be alerted immediately.

- Treatment of ICH is supportive. Fully 70% of patients with ICH will die from the neurologic insult within 72 hours; bleeds of more than 5-cm diameter in the cerebrum and more than 3-cm diameter in the cerebellum are usually immediately fatal. Hemorrhage contained only to the cerebellum may be amenable to neurosurgical drainage. Patients with a Glasgow Coma Score of 9 or less will require intubation and ventilation. Blood pressure should not be lowered excessively in these patients.

- Treatment of SAH is both medical and surgical. Patients may require lumbar puncture to confirm the diagnosis if unenhanced CT scanning is nondiagnostic. Intubation and ventilation of patients with a Glasgow Coma Score of 9 or less are appropriate; all patients will require urgent neurosurgical consultation. Patients with increasing lethargy may benefit from urgent ventriculostomy, whereas patients with a well-localized aneurysm may benefit from surgical interruption of the aneurysm by either clipping or angiologically directed coil occlusion.

Blood Pressure Considerations

- Acute stroke produces elevated blood pressure in 80% of patients. Regardless of the treatment for stroke, blood pressure must be monitored. Minimal or moderate elevations in pressure require no specific therapy. If mean arterial pressure (formula: mean arterial pressure = diastolic BP + (systolic BP − diastolic BP)/3) is greater than 130 mm (normal range: 80–100), or systolic pressure is greater than 240 mm, then antihypertensive therapy is indicated. Treatment of systolic pressures between 180 and 230 mm or diastolic pressures between 105 and 130 mm may be indicated depending on the cause of the stroke and concurrent medical conditions such as congestive heart failure, coronary ischemia, or renal failure. Initial management of blood pressure begins with labetalol, 20 to 40 mg intravenous every 10 to 30 minutes to a maximum of 300 mg; a continuous drip of 2 mg/min may also be started for extended control. Severe hypertension unresponsive to labetalol will require nitroprusside infused at 0.5 to 2.0 µg/kg/min. Rapid reductions in blood pressure are unnecessary, and maintaining upper limits of systolic pressure at 200 to 220 mm and diastolic pressure at 100 to 120 mm is acceptable.

Anticoagulation

- The use of intravenous or subcutaneous heparinoids in acute stroke is controversial and may have adverse effects including latent intracranial hemorrhage. Indications for use of heparinoids in acute stroke are few and really include only a cardioembolic event or prevention of subsequent venous thromboembolism in a predisposed patient. A nonenhanced CT scan of the brain to exclude hemorrhage is a prerequisite before starting anticoagulation; consultation with the consultant neurologist or stroke team would also be advisable.

Hyperglycemia

- Clinical studies have not supported animal model evidence that hyperglycemia enlarges infarct size. However, hypoglycemia should be aggressively sought for and treated, because hypoglycemic states may present with focal findings indistinguishable from an acute stroke. Hyperglycemia will require judicious correction with fluid and insulin therapy to prevent possible osmotic dehydration and further neurologic compromise.

Seizures
- Seizures will be present in 40% of stroke patients. They are more common in cases of hemorrhagic stroke, tend to occur in the first 24 hours after stroke, and usually manifest as a partial-type seizure. Initial stroke severity is a positive predictor of seizure activity; patients with lacunar infarcts are unlikely to have seizures, whereas those with a larger infarct or ICH/SAH are at greater likelihood of having a seizure. Emergent treatment of a seizure includes attention to airway, breathing, and circulation. Immediate control of seizure activity may be obtained with diazepam 5 to 10 mg intravenous every 5 minutes or lorazepam 1 to 2 mg intravenous every 5 minutes, followed by either phenytoin 18 mg/kg (infused at 50 mg/min) or fosphenytoin 18 PE/kg (infused at 150 mg/min). Systemic anticonvulsants should be maintained in those patients who have recurrent seizures. There is no current role for prophylactic anticonvulsant therapy in stroke patients.

Cerebral Edema
- Hypo-osmolar fluids should be avoided and isotonic intravenous therapy kept at slightly less than maintenance levels to minimize cerebral edema. Factors contributing to increased intracranial pressure such as hypoxia, hypercarbia, and hypothermia should be sought and corrected. Osmotic diuresis with mannitol is generally not indicated. Surgical decompression or evacuation of large cerebellar hemorrhages is indicated in selected cases to prevent brainstem compression.

Thrombolytic Therapy
- Tissue plasminogen activator (tPA) is used in acute ischemic stroke secondary to small- or large-vessel occlusive disease or cardioembolic stroke. In selected patients, thrombolysis provides demonstrable benefits with an acceptable risk profile. Patients with proximal MCA occlusion or extensive neurologic deficits may benefit the most. Thrombolysis may be given systemically or via a directed arterial angiographic catheter at the precise site of occlusion. Assignment of NIHSS score is important, because patients with scores more than 22 may be at risk for iatrogenic ICH if systemic tPA is used. Catheter-infused tPA is currently an investigational treatment and is available only at selected tertiary care centers. The advantages of catheter-infused tPA include not only precise administration at the site of occlusion but also an extended treatment window of 8 hours after onset of stroke symptoms. Systemic tPA has a treatment window of 3 hours after onset of stroke symptoms. Systemic tPA may be administered by the ED physician after consultation with the stroke team or consultant neurologist after reviewing the inclusion/exclusion criteria in Table 40-3.
- After inclusion/exclusion criteria are reviewed and the patient is deemed a candidate for systemic thrombolysis, informed consent should be obtained. The dose of tPA to be administered for acute ischemic stroke is 0.9 mg/kg to a maximum of 90 mg. Ten percent of the dose is given as a bolus, and the remainder is infused over 60 minutes. Subsequent administration of any other systemic antiplatelet of anticoagulant agents over the next 24 hours is contraindicated.
- **Blood pressure** must be monitored every 15 minutes for the first 2 hours after infusion, every 30 minutes for the next 6 hours, and then every 1 hour for the next 16 hours. Hypertension with systolic pressure more than 185 mm Hg or diastolic pressure of more than 110 mm Hg on two successive readings 10 to 15 minutes apart should be controlled with intravenous labetalol, 20 to 80 mg intravenous every

Table 40-3	Inclusion and Exclusion Criteria for Systemic tPA Use in Acute Ischemic Stroke

Inclusion Criteria

Ischemic stroke
    tPA can be administered within 3 h of symptom onset
    Neurologic deficit <22 by NIHSS
    Clearly defined time on onset of symptoms
Exclusion Criteria
    Evidence of ICH, SAH, or epidural/subdural bleeding
    Early CT evidence of acute infarction with surrounding edema
    Other stroke or serious head injury within preceding 3 mo
    Intracranial neoplasm, aneurysm, or AVM
    Uncontrolled hypertension not responsive within 30 min to oral or intravenous labetalol
    Rapidly improving neurologic symptoms
    History of intracranial hemorrhage
    Major surgery within the preceding 14 d
    Known bleeding diathesis
    Gastrointestinal or genitourinary bleeding within the preceding 21 d
    Arterial puncture in the noncompressible area within the preceding 7 d
    Seizure at onset of stroke
    INR >1.5 on or off Coumadin
    Heparin within the preceding 48 h with elevation of PTT
    Platelet count <100,000
    Serum glucose <50 mg/dL or >400 mg/dL

10 to 20 minutes to lower the pressure. A continuous drip at 2 mg/min thereafter may be used as necessary.

- **Complications** of thrombolysis revolve around bleeding, either in the CNS or in other organs. Hemorrhage may be either superficial or deep; the most serious hemorrhagic complication is ICH, which may occur up to 36 hours after tPA infusion. Vascular access procedures should be only performed as necessary and in locations amenable to direct pressure. Nasogastric tubes should be withheld for the first 24 hours, and bladder catheters should be avoided during the initial tPA infusion and for 30 minutes thereafter. ICH may be suspected if a significant adverse change in neurologic status, severe vomiting, or increasing headache occurs. If ICH is suspected, urgent nonenhanced CT scanning should be performed along with obtaining a CBC, PTT, and fibrinogen levels from the patient. The patient should be typed and crossed for 2 to 4 U of packed red blood cells, 4 to 6 U of fresh frozen plasma, and 1 to 2 U of platelets. Immediate neurosurgical consultation is indicated. Non-CNS hemorrhage may be treated by direct pressure at compressible sites. Bleeding in occult sites (GI tract, retroperitoneum) will require fluid resuscitation and transfusion of packed cells and fresh frozen plasma.

Newer interventional strategies: Catheter-directed intra-arterial thrombolysis is currently investigational and is available at a few selected tertiary care centers. This technique requires an angiographic suite and the availability of immediate neurosurgical intervention. Angiographic catheters are advanced into the cerebral arterial circulation via the internal carotid artery. After dye angiography has localized the occlusion, a small aliquot of tPA is infused into the clotted area. The potential of this technique is enormous, because it precisely reperfuses brain distal to the occluded vessel. Candidates for this procedure should have an NIHSS score of between 10 and 22 and should have a significant neurologic deficit. Because the tPA is administered in a directed fashion rather than systemically, the extensive exclusion criteria for systemic tPA administration does not apply so rigorously. The window for interventional treatment is currently set at 8 hours after symptom onset. Consultation with the stroke team or consultant neurologist/neurosurgeon is advisable to ascertain if the patient is a candidate for this therapy.

SYNCOPE

Syncope is a transient loss of consciousness that resolves in most cases in less than 5 minutes. Up to 50% of the population may be affected at one time or another. Presyncope (or near-syncope) is a warning of syncope and shares the same pathophysiology and differential diagnoses as syncope.

Syncope may be followed by a brief episode of seizure-like activity during which the patient may experience a clonic-type ictus involving the upper and/or lower limbs. The patient is often pale and diaphoretic. Syncopal ictus may be differentiated from a true seizure by the brevity of a syncopal seizure and the lack of a period of postictal drowsiness with a syncopal seizure. Patients may also report a prodrome of weakness, a sensation of feeling warm, or a sensation of feeling nauseated before the syncopal spell; true seizures tend to have a complex prodrome.

Syncope may be caused by cardiac or noncardiac causes. Cerebral hypoperfusion with dysfunction of the reticular activating system of the brain with loss of consciousness is the final pathway of both causes.

Cardiac Causes

These result in lack of cardiac output as a cause of cerebral hypoperfusion.

Bradyarrhythmias
- Bradyarrhythmias may be caused by exposure to a noxious stimulus with an exaggerated vagal response (common in young persons); heart block of Mobitz type II or third-degree block; drugs causing excessive AV nodal block such as digoxin, beta-blockers, diltiazem, verapamil, sotalol, or amiodarone; or conducting system disease secondary to ischemia, diabetes, cardiomyopathy, or toxins.

Tachyarrhythmias
- Tachyarrhythmias may be of supraventricular or ventricular origin: rapid atrial fibrillation or flutter without a controlled ventricular response, reentrant atrial tachyarrhythmias such as paroxysmal atrial tachycardia or multifocal atrial tachycardia, bypass tract arrhythmias such as Wolff-Parkinson-White syndrome, ventricular tachycardia or fibrillation, or ventricular torsades de pointes.

Obstruction to Cardiac Outflow
- Obstruction to cardiac outflow includes valvular stenotic lesions, especially mitral and aortic stenosis; hypertrophic cardiomyopathy; intra-atrial or intraventricular myxomata or thrombi that cause decreased outflow because of a ball-valve effect; and pericardial disease.

Ischemic Causes
- Ischemic causes involve coronary disease leading to myocardial hypoperfusion and resultant loss of pump function or ischemic arrhythmia.

Neurocardiogenic Syncope
- Neurocardiogenic syncope is a poorly understood condition that affects some people. Current theory identifies oversensitive stretch receptor in the left ventricle with resultant blood pooling, increased vagal tone, and bradycardia as the root cause of the syncopal episode. Patients tend to be in the erect position when they have syncope. Diagnosis is made via tilt-table testing.

Noncardiac Causes

Noncardiac causes include conditions resulting from vascular, metabolic, neurologic, otologic, or hematologic conditions.

Vascular Conditions
- Vascular conditions include carotid occlusion caused by entrapment under an accessory rib, spasm caused by hyperactive baroreceptors, or thromboembolic disease from a carotid source; and drugs inhibiting vascular tone such as beta-blockers, calcium channel blockers, or alpha-adrenergic blockers.

Metabolic Conditions
- Metabolic conditions include diabetes mellitus with hypoglycemia, adrenal failure (Addison disease) with resultant salt and water depletion, hypothyroidism, starvation ketosis, and extreme hyponatremia caused by water intoxication or the syndrome of inappropriate secretion of antidiuretic hormone.

Neurologic Conditions
- Neurologic conditions include stroke caused by thromboembolic disease in the carotid or vertebrobasilar circulation, degenerative neurologic conditions causing loss of autonomic function and decreased sympathetic tone throughout the body with resultant loss of vascular tone (Shy-Drager syndrome, myasthenia gravis, chronic degenerative polyneuropathies, advanced age, and heavy metal poisoning).

Vasovagal Syncope
- Vasovagal syncope (common faint) refers to a transient loss of consciousness caused by cerebral ischemia that results from reduced blood flow to the brain. This alteration in consciousness recurrently affects 3.1% of men and 4.5% of women and seems to demonstrate a familial trend.
- **Pathophysiology:** In the classic case, an individual is exposed to an intense emotional experience, the sight of blood, or other painful or emotional stimuli. This is followed by a brief period of alertness by the patient, and an elevation of blood pressure, pulse, and respiratory rate. This initial response is followed by a strong vagal response that causes a decrease in blood pressure and a slowing of the heart rate. These responses lead to decreased cerebral perfusion and resultant syncope. Classically, the patient, if seen soon after the event, will have bradycardia, hypotension, and pallor.
- The **diagnosis** of vasovagal syncope depends on the association of a compatible history with evidence of bradycardia and hypotension in an individual who is not otherwise influenced by drugs that may slow the heart rate in the face of hypotension (e.g., beta-blockers). Frequently, however, the diagnosis of vasovagal syncope can be made only after the exclusion of other causes, particularly those that result in a loss

of intravascular fluid volume, dysrhythmias, anaphylaxis, sepsis, or seizures. Patients should have a physical evaluation for injury, postural hypotension, cardiac dysrhythmias, and gross neurologic abnormalities. A rectal examination for occult blood will help to rule out gastrointestinal bleeding. Mucous membrane moistness and skin turgor will help exclude dehydration. If dysrhythmias or a myocardial event is suspected, an ECG should be obtained. A CBC and determination of electrolytes and BUN will help exclude hemorrhagic and volume depletion states. Women of childbearing age should have a pregnancy test, and if positive, ectopic pregnancy should be considered.

- **Treatment** in the majority of individuals is supportive only. Vasovagal syncope is self-limited, and after a brief period of observation, patients may be discharged with the instructions to sit or lie down if the symptoms recur. It is unusual for vasovagal syncope to occur in a supine patient, because cerebral perfusion is maintained with recumbency.

Otologic Conditions
- Otologic conditions of the inner ear can result in vertigo and an exaggerated vagal response with subsequent syncope.

Hematologic Conditions
- Hematologic conditions that result in anemia or hypovolemia can cause syncope.

Emergency Department Workup of Syncope

- A clear history of exposure to a noxious stimulus with an exaggerated vagal response causing syncope in a patient with no significant physical findings is reassuring and may terminate the evaluation.
- In other patients, especially older individuals or those with co-morbid conditions such as ischemic heart disease or diabetes, the syncope workup should also include postural blood pressures, rectal examination for occult blood, CBC, electrolytes, BUN, creatinine, PTT/INR, blood sugar, ECG, and a chest radiograph. Further studies such as cardiac enzymes or CT scanning of the head should be reserved for patients whose history or physical examination suggests causes of infarction or stroke.

Treatment

- Treatment of syncope is based on cause. Patients who are suspected of having other than a simple cause for their syncope require attention to their airway, breathing, and circulation. If the airway is stable, oxygen should be provided to maintain SaO_2 at more than 95%. An intravenous drip of normal saline should be started to expand intravascular volume and replenish body salt. If hypoglycemia is suspected, then perform a rapid bedside fingerstick glucometer measurement and give 25 to 50 mL of D50W. Bradyarrhythmias may require volume maintenance and possibly atropine 0.1 to 0.5 mg intravenous or external pacing if symptomatic. Tachyarrhythmias may require urgent termination by chemical means (intravenous adenosine, diltiazem, procainamide, or amiodarone); if this is unsuccessful and/or the patient remains symptomatic, emergent cardioversion should be used.
- Older patients, unreliable patients, patients with significant co-morbid illnesses (especially cardiomyopathy), patients who are drug toxic, or those with an unclear or complex cause may require observation or admission with cardiac monitoring.

Dizziness

The symptom of dizziness encompasses several pathophysiologic entities: light-headedness accompanying orthostatic hypotension, generalized weakness, presyncope, and true vertigo may all be interpreted by the patient as "dizziness." For this reason, a careful history and detailed cardiologic and neurologic examinations are essential to evaluate these patients adequately.

COMMON CAUSES OF DIZZINESS

- Orthostatic hypotension (caused by gastrointestinal bleeding, dehydration, medications)
- Cardiac arrhythmias causing symptomatic hypotension
- Labyrinthitis*
- Benign positional vertigo*
- Hyperventilation

LESS COMMON CAUSES OF DIZZINESS NOT TO BE MISSED

- Cerebellar hemorrhage
- Cerebellopontine angle tumor
- Brainstem or cerebellar infarction

OTHER CAUSES OF DIZZINESS

- Vestibular neuronitis*
- Ménière syndrome*
- Syphilitic labyrinthitis

HISTORY

- It is essential to determine at the outset whether the patient's report of "dizziness" represents light-headedness or true vertigo. When light-headedness is present, patients will report feeling "faint" or light-headed on standing or walking, as if they are about to pass out. Conversely, one may elicit a history of true vertigo by determining that the room or the patient appears to spin or rotate; these latter truly vertiginous symptoms may be positional to the extent that they are precipitated or worsened by head turning or head motion. A history of chronic headache worsening in association with hearing loss suggests a **cerebellopontine angle tumor**. The sudden onset of headache associated with vertigo, nausea, vomiting, and difficulty standing

---

*Discussed in this chapter.

or walking should suggest a **cerebellar hemorrhage**. The major central nervous system illness associated with the sudden onset of vertigo is acute intracerebellar hemorrhage; this entity must be suspected and recognized early to minimize patient morbidity and mortality. Nausea and vomiting are routinely associated with vertigo caused by **vestibular neuronitis, labyrinthitis, benign positional vertigo**, or **Ménière syndrome.** Tinnitus, associated with hearing loss, and vertigo suggest Ménière syndrome, especially if the symptoms of vertigo are chronic and episodic.

PHYSICAL EXAMINATION

- Orthostatic changes in pulse and/or blood pressure obtained after 2 minutes in either the sitting or the standing position suggest intravascular volume depletion or **orthostatic hypotension** as a cause for light-headedness; this is commonly interpreted and reported as "dizziness" by the patient. A 10% to 15% increase in pulse or decrease in diastolic blood pressure is considered significant, although an increase in pulse of 30 bpm is more specific.

- **Nystagmus** on lateral gaze, hearing loss, other cranial nerve abnormalities, or positional changes associated with true vertigo all suggest a **labyrinthine, eighth nerve**, or **central nervous system** process; distinguishing among these causes of true vertigo requires a careful neurologic evaluation. Abnormalities of the fifth, seventh, ninth, and tenth cranial nerves in association with rotational vertigo and headache suggest a **cerebellopontine angle tumor**.

- **Benign positional vertigo** is extremely common. Patients often report symptoms associated with turning the head quickly, or in a specific direction, while in bed or upon standing; vertigo and nausea usually last only seconds. **Bárány test** helps document the presence of benign positional vertigo as a cause for the patient's symptoms and is performed by rapidly moving the patient from the sitting to the supine position while simultaneously turning the head to the extreme left or right and noting the appearance of end-gaze nystagmus in that position. Patients with benign positional vertigo demonstrate end-gaze nystagmus and report nausea and vertigo primarily in one position. As noted, symptoms usually last only seconds.

- In patients with brainstem-posterior fossa disorders (acoustic neuroma, vertebrobasilar ischemia, multiple sclerosis), nystagmus typically lasts for more than 1 minute and occurs in multiple positions.

- Patients with **cerebellar hemorrhage** may have severe headache and protracted vomiting, may refuse to get out of bed, and may be unable to walk or stand. Ipsilateral facial paresis and gaze palsy may be noted as well.

DIAGNOSTIC TESTS

- Hypernatremia, contraction alkalosis, an increased blood urea nitrogen (BUN), and a mildly increased hematocrit all suggest intravascular volume depletion. Anemia from occult blood loss may be noted in patients with chronic gastrointestinal bleeding, and a stool guaiac may be positive. Patients with acute upper gastrointestinal bleeding resulting in resting or postural hypotension frequently have normal hematocrits and guaiac-negative stool; hence, these tests must not be used to exclude gastrointestinal bleeding. Hypocalcemia and hypoglycemia may be associated with the sensation of true vertigo. An emergency computed tomography scan should be obtained, along with urgent neurosurgical consultation in patients with suspected intracerebellar hemorrhage.

CLINICAL REMINDERS

- Record postural vital signs to exclude orthostatic hypotension reported as "dizziness."
- Replenish volume losses in patients who are hypotensive as a result of dehydration.
- Obtain an electrocardiogram (ECG) in patients who are hypotensive or of the age and risk factor history for coronary artery disease.
- Pass a nasogastric tube, and obtain a stool guaiac and a complete blood count (CBC) to rule out gastrointestinal bleeding in patients with postural changes in pulse and/or blood pressure.
- Maintain a low threshold for emergently excluding cerebellar hemorrhage in patients with a suggestive history or examination.

SPECIFIC DISORDERS

Labyrinthitis

- Labyrinthitis often results from a presumed viral infection of the inner ear; it may occasionally be caused by extension of bacterial middle ear infection. In addition, cholesteatoma formation secondary to middle ear infections may produce labyrinthitis. Labyrinthine fistulas may also develop as a result of erosion secondary to chronic infection or cholesteatoma.

Diagnosis
- The patient usually reports true vertigo, which may be intermittent or, if the labyrinthitis is severe, constant. Nausea and vomiting are common on initial presentation. If the patient notes that vertigo occurs when a finger is placed in the external canal of the affected ear, a labyrinthine fistula should be suspected.
- On physical examination, the affected ear may be unremarkable or a purulent discharge, evidence of otitis, or a cholesteatoma may be noted. Conductive hearing loss is often present in patients with concomitant middle ear infections or labyrinthine fistulas.

Treatment
- Meclizine hydrochloride, 25 mg orally three times daily for 7 to 10 days, is often helpful for the relief of vertiginous symptoms. Some clinicians also recommend diazepam 5 mg orally three times daily. Patients who are nauseous or vomiting will often benefit from prochlorperazine (Compazine), 10 mg intravenous or 25 mg per rectum, or promethazine (Phenergan) 12.5 to 25 mg every 4 hours orally or intravenous. In patients with symptoms worsened or precipitated by head motion, a period of bed rest and avoidance of rapid head turning should be advised. If a bacterial middle ear infection or a fistula accompanies the labyrinthitis, otolaryngologic consultation is indicated before discharge.

Benign Positional Vertigo

Diagnosis
- Patients with benign positional vertigo usually experience severe vertigo precipitated by movement of the head in one particular direction. These episodes usually last 1 to 3 minutes and are often first noted at night with movement or head turning. Most

commonly, symptoms occur without previous illness, but occasionally the patient has had a recent upper respiratory tract infection. Headache is **not** an expected symptom.

- The physical exam is generally within normal limits, horizontal nystagmus may be appreciated, and the Bárány test described in "Physical Examination" is positive.

Treatment

- Patients with benign positional vertigo may be treated with meclizine hydrochloride, 25 mg every 8 hours as needed. In patients with vomiting, prochlorperazine (Compazine), 10 mg intravenous or 25 mg per rectum, or hydroxyzine, 25 to 50 mg intramuscular, may be used. The patient should also be instructed to avoid positions and head movements that initiate vertiginous symptoms. An occasional patient will require admission for stabilization and intravenous fluid replacement.

Vestibular Neuronitis

- Vestibular neuronitis is generally felt to be of viral origin and often appears in epidemic form. Patients report unsteadiness of gait and vertiginous symptoms for a few days to several weeks without a change in auditory acuity.
- On physical examination, patients demonstrate normal auditory acuity with a normal otologic examination; occasionally, spontaneous nystagmus is noted. This illness is self limited and only requires symptomatic treatment as described in "Benign Positional Vertigo."

Ménière Syndrome

- Patients with Ménière syndrome report episodic dizziness associated with tinnitus and progressive hearing loss; this illness also has a labyrinthine origin. The pathologic changes in Ménière syndrome are said to consist of endolymphatic system dilation producing eventual degeneration of vestibular and cochlear hair cells.

Diagnosis

- Tinnitus and deafness may be absent during the initial attacks of vertigo, but they invariably appear as the disease progresses; symptoms often dramatically increase in severity during acute attacks.
- Nystagmus, unsteadiness of gait, and decreased auditory acuity are noted. Typically, the hearing deficit is unilateral and progressive; when total deafness develops, vertiginous episodes cease.

Treatment

- Treatment is initially directed at symptoms and most commonly involves bed rest with the patient urged to assume positions that minimize vertigo; meclizine, 25 mg four times daily, is useful in some patients. If attacks persist despite treatment and are severe, permanent relief may be achieved by surgical ablation of the labyrinth or intracranial interruption of the vestibular portion of the eighth nerve. Otolaryngologic referral is recommended.

Orthostatic Hypotension

- Orthostatic hypotension refers to the drop in blood pressure when a patient moves from a sitting or lying position to an upright position. Any volume depletion from the intravascular space may cause orthostatic hypotension, whether it is caused by vomiting, diarrhea, hemorrhage, restricted intake, diuresis, or endocrine disturbances such as adrenal insufficiency. When the cause of volume depletion is not evident, one must suspect gastrointestinal bleeding or bleeding from an ectopic pregnancy or aortic aneurysm. Orthostatic hypotension particularly affects those older than 65 years of age. This comes in part from cardiovascular deconditioning. Additionally, the reflex control of arterial blood pressure that occurs in healthy individuals may be altered by a wide variety of conditions including multiple sclerosis, spinal cord injuries, Landry-Guillain-Barré syndrome, syringomyelia, tabes dorsalis, alcoholic neuropathy, diabetic neuropathy, Wernicke syndrome, porphyria, amyloidosis, and drugs such as diuretics, antihypertensives, vasodilators, sedatives, hypnotics, antidepressants, and tranquilizers.

- The **diagnosis** of orthostatic hypotension is made by measuring postural vital signs and looking for an abnormal decrease in blood pressure when the patient assumes an upright position. The definitive diagnosis of the cause of the orthostatic hypotension may be made in most cases by history and physical examination. Tests that may help in the diagnosis include CBC, electrolytes, BUN, creatinine, stool for occult blood, and ECG. Tests specific for ectopic pregnancy and evaluation for an abdominal aortic aneurysm may also be helpful in certain patients.

- The specific **treatment** for orthostatic hypotension should be directed toward the underlying cause.

42 Headache

Headache is a common complaint in emergency practice. The differential diagnosis ranges from benign self-limiting conditions to life-threatening emergencies. The clinical challenge is to provide relief to those patients who suffer from primary headache syndromes (the majority) but detect those headaches that are due to potentially fatal or permanently disabling causes.

COMMON CAUSES OF HEADACHE

- Tension headache*
- Migraine headache*
- Cluster headache*
- Sinusitis*
- Trauma/posttrauma

LESS COMMON CAUSES OF HEADACHE NOT TO BE MISSED

- Subarachnoid hemorrhage (SAH)*/cerebellar hemorrhage*
- Meningitis* or encephalitis
- Brain tumor/mass effect
- Acute narrow-angle glaucoma
- Thromboembolic cerebrovascular accident
- Temporal arteritis*
- Carbon monoxide poisoning

OTHER CAUSES OF HEADACHE

- Benign intracranial hypertension
- Uveitis
- Hypoglycemia
- Trigeminal neuralgia
- Central venous sinus thrombosis

HISTORY

- Headache caused by **tension** is frequently bilateral, is described as "band-like," commonly occurs at the end of the day, and is often relieved with rest.

---

*Discussed in this chapter.

- **Migraine** headaches are usually unilateral but commonly alternate sides. Attacks of migraine or vascular headache are often preceded by or associated with nausea, vomiting, or an aura, which includes scintillating scotomata, loss of the peripheral field of vision, and other disturbances of visual perception. Occasionally, patients with migraine report associated neurologic deficits, including hemiparesis and cranial neuropathies. These phenomena are attributed to cerebral vasospasm with resulting ischemia and generally improve without residual deficit.
- The **cluster headache** is a form of vascular headache that usually localizes to the periorbital area, occurs in "clusters" every few weeks to months, and may be accompanied by unilateral tearing and conjunctival injection and occasional visual disturbances.
- Patients with headaches secondary to **sinusitis** may report pain over or surrounding the involved sinus and may complain of purulent nasal discharge or symptoms of a recent upper respiratory tract infection.
- The headache associated with **subarachnoid hemorrhage** is classically described as sudden onset and the "worst headache of one's life" and may be associated with neck aching or stiffness or an initial loss of consciousness.
- **Meningitis/encephalitis** produces dull, constant headaches, as do **brain tumors**; the latter are occasionally associated with the report of headaches on awakening, which may accompany specific progressive neurologic signs or symptoms.
- Patients with **cerebellar hemorrhage** generally have a history of hypertension or are noted to be hypertensive at presentation; they experience a sudden-onset, severe, occipital headache associated with nausea, vomiting, and inability to walk or stand. Some patients report vertiginous symptoms as well.

PHYSICAL EXAMINATION

- **Photophobia** is a common finding in patients with vascular headaches and meningitis; tension headaches also may be associated with photophobia.
- **Percussion tenderness** over the involved sinus and a decrease in sinus **transillumination** are often noted in sinusitis.
- **Neck stiffness** may accompany SAH and meningitis, and both of these disorders may cause fever and an abnormal mental status.
- Signs of increased intracranial pressure from subarachnoid or intracerebral hemorrhage, purulent meningitis, or brain tumor may be detected on **funduscopy.**
- **Focal neurologic deficits** may be detected in patients with brain tumors, migraine, subarachnoid or intracerebral hemorrhage, and, rarely, meningoencephalitis.
- Uveitis causes an **acutely red and painful eye** with a characteristic ciliary or perilimbal flush; narrow-angle glaucoma may be associated with corneal clouding, decreased visual acuity, and, most distinctively, increased intraocular pressure on tonometry.
- Patients with cerebellar hemorrhage are typically nauseous, vomiting, and **unable to stand or walk without assistance.** In addition, paresis of conjugate ipsilateral gaze, ipsilateral sixth nerve weakness, and forced conjugate deviation of the eyes are occasional accompanying signs. Although the mental status of such patients may initially be normal, it may rapidly deteriorate.

EMERGENCY DIAGNOSTIC TESTS

- A **complete blood count** often reveals a leukocytosis in patients with **meningitis,** often with an increase in polymorphonuclear and band forms.

- **Sinus roentgenograms** or **sinus computed tomography** (CT) may demonstrate mucosal thickening, opacification, and/or air-fluid levels in the affected sinus or sinuses.
- In 90% to 95% of patients with SAH, the **CT** scan of the brain will reveal evidence of bleeding. If SAH is likely but the CT scan is negative, a **lumbar puncture** must be performed to exclude a hemorrhage.
- When meningitis or encephalitis is suspected, a **lumbar puncture** must be performed.
- A **CT scan** of the head should be obtained prior to **lumbar puncture** in patients with an abnormal mental status, evidence of increased intracranial pressure, immunocompromised or focal neurologic deficits.

CLINICAL REMINDERS

- Perform a lumbar puncture in any patient suspected of having meningitis. If immunocompromised, clinical signs of focality or increased intracranial pressure are noted, obtain a noncontrast CT first.
- If SAH is suspected, CT alone is not adequate to exclude hemorrhage. CT must be followed by lumbar puncture to definitely exclude SAH.

SPECIFIC DISORDERS

Tension Headache

- Tension headache is the most common cause of headache but must be diagnosed by exclusion. Patients often report a "band-like" tightness about the head that is often worse toward the day's end, especially in the setting of stress at work or home. Headaches typically occur posteriorly, cervically, or temporally, where muscle spasm may be prominent and palpable. The physical examination and laboratory studies are normal. Occasionally, a trigger point may be elicited on examination of the occipital area or neck. Patients usually find relief from mild analgesics, including acetaminophen or NSAIDs. Social or psychological consultation may be required if headaches become persistent or severe.

Migraine Headache

- Migraine headaches are a form of vascular headache, which result from cerebral vasospasm followed by vasodilation. Although a variety of factors, including food (nuts, coffee, chocolate), alcohol, and stress have been implicated as precipitants, the causal role of these agents in migraine remains unclear. It is the dilatory phase that is responsible for the headache and toward which acute pharmacotherapy is directed; prophylactic therapy is aimed at both phases. The vasospastic phase is occasionally accompanied by neurologic deficits, and it is this pathophysiologic event that is responsible for the prodrome.

Diagnosis
- Patients with migraine headache typically report unilateral discomfort, the side of which may alternate with each episode. The migrainous prodrome in its classic form includes nausea, vomiting, and a visual or perceptual aura that may include "lightning-like" images, scintillating scotomata, or loss of the peripheral field of vision, all of which usually disappear with the onset of the headache. The headache itself is quite severe, often throbbing, and associated with profound photophobia.

- Despite the severity of symptoms, the physical examination usually is unrevealing. Rarely, patients have true focal neurologic deficits accompanying the aura or headache (*complex migraine*), which usually improve and disappear as vasospasm subsides. Very rarely, a patient with a history of migraine headache may present with an isolated neurologic deficit *without* headache; aura may be noted in these patients and is important diagnostically.

Diagnostic Tests
- The diagnosis of migraine headache cannot be confirmed or excluded with any laboratory test; all basic studies typically are normal.

Treatment
- In the **acute phase,** patients appear quite ill and require prompt treatment. During the aura or prodromal period or immediately after the onset of headache, patients may be treated with one of the following regimens to abort the onset of headache.
  - Prochlorperazine (Compazine) or metoclopramide (Reglan) 10 mg IV with IV fluids. May be repeated as necessary. Occasionally, patients get akathisias in response to the medication, which is rapidly reversed by diphenhydramine (Benadryl) 25 mg IV.
  - Ergotamine tartrate and caffeine (Cafergot) tablets, one or two immediately, repeating each hour up to five per attack as needed.
  - Ergotamine tablets (2 mg), one immediately, repeating each 30 minutes up to three per attack as needed.
  - Sumatriptan (Imitrex), 6 mg subcutaneously, repeating in 60 minutes as needed (note contraindications discussed later).

  Medications (2), (3), and (4) are contraindicated in pregnancy, coronary or peripheral artery disease, and significant hepatic or renal disease. Sumatriptan is also contraindicated in uncontrolled hypertension and basilar or hemiplegic migraine. When sumatriptan is used, ergotamines should be avoided for 24 hours.

  If this is unsuccessful, patients may be treated with hydromorphone 1 to 2 mg IM or IV or another narcotic of choice. Patients with mild discomfort and insignificant vomiting after treatment may be treated with an NSAID for several days. Symptomatic bed rest and a cool compress to the forehead and face are also commonly advised. Typically, if the patient falls asleep, the headache subsides.

Cluster Headaches
- Cluster headaches are a form of vascular headache that occur in a group or cluster with long headache-free intervals between attacks. Typically, the headache is periorbital and, in addition to the common prodromal symptoms associated with the other vascular headaches, may be accompanied by unilateral lacrimation, rhinorrhea, subjective nasal congestion, and, occasionally, ptosis and miosis. Patients presenting very early may be treated similar to those with migraine headaches, although termination of the headache is less successful. In some patients, treatment with hydromorphone or another narcotic analgesic may be required.

Acute Sinusitis
- Acute sinusitis frequently presents with localized headache or facial pain overlying and surrounding the involved sinus or sinuses. Systemic symptoms, such as

fever and chills, are often present, and many patients report postnasal discharge, previous or ongoing upper respiratory tract infection, and posture-related changes in discomfort. Frequently, a history of pain or the sensation of pressure on awakening is reported, which resolves as the morning progresses, presumably as a result of posture-related drainage of the involved sinus.

- Physical examination may reveal localized facial tenderness with percussion or palpation over the involved sinus or sinuses; overlying erythema and edema are occasionally noted. Often, asymmetry with percussion is noted between the involved and uninvolved sides. Purulent material may be visualized surrounding the nasal turbinates, in which case a culture should be obtained. In addition, reduced transillumination of the involved area may be noted.
- Common organisms in acute sinusitis are *Streptococcus pneumoniae* and *Haemophilus influenzae,* although those in chronic sinusitis include both of those plus *Staphylococcus aureus,* Gram-negative rods, and anaerobes.
- Radiologic assessment with roentgenograms or facial CT may demonstrate opacification, an air-fluid level, or mucosal thickening; frequently, however, roentgenograms are within normal limits.
- Treatment should be initiated with an appropriate antibacterial agent. The recommended antibiotics for acute sinusitis are amoxicillin-clavulanate, cefuroxime, or trimethoprim-sulfamethoxazole. These should be given along with a systemic and topical decongestant. Administer the antibiotic for 10 days. Nasal steroids may reduce inflammation. Patients with severe discomfort should receive an analgesic for 3 to 4 days, and follow-up should be advised in 5 to 10 days.

Subarachnoid Hemorrhage

- Most SAHs result from trauma and are self-limited. Atraumatic SAH is typically caused by rupture of a berry aneurysm or a leaking arteriovenous malformation. Berry aneurysms commonly occur at sites of vascular bifurcation, with the origin of the anterior communicating and the middle cerebral arteries being the most common locations. Vascular malformations are less common and have no typical anatomic predilection. Blood in the subarachnoid space may cloud consciousness, produce neck stiffness given its meningeal-irritating properties, and, most importantly, increase intracranial pressure.

Diagnosis

- Classically, the headache associated with an acute SAH is described as the worst of one's life. The onset is typically abrupt and may be associated with nausea and vomiting; depending on the site of rupture, focal neurologic deficits may be apparent on initial presentation.
- Patients with a leaking aneurysm may present with only a headache (sentinel hemorrhage). It is imperative to diagnosis this small hemorrhage because the aneurysm remains and is at extremely high risk of rupture with devastating consequences.
- Physical examination, including mental status, may be completely normal. An abnormal mental status ranging from mild lethargy to frank coma, subhyaloid hemorrhages on funduscopy, neck stiffness, and focal neurologic findings may be noted.

Diagnostic Tests

- CT or lumbar puncture is essential for confirming the diagnosis. In patients with SAH, CT may be negative in approximately 10%, depending on the amount of bleeding present and the interval between the onset of bleeding and imaging. When this diagnosis is suspected, patients with a negative CT scan should undergo lumbar puncture. Cerebrospinal fluid (CSF) findings indicative of SAH show increased red blood cells. A false-positive result can occur when a traumatic tap is obtained; this is suggested by an absence of xanthochromia. The latter, a yellow color imparted to the supernatant of centrifuged CSF, results from the breakdown of red blood cells in the CSF and is only present with SAH.

Treatment
- Emergency treatment consists primarily of reducing increased intracranial pressure and initiating measures to prevent rebleeding. If evidence of increased intracranial pressure is present, mannitol (1 g/kg intravenous) and dexamethasone (0.1 mg/kg intravenous) should be administered; intubation and hyperventilation to produce an arterial Pco_2 between 25 and 30 mm Hg will also lower intracranial pressure and is indicated in selected patients. The treatment of choice is surgical or endovascular repair. Hypotension should be avoided, and only extreme elevations in blood pressure (more than 130 mm Hg diastolic) should be treated. In addition, patient activity should be limited and therapy begun with nimodipine, a calcium channel blocker, at 60 mg orally every 4 hours, which has been shown to reduce the incidence of associated cerebral vasospasm. In all patients, prompt neurosurgical or neurologic consultation should be obtained.
- Under the best of circumstances and with the most meticulous attention to therapy, **mortality** still remains high, making this a most lethal event in otherwise healthy, often young individuals.

Meningitis

- Meningitis has multiple causes; both infectious and noninfectious. Of the infectious causes of meningitis, bacterial causes are both the most serious and treatable, and their early diagnosis is critical. Specific bacterial causes are somewhat age dependent. Neonates are commonly infected with *Escherichia coli*, whereas infants and young children acquire *S. pneumoniae*, *H. influenzae*, or meningococcal organisms. Those between the ages of 7 and 50 can become infected by *S. pneumoniae*, meningococcus, and *Listeria monocytogenes*. Meningococcus also typically causes meningitis in young adults and, because of its somewhat insidious onset but fulminant course, remains a major cause of morbidity and mortality in this age group. Elderly and debilitated patients are most commonly infected with the pneumococcus, and rarely coliforms. Other infectious causes of meningitis and, more specifically, meningoencephalitis include viral agents such as the mumps, measles, herpes simplex, arboviruses, and the acquired immunodeficiency syndrome virus. Typically, the arboviruses are transmitted by insect vectors (flies), are contracted in endemic fashion throughout the late summer, and tend to disappear with the first frost. *Cryptococcus neoformans* is an infectious cause of chronic meningitis seen in otherwise normal persons as well as in immunocompromised individuals.

Diagnosis
- Many patients with infectious meningitis present with a prodrome of 1 to 3 days' duration, suggesting an upper respiratory tract infection. These relatively nonspecific findings are followed by fever, malaise, nausea, lethargy, headache, neck stiffness, and photophobia. Young children and neonates present a special diagnostic problem, because mild lethargy or a disinterest in feeding may be the only symptoms.

For this reason, the emergency physician must maintain a high index of suspicion in the very young to maximize diagnostic sensitivity.

- **The physical examination** of patients with suspected meningitis may demonstrate only mild lethargy and fever. Signs of meningeal irritation, including positive Kernig and Brudzinski signs, may be noted. Findings consistent with increased intracranial pressure may be seen, especially in patients with a significantly purulent meningeal reaction or in those presenting somewhat later in their course. Again, neonates may show no signs of meningeal irritation and may simply appear lethargic, irritable, or febrile on examination.

Diagnostic Tests

- The essential diagnostic test in patients with suspected meningitis is the lumbar puncture.
- When practical, opening pressure should be determined and CSF removed for **(tubes number 1 and 4)** a cell count and differential, a total protein and glucose level **(tube number 2)**, a VDRL or RPR, Gram stain, and a culture for bacterial organisms **(tube number 3)**. In addition, in patients with suspected fungal meningitis (i.e., immunocompromised patients or patients with a chronic meningitis syndrome), an India ink preparation should be examined and toxoplasma titers and cryptococcal antigen titers measured.
- The typical CSF finding in patients with bacterial meningitis includes an opening pressure greater than 180 mm H_2O, a CSF pleocytosis with a predominance of polymorphonuclear leukocytes, hypoglycorrhachia (<40% of a simultaneous serum glucose provided the serum glucose is <250 mg/dL), and an increased CSF protein (more than 45 mg/dL). Viral infections tend to produce a lymphocytic pleocytosis and, except in the case of mumps meningitis, do not depress CSF glucose levels. It should be noted, however, that a number of viral meningitides may be associated with an early, predominantly polymorphonuclear CSF formula. A Gram stain of centrifuged CSF is also essential because culture results are not available for 48 to 72 hours. Identification of the offending bacterial organism may permit the institution of more specific therapy. In addition to bacterial cultures of the CSF, in immunocompromised patients or those with chronic symptoms, fungal cultures and smears should be requested. At the present time, there is no role for viral cultures; the diagnosis of viral infection is made by antibody titer analysis in most patients or temporal lobe biopsy when herpes simplex virus is suspected. Cryptococcal meningitis may be diagnosed by India ink analysis of the CSF, CSF cryptococcal antigen titer analysis, or both.
- Although it is true that even when the neurologic examination is meticulous and unremarkable, posterior fossa events may produce acute herniation with lumbar puncture, one should **never** delay cautious lumbar puncture needlessly in patients in whom it is essential. On measuring the opening pressure, if readings greater than 250 mm H_2O are obtained, the spinal needle should be kept in place and turned off to the atmosphere with a three-way stopcock, the patient's head should be placed at a level lower than the lumbar spine, and intravenous mannitol (1.0–1.5 g/kg) should be administered immediately. Once a decrease in the CSF pressure to a safe range is achieved, the spinal needle may be removed. In all cases, however, sufficient CSF should be removed to obtain a cell count and differential, Gram stain, and culture.

Treatment

- Antibacterial therapy depends on the patient's clinical condition, the CSF findings, and the results of the Gram stain of centrifuged CSF. More often than not, a specific bacteriologic diagnosis will be unavailable after the initial evaluation, and patients who are ill require that empirical antibiotic therapy be instituted immediately, as noted below in Table 42-1.

- **Neonatal meningitis** (infants younger than 1 month of age) is generally caused by group B or D streptococci, Enterobacteriaceae, or *Listeria*. For these neonates, use the following:
  - **In term neonates younger than 1 week old,** ampicillin, 50 mg/kg intravenous every 12 hours, *plus* cefotaxime 200 mg/kg/day divided into every 6-hour doses *or* gentamicin, 5 mg/kg/day intravenous in two divided doses.
  - **In term neonates older than 1 week,** ampicillin, 50 to 100 mg/kg intravenous every 8 hours, *plus* cefotaxime 50 mg/kg every 8 hours plus gentamicin, 7.5 mg/kg/day in three divided doses.

Table 42-1	Age Groups with Corresponding Common Causes of Meningitis and Recommended Empiric Treatment	
Age Group	**Common Organisms**	**Recommended Therapy Until Culture Results Available**
Infants aged 1–3 mo	*Streptococcus pneumoniae* *Neisseria meningitides* *Haemophilus influenzae* Group B or D streptococci Enterobacteriaceae *Listeria monocytogenes*	Ampicillin plus cefotaxime plus dexamethasone or ceftriaxone plus gentamicin plus dexamethasone
Infants and children to age 7 y	*S. pneumoniae* *N. meningitides* *H. influenzae*	Either cefotaxime or ceftriaxone plus vancomycin[a] plus dexamethasone
Age 7–18 y	*S. pneumoniae* *N. meningitides* *L. monocytogenes*	As above
Adults 18–50 y	*S. pneumoniae,* *M. meningitides*	Either ceftriaxone or cefotaxime plus vancomycin[a]
Older adults (>50 y)	*S. pneumoniae* *H. influenzae* *N. meningitides* *L. monocytogenes* Gram-negative rods (enteric)	Either cefotaxime or ceftriaxone plus ampicillin plus vancomycin[a] *plus* dexamethasone

[a]Note that Vancomycin has been added to these regimens to cover drug-resistant *S. pneumoniae*.

- Infants and children receiving antibiotics for suspected or proven bacterial meningitis may benefit from concomitant treatment with corticosteroids (dexamethasone) 0.4 mg/kg every 12 hours intravenous for 2 days starting 15 to 20 minutes before antibiotics. The use of this anti-inflammatory agent reduces the incidence of some complications (particularly deafness), presumably by reducing the inflammatory response to the bactericidal action of antibiotics.
- Once culture and sensitivity testing are complete, a more specific antibiotic may be chosen.
- The therapy of meningoencephalitis secondary to herpes simplex virus includes the use of intravenous acyclovir 10 mg/kg intravenous infused over 1 hour every 8 hours for 10 to 14 days.
- Amphotericin 0.5 to 0.8 mg/kg/day intravenous and 5-fluorocytosine 37.5 mg/kg every 6 hours intravenous are used in the therapy of cryptococcal meningitis; appropriate consultation is required along with careful monitoring of both renal function and the white blood cell count.
- Consideration should also be given to additional causes of meningitis such as tuberculosis, syphilis, Lyme disease, and HIV-related infectious processes.
- **Prophylaxis** of intimate contacts of the patient with meningococcal meningitis, those who share a household with the patient, and those who directly and continually cared for the patient in the hospital warrant prophylactic therapy.
  - **Children.** Younger than 1 year old: rifampin, 5 mg/kg every 12 hours for four doses; 1 to 12 years old: rifampin, 10 mg/kg every 12 hours for four doses or ceftriaxone 125 mg intramuscular as a single dose (for children younger than age 15 years).
  - **Adults.** Rifampin, 600 mg every 12 hours for four doses *or* ciprofloxacin, 500 mg, in one daily dose or ceftriaxone 250 mg intramuscular as a single dose.

Cerebellar Hemorrhage

- Acute cerebellar hemorrhage is most commonly caused by hypertension-induced rupture of arteries within brain tissue rather than those on the brain surface adjacent to the subarachnoid space. The extravasation that results from rupture forms an oval or circular mass, which disrupts tissue as it increases in volume.

Diagnosis

- Symptoms in patients with cerebellar hemorrhage usually evolve over a period of hours; when compared with other forms of intracerebral hemorrhage, loss of consciousness at the outset is rare. Headache occurs in approximately one half of patients and nuchal rigidity less commonly. Repeated vomiting is the hallmark of cerebellar hemorrhage, as is the occipital location of the headache, vertigo, and difficulty walking or standing.
- The physical examination often reveals paresis of conjugate lateral gaze to the side of the bleed, forced conjugate deviation of the eyes to the side opposite the bleed, and ipsilateral sixth nerve weakness. At the outset, little or no evidence of cerebellar dysfunction may be apparent; only a minority of patients manifest nystagmus or cerebellar ataxia. Ocular "bobbing," blepharospasm, involuntary closure of one eye, skew deviation, mild ipsilateral facial weakness, a diminished ipsilateral corneal reflex, dysarthria, and dysphagia may also be noted early in the course. As hours pass, and occasionally rather suddenly, the patient becomes stuporous and then comatose as a result of progressive brainstem compression, by which time successful reversal of the syndrome by surgical intervention becomes less likely.

Treatment
- The diagnosis is best confirmed by emergency CT scan while urgent neurosurgical consultation, along with standard measures to reduce intracranial pressure, if elevated, are implemented. In contrast to other forms of hypertensive intracerebral hemorrhage, after the diagnosis is made, acute cerebellar hemorrhage is readily amenable to surgical evacuation of the clot; such therapy is the clear treatment of choice when hemorrhage is diagnosed within the first 2 days of the illness, and all efforts should be made rapidly to exclude or confirm this diagnosis whenever suspected. The control of hemorrhage by acutely lowering blood pressure has not met with significant success, and given the profound fluctuations in blood pressure accompanying many intracerebral catastrophes, the administration of such agents in acute cerebellar hemorrhage is not usually recommended.

Temporal Arteritis (See section "Temporal Arteritis and Polymyalgia Rheumatica," in Page 393, Chapter 43).

Weakness

The patient who presents to the emergency department complaining of generalized weakness or of vague, poorly defined symptoms often poses a major diagnostic dilemma. A thorough history and physical examination are essential. A chest radiograph, complete blood count (CBC), measurement of electrolytes, blood sugar, blood urea nitrogen (BUN), and erythrocyte sedimentation rate (ESR) are useful initial tests in these patients. More specific studies may be ordered depending on the historical and physical findings.

COMMON CAUSES OF WEAKNESS

- Anemia
- Infection/fever
- Hypotension (including shock)
- Diabetes mellitus
- Dehydration

LESS COMMON CAUSES OF WEAKNESS NOT TO BE MISSED

- Myocardial infarction
- Shock
- Hypoglycemia
- Guillain-Barré syndrome*
- Myasthenia gravis*
- Hypoxemia
- Botulism*

OTHER CAUSES OF WEAKNESS

- Congestive heart failure
- Occult malignancy
- Tuberculosis
- Infective endocarditis*
- Infectious mononucleosis
- Electrolyte disturbances*
- Periodic paralysis
- Steroid-induced myopathy
- Eaton-Lambert syndrome
- Organophosphate poisoning

---

*Discussed in this chapter.

- Hypothyroidism
- Adrenal insufficiency*
- Hyperparathyroidism
- Pituitary insufficiency
- Polymyositis and dermatomyositis*
- Temporal arteritis and polymyalgia rheumatica*
- Cerebrovascular accident
- Depression

SPECIFIC DISORDERS

Guillain-Barré Syndrome

- Acute idiopathic ascending polyneuritis, or the Guillain-Barré syndrome, often occurs in the setting of a viral infection and usually begins insidiously. Patients may report weakness, lassitude, or fatigue and are found to have decreased strength primarily in the distal muscle groups. Weakness is typically symmetric and begins in the lower extremities, **ascending** to involve the upper extremities and most importantly the respiratory muscles. Rarely, the upper extremities may be involved first, and in exceptional circumstances, the facial and extraocular muscles may be involved. Although sensory function is normal and atrophy absent, decreased or absent deep tendon reflexes are commonly noted. Laboratory studies are not particularly helpful (except to exclude some potential diagnoses such as hypokalemia, etc.); however, a small number of patients will exhibit an increased cerebrospinal fluid protein and a moderate lymphocytic or monocytic pleocytosis.
- Patients in whom the diagnosis of Guillain-Barré syndrome is suspected should be admitted and closely monitored for changes in vital capacity. Dramatic decreases in pulmonary function resulting in respiratory failure can occur rapidly and without warning. When the vital capacity falls below 10 mL/kg, assisted ventilation is indicated. The use of corticosteroids is controversial; a number of dramatic responses have been reported, and on this basis, a trial of prednisone is often undertaken. Intravenous IgG may be helpful if begun within 14 days of the onset of symptoms, and plasmapheresis may help if begun within 7 days of the onset of symptoms. Urinary retention, wide swings in blood pressure associated with profound diaphoresis, and paroxysmal bradyarrhythmias may be noted with involvement of the autonomic nervous system.

Botulism

- Classic food poisoning results from the ingestion of *Clostridium botulinum* toxin, which is often found in home-canned or smoked foods. Toxins elaborated by the organism block the release of acetylcholine from nerve terminals, resulting in early involvement of the central nervous system.
- The sudden onset of weakness, respiratory paralysis, diplopia, dry mouth, dysphagia, and dysphonia are often noted. Symptoms begin 12 to 48 hours after ingestion. Unlike the Guillain-Barré syndrome, the symptoms and signs of botulism usually appear in a **descending fashion** and may be heralded by nausea and vomiting.
- Once the diagnosis of botulinum is suspected, the Centers for Disease Control and Prevention in Atlanta (404-639-3311 or 404-639-2888) should be contacted for acquisition of pentavalent botulinus antitoxin. Adequate ventilation and oxygenation must be maintained; intubation and mechanical ventilation should be instituted if necessary and nutritional support provided parenterally in patients

with abnormalities of swallowing. If ventilation can be maintained or adequately supported, mortality improves significantly from that of 50% to 70% in untreated patients.

- Infants afflicted with botulism present with weakness and generalized hypotonicity; these symptoms, although vague, should suggest the diagnosis, which may be confirmed by electromyography.

Infective Endocarditis

- **Acute endocarditis** runs a fulminant course in which patients become rapidly ill and present with rigors, high fever, and signs of impending vascular collapse. Suggestive physical findings include conjunctival, subungual, oral, or dermal petechiae; Janeway lesions; Osler nodes; retinal hemorrhages, exudates, or Roth spots; splenomegaly; and, in most patients, a heart murmur. Hematuria is noted in more than half of patients. Embolic phenomena are common and include large vessel embolization (cerebral, renal, coronary) and septic pulmonary emboli resulting from right-sided endocarditis. Cerebral emboli may produce seizures, confusion, multiple focal deficits, or hemiplegia.
- More invasive bacterial organisms, such as staphylococci, typically produce an acute, fulminant form of endocarditis in which a totally normal endocardial surface may serve as the substrate for initial infection. Patients commonly present with low-grade fever, malaise, anorexia, weight loss, and generalized weakness; low back pain, headache, and arthralgias are often reported as well.
- **Subacute endocarditis** usually results from infection with less virulent organisms such as *Streptococcus viridans* and is responsible for presentations that are both varied and subtle. Bacteremia resulting in endocardial infection usually originates from the upper airway, genitourinary tract, gastrointestinal tract, or skin. Subacute endocarditis usually occurs in the context of a previously damaged heart valve or a congenital intracardiac lesion.
- The diagnosis of infective endocarditis rests on a high degree of suspicion and the results of blood cultures; specifically, with certain exceptions, persistent bacteremia must be documented. Exceptions include patients treated with antibiotics or those infected with a particularly fastidious organism. Additional laboratory findings include anemia, a mild to moderate leukocytosis, a significantly elevated ESR, a positive latex fixation test, hematuria, proteinuria, circulating immune complexes, and antiteichoic acid antibodies when *Staphylococcus aureus* is the causative agent. Echocardiography may be useful diagnostically by defining valvular vegetations when these approach at least 2 mm in diameter and in detecting flail valvular leaflets, ruptured chordae tendineae, and regurgitant lesions.
- The major complications of infective endocarditis include progressive valvular dysfunction, congestive heart failure (CHF), embolic events, myocardial abscess formation that may extend into the conduction system producing conduction abnormalities, and mycotic aneurysm formation.
- Treatment includes 4 to 6 weeks of appropriate intravenous antibiotics, although shorter course regimens are advocated for some patients with certain, specific infections. Because culture results will not be available to the emergency physician, when endocarditis is suspected and there are signs of cardiac failure or systemic emboli, empirical treatment may need to be initiated. If the patient is not in failure or has no signs of embolization, empirical therapy may be delayed until multiple blood cultures have been obtained. The organisms and empirical treatment for infected

native valves differ from those of artificial valves. Native valves are frequently infected with *S. viridans,* enterococci, *S. aureus, Staphylococcus epidermidis* and the HACEK group (*Haemophilus, Actinobacillus, Cardiobacterium, Eikenella,* and *Kingella*), whereas prosthetic valves are infected by those same organisms plus Gram-negative aerobes. Empirical treatment for infected native valves includes vancomycin 15 mg/kg every 12 hours intravenous plus gentamicin 2 mg/kg loading dose followed by 1 mg/kg every 8 hours intravenous *or* nafcillin 2 g intravenous every 4 hours plus ampicillin 2 g intravenous every 4 hours plus gentamicin 2 mg/kg loading dose, then 1 mg/kg intravenous every 8 hours. Infected prosthetic valves may be treated with vancomycin 15 mg/kg intravenous every 12 hours (maximum dose of 1 g) plus gentamicin 2 mg/kg intravenous loading dose followed by 1 mg/kg every 8 hours, plus rifampin, 600 mg, orally daily.

Myasthenia Gravis

- Autoantibodies directed against the acetylcholine receptor are believed to be responsible for the clinical expression of myasthenia gravis. The bulbar muscles are predominantly affected; weakness in these muscles produces diplopia, facial weakness, and ptosis as well as difficulty with chewing, speaking, swallowing, and, in the most severe cases, breathing. Patients typically also report marked fatigue.
- Particularly when the condition is newly diagnosed, sudden respiratory insufficiency may occur. In these patients, parenteral neostigmine may be given in 1-mg increments over 1 minute up to 3 mg in 1 hour or until an adequate response is obtained. Assisted ventilation may become necessary and should be initiated as needed.
- Overtreatment with the cholinergic drugs (such as pyridostigmine) in some patients may precipitate a so-called **cholinergic crisis**; this is characterized by progressive or worsening weakness and may be difficult to differentiate from a true myasthenic crisis. In these patients, edrophonium, 10 mg intravenous (Tensilon test), may be used diagnostically and therapeutically and will improve muscle strength in patients with myasthenic crisis but will have no significant effect in those with cholinergic crisis. Myasthenia gravis patients with cholinergic crisis should be admitted to the hospital for respiratory care and observation.
- Less acutely ill patients are typically treated with pyridostigmine (0.6–1.5 g/day at adequately spaced intervals), thymectomy in patients younger than 60 years of age, and corticosteroids as needed (such as prednisone 50–100 mg daily).

Electrolyte Disturbances

Hyperkalemia

Hyperkalemia may occur in patients with renal failure, adrenal insufficiency, primary hypoaldosteronism, hemolysis, acidosis, trauma involving significant muscle destruction, and familial hyperkalemic periodic paralysis. Treatment with an aldosterone-antagonist diuretic, such as spironolactone or triamterene, may also elevate the serum potassium. **Spurious hyperkalemia** may be seen in patients with significant thrombocytosis or leukocytosis or in those with hemolysis induced by aspirating blood too rapidly through a small-caliber needle.

- Cardiac irritability and peripheral muscle weakness are the major clinical manifestations of hyperkalemia. Electrocardiographic (ECG) findings include peaking or "tenting" of the T waves (especially in the precordial leads), ST-segment depression, reduced R-wave amplitude, PR-segment prolongation, heart block, atrial asystole, sinoventricular rhythm, widening of the QRS complex, ventricular fibrillation, and asystole. Minor ST-T–wave changes are typically noted as the serum potassium level reaches 7 mEq/L, and ventricular fibrillation and asystole are noted when levels reach 9 to 10 mEq/L.

- Treatment depends on the extent of serum potassium elevation and the electrocardiogram.
  - Patients with **serum potassium levels in the range of 5.5 to 6.1 mEq/L** require only careful observation and elimination of any precipitating factor or factors.
  - **Patients** with **serum potassium levels in the range of 6.1 to 8.0 mEq/L** require continuous ECG monitoring and the institution of pharmacologic intervention. Potassium can be temporarily shifted into the cell, lowering serum levels, with one ampule of 50% dextrose, one ampule of sodium bicarbonate, and 10 U of regular insulin rapidly administered by intravenous push, as well as nebulized albuterol. Cation exchange resins such as oral sodium polystyrene sulfonate (Kayexalate), 20 g in 30 mL of 50% to 70% sorbitol reduce total body potassium. If the patient cannot tolerate oral intake, 50 g of Kayexalate in 200 mL of tap water should be administered as a retention enema. The oral dose may be repeated every 6 to 8 hours as needed, and the enema may be repeated as needed every 1 to 2 hours. Repeated treatments must of course be based on frequently determined serum potassium levels. Because sodium polystyrene sulfonate works by exchanging sodium for potassium, patients vulnerable to sodium-induced volume overload should be treated cautiously with this agent. The concomitant administration of intravenous furosemide (20 mg for patients not on furosemide or one third to one half of the daily oral dose for those chronically treated with this agent) may decrease the risk of volume overload.
  - Patients with **serum potassium levels greater than 8.0 mEq/L** must be aggressively treated both to eliminate immediately the untoward effects of hyperkalemia on the heart and to reduce total body potassium. In patients with serious cardiac arrhythmias, 10 mL of 10% calcium gluconate may be given intravenously over 2 to 5 minutes; continuous ECG monitoring is advised, and the dose may be repeated in 5 minutes as needed. Simultaneously with the administration of calcium, one ampule of 50% dextrose, one ampule of sodium bicarbonate, and 10 U of regular insulin may be rapidly administered by intravenous push. Because these maneuvers simply redistribute potassium and thereby fail to reduce total body stores, sodium polystyrene sulfonate should be administered, as well, as discussed. Hemodialysis may be required for some patients. Patients requiring intravenous calcium for the control of cardiac irritability in the context of hyperkalemia who are on a digitalis preparation must be cautiously monitored because the administration of calcium in this setting may precipitate digitalis toxicity.

Hypokalemia

Hypokalemia is most often associated with gastrointestinal losses, including vomiting, diarrhea, and nasogastric suctioning, as well as intentional or surreptitious diuretic use and as a result of a variety of hormonal disturbances, particularly mineralocorticoid excess (including steroid therapy).

- Muscle weakness is the most commonly reported clinical manifestation of hypokalemia; however, nausea, vomiting, emotional lability, and polydipsia may also be noted. Muscle weakness is associated with serum potassium levels in the range of 2.0 to 3.0 mEq/L and represents a total body deficit of approximately 300 mEq. Reduction of serum potassium to less than 2.0 mEq/L is associated with areflexia and flaccid paralysis, although in clinical practice such profound hypokalemia is unusual; a total body deficit of 500 mEq is present in these patients.

- Hypokalemia may elicit or enhance cardiac irritability, particularly in patients maintained on or intoxicated with a digitalis preparation, and it is in this context that the emergency replacement of potassium may become most crucial.
- **Treatment.** In patients with only modest depression of serum potassium, oral replacement alone will be adequate, and a variety of preparations are available for this purpose. When repletion of potassium is more urgently required, only the intravenous route should be used, and it is generally recommended that replacement not exceed 10 to 20 mEq/h. In extreme circumstances, 10 mEq of potassium chloride may be added to 50 mL of normal saline and administered intravenously over 10 to 15 minutes; this may be repeated as necessary, but should not exceed 40 mEq/h. Alternatively, 40 mEq may be added to 500 mL of normal saline or 5% D/W and administered more slowly, at a rate dictated by the patient's clinical status. In patients able to tolerate more fluid, supplemental potassium may be administered in a larger volume and given through a proximal or central intravenous catheter to reduce local discomfort and the incidence of subsequent chemical phlebitis. Potassium must be replaced more slowly in patients with renal insufficiency.

Hypernatremia

Hypernatremia may result from gastrointestinal, cutaneous, or renal free water losses, adrenal hormone excess, or lack of access to or inability to obtain free water. The development of diabetes insipidus after head injury or insult (such as pituitary neurosurgery) may also be associated with significant hypernatremia. Occasionally, the treatment of patients with osmotic agents, such as mannitol, may precipitate hypernatremia.

- Clinically, patients may present with subtle changes in mental status, confusion, lethargy, or coma. In many patients, symptoms and signs are more often related to severe volume depletion and include weakness, lassitude, fatigue, and, occasionally, frank hypovolemic shock.
  - **Treatment.** When resting or postural hypotension is present, repletion of intravascular volume is a first priority and is undertaken with isotonic saline at a rate determined by the patient's clinical condition. After repletion of intravascular volume with a return of normal hemodynamic and renal function, serum electrolytes are then determined and the deficit in free water corrected as outlined.
- Repletion of free water is based on the calculated body water deficit:

  Body water deficit = (0.6 × ideal body weight in kilograms) − ([0.6 × body weight in kilograms × 140]/the patient's serum sodium)

- The calculated body water deficit is that amount of free water required to restore the serum sodium to normal. Correcting the deficit too rapidly may result in cerebral edema, seizures, lethargy, and worsening of the patient's clinical condition. For this reason, we recommend replacing approximately one half of the total deficit over the initial 18 to 24 hours and administering the remainder over the subsequent 1 to 2 days. In patients with serum sodium levels greater than 160 mEq/L, such replacement should be accomplished intravenously using a solution of 5% D/W. Reassessment of serum electrolytes at 6-hour intervals is essential during the repletion process to ensure appropriate maintenance of total electrolyte balance.

Hyponatremia

Hyponatremia may be associated with states of normal, increased, or depleted total body water. The differential diagnosis of hyponatremia is extensive (Table 43-1). Artifactual hyponatremia may result from laboratory error, hyperlipemia, and

Table 43-1	Causes of Hyponatremia

Dehydration
Congestive heart failure
Cirrhosis
Nephrotic syndrome
Acute renal failure with oliguria
Adrenal insufficiency
Psychogenic polydipsia
Chronic renal failure
Inappropriate secretion of ADH
Hypothyroidism
Medications
  Narcotics
  Barbiturates
  Chlorpropamide (Diabinese)
  Tolbutamide (Orinase)
  Vincristine (Oncovin)
  Cyclophosphamide (Cytoxan)
  Thioridazine (Mellaril)
  Fluphenazine (Prolixin)
  Carbamazepine (Tegretol)
  Amitriptyline (Elavil)
  Thiothixene (Navane)
  Many diuretics
Artifactual hyponatremia (see text)

hyperproteinemia. Finally, the presence of additional solute within the intravascular space may lower the measured serum sodium; this is seen most commonly in patients treated with mannitol or in those with hyperglycemia—serum sodium decreases 5 mEq/L for each 180 mg/dL increase in the serum glucose.

- The clinical manifestations of hyponatremia include mental status changes such as restlessness, irritability, and confusion (occurring when the serum level approaches 120 mEq/L), with seizures and coma evolving as the serum level approaches 110 mEq/L. Although mild hyponatremia is frequently noted in patients seen in the emergency department, particularly those taking diuretics, it is infrequently associated with symptoms and does not usually require emergent intervention. Patients with significant or symptomatic hyponatremia, in whom the cause is not apparent, require a thorough evaluation to determine the cause.

- **Treatment.** In most patients, correction of hyponatremia should be gradual so as to avoid both acute volume overload and/or **central pontine myelinolysis.** If mild symptoms and only a moderate deficit of sodium exist, normal saline may be used for replacement; 3% saline is advised for patients with more significant symptoms or severe deficits and may be administered as 75 to 100 mL/h for 2 to 4 hours, during which time serum electrolytes should be checked hourly. The infusion is discontinued when the serum sodium level reaches 120 mEq/L. For **dilutional hyponatremia associated with inappropriate antidiuretic hormone (ADH) secretion** (SIADH),

Table 43-2	Common Causes of Hypercalcemia

Primary hyperparathyroidism
Secondary hyperparathyroidism
Neoplastic disorders: especially multiple myeloma and breast cancer
Sarcoidosis
Milk-alkali syndrome
Vitamin D intoxication
Adrenal insufficiency
Hyperthyroidism
Immobilization (particularly in the elderly)
Thiazide diuretic use

water restriction is essential and is the treatment of choice; in addition, furosemide and normal saline may be used in conjunction to promote free water excretion. In more refractory, chronic cases of SIADH, demeclocycline (300–600 mg twice daily) has proved effective in promoting a free water diuresis. The **edematous patient** with hyponatremia must be treated with water restriction and interventions that improve renal perfusion; these vary depending on the cause (e.g., afterload reduction in patients with CHF, bed rest in patients with cirrhosis). The use of hypertonic saline in these patients is not advised.

Hypercalcemia
Some common causes of hypercalcemia are listed in Table 43-2.
- Clinically, polyuria, polydipsia, nausea, vomiting, and anorexia are noted with mild to moderate elevation of the serum calcium level. A variety of neurologic symptoms are noted as well, including **proximal muscle weakness,** abnormalities of memory and cognition, depression, changes in personality, emotional lability, and muscle fasciculations; in extreme cases, coma ensues. A shortened corrected QT interval is noted on the electrocardiogram in some patients.
- Treatment should be directed toward the underlying cause; however, the initial emergency management of severe or significantly symptomatic hypercalcemia, regardless of cause, remains the same. Restoration and expansion of the intravascular volume with isotonic saline and the concomitant administration of furosemide will induce a calcium diuresis caused by the coupling of sodium and calcium excretion at the proximal tubule. Mithramycin, steroids, calcitonin, and indomethacin have also been used in selected patients with variable results.

Hypocalcemia
Hypocalcemia may be associated with hypoparathyroidism, hyperphosphatemia, the malabsorptive states, hypomagnesemia, chronic renal failure, renal tubular acidosis, malnutrition, acute pancreatitis, and vitamin D resistance or deficiency (Table 43-3). In addition, hypoalbuminemia produces a reduction in the measured serum calcium, although the corrected ionized serum calcium may be normal and patients are asymptomatic. Hypocalcemia in the setting of hypomagnesemia (i.e., serum magnesium <1 mEq/L) is related to a reduction in parathyroid hormone secretion and a reduced effectiveness at the kidney.

Table 43-3	Common Causes of Hypocalcemia

Hypoparathyroidism
Hyperphosphatemia
Malabsorptive states
Hypomagnesemia
Chronic renal failure
Renal tubular acidosis
Malnutrition
Acute pancreatitis
Vitamin D resistance or deficiency
Hypoalbuminemia (see text)

- Clinically, patients with hypocalcemia may report distal extremity numbness and tingling; latent tetany may be demonstrated with Chvostek sign (twitching of the perioral or perinasal muscles in response to gentle tapping over the facial nerve) or Trousseau's sign (the elicitation of carpal spasm after 3 minutes of ischemia produced by inflating a tourniquet above systolic pressure on the upper extremity. The ECG may demonstrate a prolonged corrected QT interval in some patients (Table 43-4). In all patients with hypocalcemia, serum albumin, magnesium, phosphate, creatinine, BUN, vitamin D, electrolytes, and amylase should be determined.
- Treatment depends on the specific cause; however, patients with severe or symptomatic hypocalcemia require intravenous calcium. Calcium gluconate may be added to 5% D/W and given intravenously at 0.01 to 0.5 mL/kg/h. Urgent replacement can be accomplished with 20 to 30 mL of 10% calcium gluconate intravenous given over 10 to 15 minutes, followed by a continuous infusion as described above. In patients with severe coexistent magnesium deficiency, which may contribute to hypocalcemia, 2 mEq/kg of magnesium sulfate may be administered in 5% D/W over 6 to 8 hours. Less severe deficiencies of this ion may be treated with oral magnesium supplementation as magnesium oxide, 250 to 500 mg two to four times daily.

Adrenal Insufficiency

- Acute adrenal insufficiency or Addisonian crisis may be seen in patients with undiagnosed adrenal or pituitary insufficiency, in those with inadequately treated adrenal insufficiency, or as a result of acute adrenal destruction from overwhelming sepsis or massive intra-adrenal hemorrhage in association with anticoagulant therapy. Carcinomatous involvement of the adrenal gland, usually secondary to breast or ovarian cancer, remains an additional cause. More commonly, patients maintained on chronic steroid therapy with or without a prior diagnosis of adrenal or pituitary insufficiency present acutely with adrenal crisis; crises typically occur at times of stress or concurrent systemic illness. It must be emphasized that the diagnosis of adrenal insufficiency is a clinical one; **treatment must be initiated in virtually all patients before laboratory confirmation of a reduced serum cortisol level.**
- Patients with adrenal insufficiency present with nausea and vomiting, abdominal pain, weakness, fever, and often-severe dehydration; shock is present in approximately 25% of patients. Hyperpigmentation of the skin and mucous membranes (especially

Table 43-4	ECG Changes Caused by Electrolyte Disturbances					
Imbalance	P Wave	PR Interval	QRS	ST Segment	T Wave	QT Interval
Hyponatremia (20% deficit)			Duration and voltage increased	Displaced opposite to QRS	Morphology opposite to QRS	Shortened
Hypernatremia			Duration and voltage decreased			Lengthened
Hypopotassemia 3–3.5 mEq/L	Increased duration and voltage	Negative displacement	Increased voltage	Negative displacement	Increased low duration, amplitude	
2 mEq/L					Increased duration Morphology: negative or positive with straight rising limb	Shortened
5–7 mEq/L		Incomplete AV block	Over 0.12 s, decreased voltage		Decreased duration Morphology: tall and peaked T more prominent in V_1 than normally	
Hypocalcemia				Duration lengthened	Peaked or negative in precordial leads Duration diminished	Lengthened
Hypercalcemia				Duration shortened	Decreased or normal duration	Shortened

AV, atrioventricular.

about the joints and bite line of the oral mucosa) may be noted in patients with primary adrenal failure; this is due to increased levels of adrenocorticotropic hormone and melanocyte-stimulating hormone. Much more common, however, are patients with *secondary* adrenal suppression or failure; these patients fail to manifest hyperpigmentation. In addition, signs of Cushing syndrome may be noted in patients maintained on chronic steroid therapy. Although the mental status is variable, lethargy is common at presentation. Importantly, in patients with adrenal insufficiency in the context of chronic steroid use, substantial mineralocorticoid function may be preserved, and consequently, it is not surprising that dehydration and hypotension are less common and less severe.

- **Hyponatremia, hyperkalemia, hypoglycemia, and eosinophilia** may be noted on laboratory analysis and should suggest the diagnosis of adrenal insufficiency when other signs are present. Blood should be obtained for routine studies including a CBC, and measurement of BUN, blood sugar, electrolytes, serum cortisol, and thyroid-stimulating hormone levels.

  - **Treatment.** Patients with hypotension obviously require isotonic fluid replacement with 5% dextrose in normal saline. Dextrose (glucose) should be administered with saline because hypoglycemia frequently coexists at presentation and, with volume replacement and correction of acidosis, intracellular movement of glucose occurs; additionally, oral intake may initially be restricted secondary to nausea, vomiting, or lethargy.

  - In addition, intracellular potassium movement accompanies glucose transport and may lead to hypokalemia as volume repletion occurs; when it is determined that renal function is normal, potassium may be added to the infusion.

  - Corticosteroid therapy of patients with acute adrenal insufficiency should include the immediate administration of hydrocortisone (Solu-Cortef), 100 mg intravenous and a continuous infusion of hydrocortisone, providing 200 mg over 24 hours, should be instituted. The long-term management of any acute crisis will involve the identification and treatment of any precipitating factors, the institution of oral glucocorticoid therapy, and if indicated, mineralocorticoid therapy as well, once resumption of oral intake occurs.

Polymyositis and Dermatomyositis

- Patients with the related autoimmune disorders of polymyositis and dermatomyositis present with several weeks to months of progressive, **symmetric proximal muscle weakness.** Maneuvers stressing these muscle groups, such as climbing stairs, combing the hair, or rising from a chair, become difficult early in the course of these illnesses and are often spontaneously described by the patient as increasing problems. Some patients will also report that activities requiring a sustained head position are difficult; weakness of pharyngeal muscles may produce abnormalities of swallowing. In addition to these symptoms, patients with dermatomyositis also report a rash, which may occur either before or after the development of muscle weakness.

- Weakness of the neck, shoulder girdle, and proximal hip muscles is noted. Mild tenderness to palpation is reported in some patients, and deep tendon reflexes are occasionally slightly reduced. In dermatomyositis, a heliotropic rash (lilac or violaceous discoloration of the skin of the eyelids, nasal bridge, and forehead) may be noted, as are Gottron papules (extensor surface skin nodules overlying the interphalangeal joints of the hands).

- The diagnosis of polymyositis or dermatomyositis is confirmed on the basis of an elevated serum creatine phosphokinase and aldolase, an abnormal muscle biopsy, and an abnormal electromyographic study. The ESR is not particularly helpful because it may be either elevated or normal; when significantly elevated, the diagnosis of polymyalgia rheumatica should be considered.
- Treatment includes steroids, nonsteroidal antiinflammatory agents, and physical therapy. Because approximately 10% of patients with polymyositis or dermatomyositis develop these disorders as paraneoplastic phenomena, an evaluation for an occult malignancy should be instituted in all patients.

Temporal Arteritis and Polymyalgia Rheumatica

- The rheumatologic disorders of temporal arteritis and polymyalgic rheumatica commonly coexist (~30% of patients with temporal arteritis develop polymyalgia rheumatica, and vice versa) and virtually always affect patients older than 50 years of age.
- Patients with **temporal arteritis** complain of a unilateral, throbbing headache, local skin tenderness or hypersensitivity, a variety of visual symptoms, jaw claudication, and generalized fatigue, often with fever. Loss of temporal artery pulsations, focal thickening, and local tenderness may be noted on physical examination. A markedly elevated ESR is noted in most patients, often approaching 100 mm/h. Because temporal artery biopsy is both diagnostic and relatively benign, and because the risk of sudden, **irreversible blindness** from ophthalmic artery involvement is unpredictable, emergency surgical consultation for biopsy should be obtained when this diagnosis is suspected and intravenous corticosteroids (methylprednisolone 1000 mg IV) administered immediately, which will not affect the results of temporal artery biopsy if the biopsy is promptly undertaken. The initial dose of steroid is followed by oral therapy with 60 mg/day of prednisone, slowly tapering over several months. Alternate-day steroids are not effective treatment for patients with this disorder.
- **Polymyalgia rheumatica** often develops abruptly, more commonly in women than in men. Pain and stiffness of the pelvis and shoulder girdle in association with fever, malaise, and weight loss are noted. A markedly elevated ESR and anemia may be seen as well; these patients also respond to corticosteroids, which should be initiated as 40 mg/day of prednisone, slowly tapering over several months. Alternate-day steroids are not effective in this illness. Electromyography, serum muscle enzymes, and muscle biopsy are normal.
- In **both temporal arteritis and polymyalgia rheumatica,** continued therapy is predicated on the ESR and the patient's symptoms. Once the ESR has reached the normal range, blindness rarely occurs. Therapy may be discontinued once disease activity subsides, usually after 9 to 18 months.

PART 9

Musculoskeletal and Soft-Tissue Disorders

44 Abscesses

GENERAL CONSIDERATIONS

Cutaneous abscesses requiring drainage are commonly encountered in the emergency department and are best treated with routine incision and drainage. Antibiotic therapy alone is an inadequate treatment strategy. Frequent errors include
- Making an inadequate incision for complete initial or continued drainage
- Failing to stress the need for 24- to 48-hour follow-up in patients with significant abscesses requiring drain replacement and reassessment
- Failing to institute antibiotic treatment or recommend hospital admission in patients with significant cellulitis, systemic evidence of infection, or compromise of the immune system (including diabetes mellitus)

Local cutaneous infection without fluctuance will not benefit from incision and drainage, and this presentation is common. Although local induration and pain with palpation are expected along with other signs of infection, true fluctuance or the perception that free pus is contained within the tissues is not present in this group of patients. These patients should be instructed to apply heat to the area four to six times per day, receive an appropriate antistaphylococcal antibiotic such as dicloxacillin or cephalexin, and be reevaluated in 24 to 48 hours; patients should be told that at that time the abscess may be ready for incision and drainage. Consideration should be given to antibiotic coverage against the emerging community-acquired methicillin-resistant Staphylococcus aureus, such as TMP/sulfa, but only if antibiotics are indicated. We have divided our discussion into nonfacial and facial abscesses because of important differences in the approach to these two groups of patients.

NONFACIAL ABSCESS

Our approach to patients with fluctuant, nonfacial abscesses is as follows:
- The area overlying and surrounding the abscess is prepared with povidone-iodine (Betadine) and draped in the usual fashion.

- Systemic analgesia may be considered, given the poor efficacy of local anesthesia in the acidic medium of the purulent cavity.
- Local anesthesia may be provided in a number of ways depending on the size and depth of the abscess and the depth of tissue through which one must incise. *Large abscesses* that will require some exploration to lyse internal adhesions or loculations are best treated with circumferential field anesthesia. This is performed with 1% lidocaine instilled first superficially and proximally and to the approximate presumed depth of the abscess. Moving circumferentially around the area in a similar manner, a field of anesthetic agent that isolates the area of involvement is laid down. It is important to remember that field anesthesia may require 5 to 10 minutes for the area to become anesthetized. *Small- to moderate-sized abscesses* are adequately anesthetized simply by directly instilling the anesthetic agent along the tract to be incised.
- Actual incision should proceed along normal skin lines to minimize subsequent scar formation; abscesses occurring in cosmetically significant locations are discussed in "Facial Abscesses." The incision should be of adequate length to allow exploration and disruption of any loculations or adhesions within the abscess cavity and to allow initial and, just as importantly, subsequent drainage of the abscess over the next several days.
- After incision, as much purulent material should be removed as possible, and, in patients with evidence of systemic infection, significant surrounding cellulitis, or abnormalities of immune function, aerobic and anaerobic cultures and sensitivity should be obtained.
- When deep abscesses (which have a tendency to close prematurely) occur in cosmetically *insignificant* locations, a small wedge of tissue may be excised along the line of incision to facilitate drainage over the subsequent 3 to 7 days; this is particularly helpful in the patient who is unlikely to seek follow-up or unlikely or unable to comply with posttreatment instructions regarding the regular opening and soaking of the abscess.
- Iodoform gauze or a Penrose drain of sufficient size should be inserted through the incision to separate the wound edges and thereby allow further drainage of the abscess; if premature closure of the skin occurs, reaccumulation of the abscess is inevitable.
- Patients who appear systemically ill with high fever or rigors, those with extensive abscesses (usually involving the perianal area), or those with AIDS, diabetes, or other abnormalities of immune function should be considered candidates for hospital admission and surgical consultation; an appropriate antistaphylococcal antibiotic should be instituted early and intravenously.
- Follow-up is somewhat dependent on the size and location of the abscess, the adequacy of drainage, whether significant surrounding cellulitis or high fever is present, and the anticipated compliance of the patient. Patients with large or deep abscesses, those with significant surrounding cellulitis or fever, and those in whom compliance with respect to drain removal, opening of the skin, and soaks remains questionable should be seen in 24 hours for drain removal or replacement and reevaluation; patients with perianal or perineal abscesses, which are often large, should generally be reexamined at this time as well because drain replacement will often be required. Patients who do not require hospital admission but have modest surrounding cellulitis or low-grade fever may be treated with an appropriate antibiotic for 3 to 5 days.

Patients with relatively small abscesses that are adequately drained and in whom surrounding cellulitis and evidence of systemic infection are minimal and absent, respectively, may be instructed to remove the drain in 24 hours and, thereafter, to open the skin manually, express any purulent or bloody material, and soak the wound for 15 to 20 minutes at 4- to 6-hour intervals. A dry, sterile dressing should be applied to the wound after incision and after each soaking. Patients should be told that this routine must be continued for 4 to 7 days, after which time the aggressiveness of opening the abscess may be reduced, provided resolution is progressing. An appropriate analgesic should be provided to patients for 24 to 36 hours if needed.

FACIAL ABSCESSES

In patients with cosmetically significant, large facial abscesses, we generally suggest plastic surgical consultation, since definitive incision and drainage will be required; needle aspiration may be undertaken and may be effective in patients with minor but fluctuant collections. When obvious fluctuance is not present, which is common on the face, an appropriate antibiotic, such as dicloxacillin or cephalexin and/or TMP/sulfa, and the application of heat at 4-hour intervals are recommended and will usually result in resolution. When fluctuance is present and needle aspiration is elected, after the area is prepared, an 18- or 16-gauge needle should be used to enter the abscess cavity and any purulent material aspirated and sent for culture and sensitivity; an appropriate antistaphylococcal antibiotic should be instituted in high doses, and the application of heat every 4 hours for 15 to 20 minutes emphasized. Patients should be advised that formal incision may be required in 24 to 48 hours, and surgical follow-up at that time is advised. Given the risk of suppurative, cavernous or other venous sinus thrombophlebitis in the brain, facial cellulitis or abscesses involving the general area of the nose and orbit require aggressive treatment; this includes a lowered threshold for surgical consultation, hospital admission, and intravenous antibiotics.

45 Back Pain

Patients presenting with back pain following trivial or unrecalled trauma are considered here, along with a variety of nontraumatic etiologies. This chapter does not include spinal cord injuries or fractures of the spine.

COMMON CAUSES OF BACK PAIN

- Musculoligamentous strain or sprain*
- Ruptured or herniated intervertebral disk*
- Osteoarthritis of the spine*
- Renal or ureteral colic*
- Pleural-based posterior pneumonitis*
- Pleurodynia*
- Rib fracture*

LESS COMMON CAUSES OF BACK PAIN NOT TO BE MISSED

- Pneumothorax*
- Leaking abdominal aortic aneurysm*
- Aortic dissection*
- Pulmonary embolism*
- Pyelonephritis*

OTHER CAUSES OF BACK PAIN

- Herpes zoster*
- Pancreatitis
- Cholecystitis
- Penetrating duodenal ulcer
- Malignancy*
- Metabolic bone disease*
- Spinal stenosis*
- Vertebral osteomyelitis*
- Epidural abscess

---

*Discussed in this chapter.

HISTORICAL FEATURES

Historical features that may be helpful in the differentiation of the various causes of back pain include the following:

- **Musculoskeletal pain** usually begins suddenly and in clear relation to physical exertion (e.g., bending, lifting, climbing), is not pleuritic, and is reproduced by activities or maneuvers that stress the particular area.
- The sudden onset of back or thoracic discomfort made worse by inspiration and associated with shortness of breath suggests **pleurodynia, pneumothorax,** or **pulmonary embolism**; these diagnoses must be excluded in all such patients. Pleural-based **pneumonia** is also suggested by these symptoms, and many such patients also report fever, chills, cough, and sputum production. Predisposing factors for the development of thromboembolic disease should be investigated, and if present, the possibility of **pulmonary embolism** should be considered. It is important to note that, since the kidney normally descends during inspiration, patients with **pyelonephritis, perinephric abscess,** or **renal or ureteral colic** frequently report a pleuritic component to their discomfort.
- A prior history of dysuria, frequency, fever, and chills further suggests the diagnosis of **pyelonephritis**. Back pain that radiates or is vaguely referred to the lower abdomen, testicle, or labia is commonly noted in patients with ureteral colic.
- **Herpes zoster** (shingles), when involving the thoracic or lumbar spinal nerve roots, may produce a number of puzzling back symptoms, even before the development of any rash. Patients may complain of a severe, often lancinating pain, usually beginning in the back and radiating anteriorly, frequently along the course of a rib. Patients without an initial rash will, within several days, develop first erythema and papules, and eventually typical vesicles in the affected distribution.

Frequently, considerable confusion occurs as to whether a patient's pain is truly pleuritic in nature. If so, a number of diagnostic possibilities gain importance. Much of the thoracic and periscapular musculature is involved in deep inspiration; certainly, such muscle groups, if injured or inflamed, will produce discomfort during inspiration and may prompt a designation of such pain as "pleuritic." Such a designation, although technically correct, is diagnostically misleading unless efforts are made to separate pulmonary from extrapulmonary etiologies of pleuritic pain. In addition, most activities requiring some degree of minimal effort, such as sitting up or bending over, are preceded by an inspiratory effort; this fact becomes extremely important both historically and during the examination of the patient in differentiating movement- or posture-related muscular pain from potentially more significant causes of genuine pulmonary, pleuritic discomfort.

PHYSICAL EXAMINATION

- Pain that can be reproduced or increases during quiet, slow inspiration should be considered pulmonary (and occasionally renal) unless proved otherwise.
- Local tenderness with palpation and coarse crepitus auscultated on inspiration over a rib suggests **rib fracture**.
- In the patient with **pneumothorax**, breath sounds may be normal, reduced, or absent.
- Tenderness with percussion over the renal area suggests **pyelonephritis, perinephric abscess, or renal or ureteral colic.**

Table 45-1		Symptoms and Signs of Lower Back Disk Herniation			
Interspace	Nerve	Pain/ Paresthesia	Motor Loss	Sensory Loss	Reflex Loss
L3-4	L4	Anterior thigh, inner shin	Quadriceps	Anterome- dial thigh down to inner shin	Knee jerk
L4-5	L5	Outer side of back of thigh, outer calf, dorsum of foot to first toe	Extensor hallucis longus	Outer side of calf and first toe	None
L5-S1	S1	Back of thigh to foot and lateral toes	Gastrocne- mius	Outer side of calf, lateral foot and toes	Ankle jerk

- Rales may be appreciated in patients with **pneumonitis, pleurodynia, and pulmonary embolism;** evidence of consolidation suggests pneumonia. A pleural friction rub may be heard in patients with any of these complaints.
- Calf tenderness or swelling should be sought and if present, in association with pleuritic back pain, makes the diagnosis of **pulmonary embolism** likely. It is important to remember, however, that calf swelling or tenderness is noted in no more than 40% of patients with pulmonary embolism.
- A rash may indicate **herpes zoster** infection, although, as noted, symptoms may precede the rash by several days. Skin hypersensitivity along the suspected dermatome or a subjective difference in sensitivity when sides are compared is suggestive of this diagnosis. In patients with evolving herpes zoster, initial erythema is followed by the development of typical papules and vesicles.
- Localized muscle spasm and occasional tenderness are found in patients with **muscular injury,** sprain, and disk injury.
- If lower extremity reflexes are focally and unilaterally absent or decreased, potentially serious root injury is suggested, and subspecialty consultation should be considered. Abnormalities of sensation may be determined and may provide evidence for a specific nerve root syndrome as well (Table 45-1). Passive straight-leg raising with the knee extended places traction on the lumbosacral roots and may increase back discomfort in patients with root compression syndromes. The specificity of the straight-leg-raising test is enhanced if the lumbosacral discomfort occurs on the side *opposite* the raised leg (the so-called crossed-leg-raising test).
- A careful abdominal examination should be performed to exclude primary abdominal disorders associated with referred discomfort to the back (see Chapter 26).

DIAGNOSTIC TESTS

Chest X-Ray

An upright, end-expiratory chest x-ray excludes the diagnosis of pneumothorax. Aortic widening, as well as evidence of consolidation, will be noted in patients with thoracic aortic dissection and lobar pneumonitis, respectively.

Lumbosacral Spine X-Rays

Indications for lumbosacral spine x-rays include
- Significant motor vehicle or industrial accidents or other trauma
- Those with neurological deficits
- Extremes of age
- Those with significant comorbities such as prostate cancer

In the older patient with major back complaints, it is important to demonstrate radiologically normal bony architecture and thus exclude malignant or severe degenerative processes involving the spine.

Chest CT Angiogram/VQ Scan

Unfortunately, measurements of oxygen saturation by pulse oximetry or arterial blood gases are not particularly helpful in the diagnosis of pulmonary embolism; similarly, the chest x-ray and electrocardiographic findings are nonspecific and insensitive in pulmonary embolism. Most authorities agree that the diagnosis of pulmonary embolism, in the absence of pulmonary angiography, can be excluded in only the following settings: the physician's level of clinical suspicion is low *plus* a negative CT angiogram of the chest (if the patient's renal function is enough to handle an IV contrast dye load) or a completely normal (not low-probability) lung scan is obtained.

Urinalysis

A clean-voided urine specimen for urinalysis will demonstrate hematuria in most patients with renal or ureteral colic; patients with pyelonephritis have pyuria as well.

SPECIFIC DISORDERS

Musculoligamentous Strain or Sprain

Muscular strains and minor ligamentous sprains are among the most common complaints in emergency medicine. These injuries may occur in relation to an unusual period of strenuous activity, an episode of lifting, prolonged sitting in a single position, or sudden deceleration, or they may occur totally unrelated to any such events or activity. Musculoligamentous strains are common in the industrial population, and many patients report multiple prior episodes.

Clinical Presentation
Diagnosis is based on the patient's history and relative confinement of discomfort to the back, usually the lower lumbar area, with occasional referral to the buttocks or proximal thighs. Muscle spasm may be prominent and may be palpable in the affected area. Stressing the particular area may accentuate the patient's discomfort and is diagnostically important to demonstrate. Examination of sensory and motor function in the lower extremities should be undertaken; these functions are expected to be normal in patients with simple strain or sprain.

Diagnostic Tests
Depending on the nature of the patient's injury, lumbosacral spine x-rays may be indicated. Radiologic confirmation of normal bony architecture is generally recommended in the following patients:
- Patients who are elderly, generally over 70
- Patients over 55 who have minor injuries
- Patients with osteoporosis
- Those extremely symptomatic

- Those who present after significant industrial or motor vehicle accidents or other major trauma.
- Those on chronic steroid therapy

Treatment

Treatment involves providing symptomatic relief given the generally self-limited nature of most musculoligamentous injuries of the back:

- A short period of activity limitations, to include limits on bending or lifting, usually 1 to 3 days
- Sleeping on a firm mattress
- Local heat may be beneficial.
- An appropriate analgesic based on symptoms; NSAIDS are generally prescribed; an abbreviated course of narcotic analgesics may be appropriate for severe pain.
- Muscle relaxants when evidence of spasm is present are currently recommended.
- Slight flexion of the hip with the patient supine will often substantially relieve spasm-related discomfort; this may be accomplished simply by placing one or two pillows under the patient's knees.

Follow-up

Follow-up should be recommended at approximately 5 to 7 days; the patient should be instructed to seek care earlier should bowel or bladder dysfunction or leg weakness or numbness develop.

Ruptured or Herniated Intervertebral Disk

Patients with ruptured intervertebral disks may present acutely with the sudden onset of severe back and/or leg pain or chronically after several days, weeks, or months of symptoms. Most often no injury is recalled; however, occasional patients will note the onset of symptoms after minor trauma or a particular maneuver.

Herniations most often occur at the level of L5-S1, L4-5, or L3-4 and produce, in addition to local back pain, radicular symptoms involving the S1, L5, and L4 nerve roots, respectively. Posterior degeneration of the annulus fibrosis allows either protrusion or actual expulsion of disk material posteriorly, thereby compressing nearby spinal roots. In addition to back and leg pain, which may be excruciating, many patients report paresthesias, involuntary spasms, twitching, and fasciculations in the involved area. Both hypersensitivity and hyposensitivity may be demonstrated during the sensory examination.

Clinical Presentation

Diagnosis is based on the history and evidence of particular nerve root dysfunction:

- Patients with **S1 compression** or irritation from L5-S1 herniation most often report back, posterior thigh and calf, and plantar foot discomfort; pain or dysesthesias may be referred to the fifth toe. The ankle jerk may be depressed, and weakness, if present, involves plantar flexion of the foot and toes.
- Patients with **L5 compression** secondary to L4-5 disk disruptions produce back, lateral thigh and calf, dorsal foot, and first or second toe discomfort. In addition, weakness may be demonstrated in the dorsiflexors of the foot and toes.
- Patients with **L4 compression** secondary to L3-4 disk disruptions produce quadriceps weakness and a depressed knee jerk.

Diagnostic Tests

Plain films of the lumbar spine are generally indicated in patients with radicular symptoms, and although such films are usually normal, narrowing of the involved interspace may be noted. Although the definitive diagnosis is made by computed tomography (CT) or magnetic resonance imaging (MRI), these studies are not indicated acutely unless motor loss is significant or progressive.

Treatment
Treatment depends on the patient's symptoms and the presence or absence of weakness.
• Some patients require admission to the hospital for treatment. These include patients with
  • An inability to cope at home due to environmental reasons, social reasons, or pain unrelieved by oral medications
  • Severe or worsening neurologic deficits
  • Cauda equina syndrome
    The **cauda equina syndrome** is uncommon but can be the result of a large, midline disk herniation at the L4-5 or L5-S1 level. In addition to radicular pain, the patient experiences back pain, perianal pain, overflow urinary incontinence, impotence, and numbness of the feet and perianal area. Frequently, the anal and bulbocavernosus reflexes are lost. This is a potential surgical emergency in which prompt decompression can reverse the neurologic loss, maintain bladder tone, and reverse paresis. The definitive diagnosis is made by MRI, CT scanning, or myelography.
• **Outpatient therapy** involves a short period of limitation of activities, usually 1 to 3 days, local heat, and analgesics. Most patients will benefit symptomatically from flexion of the hip on the involved side; this is most easily accomplished by placing one or two pillows under the knee and thigh. Many physicians prescribe muscle relaxants, although we have not found these to be particularly useful. A short course of a nonsteroidal anti-inflammatory agent such as ibuprofen is often helpful. A short course of narcotic analgesics may be necessary.

Follow-up
Early follow-up is essential, as are instructions to seek care promptly should bowel or bladder dysfunction or significant weakness develop.

Osteoarthritis of the Spine

Osteoarthritis may involve the lumbar spine, may produce significant pain and stiffness in the involved area, and may infrequently be associated with spinal root, cauda equina, or actual spinal cord compression if appreciable stenosis of the spinal column develops.

History
Most patients are middle-aged or elderly and have had symptoms for days or weeks, although many patients will relate the onset of symptoms to a particular recent activity or injury.

Diagnostic Tests
It is well recognized that symptoms in patients with osteoarthritis bear little relationship to the radiologic appearance of the spine. Many patients will be totally asymptomatic despite extensive radiologic evidence of disease, while other patients will report severe, disabling symptoms with only minimal observable changes. Thus, a causal relationship between radiologically demonstrated osteoarthritis and acute back pain is often unjustified. In fact, many patients with back pain and radiologic evidence of degenerative changes will be found to have simple musculoligamentous injuries.

Treatment

A short course of activity limitation and local heat are generally sufficient in most patients. Analgesics may be necessary and helpful in some patients, and a course of a nonsteroidal anti-inflammatory agent such as ibuprofen is recommended. A short course of narcotic analgesics may be necessary.

Renal or Ureteral Colic

Clinical Presentation

The classic patient with renal or ureteral colic presents acutely to the emergency department with severe, unilateral back or abdominal pain (or both), often associated with severe nausea and vomiting, with pain often radiating to the ipsilateral lower quadrant, testicle, or labia. Patients are extremely uncomfortable, restless, often agitated, appear unable to find a comfortable position on the stretcher, and may be both pale and diaphoretic. Tenderness over the involved kidney or asymmetry with percussion may or may not be noted; abdominal discomfort is commonly demonstrated and may be impressive, but signs of peritoneal inflammation are not generally present (rebound tenderness, guarding). Hematuria is usually present, which may be gross or microscopic. The testes should be examined to exclude torsion, infection, or inguinal hernia. In women, a pelvic exam in conjunction with HCG determination should be performed to exclude pelvic infection, ovarian torsion, or ectopic pregnancy. CT scan without contrast has become the imaging study of choice not only for its ability to diagnose stones in the genitourinary tract but also for its ability to rule out other diagnoses that may mimic renal colic, most importantly abdominal aortic aneurysm. Ultrasound is the initial imaging of choice in the pregnant patient.

Unfortunately, a number of variations in this classic scenario make the diagnosis of renal or ureteral colic difficult in many patients. For example, referred pain to the testicle or labia is often absent. Vomiting may completely dominate the initial presentation and may be associated with severe abdominal and little or no back pain. Abdominal symptoms and findings may simulate other disorders associated with biliary, peptic ulcer, appendiceal, or gynecologic problems; many patients will have convincing abdominal tenderness on examination particularly in areas overlying the obstructed or distended ureter. Ten percent of stones are radiolucent and therefore will not be seen on routine abdominal x-rays. In addition, some patients will not volunteer information relating to testicular or vulvar pain; this is perhaps partly a function of the relatively less severe discomfort in these areas as well as the tendency of these symptoms to be both poorly localized and not reproducible by palpation.

The diagnosis of renal or ureteral colic thus requires a very high degree of suspicion and a knowledge of the classic and unusual clinical presentations. Two features that deserve mention and often provide an initial clue to the diagnosis are the presence of severe diaphoresis and restlessness. By history, patients report that when the pain was severe, they were unable to find a comfortable position or "walked the floors"—very much unlike the patient with peritoneal irritation who lies still. In addition, one often finds that the patient is extremely diaphoretic, anxiously pacing about the examining room awaiting the arrival of the physician, or moving about on the stretcher. These observations have proved to be somewhat unique and are therefore important diagnostic clues in the patient with other, less classic symptoms.

Treatment

Pain Control

In most patients, the diagnosis of renal or ureteral stones is clinical and is most often based on the patient's history, examination, and a urine dipstick that demonstrates hematuria; pain relief should not be delayed pending absolute confirmation of the diagnosis. Most patients will require narcotic analgesics such as hydromorphone 1 mg IV or IM with antiemetics as needed for nausea and/or vomiting. Ketorolac, 30 mg, IV, or 30 to 60 mg IM can be given concurrently and is often helpful. No clear benefit to IV fluids has been shown although it may be helpful in patients with enough vomiting to create dehydration.

Admission

Admission is generally considered for the following patients:

• Patients with severe or persistent pain or vomiting despite treatment
• Patients with severe and persistent symptoms in whom a definitive clinical diagnosis of renal or ureteral colic cannot be made
• Patients with infection and ureteral obstruction (emergent urological consultation recommended)
• Patients with a solitary obstructed kidney
• Patients who are significantly dehydrated secondary to persistent vomiting
• Patients with urinary extravasation
• Lower threshold for patients with large stones unlikely to pass spontaneously (>6 mm), renal insufficiency, high-grade obstruction, intrinsic renal disease, significant comorbidities

Out-Patient Treatment

Patients not considered as being in one of the admission categories described may be discharged with instructions to return to the ED if fever, persistent vomiting, or increasing pain unrelieved with discharge medications is noted. Patients should be prescribed analgesics for 2 to 3 days and instructed to strain the urine and retain any passed stones for analysis. Oral hydration is advised. Patients who pass a stone in the ED require no specific treatment other than follow-up with their primary care physician. Frequently, both in patients with a clinical diagnosis of ureteral stone and in patients with radiographically demonstrated stones, symptoms suddenly disappear. Unfortunately, it cannot be concluded in such patients that passage of the stone into the urinary bladder has occurred. Resolution of pain may reflect analgesic therapy or changes in location or orientation of the stone such that spasm or obstruction is eliminated. Patients should be advised that symptoms may recur and that final passage of the stone may be uncomfortable. A majority of stones greater than 6 mm are unlikely to pass spontaneously and may need mechanical removal, making follow-up with a urologist important. Urologic follow-up is suggested even in the asymptomatic patient to ensure ureteral patency.

Acute Pyelonephritis

Acute pyelonephritis is an acute infectious process involving the renal interstitium frequently associated with bacteremia and often presenting with acute back pain, high fever, rigors, headache, nausea, vomiting, and occasionally diarrhea. Most patients are women, and many will report symptoms suggestive of prior or recent cystitis. Interestingly, since the kidney normally descends during inspiration, many patients will report a pleuritic component to their discomfort, which in some patients may be a prominent part of their symptom complex.

Clinical Diagnosis

The clinical diagnosis is based on the patient's history, clinical presentation, the finding of unilateral or bilateral percussion tenderness over the involved kidney (or kidneys), and evidence of bacteria in freshly obtained, uncentrifuged urine. Varying degrees of pyuria, including white blood cell casts, and hematuria may be noted. It must be remembered that a number of factors such as recent antibiotic therapy, coexistent ureteral obstruction, and extreme urinary acidity or hyperosmolality will substantially alter the expected microscopic findings.

A urine sample should be collected and Gram stain, urinalysis, and culture and sensitivity obtained.

Disposition and Treatment

Disposition and treatment are determined by the patient's clinical condition.
- Admission should be considered for the following patients:
  - Patients who appear toxic or systemically ill
  - The elderly patient with inability to provide reasonable care at home
  - Patients with intractable pain or vomiting unrelieved by analgesics
  - Pregnant patients
  - Patients with urinary obstruction or indwelling catheters
  - Immunosuppressed patients
  - Those not responding to outpatient treatment

  Admitted patients require intravenous fluid replacement, intravenous antibiotics, often an effective analgesic and antiemetic, and measures to reduce fever if appropriate. Patients who are ill with presumed bacteremia require management of fluid status, often pressors, and initial intravenous antibiotic therapy with a fluroquinone (e.g., ciprofloxacin), ampicillin plus an aminoglycoside (e.g., gentamicin), a third-generation cephalosporin (e.g., ceftriaxone), or an extended spectrum penicillin with a β-lactamase inhibitor (e.g., ticarcillin/clavulanate). When culture and sensitivity results are available, a potentially more efficacious antibiotic regimen may be instituted.
- Patients with factors known to predispose to treatment failure or with resistant organisms may require more aggressive initial therapy. Such factors include multiple prior episodes of pyelonephritis, coexistent calculi or obstruction, abnormalities of immunity, and previously demonstrated resistant organisms.
- For **outpatient therapy**, a 12- to 14-day course of ciprofloxacin (500 mg b.i.d.) or another fluoroquinone is likely adequate with follow-up of culture results important to guide any necessary treatment alterations. Patients should be instructed to finish the entire course of medication despite improvement in clinical status. Liberal intake of fluids is encouraged. Patients with discomfort but without other indications for admission may be provided an appropriate analgesic for 2 to 4 days, during which time symptoms should subside. Patients with low-grade fever should be instructed to take acetaminophen as needed. Follow-up in 3 to 4 days is indicated for all patients.
- **Recurrent episodes** of pyelonephritis in women and initial episodes in young men generally require urologic evaluation to exclude important and potentially correctable anatomic abnormalities.

Pneumonia

Patients with evolving pneumonia occasionally present with severe, sudden, unilateral back pain, which is often pleuritic and associated with minimal or absent cough or sputum production and without fever. Physical examination may be unremarkable or may demonstrate fine rales in the involved area. Although many patients are quite ill at the time of presentation, chest x-rays may be normal initially. Cough, high fever, rigors, purulent sputum (often containing pneumococci), and the typical physical and radiologic evidence of pulmonary consolidation will develop over 6 to 12 hours in many of these patients (see Chapter 19, "Pneumonia").

Malignancy

Patients may present with back pain and no history of trauma. If the patient is elderly or has a history of malignancy (especially of certain types), metastasis or malignancy of the vertebral column should be suspected. Typically, the pain is unrelieved by rest or lying down, is worse at night, is continuous, and may be associated with systemic complaints. Primary malignancies include multiple myeloma, whereas metastatic malignancies come generally from malignancies of the prostate, breast, lung, kidney, or thyroid. The diagnosis may be suggested by radiography, but at least one quarter of the bone must be lost before plain x-rays are able to detect the lesion. Even then, the lesion may only be suspected because of the collapse of a vertebral body. Bone scans and MRI are more sensitive in diagnosing vertebral malignancies. If the diagnosis is suspected and the patient is ambulatory, the patient should be referred for prompt outpatient follow up and further diagnostic studies.

Metabolic Bone Disease

Osteoporosis is the most common metabolic bone disease in the United States, and the bones of the spine and pelvis are the most common site. Women are more commonly affected than men (more than 50% by the age of 45). When osteoporosis becomes advanced, vertebrae may collapse because there is an insufficient amount of bone to maintain the structural weight-bearing integrity of the spine. There are multiple causes of osteoporosis, but most are of unknown etiology. Decreases in estrogen and activity levels, and insufficient amounts of dietary calcium contribute to the process. Patients who present with back pain and osteoporosis may demonstrate vertebral collapse on x-ray. Such patients should be treated with analgesia and a brief period (3 days or less) of bed rest, with follow-up by a primary physician who can evaluate the cause further and can prescribe hormonal, dietary, and activity therapy as needed. Percutaneous vertebroplasty is a promising emerging treatment option.

Spinal Stenosis

Patients with spinal stenosis typically are over 60 years old and experience pain in both legs exacerbated by walking and relieved by resting (pseudoclaudication). They may also have low back pain and buttock pain. Some patients may have pain on only one side. As the lumbar spine is flexed, they find relief of the pain and sometimes comment that they find it easier to walk uphill than downhill. This problem is caused by a narrowing of the bony spinal canal and compression of the cauda equina. This problem should be suspected in patients over age 65 who have the onset of radiculopathy. Spinal stenosis is reported to be the most common cause of radiculopathy in this age group. All such patients should be referred for orthopaedic consultation.

Vertebral Osteomyelitis

Vertebral osteomyelitis generally develops from hematogenous spread, especially of *Staphylococcus aureus*. Diabetics are prone to the development of vertebral osteomyelitis, as are patients who have had spinal surgery, intravenous drug abusers (*Pseudomonas* and *Serratia*), patients with sickle cell disease (*Salmonella*), and patients who have had urinary tract manipulations (Gram-negative organisms). As the infection develops, bone may be destroyed that can lead to collapse of vertebral bodies and paralysis.

Diagnostic Studies

X-rays may show moth-eaten vertebral body end plates, narrowing of the disk spaces, swelling of paravertebral tissues, and osteoporosis of the involved vertebral body. CT scans may help define the area involved, but bone scans are frequently needed to delineate "hot" areas. MRI is also useful. White blood cell counts and the sedimentation rates are generally elevated. The sedimentation rate may be greater than 100 mm/h. Needle aspiration may be necessary for obtaining culture material, but blood cultures will sometimes reveal the organism.

Treatment

Treatment requires long-term intravenous antibiotics and bed rest.

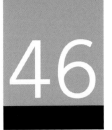

Extremity Pain and Swelling—Atraumatic

Pain in or swelling of one or both extremities may be caused by a variety of both acute and chronic disorders, many of which require prompt and accurate diagnosis if morbidity and, in some cases, mortality are to be minimized. In this chapter, we discuss extremity pain and/or swelling that is either atraumatic or results from relatively insignificant trauma.

UPPER EXTREMITY

INTRODUCTION

Many disorders, both local and distant from the arm, may produce arm pain. The physician must remember that cardiac ischemic pain may present with shoulder, arm, or forearm pain *unassociated* with chest discomfort; local symptoms that are not affected by movement or palpation of the arm should suggest a remote cause (cervical spine, cardiac ischemic disease). Importantly, cervical trauma resulting in arm pain may be trivial or initially unrecognized and may be unassociated with neck discomfort.

COMMON CAUSES OF UPPER EXTREMITY PAIN

- Muscle strain
- Bursitis or tendinitis*
- Lateral epicondylitis (tennis elbow)*
- Cervical spondylosis*
- Arthritis
- Synovial cyst or ganglion*

LESS COMMON CAUSES OF UPPER EXTREMITY PAIN NOT TO BE MISSED

- Cardiac ischemic pain*
- Occult cervical spine injury

OTHER CAUSES OF UPPER EXTREMITY PAIN

- Nerve compression syndromes*
- Hand infections*
- Superficial thrombophlebitis*
- Osteomyelitis
- Thoracic outlet syndrome*
- Herpes zoster (shingles)

---

*Discussed in this chapter.

SPECIFIC DISORDERS

Cervical Spondylosis

Cervical spondylosis refers to degenerative changes of the cervical spine; these include osteophyte formation, thickening of associated spinal ligaments, and narrowing of the intervertebral disk space. Although these changes are commonly noted in asymptomatic patients, they may also be associated with a variety of clinical presentations.

Distinction should be made between compression of the cervical spinal cord, resulting in myelopathy, and compression of spinal nerve roots, resulting in radiculopathy. Both syndromes may result from bony osteophyte formation and ligamentous hypertrophy. Both may produce symptoms as a result of minor or major cervical trauma.

Myelopathy

Myelopathy most often occurs in patients with a presumptive congenital narrowing of the cervical spinal canal. Symptoms related to myelopathy include mild upper extremity weakness, atrophy, hyperreflexia in the lower extremities, and extensor plantar responses.

Radiculopathy

Patients with radiculopathy present with symptoms referable to the particular nerve root that is compressed; most commonly C6 and C7 are involved and result in neck, parascapular, and arm pain, all of which may be accentuated or precipitated by movement of the head or neck. Motor abnormalities, including weakness and diminution or loss of reflexes, may be noted in the biceps, brachioradialis, and triceps muscles. Sensory loss may involve the radial aspect of the thumb or index and long fingers (see Table 46-1).

Diagnostic Studies

The demonstration of cervical spondylotic changes by plain radiography cannot be considered diagnostic, given the extremely high incidence of asymptomatic patients. Such radiographic abnormalities, however, when correlated with physical findings, are suggestive. The diagnosis of cervical myelopathy requires demonstration that the cervical canal is less than 10 mm in diameter; this dimension may be measured by magnetic resonance imaging (MRI) or computed tomography imaging, which can usually be done nonemergently.

Treatment

Patients in whom the diagnosis of myelopathy is considered should be discussed with the orthopaedic or neurosurgical consultant before disposition; this is particularly true when trauma has precipitated or worsened symptoms or when motor loss is suspected. Patients with cervical radicular symptoms should be treated with immobilization of the neck in a soft cervical collar and several days of activity limitations; nonsteroidal anti-inflammatory agents, local heat, muscle relaxants, and analgesics as needed are generally recommended as well. When motor abnormalities are noted, consultation before disposition is recommended.

Cardiac Ischemic Pain

The syndromes of myocardial ischemia are discussed in detail in Chapter 23; a brief note is made here to suggest that these are important considerations in the differential diagnosis of patients presenting with isolated arm or shoulder pain.

Table 46-1	Lateral Cervical Disk Herniation Syndromes			
Involved Nerve	Herniation Interspace			
	C4-5	C5-6	C6-7	C7-T1
	(C5)[a]	(C6)[a]	(C7)[a]	(C8)[a]
Pain and aspect paresthesia distribution	Neck, shoulder, upper arm	Neck, shoulder, lateral arm, radial aspect of forearm, thumb and index finger	Neck, lateral aspect of arm, ring and index fingers	Ulnar aspect of forearm and hand
Motor loss	Deltoid, biceps	Biceps	Triceps, extensor carpi ulnaris	Intrinsic muscles of hand, and wrist extensors
Reflex loss	Biceps	Biceps	Triceps	None
Sensory loss	Shoulder	Thumb, index finger, radial forearm, lateral arm	Index and middle fingers, radial forearm	Ulnar side of ring finger, little finger

[a]Involved N.

Adapted from Samuels MA. *Manual of neurologic therapeutics*, 2nd ed. Boston: Little, Brown and Company; 1982:77, with permission.

Diagnosis

As noted previously, isolated discomfort involving the upper or lateral shoulder, arm, or forearm may be reported as the initial and only complaint in patients with cardiac ischemia. A history of discomfort beginning or worsening with exertion is occasionally present but cannot be relied on to exclude or make less likely the possibility of cardiac pain. Diagnostically, a critically important finding is that neither movement of the extremity nor palpation elicits or worsens the patient's discomfort; when this is the case, local causes are unlikely. Unfortunately, in most patients, the **electrocardiogram (ECG) will not exclude** the possibility of cardiac ischemic pain, because it is recognized that as many as half of all patients presenting to the emergency department (ED) with an acute myocardial infarction may have a normal ECG when first evaluated.

Treatment

When the clinician suspects the diagnosis of cardiac ischemic pain, further workup and admission are indicated.

Bursitis and Tendinitis of the Shoulder

A variety of structures surrounding and supporting the shoulder may become acutely inflamed and thereby symptomatic. The supraspinatus tendon, the subacromial/subdeltoid bursa, and the long head of the biceps are most commonly involved.

Diagnosis

When these structures are inflamed, severe discomfort is described, often perceived as more severe at night and preventing sleep. Pain is clearly enhanced both by palpation and by passive or active motion of the shoulder. Discomfort commonly radiates superiorly toward the neck and distally toward the elbow. Radiologically, local deposits of calcium may be noted.

Treatment

Treatment includes an initial but abbreviated period of immobilization in a sling (2–3 days at most) and the institution of anti-inflammatory agents. Patients should be instructed to remove the sling each day for bathing and at night to prevent the development of shoulder (adhesive capsulitis) or elbow stiffness. Daily, gentle range-of-motion exercises are recommended to minimize the development of adhesive capsulitis. The use of a nonsteroidal anti-inflammatory agent such as ibuprofen and an analgesic for particularly symptomatic patients is reasonable and effective treatment. If discomfort is well localized, and infection has been excluded, a local injection of a long-acting steroid preparation, such as methylprednisolone acetate, 40 mg, combined with an anesthetic agent, such as 2 mL of 1% or 2% lidocaine or 1 to 2 mL of bupivacaine, is also effective; this modality is frequently reserved for patients failing a course of anti-inflammatory agents. No more than one or two such injections (the initial injection should be given 2 weeks to be effective) should be given in the ED; orthopaedic referral is preferred at this point. Patients receiving an injection should be told that although the anesthetic will acutely alleviate discomfort, pain will recur and last for approximately 12 to 36 hours, after which time the effect of the steroid becomes apparent. Referral should be advised in 5 to 7 days to assess progress and institute range-of-motion exercises.

Lateral Epicondylitis (Tennis Elbow)

Diagnosis

Patients with lateral epicondylitis usually provide a history of repetitive or excessive use of the muscles of the wrist or forearm; however, often no such history is present. On examination, tenderness of the lateral epicondyle is noted with palpation, which is accentuated by extension of the wrist, particularly against resistance. Passive range of motion of the elbow is normal.

Treatment

Treatment involves prohibiting maneuvers that result in use of the forearm and wrist extensors; providing a sling, which should be removed for bathing and at night; and instituting a course of oral nonsteroidal anti-inflammatory agents. A variety of splint-type devices are available (these are referred to as "tennis-elbow bands or wraps"), which when applied result in mild compression of the muscles in the forearm, in this case the forearm or wrist extensors, thereby reducing transmitted force to the epicondyle. Radiologic assessment of the elbow is indicated in most patients to exclude displacement, which, if present, may require operative reduction and fixation. Although the local injection of corticosteroids is effective, this treatment should be reserved for patients not responding to more conservative therapy.

Medial Epicondylitis

Patients with medial epicondylitis present with discomfort localized to the medial epicondyle, clearly accentuated by valgus stress applied to the elbow joint. This entity is common in baseball pitchers, golfers, and individuals playing racquet sports; it is also referred to as golfer's elbow or little league elbow. The disorder results from a variety of overuse scenarios, including simple muscle and ligament strain, tendinitis, and actual avulsion fractures of the epicondyle and the subchondral bone of the radial head may be seen as well.

Diagnosis
In most patients, an x-ray should be obtained to exclude avulsion fractures of the epicondyle or displacement. Ulnar nerve irritation is commonly associated with the above syndromes and may be symptomatic.

Treatment
Treatment includes rest, by prohibiting activities resulting in symptoms, local heat, and prescribing of an anti-inflammatory agent. A variety of splint-type devices are available ("tennis-elbow bands or wraps"), which when applied result in mild compression of the muscles of the forearm, in this case the forearm flexors and major pronator, thus reducing transmitted force to the epicondyle. Patients should be referred to an orthopaedic surgeon, since refractory cases may require immobilization in a long-arm splint or cast with the forearm in pronation. Local injection with a corticosteroid may also be recommended in particularly refractory or symptomatic cases but must be undertaken with caution due to the proximity of the ulnar nerve. Patients with fractures or displacement of the epicondyle should be referred to an orthopaedic surgeon for prompt follow-up.

Olecranon Bursitis
Diagnosis
Patients with olecranon bursitis present with severe pain overlying the olecranon; a history of chronic overuse or recent injury to the area is often present. On physical examination, the posterior elbow is exquisitely tender to palpation and often markedly inflamed with increased warmth and erythema; the thickened, fluid-filled or "boggy" olecranon bursa is easily appreciated. *Suppurative bursitis must always be considered* when penetrating or other trauma has preceded the onset of symptoms or when evidence of systemic infection is present; under these circumstances, sterile aspiration of the bursa is indicated. In addition, the possibility of gouty bursitis can be addressed with the analysis of aspirated bursal fluid.

Treatment
Treatment includes the use of a sling, which should be removed for bathing and at night, and the institution of a nonsteroidal anti-inflammatory agent. Patients should be advised that if symptoms have not improved in 5 to 10 days, aspiration and possible steroid injection may be required; orthopaedic follow-up at this time is therefore advised. Analgesics are often required during the initial 2 to 3 days of treatment.

Superficial Thrombophlebitis
Superficial thrombophlebitis may occur spontaneously or in association with trauma, recent venipuncture, or the intravenous administration of medication (e.g., most commonly the in-hospital administration of diazepam or potassium or out-of-hospital illicit drug use).

Diagnosis
Patients usually complain of a dull ache in the involved area; physical findings include local induration, erythema, and tenderness. Tenderness is often found to extend

proximally along the course of the involved, indurated vein; true fluctuance is rarely present, but when it is noted, suppurative thrombophlebitis should be suspected. In patients with idiopathic or drug-induced thrombophlebitis, the inflammatory process generally subsides within 5 to 7 days with treatment, but a firmly palpable cord remains for a longer period. Edema and deep pain involving the arm do not occur unless deep venous or suppurative thrombophlebitis coexists.

Suppurative Thrombophlebitis

In patients with recent venipuncture, intravenous catheter placement, medication administration, or illicit intravenous drug use, the possibility of **suppurative thrombophlebitis** must be considered. Fortunately, in patients with recent venipuncture, intravenous catheter placement, or in-hospital medication administration, thrombophlebitis is most often irritative or chemical in nature rather than infectious. These patients require only routine symptomatic treatment as outlined below. However, because it is virtually impossible to exclude completely the diagnosis of suppurative phlebitis, a re-examination in 24 to 48 hours is indicated. Patients with high fever, leukocytosis, evidence of systemic illness, bacteremia, local fluctuance, cellulitis, or an appropriate history require that suppurative phlebitis be excluded, and to this end, general or vascular surgical consultation at the time of presentation is appropriate. If confirmed, patients will require admission, intravenous antibiotics, and early surgical intervention.

Treatment

In patients with irritative or chemical phlebitis, only local and symptomatic measures, including moist heat, elevation, and a short course of an appropriate anti-inflammatory agent, are necessary.

Synovial Cyst or Ganglion

Synovial cysts most often occur at the wrist, may be either dorsal or volar, and are made more obvious by flexion or extension of the involved joint, these maneuvers simply serving to tent the skin over the lesion.

Diagnosis

Many patients are asymptomatic, although occasionally aching discomfort accentuated by pressure over the area is reported, often in association with minor trauma or overuse of the involved joint. By palpation, synovial cysts are somewhat firm and nodular, and when trauma or overuse has preceded or precipitated symptoms, evidence of mild inflammation may be noted. Most such lesions are small—approximately 1 cm—and may also be found in association with the tendon sheaths of the distal lower extremity. Pathologically, lesions consist of a wall of tough fibrous material, often containing synovial cells and filled with a fluid rich in glycosaminoglycans.

Treatment

When evidence of inflammation is present, treatment includes reassurance, immobilization of the joint, and a course of an anti-inflammatory agent. Patients without signs or symptoms of inflammation require only orthopaedic referral at an interval determined by the patient's symptoms. Surgical removal may be elected if significant symptoms persist.

Pronator Teres Syndrome

Pronator teres syndrome results when the **median nerve** is compressed below the elbow as it passes through the two heads of the pronator teres muscle.

Diagnosis

Repetitive trauma to the area is often reported, as is an occupation or activity requiring weight bearing on this area of the forearm. In addition to symptoms related to median nerve compression, forearm pain is reported, and local tenderness to palpation is noted. Physical findings are somewhat similar to those found in patients with the carpal tunnel syndrome; however, in addition, weakness of distal thumb flexion is noted because the flexor pollicis longus derives its innervation proximal to the wrist.

Treatment

Treatment depends on the extent of symptoms and whether motor function is impaired. Orthopaedic referral is recommended.

Thoracic Outlet Syndrome

Thoracic outlet syndrome results from pressure on the lower roots of the **brachial plexus** as they pass over the cervical rib or through the thoracic outlet between the first rib and the scalenus anticus muscle. Given the close anatomic relation between the brachial plexus and the subclavian vessels in this area, vascular rather than neural compromise may produce an ischemic brachial neuropathy with similar symptoms. Other causes of brachial neuropathy must always be considered and excluded; these include a ruptured or prolapsed cervical disk, cervical spondylosis, and the carpal tunnel syndrome.

History

Most patients will be young to middle-aged women who report a vague or ill-defined ache involving the hand or forearm; pain is sometimes noted to involve the upper arm and neck. Symptoms are usually precipitated or exacerbated by activities requiring repetitive movements of the upper limbs, especially above the head. Accentuation of symptoms at night is common, and some patients report that the entire limb feels numb; paresthesias and weakness involving the fingers and hand are also commonly reported. A "whiplash" injury precedes the onset of symptoms in some patients.

Physical Examination

When the arm is abducted to 90 degrees and externally rotated, patients with thoracic outlet obstruction may develop typical paresthesias and numbness with immediate resolution of symptoms once the arm is returned to the side; with abduction, a bruit may also be auscultated in the supraclavicular fossa. Loss of the radial pulse with the arm abducted (positive Adson test), once considered the diagnostic hallmark of the syndrome, is often noted in asymptomatic individuals. Nerve conduction studies are sometimes helpful in supporting the diagnosis or suggesting other cause. Arteriography is sometimes used to establish the diagnosis, most often before surgery.

Treatment

Treatment is initially symptomatic, with avoidance of heavy lifting and repetitive movements of the upper extremities, particularly above the head. Patients should also be instructed not to sleep with their arms above the head. A sling can be tried on the affected arm, which should be removed for sleeping. Physical therapy and warm compresses to the shoulder are sometimes symptomatically helpful; muscle relaxants can be tried as well. Surgical treatment usually involves resection of a cervical rib or fascial bands; surgery is normally reserved for patients with severe symptoms who fail a course of conservative therapy or for those with embolization or actual arterial occlusion.

Tendinitis of the Wrist and Thumb

Most commonly, in the distal upper extremity, the extensor tendons of the wrist and fingers and the long abductor and short extensor of the thumb become inflamed and result in acute tendinitis; the latter condition involving the thumb is referred to as **de Quervain tenosynovitis.**

Diagnosis

In many patients with tendinitis around the wrist or fingers, a history or occupation involving repetitive motion of the joint is elicited and has preceded the development of symptoms; this history is absent in approximately 50% of patients. Most patients report poorly localized discomfort to the area of the involved tendon or tendons; such discomfort, however, is clearly worsened by passive or active movement of the involved tendon, and this remains a key diagnostic point. Increased warmth, overlying erythema, and occasionally palpable crepitus are noted; crepitus is appreciated by palpation directly over the involved tendon with active or passive motion. Patients with de Quervain tenosynovitis report discomfort at the radial styloid often radiating into the thumb and forearm. Discomfort may be increased by flexion and apposition of the thumb and fifth finger.

Treatment of Tendinitis

Treatment of tendinitis involves immobilization of the involved joint with a splint, use of a nonsteroidal anti-inflammatory agent, and elevation. Use of the joint should be prohibited, and follow-up is suggested at 5 to 7 days to evaluate the patient's response to treatment. Patients should be advised to remove the splint each day for bathing and gentle range-of-motion exercises to prevent the development of joint stiffness. If treatment is unsuccessful, locally administered steroids may be effective.

Carpal Tunnel Syndrome

Median nerve compression at the wrist caused by the transverse carpal ligament is common and usually occurs in women.

History

Carpal tunnel syndrome is most often unassociated with trauma, and patients report the gradual onset of primarily nocturnal hand, wrist, and forearm pain often accompanied by numbness or dysesthesias. Pain is sometimes better localized to the volar first or second fingers. Patients are commonly awakened from sleep and report relief of symptoms by shaking or elevating the hands. Bilateral involvement is occasionally reported, but more often only one upper extremity is involved. The incidence is increased in pregnancy and associated with birth control pill use.

Physical Examination

On physical examination, sensation to pinprick is reduced on the volar (palmar) aspect of the index finger; frequently, a subjective difference between the two hands can be demonstrated. Mild atrophy of the thenar eminence is noted in some patients, and thumb adduction is often slightly weakened. The diagnostic impression of carpal tunnel syndrome can be further supported if holding the patient's wrist in flexion (Phalen test) for 60 seconds reproduces symptoms and placing the wrist in the neutral position relieves symptoms. Tinel sign (light tapping over the median nerve as it crosses under the carpal ligament) may also elicit symptoms (tingling in the fingers in the median nerve distribution) and is useful diagnostically.

Diagnostic Tests

Radiologic assessment should be undertaken when trauma has preceded the onset of symptoms, because carpal displacement and Colles fractures have both been associated with the development of the carpal tunnel syndrome. More commonly, tenosynovitis localized to the wrist flexors is responsible. The diagnosis can be confirmed by electromyography.

Treatment

Treatment is determined by the extent of symptoms and whether motor loss is present; patients with abnormalities of motor function in the distribution of the median nerve require prompt orthopaedic consultation for possible decompression. Other patients should be treated with wrist immobilization by splinting in the neutral position; patients should remove the splint once each day for bathing, but it should otherwise remain applied. Wearing the splint during sleep, particularly during the first 3 to 5 days of therapy, and keeping the involved extremity elevated as much as possible should be emphasized. An initial trial of a nonsteroidal anti-inflammatory agent is recommended; treatment with steroids or definitive repair (release of the transverse carpal ligament) or both may be undertaken subsequently in selected patients. Follow-up in patients without motor loss should be advised in 7 to 10 days.

Medical Evaluation

A medical evaluation should be considered to exclude various medical conditions frequently associated with carpal tunnel syndrome; these include diabetes mellitus, rheumatoid arthritis, hypothyroidism, multiple myeloma, acromegaly, amyloidosis, nephrosis, sarcoidosis, and tuberculosis.

Trigger Finger and Thumb

Diagnosis

Patients with trigger finger or thumb report "sticking" or "locking" of the involved digit in mid flexion—with greater effort, a "snap" is heard or sensed as flexion is completed. Very often, the patient is unable to reextend the digit without recruiting other fingers. In an occasional patient, repetitive trauma to the flexor apparatus of the involved digit will be reported; however, more often no such history is obtained. Pathologically, the flexor tendon and its associated sheath are inflamed and thickened, the flexor tendon becoming focally swollen in such a way that increased resistance to movement through the sheath with subsequent locking is noted.

Treatment

Treatment involves minimizing use and trauma to the digit, splinting the digit in a position of function, instituting an appropriate anti-inflammatory agent, and arranging orthopaedic referral in 5 to 7 days. Patients should be instructed to remove the splint each day for bathing but should be cautioned to avoid regularly "testing" the digit's range of motion. Local instillation of steroids into the tendon sheath is often successful if improvement has not occurred by 5 to 7 days. Surgical release remains an option in selected patients unresponsive to other measures.

Paronychia

Classically, paronychial infections produce a well-localized, fluctuant abscess exterior and adjacent to the nail; these are exquisitely tender and surrounded by varying amounts of erythema and swelling. Often, when some delay has occurred before presentation, the central or overlying tissue may be necrotic and will appear white or gray.

- **When fluctuance or local abscess is not present,** treatment includes soaks four to six times per day, an appropriate antistaphylococcal antibiotic, and follow-up as needed in 3 to 5 days. Patients with significant surrounding or advancing cellulitis, systemic evidence of infection, or abnormalities of immune function should be treated aggressively with antibiotics for the subsequent 5 to 7 days and have close follow-up in 48 hours. Patients should be told that over the next several days the infection will either resolve or become localized and then require incision and drainage. Chronic paronychial infections should raise the possibility of candidal infection.

- **Local fluctuance** is frequently noted and indicates the need for prompt drainage of the abscess. Initially, one must determine whether infection has originated or extended under the nail; if so, removing this section of the nail, in addition to draining any other more superficial collections, is advised. In most patients, extension under the nail is not present, and the abscess can clearly be observed and palpated adjacent and exterior to the nail; in these patients, nail removal is not indicated.

- **Anesthesia** for drainage is easily provided by digital block with 1% or 2% lidocaine **without epinephrine** or proximal field instillation; the former is generally preferable. In an occasional patient, however, particularly one with overlying or central necrosis of the "roof" of the abscess, incision, removal of the roof of the abscess, and drainage may be undertaken without the additional discomfort of anesthesia. In this case, the area typically appears white or necrotic and there is no sensation to light pinprick. Even for patients without this central necrosis, the digital block is considered by some to represent a more painful experience than the quick incision required for simple drainage.

- Very often, when the collection is immediately **adjacent to the skin edge,** simply inserting a 16-gauge needle or the tip of a sharply pointed scalpel between the nail and the skin edge will provide temporary drainage. In these patients, drainage can be facilitated by placing a small wick, such as the end or corner of a one-quarter-inch plain gauze along the needle track, which can be removed in 12 to 24 hours; drain insertion, even as noted, is often not possible because of the small size of the cavity. Patients should be instructed to retract the pericuticular skin before and during soaks four to six times per day and to express any bloody or purulent material; the rationale for this should be explained to the patient and will enhance compliance and the probability of resolution without a need for further intervention. Practically, we find that simple needle drainage, with or without temporary wick insertion, will result in relatively frequent recurrences; this seems to be true even when soaks are frequent and when initial drainage was considered complete. For this reason, in patients with pericuticular abscesses that are drained by needle, the removal of a small wedge of necrotic tissue contiguous with the abscess cavity and adjacent to the skin edge will ensure initial drainage of the abscess for 48 to 72 hours, makes skin retraction prior to soaks easier for the patient, and reduces the probability of recurrence.

- When the abscess is **located away from the skin edge** and is therefore not clearly amenable to needle drainage, incision and the removal of a small section of the overlying, central, or necrotic "roof" area of the abscess is similarly useful; the latter will ensure continued drainage and decrease the probability of reaccumulation or recurrence. Patients should be instructed to remove any clotted material from the opening of the abscess, to express any clotted material from the opening of the abscess, to express any purulent or bloody material, and to begin soaks for 15 to 20 minutes in warm water, all repeated four to six times per day. Soaks should be continued for 5 to 7 days or until resolution is complete. Note that antibiotics are not required for treatment of an uncomplicated paronychia.

Felon

Infection involving the distal volar (palmar) pulp space of the finger is called a felon. Treatment has changed over the years, probably reflecting the emergence of more effective antistaphylococcal agents. The general trend is to reserve previously advocated surgical procedures, many of which were associated with significant complications, for patients refractory to medical therapy.

- If diagnosed early, patients with mild involvement, no clear fluctuance, and no systemic evidence of infection may be treated with 5 to 7 days of an oral antistaphylococcal antibiotic, heat, elevation, and a reexamination in 24 hours. Oral antibiotics include amoxicillin-clavulanate, a cephalosporin, clindamycin, or a macrolide. Patients without improvement should have a hand surgery consultation and may require hospital admission and intravenous antibacterial therapy.
- An occasional patient, either initially or at follow-up, will manifest evidence of the abscess pointing anteriorly or volarly (or palmarly). In these patients, a relatively confined volar or palmar incision will adequately drain the abscess and, in conjunction with antibacterial therapy, soaks, heat, and elevation, may eliminate the need for other more extensive procedures.
- When evidence of vascular compromise is noted (as a result of swelling), or when systemic symptoms are present, hospital admission, intravenous antibiotics, and early surgical consultation are required.

Closed Space and Tendon or Tendon Sheath Infections

Infection, however subtle, involving the thenar or hypothenar eminence, the web spaces of the hand, or the palmar space must be treated extremely aggressively if significant local morbidity is to be avoided. In most patients, hand surgery consultation should be obtained prior to disposition; hospital admission and intravenous antibiotics may be indicated.

Diagnosis

Classically, patients with flexor-tendon involvement will present with the finger held in slight flexion; passive or active movement of the finger is resisted and is associated with severe discomfort. Erythema, swelling, and tenderness are usually noted along the course of the tendon. Such infections may rapidly ascend to involve the closed spaces of the hand as discussed; subspecialty consultation should be obtained when this diagnosis is suspected or established.

Treatment

Hospital admission, intravenous antibiotics, heat, and elevation along with early incision and drainage generally are the treatment of choice. Extensor tendon involvement, although more amenable to medical treatment, should similarly be discussed with the subspecialist before disposition.

Common Warts

Warts represent a cutaneous tumor arising in the epidermis as a result of infection with the human papillomavirus. Children are most commonly affected.

Diagnosis

Flesh-colored, painless papules, usually scattered on the hands or fingers, are characteristic. Lesions may become painful when pressure is exerted over them or when infection occurs.

Treatment

Treatment with cryosurgery (liquid nitrogen) or light electrodesiccation and curettage is associated with minimal discomfort and scarring and is the recommended approach; referral to a dermatologist is appropriate.

LOWER EXTREMITY

COMMON CAUSES OF LEG PAIN AND SWELLING

- Congestive heart failure
- Portal hypertension
- Sciatica
- Meralgia paresthetica*
- Trochanteric bursitis*
- Toxic synovitis of the hip*
- Cellulitis*
- Arthritis
- Deep venous thrombosis*
- Superficial thrombophlebitis*
- Chronic venous insufficiency*
- Bursitis of the knee*
- Chondromalacia patellae*
- Ruptured Baker cyst
- Osgood-Schlatter disease*
- Gastrocnemius muscle tear*
- Achilles tendon strain or rupture*
- Plantaris tendon rupture*
- Achilles tenosynovitis*

LESS COMMON CAUSES OF LEG PAIN AND SWELLING NOT TO BE MISSED

- Acute arterial insufficiency*
- Pregnancy
- Slipped capital femoral epiphysis*
- Adductor muscle strain*
- Osteomyelitis
- Pelvic neoplasms
- Legg-Calvé-Perthes disease
- Filariasis
- Hypoalbuminemia (secondary to liver dysfunction or nephrotic syndrome)
- Milroy disease (hereditary lymphangiectasia)
- Morton neuroma*

HISTORY

Bilateral

A history of chest discomfort or symptoms of left-sided heart failure, such as dyspnea on exertion, paroxysmal nocturnal dyspnea, or orthopnea, suggest **congestive heart failure** as a cause for leg swelling, which is typically bilateral. A history of chronic alcohol ingestion with a recent history of increasing abdominal girth associated with bilateral lower extremity edema suggests **portal hypertension. Pregnancy** is often associated with bilateral edema; this results from compression of venous and lymphatic vessels in the pelvis and also from the effect of progesterone on vascular smooth muscle, producing venodilation with consequent valvular incompetence. The non-steroidal anti-inflammatory agents, along with a variety of antihypertensive medications, may produce bilateral peripheral edema; this is typically noted at the end of the day after therapy with one of these agents is started, or associated with the initiation of a higher dose. Intra-abdominal and intrapelvic neoplastic processes, particularly **lymphoma,** may cause either unilateral or bilateral peripheral edema.

Unilateral

Pregnancy also predisposes to venous thromboembolism; because of its potentially devastating consequences, great caution must be exercised when these patients are evaluated. A history of palpitations, recent myocardial infarction, rheumatic heart disease, or atrial fibrillation associated with the sudden onset of leg pain and pallor should suggest an **acute embolic event.** A history of previous deep venous thrombophlebitis, recent immobilization (e.g., prolonged bed rest, sitting, lower extremity casting, or standing), and birth control pill use all predispose to **deep venous thrombosis.** Recent trauma, a history of diabetes, fever, and local discomfort are noted in patients with cellulitis, which is typically unilateral.

Hip Pain in Children and Adolescents

The differential diagnosis is extensive; one must consider **septic arthritis, slipped capital femoral epiphysis** (which may cause hip or knee pain or limp after trivial or unrecalled trauma), **osteomyelitis, toxic synovitis,** and **early Legg-Calvé-Perthes disease** (idiopathic, avascular necrosis of the proximal femoral epiphysis).

Thigh pain

Meralgia paresthetica, a relatively common disorder, produces vague but often moderately severe discomfort or dysesthesias (or both) in the lateral and anterior thigh. Symptoms occur as a result of compression or entrapment of the lateral femoral cutaneous nerve. This disorder is typically more common in women, many of whom have a history of diabetes, obesity, recent weight gain, pregnancy, or occupations requiring periods of prolonged sitting.

Knee Pain

Patients with **bursitis involving the knee** most often report several days of progressive discomfort, which may involve any of the bursal structures surrounding the knee; pain is increased with movement. Adolescents, particularly those involved in any variety of athletic pursuits, who report gradually increasing discomfort over the anterior, proximal tibia, should be suspected of having **Osgood-Schlatter disease.** Not infrequently, a contusing injury results in increased discomfort and brings the patient to the ED. **Chondromalacia patellae** most often affects young women, who typically report vague discomfort localized to the area of the knee and inferior patella; pain is classically increased by walking up stairs and is unassociated with trauma.

Calf/Lower Leg Pain

The sudden onset of unilateral, often severe, posterior popliteal or proximal calf pain and swelling associated with significant activity should suggest rupture of a **Baker cyst; gastrocnemius muscle tear, plantaris tendon rupture,** and **Achilles tendon strain or rupture** are also suggested by this history. A ruptured Baker cyst is an important entity because its symptoms and signs may simulate deep venous thrombosis of the calf. Important differential points include the observation that many patients with ruptured Baker cysts report chronic, but often vague, symptoms referable to the popliteal fossa prior to rupture, and at the onset of rupture, a "tearing" sensation involving the upper calf is frequently reported. It is also important to note that a significant number of patients with a ruptured Baker cyst have accompanying DVT, presumably induced by proximal venous compression. Patients with **partial rupture of the gastrocnemius muscle, Achilles tendon strain or rupture,** and **plantaris tendon rupture also** report the sudden onset of severe pain usually (but not always) associated with activities that stress the involved muscle or tendon. Such maneuvers include, for example, pushing a stalled car, charging the net at tennis, or beginning a foot race.

PHYSICAL EXAMINATION

The presence of ascites, jugular venous distention, an S_3 gallop, or signs of pulmonary edema suggest right or **left ventricular failure.** Ascites without jugular venous distention and evidence of estrogenization (palmar erythema, spider angiomata, gynecomastia, and testicular atrophy) suggest chronic liver disease and **portal hypertension** as a cause for peripheral edema. Diffuse anasarca, especially with periorbital edema, is seen most commonly in nephrosis. Weight loss associated with the gradual development of lower extremity edema (especially when unilateral) suggests an **intra-abdominal mass.**

The sudden onset of local pallor, coolness, and cyanosis are seen in **acute arterial occlusion;** if peripheral pulses persist, small vessel thrombi (seen in diabetics) or small emboli (e.g., cholesterol emboli from ulcerated, proximal plaques) may have occurred. Discomfort along the distal inguinal crease or proximal medial leg accentuated by adduction of the leg against resistance suggests **adductor muscle strain** and commonly follows hyperabduction injuries.

In patients with **meralgia paresthetica,** reduced sensation to pinprick in the region of the lateral or anterolateral thigh or the subjective impression of asymmetry after cutaneous, simultaneous stimulation of both anterolateral thighs may be noted. Pain with palpation involving the lateral hip and its accentuation with external rotation (Patrick or "Fabere" test) are noted in patients with toxic synovitis; most such patients are children, usually boys, between 5 and 10 years of age, and low-grade fever may be noted. Similarly, patients with a slipped capital femoral epiphysis present with hip or knee pain and limp after mild or unrecalled trauma; discomfort is typically increased with internal rotation, and the diagnosis is confirmed radiologically with lateral frog-leg views of the hips.

A tense, tender, erythematous thigh or calf with a palpable cord and a positive Homans sign (calf pain on forced dorsiflexion of the ankle) are sometimes noted in patients with **DVT;** in approximately 50% of patients, however, these signs are absent or misleading. In some patients with calf thrombophlebitis, a prominent venous pattern may be noted on the dorsal surface of the involved leg (Pratt sign). In extreme cases associated with proximal obstruction of the deep femoral and iliac venous systems, edema and cyanosis may develop rapidly, producing phlegmasia alba dolens (milk leg) or, with loss of peripheral pulses and the evolution of ischemic changes, phlegmasia cerulea dolens. Simple superficial venous varicosities may produce peripheral edema and venous valvular incompetence, especially after previous episodes of DVT.

Pain, increased warmth, and varying amounts of erythema occurring in the prepatellar, infrapatellar, medial inferior knee, or popliteal fossa area suggest **acute bursitis,** the discomfort of which is increased by movement of the knee. Importantly, when evidence of skin disruption is noted in association with bursal inflammation, the possibility of suppurative bursitis must be considered.

Fever and a tender, locally erythematous area involving the limb and accompanying lymphangitis or lymphadenopathy are noted in patients with **cellulitis.**

Plantaris tendon rupture and proximal tears of the gastrocnemius muscle produce pain and swelling localized to the middle calf. Importantly, discomfort in patients with gastrocnemius tears is routinely enhanced with plantar flexion of the foot against resistance, while this is less common in patients with plantaris tendon rupture; this simple maneuver may represent an important diagnostic distinction. **Partial tears of the Achilles tendon** must be accurately diagnosed although, unfortunately, these injuries often produce subtle findings; failure to diagnose partial tears may result in complete disruption should normal activity be resumed. Discomfort, which may be mild, is localized to the tendon and is often increased by plantar flexion of the foot against resistance. A palpable "step-off" or loss of normal tendon contour may be noted as well unless local hematoma or swelling obscures this finding.

DIAGNOSTIC TESTS

A chest radiograph will support the diagnosis of congestive heart failure. Abdominal or pelvic ultrasonography is useful to define any intra-abdominal or intrapelvic processes that may produce leg swelling or pain. In addition, ultrasonography may also reveal a cirrhotic-appearing liver, splenomegaly, and ascites in patients suspected of portal hypertension. Acute arterial occlusion, of course, is diagnosed by Doppler flow studies and confirmed angiographically, if necessary.

Radiologic evaluation of the hip is indicated in most children and adolescents presenting with hip or knee pain or limp; the diagnosis of **slipped capital femoral epiphysis** will be confirmed with lateral frog-leg views, which most often demonstrate posterior and inferior displacement of the femoral epiphysis. **Osteomyelitis of the hip,** although uncommon, may also be suggested radiographically. **Osgood-Schlatter disease** may or may not be associated with significant radiologic findings; when present, irregularity or prominence of the tibial tuberosity or frank avulsion may be noted and is diagnostic. A **Baker cyst** may be demonstrated by ultrasonography or arthrography.

Doppler ultrasound (duplex scanning) and impedance plethysmography (IPG) of the lower extremities are useful in documenting DVT of the thigh, with a sensitivity and specificity in the 90% range; both tests are far less sensitive in documenting calf vessel involvement. In patients considered unlikely to have DVT, a negative D-dimer test (which is highly sensitive, but relatively nonspecific) makes the diagnosis of DVT significantly less likely and some authorities suggest that further studies are not required in this setting. It is less helpful in patients for whom clinical suspicion for DVT is moderate or high. Radionuclide venography is useful for documenting calf vein thrombosis. Although the venogram is the definitive test for the diagnosis of DVT, it is itself occasionally complicated by phlebitis. MRI has excellent sensitivity and specificity, both for proximal and for distal clot, is unassociated with complications, and may replace venography as the definitive diagnostic test for DVT.

SPECIFIC DISORDERS

Acute Arterial Occlusion

Acute arterial occlusion may occur as a result of embolism or in situ thrombosis. The source of emboli may be a thrombus or myxoma originating within the heart, an endovascular infection, or an atherosclerotic or thrombosed site proximal to the occlusion. Symptoms are determined by the suddenness and location of the occlusion, whether infarction occurs, the degree of collateral circulation, and the presence and extent of arterial spasm. Although pain is the major symptom, paresthesias, coldness, and progressive loss of sensation and muscle strength are common. The physical findings of absent peripheral pulses; cool, pale skin; and decreased venous filling with extremity dependence complete the picture. Cholesterol emboli classically produce purple toes or livedo reticularis with intact distal pulses; these typically originate from a more proximal ulcerated plaque. When acute arterial occlusion is suspected, emergency vascular surgical consultation and angiography should be obtained. When the diagnosis is in doubt, pulses can be evaluated at the bedside via Doppler analysis, and, if necessary and time permits, the diagnosis can be confirmed via duplex scanning.

Superficial Thrombophlebitis

Superficial thrombophlebitis may occur spontaneously in pregnant or postpartum women; in patients with superficial, lower extremity varicosities; or in association with trauma, recent venipuncture, or the intravenous administration of medications (e.g., most commonly the in-hospital administration of diazepam or potassium or illicit drug use).
- **Diagnosis:** In the lower extremity, the long saphenous vein is most commonly involved; importantly, superficial thrombophlebitis occurring above the knee is accompanied by DVT in approximately 20% of patients. Patients usually report a dull ache in the involved area; physical findings include local induration, erythema, and tenderness. Tenderness is often noted to extend proximally along the course of the involved, indurated vein; true fluctuance is rarely present, but when noted, suppurative thrombophlebitis should be suspected. In patients with idiopathic thrombophlebitis, the inflammatory process generally subsides within 5 to 7 days with treatment, but a firmly palpable cord remains for a longer period. Importantly, edema and deep pain involving the calf do not occur unless deep venous thrombophlebitis coexists.
- In patients with recent venipuncture, intravenous catheter placement or medication administration, or illicit intravenous drug use, the possibility of **suppurative thrombophlebitis** must be considered. This is less common in the lower extremity,

but if suspected, the workup and treatment should proceed as discussed previously in "Upper Extremity."

• **Treatment:** When a diagnosis of suppurative phlebitis is unlikely, only local and symptomatic measures, including moist heat, elevation, and a short course of an appropriate anti-inflammatory agent, are necessary.

Meralgia Paresthetica

Meralgia paresthetica is a sensory neuropathy resulting from compression of the lateral femoral cutaneous nerve at the level of Poupart ligament or in the fascia lata.

History

Patients may present acutely with pain and paresthesias involving the lateral and, occasionally, anterior proximal thigh. Symptoms are unilateral, and the disorder affects women more commonly than men; it is also often associated with diabetes mellitus. Recent weight gain or pregnancy may be reported and may be pathophysiologically pertinent. This disorder is most often confused with trochanteric bursitis (see "Trochanteric Bursitis," below), particularly when isolated lateral thigh symptoms predominate.

Physical Examination

Although physical findings are often subtle, reduced or altered sensation to pinprick or light touch is usually demonstrable in the distribution of the lateral femoral cutaneous nerve (anterolateral thigh). Frequently, a qualitative difference between the affected and unaffected sides will be noted with sensory testing. Motor function of the lower extremity is normal, and for a complete evaluation, the area of the inguinal ring should be examined in the upright position to exclude hernia.

Treatment

Treatment involves reassurance and a short course of a nonsteroidal anti-inflammatory agent. Weight loss should be encouraged, and prolonged sitting or repetitive bending at the waist should be discouraged. Application of local heat may be helpful in some patients; surgical extirpation of the nerve is an option used only after routine measures consistently fail.

Trochanteric Bursitis

Trochanteric bursitis results from inflammation of the trochanteric bursa and is usually seen in overweight individuals 30 to 50 years of age. Trochanteric bursitis is somewhat more common in persons with previous episodes of calcific tendinitis or bursitis of the shoulder, and vice versa.

Diagnosis

The patient usually relates lateral proximal thigh discomfort made worse with movement. The physical examination reveals tenderness to palpation over the trochanteric bursa and accentuation of discomfort with external rotation of the hip; sensory and motor testing are normal. Diagnostically, sensation is normal and symmetric in the distribution of the lateral femoral cutaneous nerve; this finding is of importance to help distinguish trochanteric bursitis from meralgia paresthetica (see "Meralgia Paresthetica").

Treatment

Treatment involves the application of local heat, several days of inactivity, and the use of an oral nonsteroidal anti-inflammatory agent for 7 to 10 days. Injection of a long-acting, nonabsorbable steroid (methylprednisolone acetate [Depo-Medrol], 40 mg) accompanied by 1 to 2 mL of 1% to 2% lidocaine (Xylocaine) or 1 to 2 mL of bupivacaine (Marcaine) may be undertaken in patients with particularly refractory symptoms.

Toxic Synovitis of the Hip

Toxic synovitis of the hip is a transient, self-limited phenomenon occurring primarily in children (mostly boys) between the ages of 5 and 10 years, who present with hip or knee pain and limp. Pathophysiologically, toxic synovitis of the hip is not well understood, although occasionally minor trauma or febrile illnesses precede or accompany the onset of symptoms.

Diagnosis

By physical examination, low-grade fever, limitation of motion as a result of local muscle spasm, accentuation of discomfort with movement of the leg, and minor joint swelling may be noted; the extremity is most often internally rotated, adducted, and somewhat flexed. The differential diagnosis in these patients should include septic arthritis, osteomyelitis, slipped femoral capital epiphysis, and early Legg-Calvé-Perthes disease. In patients with toxic synovitis, the involved hip appears normal when observed radiologically.

Treatment

When septic arthritis and osteomyelitis are unlikely or excluded, treatment involves several days of bed rest, acetaminophen or NSAID for discomfort, and orthopaedic follow-up in 3 to 5 days if symptoms are not resolving.

Slipped Femoral Capital Epiphysis

Slipped femoral capital epiphysis is most common in children and adolescents who, after minor or unrecalled trauma, present with hip, groin, or knee pain or limp; many patients are obese and bilateral involvement can occur. On physical examination, discomfort increases with internal rotation of the hip and the leg is typically externally rotated. Typically, the femoral epiphysis is displaced posteriorly and inferiorly and is so observed radiologically on AP and lateral views of the pelvis and hips. Lateral views are taken in the frog-leg position with the hips flexed 90 degrees and abducted 45 degrees. Complications include avascular necrosis of the femoral head and premature fusion of the epiphyseal plate. Prompt orthopaedic consultation is appropriate when the diagnosis is suspected or confirmed; patients will require admission, immobilization of the affected hip, and surgical repair.

Adductor Muscle Strain

Forceful or exaggerated abduction of the upper leg is the usual mechanism of adductor muscle strain and is common in gymnasts and cheerleaders; the so-called splits are a common precipitant in such patients.

Diagnosis

Pain, which is made worse by adduction of the leg against resistance, is an expected finding; pain at rest is usually reported along the distal inguinal crease or medial, proximal thigh. Avulsion fractures of the femur, often resulting from similar maneuvers, should be excluded radiologically.

Treatment

Treatment in patients with simple muscle strain includes several days of bed rest, the application of cold for 12 to 24 hours, proscription of activities resulting in discomfort for 7 to 10 days, crutches if needed, and follow-up as required.

Bursitis of the Knee

Several bursae surround the knee, any of which may become acutely inflamed and painful. Blunt trauma, which may have been trivial or unrecognized, is often reported to have preceded the onset of symptoms by several days. Occupations that involve kneeling, climbing, or other motions that repetitively flex and extend the knee may be associated with an increased incidence of bursal inflammation.

- **Physical Examination.** The prepatellar bursa located over the patella, the infrapatellar bursa located inferior to the patella, the anserine bursa located medially between the tibial plateau and the pes anserinus, and the medial gastrocnemius bursa located in the posterior popliteal fossa may all become acutely inflamed. Local swelling, overlying warmth, erythema, and discomfort are noted. Enlargement of the medial gastrocnemius bursa is commonly referred to as a **Baker cyst** and is more common in patients with intrinsic joint disease.

- Importantly, when trauma has preceded the onset of symptoms and has involved a penetrating injury or when evidence of local cellulitis or systemic infection is present, **suppurative bursitis** must be excluded. This is done by sterile aspiration of the bursa, with synovial fluid analysis which includes cell count and differential, Gram stain, and culture and sensitivity. Patients with suppurative bursitis require orthopaedic consultation and may require hospitalization, antibiotics, and formal incision or aspiration and drainage. Gout and pseudogout, which may simulate acute bursitis, must also be included in the differential diagnosis in most patients, and aspirated bursal fluid should therefore be analyzed for the presence of crystals.

- When infection is excluded or unlikely, **treatment** includes prohibition of activities or maneuvers that cause the bursa to move, local heat, and the institution of an oral nonsteroidal anti-inflammatory agent. Limitation of activities should be advised for most patients, and if activity is necessary, crutches should be recommended; orthopaedic referral at 5 to 7 days is appropriate.

Chondromalacia Patellae

Diagnosis
Young women are most commonly affected; these patients report vague discomfort localized to the knee, unassociated with trauma, however almost uniformly made worse by climbing stairs. The results of the physical examination are normal except for an occasional patient with pain and crepitus associated with downward and lateral movement of the patella. Radiologically, the knee is normal; pathologically, roughening of the articular cartilage of the patella is noted.

Treatment
Treatment includes immobilization, the institution of anti-inflammatory agents, and a formal physical therapy program designed to strengthen the quadriceps muscle.

Osgood-Schlatter Disease

Osgood-Schlatter disease is seen most often in adolescents, most of whom are athletic, and presumably results from a traction-type injury to the tibial tubercle at the site of insertion of the patellar tendon.

Diagnosis
Chronic symptoms are common; however, minor trauma to the area may cause the sudden onset or worsening of symptoms. Point tenderness is noted over the tibial tubercle, which may be inflamed as evidenced by local swelling, mild erythema, and

increased warmth. Radiologically, a lateral view of the proximal tibia may be normal and may demonstrate irregularity or prominence of the tibial tuberosity, or in some patients, an actual avulsion of the tuberosity may be noted.

Treatment
Treatment is determined by the patient's symptoms. Initially, in most patients, activities requiring repetitive knee extension such as running and jumping should be prohibited for 3 to 4 weeks. Nonsteroidal anti-inflammatory agents are useful and should be instituted along with crutches for patients with severe symptoms or evidence of inflammation. Ice may be applied initially to the area and may also be helpful. Immobilization of the knee and orthopaedic referral in 5 to 7 days is appropriate.

Chronic Venous Insufficiency

Chronic venous insufficiency of the lower leg generally develops as a result of valvular incompetence producing progressive venous stasis. Previous DVT may contribute to this development. In these patients, deep veins become functionally incompetent after local valves are destroyed; thus, blood is then shunted under high pressure to the superficial venous system. This constant transmission of high venous pressure through the perforating and superficial veins produces a variety of secondary changes, including local hemorrhage, fat necrosis, edema, lymphatic damage, and skin ulceration. Superficial venous dilation occurs, producing stasis and varicosities.

Diagnosis
Progressive edema and, later, secondary changes in the skin characterize the chronic venous insufficiency states. Pruritus, a dull discomfort worsened by standing, ulceration, and pain are common symptoms. Thin, shiny, atrophic skin often associated with brown pigmentation evolves. Recurrent ulcerations are common, primarily in the medial or anterior ankle; varicosities, eczema, and superficial dermatitis are also frequently noted.

Treatment
Treatment includes leg elevation, avoidance of long periods of standing, and the use of elastic stockings. Dermatitis may be treated with elevation and compresses of Burow solution; antibiotics are indicated if signs of infection are present. Surgical evaluation regarding the need for definitive treatment of varicose veins should be considered if conservative measures fail.

Deep Venous Thrombosis

Venous thrombosis of the lower extremity develops approximately 80% of the time in the deep veins of the calf and, in the remainder, in the femoral and iliac system. Clinical thrombosis will develop in a significant number of patients undergoing major surgery, particularly those undergoing total hip replacement. Risk factors include prior thromboembolism or DVT, a family history of DVT, tobacco use, trauma or surgery involving the extremity, any of the hypercoagulable states (oral contraceptives use, pregnancy, malignancy, nephrotic syndrome, sepsis, ulcerative colitis, specific protein deficiencies or mutations [S, C, or antithrombin III] deficiences, or Factor V Leiden mutation), and stasis (prolonged sitting or air travel, bed rest, casting of the lower extremity, low-flow states engendered by congestive heart failure or pulmonary hypertension, or neurologic disorders affecting mobility).

Clinical Presentation

Patients with deep venous thrombophlebitis may complain of a dull ache, a tight feeling, or frank pain in the calf or thigh accentuated by walking. Physical findings are misleading, unreliable, or absent in approximately one half of patients. If present, findings include swelling of the involved calf or thigh, local erythema and tenderness, distention of superficial dorsal collaterals (Pratt sign), pain in the calf with forced dorsiflexion of the ankle (Homans sign), and low-grade fever. If the femoral and iliac veins are involved, swelling in the extremity may be marked (phlegmasia alba dolens); if venous obstruction is severe, cyanosis and gangrene may develop (phlegmasia cerulea dolens).

Diagnostic Tests

A variety of modalities, anatomic and functional, direct and indirect, are available to the clinician in diagnosing venous disease; these include duplex ultrasound (which combines B-mode ultrasound and Doppler flow), impedance plethysmography, contrast venography, radionuclide venography, and MRI. Historically, the gold standard to which all other diagnostic modalities have been compared is contrast venography. The diagnostic modality of choice is somewhat determined by availability and the institution's experience with any given technique. All the various techniques have false-positive and false-negative results. A few generalizations can be made. Of the non-invasive tests, duplex ultrasonography, when performed by an experienced operator, has excellent sensitivity and specificity, although with some important limitations. For example, duplex scanning cannot be used reliably to exclude venous disease in patients with disease below the knee and above the groin, or in any location in asymptomatic patients; a positive test in the latter instance is sometimes used, and appropriately, to confirm the diagnosis of pulmonary embolism. When the clinical situation is suggestive of pulmonary embolism, a positive Doppler scan virtually confirms the diagnosis of pulmonary embolism. It is important to remember, however, that a negative test in the calf and above the groin, and in asymptomatic patients, is inconclusive. In these patients, other modalities must be used (contrast venography or MRI). **D-dimer analysis**, as determined by ELISA, if less than 250 ng/mL is helpful in excluding DVT (sensitivity between 80% and 90%); however, the test is nonspecific and elevated in a variety of settings (trauma, cardiovascular disease, malignancy, infection, or surgery). When combined with a normal duplex ultrasound (or IPG), a negative D-dimer determination has a negative predictive value of approximately 99% for proximal DVT. A recent study suggests an excellent negative predictive value in patients with the combination of a low index of suspicion for DVT and a negative D-dimer.

Treatment

The treatment of **isolated calf DVT** continues to be controversial; therapeutic strategies continue to evolve and improve. The goals of treatment are the lysis of clot and the prevention of pulmonary embolism and recurrent DVT. One must weigh the complications associated with anticoagulation against the complications associated with following-up the patient with untreated, calf thrombophlebitis. It is known that the incidence of recurrent DVT is significant in untreated patients; anticoagulation for 3 months largely prevents this. It is also relatively clear that the risk of significant pulmonary embolism in otherwise healthy patients with untreated, calf phlebitis, particularly those with reversible risk factors for DVT, who are now ambulatory, is very low, provided that such patients can be followed up closely for clot propagation with serial duplex ultrasound. Some centers treat all patients with isolated calf DVT; another strategy separates patients into two groups: those with a reversible or resolved risk factor for DVT, who are now fully ambulatory and who may be followed up as outpatients with duplex scanning, and those with either idiopathic DVT or associated with risk factors, which are permanent. In the first category, the risk benefit analysis may lead one to follow such patients and institute treatment if propagation of clot occurs; the second group with fixed or idiopathic DVT should be considered for anticoagulation. Some authorities suggest that patients at high risk for bleeding complications associated with anticoagulation, particularly those with reversible risk factors, may similarly be followed up (closely) for clot propagation. The issue is not fully resolved.

Otherwise healthy patients, without significant risk factors (hypercoagulability, immobility, serious cardiovascular disease, recurrent thrombophlebitis or PE), with suspected calf DVT, and having a normal duplex scan (or normal IPG), can usually be discharged from the ED but require careful follow-up, including a second scan (or IPG) approximately 5 to 7 days after discharge. A repeat scan is sometimes obtained sooner. Patients with a low clinical index of suspicion, when combined with a negative D-dimer study, are unlikely to have DVT and many authorities suggest that these patients may be discharged with close follow-up as described. Given the inherent morbidity associated with long-term anticoagulation, high-risk patients (for bleeding) should have the presence of clot confirmed or excluded via MRI before anticoagulation. In the end, the physician must weigh the risks and benefits in each patient.

Proximal DVT requires anticoagulation to prevent clot propagation and prevent pulmonary embolization; thrombolytic agents, although initially felt to represent a superior treatment strategy, particularly in regard to reducing the incidence and severity of the postphlebitic syndrome, may be best reserved for patients with extensive proximal (involving the iliac and femoral vessels) clot in whom the risk of bleeding is very low. This is, however, an area of ongoing investigation. Consultation with vascular surgery and/or interventional radiology may be helpful depending on local practice patterns. Dense iliofemoral thrombosis may fail to respond to systemically administered thrombolytic agents; local thrombolytic delivery by infusion may provide better clot lysis in proximal areas with minimal blood flow. The treatment of proximal DVT, unless patients require hospital admission for other medical or social reasons, given the availability and success of the **low molecular weight heparins (LMWHs)**, is most cost-effectively initiated in the ED with subsequent treatment provided at home. Of the available agents, enoxaparin (Lovenox) is most often selected in a dose equal to 1 mg/kg given subcutaneously every 12 hours. The LMWH agents, in comparison to unfractionated heparin, have several advantages: anticoagulation is highly predictable given standard doses, monitoring of blood levels or the patient's anticoagulation state is unnecessary, they are easily administered, and patients have significantly fewer bleeding and other (the thrombocytopenia seen with heparin does not occur) complications. Discharged patients are given an initial dose, will require additional doses every 12 hours, should be provided with the medication before discharge, and should be seen in follow-up within 12 to 24 hours by the primary care physician; the decision to use the LMWHs should be discussed with the patient's PCP, who will initiate therapy with warfarin, typically within 24 hours of ED discharge. Enoxaparin is safe in pregnancy and is the agent of choice for DVT in this setting; warfarin is contraindicated (see later).

If **treatment with heparin** is elected, an initial bolus of 80 U/kg, followed by a continuous infusion of 18 U/kg/h (see Chapter 21, Table 21-1). The dose for obese patients is calculated using the patient's ideal body weight plus 30% of weight in excess of ideal to arrive at an "effective" weight. After the initiation of heparin therapy, an activated partial thromboplastin time (aPTT) is routinely checked at 6 hours and then at 6-hour intervals with any adjustments made based on this level. An aPTT of at least 1.8- to 2.0-times control achieves adequate heparinization. Because of the incidence of early recurrent pulmonary embolism in underanticoagulated patients, efforts should be directed toward rapid and adequate heparinization within the first 6 to 12 hours; providing an initial bolus of 5,000 U fails to achieve effective anticoagulation in more than 50% of patients. Warfarin, in an initial dose of 7.5 to 10 mg orally, is typically initiated concurrently with the institution of heparin; it may be preferable to delay warfarin therapy by 24 hours after the heparin bolus, in that warfarin produces a transient, early state of hypercoagulability. Additionally, because of this, heparin should be continued for 48 hours after effective anticoagulation with warfarin; this is achieved when the INR is between 2 and 3. Warfarin is contraindicated in pregnancy (it crosses the placenta, is teratogenic, and causes bleeding in the fetus); both the LMWHs and heparin are safe in pregnancy, with enoxaparin being the drug of choice for pregnant patients with DVT.

Treatment with all agents can be complicated by **bleeding;** in patients treated with thrombolytic agents, this most often occurs from diagnostic arterial puncture sites. Simple compression of such sites will usually be adequate to control bleeding; bleeding from noncompressible sites requires that the thrombolytic agent be discontinued. It is also important to remember that the lytic state can be reversed with fresh frozen plasma and cryoprecipitate, as well as with treatment with aminocaproic acid (Amicar, 5 g intravenous is given as an initial loading dose followed by a continuous infusion of 1 g/h).

The diagnosis of **catheter-related venous thrombosis** is typically made via duplex ultrasound or contrast venography; the risk of pulmonary embolism in this setting is significant and aggressive treatment is warranted. Treatment options include anticoagulation or the selective infusion of thrombolytic agents; cases should be reviewed with the vascular surgeon who will follow up the patient.

Placement of **an inferior vena cava filter** represents an effective treatment option in selected patients; these include patients in whom anticoagulation is contraindicated or associated with bleeding complications, patients in whom venous thrombosis develops or clot enlarges in the setting of therapeutic anticoagulation, and patients with pulmonary embolization in the setting of therapeutic anticoagulation. This modality has also been suggested in patients with extensive (>5 cm), nonadherent, proximal clot because of the high rate of embolization despite medical therapy.

Gastrocnemius Muscle Tear and Plantaris Tendon Rupture

Gastrocnemius muscle tear and plantaris tendon rupture are considered together because differentiation by historical or physical criteria is often not possible and treatment is similar. The plantaris tendon is a vestigial structure with no clear function.

History

Patients with tears of the gastrocnemius muscle (which are virtually always partial) and those with plantaris tendon ruptures report the relatively sudden onset of calf pain usually precipitated by physical activity of some sort. This may simply involve running or jumping, although other maneuvers that selectively stress the involved structure, such as pushing off at the beginning of a race or charging the net at tennis, may also be responsible, although often no such history is elicited. An occasional patient with an acute plantaris tendon rupture will report an audible "snap" or "pop," which, when accompanied by calf discomfort in relation to physical activity, is highly suggestive of this entity. Both groups of patients report severe calf pain, which, especially in patients with gastrocnemius muscle tears, is accentuated by plantar flexion of the foot against resistance.

Physical Findings
Physical findings in both disorders include local calf tenderness with palpation, often extensive swelling, and ecchymoses, and in many patients, presenting somewhat later, ankle swelling, warmth, and layering of blood just below the malleolus are noted. When swelling and hemorrhage are extensive, local vascular perfusion may become compromised, producing rapidly evolving ischemia of the lower leg and foot; pedal pulses, the general appearance of the lower leg, skin temperature, and capillary filling should therefore be assessed in all patients with significant calf injuries. Fever may also be noted in some patients with extensive local hemorrhage and usually occurs after 2 or 3 days. Although differentiation of these two disorders has no major therapeutic advantage, many patients with plantaris tendon ruptures can relatively comfortably plantar flex the foot against resistance while those with gastrocnemius muscle tears uniformly cannot.

Treatment
Treatment for patients with plantaris tendon ruptures or gastrocnemius muscle tears is symptomatic and conservative after evolving ischemia and fibular fractures are excluded; fibular fractures may be associated with minimal discomfort and very subtle findings. 24 to 72 hours of cold application, elevation of the leg, bed rest, and the use of a nonsteroidal anti-inflammatory agent and analgesics is recommended. Crutches should be provided as dictated by the patient's symptoms. Warm compresses or soaks may be applied after 72 hours to facilitate resolution of local hemorrhage. Orthopaedic follow-up at 10 to 12 days after the injury is appropriate.

Cellulitis
Cellulitis of the lower extremity is common and may occur spontaneously or associated with minor or unrecalled trauma.

Diagnosis
Cellulitis causes local pain, swelling, increased warmth, and erythema. Systemic signs of infection are common, and a relatively clearly demarcated border of erythema is often noted. When the calf is involved, despite the presence of fever, differentiation from thrombophlebitis may be extremely difficult and, in some patients, may require that a deep venous thrombosis specifically be excluded.

Treatment
Patients with systemic signs of infection, particularly the immunocompromised patient (e.g., the diabetic), usually require hospital admission and the initiation of intravenous antibiotic therapy. Immunocompromised patients require broad-spectrum antibiotic therapy, using a second- or third-generation cephalosporin (ceftriaxone 1–2 g intravenous every day) or imipenem (500 mg intravenous every 6 hours) in severe cases; other patients may be treated with a first-generation cephalosporin (cefazolin

1 g intravenous every 6 hours) or a penicillinase-resistant penicillin (nafcillin or oxacillin 2 g intravenous every 4 hours). In patients not requiring intravenous antibiotics, dicloxacillin, 500 mg four times daily orally; azithromycin, 500 mg orally initial dose, followed by 250 mg daily for 4 days; amoxicillin-clavulanate, 875-mg amoxicillin orally every 12 hours; or EES 500 orally every 6 hours can be used. In all patients, the application of heat four to six times per day and elevation are advised, the latter being particularly important. Although organisms are not recoverable by aspiration, blood cultures may prove useful; bacteriologically, streptococcal and staphylococcal organisms are most often implicated. Consideration should be given to antibiotic coverage of methicillin-resistant *Staphylococcus aureus* (MRSA) depending on local prevalence patterns.

Achilles Tendon Strain or Rupture

Achilles tendon strains are seen in young adults, whereas actual tendon disruption occurs primarily in men, usually between the ages of 40 and 50 years.

History

Although tendon rupture may occur as a result of a direct blow to the Achilles tendon, more commonly, the tendon ruptures during a maneuver that selectively stresses it. A variety of histories demonstrating this fact is usually obtained; for example, patients report charging the net at tennis, pushing a stalled car, or starting a foot race. Many patients will report the initial feeling that they were struck from behind in the area of the distal calf, and many others report an audible "snap" or "pop" at the time of rupture. Patients' recent use of ciprofloxacin has been implicated in the predisposition to this injury.

Two important points should be emphasized: (1) pain may be excruciating with partial tears or strains of the tendon and completely absent with total disruptions, and vice versa, and (2) in some patients with total tendon disruptions, plantar flexion may be present. Given these two points, one must be very cautious when evaluating the patient with pain localized to the Achilles tendon because undiagnosed partial tears may progress with activity to complete disruption.

Physical Examination

In the **physical examination,** a palpable "step-off" in the course of the tendon or a "notch" or defect in its course suggests total disruption, as does inability to plantar flex the ankle. If 12 to 48 hours elapse between the injury and examination, however, local hematomata may "fill in" the defect and thereby obscure any palpable step-off. Local pain and its accentuation with plantar flexion are noted as well in most patients. Diagnostically, patients are typically unable to walk or stand up on their toes. Preservation of plantar flexion, either actively or passively, suggests partial rupture or strain. Absence of Achilles tendon function may be demonstrated by squeezing the gastrocnemius muscle with the patient lying prone with ankles and feet extended over the edge of the stretcher; if plantar flexion does not occur with this maneuver, (constituting a positive Thompson-Doherty test) then an important injury to the Achilles is highly likely. Although usually unnecessary, MRI will confirm the diagnosis.

Treatment

Treatment is conservative for the patient with Achilles tendon strains or suspected partial tendon tears; when a partial tear is suspected, orthopaedic consultation at the time of presentation is reasonable as plaster immobilization is often advised to prevent reinjury or total disruption. In patients with minor strains of the Achilles associated with normal motor function and minimal symptoms with stress, a period of elevation, cold application, rest, and a heel pad after symptoms have completely subsided may be advised. In patients with complete rupture, treatment is somewhat controversial, and orthopaedic referral is appropriate, because either primary surgical repair or plaster immobilization may be elected. Discharged patients will require immobilization with the foot positioned in plantar flexion and crutches.

Achilles Tenosynovitis

Occupations or athletic pursuits that repetitively result in flexion and extension of the ankle are commonly reported in patients with Achilles tenosynovitis.

Diagnosis
Pain at rest, accentuated by flexion or extension, is present. In some patients, local crepitus may be noted with passive or active motion of the ankle; overlying warmth and occasionally erythema are also noted in some patients.

Treatment
Treatment includes several days of rest or the use of crutches to immobilize the ankle, local heat, and the institution of nonsteroidal anti-inflammatory agents. A heel pad may be helpful in 5 to 7 days as symptoms are subsiding.

Heel Pain

The differential diagnosis of a painful heel includes

Plantar Fasciitis or Calcaneal Bursitis
Calcaneal bursitis and plantar fasciitis produce lateral heel pain with palpation and may be associated with minor local swelling. Practically, differentiation of these latter entities may not be possible in many patients; treatment, however, is similar and involves a brief period of immobility, elevation of the extremity, avoidance of direct pressure on the heel by the use of a heel pad if discomfort is so elicited, and a course of an anti-inflammatory agent.

Tenosynovitis or Strain of the Achilles Tendon
The diagnosis of Achilles tenosynovitis or strain should be straightforward and is described in "Achilles Tenosynovitis."

Plantar Warts
Plantar warts are noted by examination and can be exquisitely painful with palpation or deep pressure (see "Plantar Warts").

Calcaneal Spurs
Calcaneal spurs produce volar heel pain accentuated by weight bearing or direct pressure over the volar heel and are noted radiologically.

Plantar Warts

Plantar warts represent intraepidermal tumors secondary to infection with the human papillomavirus; lesions are painful when occurring in locations exposed to pressure or when infection develops. Formal excision or electrodesiccation is reserved for patients refractory to other forms of therapy such as salicylic acid pastes and other keratolytic agents applied after paring of the lesion with a scalpel. Because of the long duration of treatment necessary, patients with plantar warts are generally not treated in the

ED and are referred for outpatient therapy. If plantar warts become infected, after culturing of the wound, antistaphylococcal antibiotic coverage should be prescribed, along with rest, soaks, elevation, and follow-up in 24 to 48 hours.

Morton Neuroma

Diagnosis

Patients, most of whom are women, present with a sharp or burning pain relatively well localized to the area between and under the distal third and fourth metatarsal heads; radiation into the toes associated with walking is also commonly reported, and many patients describe the discomfort "as if a stone were in the shoe." Many patients report that elevation, rest, or rubbing the involved area results in temporarily improved symptoms. By physical examination, an area of well-defined tenderness with palpation is noted over the appropriate distal intermetatarsal area and reproduces the patient's discomfort. Pathologically, a neuroma of the interdigital nerve is noted in this location, the etiology of which is obscure.

Treatment

Treatment includes rest, the avoidance of pressure over the involved area, and an oral nonsteroidal anti-inflammatory agent. Alternatively, a steroid and bupivacaine hydrochloride (Marcaine) may be injected locally and will provide somewhat better symptomatic relief. Neither treatment modality is curative, however, and for this reason, orthopaedic or podiatry consultation in 5 to 7 days is appropriate to assess progress. Surgical removal may be elected if symptoms are refractory or recurrent.

Ingrown Toenails

The lateral or medial toenail often gradually insinuates itself into the adjacent tissues of the distal toe; pain and local infectious complications then result. Most commonly, the first toe is involved and occasionally improperly fitting shoes that compress the toes are responsible. If seen early, the lateral nail can be elevated in such a way that its projected path of growth will not reenter the tissues; this position can be sustained by placing a small, povidone–iodine-impregnated cotton pledget under the distal nail. Soaks four to six times per day, changing the pledget every 1 to 2 days to ensure nail elevation, and the avoidance of compression will usually result in resolution. More commonly, elevation of the nail is not possible because of more extensive entry into the distal tissues or associated tissue reaction. In these patients, a digital block with lidocaine, 1%, *without* epinephrine should be provided and the lateral quarter of the nail removed. Surrounding granulation tissue should be excised and the involved and adjacent areas probed with a scalpel to exclude local abscess; patients with significant surrounding cellulitis should be treated with an appropriate antistaphylococcal antibiotic. Patients should be instructed to keep the extremity elevated for 12 to 24 hours to prevent throbbing; most patients will require an analgesic for 24 to 48 hours. To avoid dressings becoming adherent to the underlying tissue, an antibacterial ointment is applied generously next to the tissue, followed by the application of a nonadherent dressing. After the initial dressing change, patients should be instructed to soak the toe three to four times per day until discomfort and any erythema have resolved. Unfortunately, recurrences are common.

47 **Joint Pain—Atraumatic**

Patients who present to the emergency department with a tender or swollen joint without a history of recent significant trauma require a careful evaluation. Although many of the disorders producing this symptom may be appropriately treated with immobilization, analgesics, and anti-inflammatory agents, the physician must ensure that bacterial infection is not present; this is true because staphylococcal, gonococcal, and pneumococcal organisms may rapidly destroy a joint if not promptly diagnosed and treated. For this reason, arthrocentesis is recommended in all patients in whom the diagnosis of septic arthritis cannot be excluded.

COMMON CAUSES OF JOINT PAIN AND SWELLING

- Degenerative joint disease (DJD; osteoarthritis)*
- Rheumatoid arthritis*
- Gout*
- Bursitis*

LESS COMMON CAUSES OF JOINT PAIN AND SWELLING NOT TO BE MISSED

- Acute bacterial arthritis (staphylococcal, gonococcal, pneumococcal)*
- Systemic lupus erythematosus
- Pseudogout*
- Acute rheumatic fever
- Toxic synovitis*
- Ruptured Baker cyst*
- Osteochondrosis*

OTHER CAUSES OF JOINT PAIN AND SWELLING

- Progressive systemic sclerosis
- Ankylosing spondylitis
- Psoriatic arthritis
- Reiter syndrome
- Neuropathic arthropathy
- Pigmented villonodular synovitis
- Synovioma
- Hemangioma
- Hemophilic arthropathy*
- Osteochondromatosis

*Discussed in this chapter.

HISTORY

A history of severe pain and swelling in a single joint, especially the first metatarsophalangeal joint or knee, intolerably uncomfortable to even the slightest pressure, suggests **gout or pseudogout.** Migrating polyarthralgia and arthritis suggest **acute rheumatic fever, rheumatoid arthritis,** or **systemic lupus erythematosus.** A history of polyserositis, nasopharyngeal ulcers, Raynaud phenomenon, alopecia, or malar rash in association with atraumatic arthralgias and arthritis suggests **systemic lupus erythematosus.** Patients with an inflamed **osteoarthritic joint** usually give a history of chronic discomfort in the involved joint increased or precipitated by use and improving with rest or immobilization. A history suggestive of venereal disease should imply either **gonococcal arthritis** or **Reiter syndrome.**

PHYSICAL EXAMINATION

Joint swelling without erythema or impressive warmth is noted in patients with **osteoarthritis.** First metatarsophalangeal arthritis (podagra) is most commonly noted in **gout,** whereas knee arthritis (gonagra) is seen more commonly in **pseudogout.** A malar rash, nasopharyngeal ulcers, and alopecia in association with arthritis are seen in **systemic lupus erythematosus.** Limitations of chest wall expansion and lumbosacral spine flexion are found in **ankylosing spondylitis,** and psoriatic skin changes may be seen in patients with **psoriatic arthritis.** Discrete papules with hemorrhagic, purple, or darkened centers overlying the extension surfaces and often associated with a urethral or cervical discharge in a patient with a history of recent sexual exposure suggest **gonococcal arthritis or tenosynovitis.**

DIAGNOSTIC TESTS

- **Radiologic examination** rarely provides a definitive diagnosis. Most commonly, the presence of soft-tissue swelling and an effusion, readily detected on physical examination, are simply confirmed radiologically. DJD, however, may be documented by roentgenograms of the involved joint. Uniform joint space narrowing, demineralization, and bony erosions suggest **rheumatoid arthritis**; linear calcium deposition within the joint space is noted in patients with pseudogout. Sacroiliac periostitis may be documented in patients with **ankylosing spondylitis,** and "pencil-in-cup" deformities are occasionally noted in the more advanced forms of **psoriatic arthritis.** Infrequently, "punched-out," radiolucent, bony tophi may be noted in advanced gout.
- The definitive diagnostic test, which should be performed in all patients presenting with an acute atraumatic synovitis or arthritis, is **arthrocentesis.** This procedure is essential to document the presence or absence of acute, destructive staphylococcal, gonococcal, or pneumococcal arthritis. When overlying cutaneous infection is not present, the peripheral joint may and should be aspirated with impunity by the physician in the emergency department. This is true except for the hip, the arthrocenteses of which should be performed by an orthopaedist with fluoroscopic guidance if necessary. Arthrocentesis should be performed after cleansing the skin and sterilizing the point at which the puncture will be made, after which the skin may then be anesthetized with lidocaine. The arthrocentesis itself follows, and the physician should attempt to remove as much fluid as possible from the joint. The fluid should

be examined for gross appearance, sent for culture and sensitivity, microscopically examined for Gram stain and cell count and differential, and glucose levels measured. Microscopic crystal analysis should also be performed with a polarizing lens to exclude gout and pseudogout. Table 47-1 indicates the results of synovial fluid analysis in each of four general classes of arthritis.

- **Additional laboratory tests** that may be useful include a sedimentation rate, antinuclear antibodies, latex fixation, antistreptolysin O titer, blood cultures, and urethral, throat, cervical, and rectal cultures for *Neisseria gonorrhoeae* when indicated. Note that serum uric acid levels have not been found to correlate with the presence of acute gouty arthritis.

CLINICAL REMINDERS

- Perform an arthrocentesis on or obtain orthopaedic consultation for all patients with an atraumatic joint effusion in whom the diagnosis of septic arthritis is possible.
- Do not administer intra-articular steroids to any patient in whom an acute infectious arthritis is suspected.
- Begin empiric intravenous antibiotics in any patient in whom the possibility of acute infectious arthritis exists once synovial and blood cultures have been obtained.

SPECIFIC DISORDERS

Degenerative Joint Disease

DJD is a chronic arthropathy characterized by degeneration of cartilage and bony hypertrophy at articular margins. The inflammatory response to these degenerative changes is usually minimal but occurs with sufficient frequency and intensity to produce common "acute-on-chronic" flairs of this disorder. DJD occurs as a primary process, most commonly affecting the distal interphalangeal joints, the first metacarpophalangeal joint, the knee, and the cervical and lumbar spines. It may also occur secondarily in response to severe or chronic articular injury.

Diagnosis
The onset of symptoms in patients with DJD is typically insidious. Joint stiffness is a prominent early feature evolving into pain on motion of the joint that is relieved with rest. The physical examination in primary DJD may reveal Heberden nodes (distal interphalangeal joint), Bouchard nodes (proximal interphalangeal joint), or crepitus of the shoulders, first metacarpophalangeal joint, and patella (seen with osteomalacia patellae in young women). Acute flairs are associated with periarticular swelling, effusion, increased warmth, and minimal or absent erythema. No signs or symptoms of an acute systemic illness are seen in chronic DJD, and laboratory tests are unrevealing. Radiologic studies typically demonstrate nonuniform narrowing of the joint space with local osteophyte formation, marginal bone lipping, dense subchondral bone, and occasionally bony cysts.

Treatment
Temporary immobilization or rest of the involved joint, the application of local heat, analgesics, and anti-inflammatory agents are all useful in providing symptomatic relief. Although at present no cure exists for the unremitting process of degeneration, conservative measures usually provide significant symptomatic relief for patients with acute exacerbations.

Table 47-1	Results of Synovial Fluid Analysis in Four Classes of Arthritis				
	Normal	**Noninflammatory**	**Inflammatory**	**Septic**	**Traumatic**
Clarity	Transparent	Transparent	Transparent-opaque	Opaque	Opaque
Color	Clear	Yellow	Yellow-white	Yellow-white	Pink-red
Viscosity	High	Low	Low	Low	High
WBC/μL	200	200–3,000	3,000–50,000	>50,000	<200
PMN (%)	<25	<25	>50	>75	<25
Glucose (mg/dL)	Equal to serum	Equal to serum	Lower than serum	Lower than serum	Equal to serum

Note that the numbers are not absolute and are guidelines only; they must be correlated with clinical suspicion.
WBC, white blood cells; PMN, polymorphonuclear leukocytes.

Rheumatoid Arthritis

Rheumatoid arthritis is a chronic, systemic disorder of unknown cause with a wide spectrum of clinical manifestations and considerable variability in both joint and extra-articular presentations. The disease affects women more commonly than men (3:1) and may begin at any age, with a peak incidence at 20 to 40 years.

Clinical Presentation

The onset of articular signs is usually gradual, with prodromal malaise, weight loss, vasomotor disturbances, and vague articular pain, swelling, or isolated morning stiffness. Characteristically, joint swelling and pain are symmetric, primarily affecting proximal interphalangeal, metacarpophalangeal, wrist, knee, ankle, and metatarsophalangeal joints. Rarely, monoarticular disease or temporomandibular joint dysfunction may be an early manifestation of the disorder. Extra-articular manifestations include subcutaneous nodules, low-grade fever, splenomegaly, lymphadenopathy, keratoconjunctivitis sicca, episcleritis, scleromalacia, vasculitis, pericarditis, pleuritis, and entrapment syndromes.

Diagnostic Tests

A moderate hypochromic, microcytic anemia is common in rheumatoid arthritis; the white blood cell (WBC) count is typically normal except in Felty syndrome, in which case leukopenia and splenomegaly are found. The latex fixation test for immunoglobulin M anti-immunoglobulin G (rheumatoid factor) is positive in approximately three fourths of patients with rheumatoid arthritis; antinuclear antibodies are also frequently present but in lower titer than in patients with systemic lupus erythematosus. Soft-tissue swelling, demineralization, and bony surface erosions are early radiographic findings; subsequently, cartilage destruction leads to uniform joint space narrowing.

Causes of Death

Among the **causes of death** in rheumatoid arthritis with which the emergency physician should be familiar are **subluxation of the cervical spine** at C1-2, **complete heart block** secondary to rheumatoid nodules of the conduction system, and cricoarytenoid joint immobility after extubation producing **vocal cord paralysis** and consequent respiratory arrest. All patients with active rheumatoid arthritis must be intubated with great care so as to minimize vocal cord and cervical spine trauma, the latter resulting in C1-2 subluxation.

Treatment

Treatment of the synovitis of rheumatoid arthritis is directed toward two goals: inducing a remission of the disease and controlling acute symptoms. Remission induction is typically attempted with methotrexate, hydroxychloroquine, gold, or penicillamine. These agents should be initiated by the rheumatologist or internist who will provide long-term care for the patient, given the serious toxicities associated with the use of each of these agents. For the initial control of acute symptoms, aspirin is the mainstay of therapy, and most adults can tolerate 4 to 6 g/day (achieving therapeutic levels of 20–30 mg/dL). Other nonsteroidal anti-inflammatory drugs (NSAIDs; indomethacin, fenoprofen, ibuprofen, naproxen, sulindac, tolmetin, and meclofenamate, among others) have also been used with success. Steroids should be used minimally, if at all, and only for a brief course when other more conservative measures fail. Intra-articular injections of poorly absorbed hydrocortisone esters (e.g., Depo-Medrol) are effective and may occasionally be required. Despite the minimal degree of systemic absorption of this steroid preparation, a single intra-articular injection often produces an improvement in both systemic symptoms and in other, uninjected but involved joints.

Gout and Pseudogout

Gout is an inherited metabolic disease characterized by hyperuricemia secondary to either overproduction or underexcretion of uric acid. Clinical gout may also be seen in association with a number of disorders including the myeloproliferative syndromes, renal failure, and the use of thiazide diuretics.

Pathophysiology

Most patients with gout are men (approximately 90%) and are usually of middle age. The tophus, a nodular deposit of monosodium urate monohydrate crystals, is the characteristic histologic lesion and may be found in cartilage, tendon, bone, kidney, and elsewhere. Phagocytosis of urate crystals in the synovial fluid, with the subsequent release by the white cell of a variety of mediators of inflammation, is believed to precipitate acute attacks. Historically, although hyperuricemia has been poorly correlated temporally with attacks of acute gout, recent studies suggest that rapid fluctuations in serum urate can occur and may indeed be responsible for precipitating attacks under conditions of urate supersaturation.

Clinical Presentation

Acute gouty arthritis is characterized by the sudden onset of pain, typically at night, usually without a precipitating cause. Events that may also lead to rapid fluctuations in the serum urate, including food or alcohol excess, surgery, infection, or diuretic use, have also been associated with attacks of acute gout. The first metatarsophalangeal joint is classically involved (podagra), the pain of which is described as so intense that even the placement of bedsheets on the foot is intolerable. Other joints may be involved, and more than one may be involved at initial presentation. The pain becomes more severe as the attack progresses, subsiding spontaneously after 3 to 4 days. Tophi are found on physical examination primarily in the pinnae and overlying the olecranon bursa. Striking erythema and warmth over the involved joint are noted, as is severe pain with palpation or movement. Pruritus and local desquamation during the recovery phase are uncommonly seen but are pathognomonic for this disorder.

Diagnostic Tests

Laboratory data are generally not useful in an acute attack. An elevated ESR or WBC is neither sensitive nor specific for an acute attack. The serum uric acid may be elevated but is often normal. Radiographic evaluation is typically normal in the acute attack but may show radiolucent, "punched-out" areas corresponding to tophi in patients with long-standing disease. **Arthrocentesis** is diagnostic, revealing, by polarizing microscope, negatively birefringent (yellow crystals on a red background) needle-shaped intracellular crystals of sodium urate.

Treatment

An acute attack of gouty arthritis may be treated in any of several ways. A NSAID such as ibuprofen or indomethacin may be administered, along with an additional analgesic, if necessary, for 5 to 7 days. Most patients require a narcotic analgesic for at least several days, during which time activity should be restricted and the involved area elevated. Patients with contraindications to NSAIDs may be given an injection of adrenocorticotropic hormone as a single 75-U intramuscular injection, which dramatically relieves attacks within 12 hours. Colchicine is another treatment option at a dose of 0.5 mg orally every 30 to 60 minutes to a maximum of 4 to 6 mg. Nausea, vomiting, and diarrhea often limit the dosage. As noted previously, regardless of the therapy chosen, patients often require an additional analgesic for several days.

All patients with a first attack of acute gout should be referred and subsequently evaluated with a serum uric acid and a 24-hour urinary urate *after* the acute attack subsides. Most patients will be found to be hypoexcretors (<600 mg/24 h) and should generally be treated with uricosuric agents, including probenecid (0.5–1.0 g/day) or sulfinpyrazone (100–300 mg/day). Overproducers should be treated with the xanthine oxidase inhibitor allopurinol, 200 to 400 mg/day. It is important to note that colchicine (0.5–0.6 mg orally twice daily) should be instituted 2 to 3 days before initiating therapy with a drug that will modify uric acid levels; otherwise, an acute attack of gout may be precipitated.

Pseudogout or Chondrocalcinosis

Pseudogout, or chondrocalcinosis, refers to the deposition of calcium pyrophosphate crystals in cartilage. This disorder is frequently familial and may be associated with diabetes mellitus, hyperparathyroidism, hemochromatosis, true gout, and ochronosis. The acute attack is precipitated by crystals from cartilage entering the adjacent synovial space. Its presentation may mimic true gouty arthritis in tempo and clinical findings, except that the knee (gonagra) is more commonly involved than the first metatarsophalangeal joint. Radiologic studies may reveal osteoarthritic changes and a linear density within the joint space representing deposition of calcium pyrophosphate. Arthrocentesis is diagnostic in that examination of the joint fluid under a polarizing microscope discloses weakly positively birefringent, rectangular intracellular crystals of calcium pyrophosphate. Treatment includes the use of anti-inflammatory agents, such as ibuprofen or indomethacin, usually providing symptomatic relief, with additional analgesics as needed.

Bursitis

Bursae facilitate the motion of tendons and muscles over bony prominences; acute bursitis may be precipitated by overuse or trauma, may be secondary to other disorders such as gout or rheumatoid arthritis, or may occur without an obvious precipitant.

Diagnosis

Attacks of bursitis may involve any one of several sites, are occasionally associated with periarticular calcification (especially about the shoulder and hip), and may be accompanied by or indistinguishable from tendinitis (especially in the shoulder). Common sites include the subacromial bursa, subdeltoid bursa, olecranon bursa, trochanteric bursa, ischial bursa ("weaver's bottom"), prepatellar bursa ("housemaid's knee"), and the anserine bursa. Physical findings include varying degrees of warmth, erythema, and the clear elicitation or enhancement of pain with movement.

Treatment

Treatment consists of immobilization, local heat, and the use of analgesics and anti-inflammatory agents. The local injection of corticosteroids (provided no signs or symptoms of infection exist) may provide prompt relief, but such treatment is usually reserved for patients unresponsive to initial therapy. If elected, methylprednisolone acetate (Depo-Medrol), 40 mg, and 1% lidocaine, 2 mL, may be injected into the involved area, with explanation to the patient that there will be relief immediately, followed by approximately 12 hours of increasing discomfort, after which the effect of the steroid becomes apparent and symptoms begin to subside. It is important to remind the patient that if the involved joint is immobilized, daily range-of-motion exercises must be performed to prevent the development of joint stiffness, especially in the shoulder.

Acute Bacterial Arthritis

Pyogenic cocci (gonococci, staphylococci, and pneumococci) are the most common organisms responsible for septic arthritis in adults. These organisms may enter the joint space directly or by hematogenous spread and are most likely to involve a previously diseased joint.

Clinical Presentation

The onset of bacterial arthritis is typically acute; chills, fever, and an acutely hot, painful joint are noted. Large, weight-bearing joints are typically involved, as are the wrists. The physical examination should include a complete evaluation of the involved joints, a thorough search of the skin for the cutaneous manifestations of gonococcal infection (discrete papules, papules with necrotic centers, and pustules), a careful periarticular search for a site of entry, and an oral, anal, and genital examination with cultures for gonococci using Thayer-Martin medium if indicated. Gonococcal infection typically produces a tenosynovitis in addition to a frank arthritis, especially involving the tendons outlining the "anatomic snuff box" (at the radial aspect of the wrist). Forced adduction of the wrist with the thumb flexed within a closed fist produces pain (a positive Finkelstein test) in patients with gonococcal tenosynovitis. Myopericarditis, perihepatitis, and meningitis may also be noted in disseminated gonococcal infection.

Diagnostic Tests

Diagnostic tests that often prove useful include a WBC and erythrocyte sedimentation rate, both of which may be elevated; blood cultures should be obtained in all patients. Cervical or urethral, anal, and oropharyngeal cultures for the gonococcus should be obtained in all patients with suspected gonococcal arthritis. Arthrocentesis typically reveals the highest of leukocyte counts, as high as $100,000/\mu L$. Synovial fluid glucose is typically depressed, and organisms may be identified in a considerable number of patients by Gram stain of the synovial fluid.

Treatment

Prompt **treatment** with systemic antibiotics is indicated in all patients with suspected acute bacterial arthritis. Frequent aspiration or formal intraoperative incision and drainage of the involved joint may be elected, as well as bed rest, immobilization, elevation, and analgesia. Orthopaedic consultation and admission to the hospital for the institution of these measures are essential. For suspected staphylococcal arthritis, oxacillin or cefazolin may be used although vancomycin is evolving as the drug of choice given the increasing prevalence of community-acquired MRSA. Gonococcal arthritis may be treated with intravenous aqueous penicillin G or, in areas with penicillin-resistant gonococci, ceftriaxone or cefotaxime. Pneumococcal arthritis may be treated with a penicillinase-resistant synthetic penicillin or aqueous penicillin G. Empiric therapy for all of the above would include both vancomycin and ceftriaxone. Therapy for 7 to 10 days typically leads to complete, uncomplicated recovery. Failure to institute therapy promptly (i.e., within 24–48 hours) may lead to irreversible articular destruction and bony ankylosis. See Table 47-2 for additional information on septic arthritis according to the age of the patient.

| Table 47-2 | Septic Arthritis |

Age	Common Organisms
Younger than 3 mo	*Staphylococcus aureus*
	Enterobacteriaceae
	Group B *Streptococcus*
	Neisseria gonorrhoeae
3 mo to 14 y	*S. aureus*
	Streptococcus Pyogenes
	Streptococcus pneumoniae
	Haemophilus influenzae
	Gram-negative bacilli
15–40 y	*N. gonorrhoeae*
	S. aureus
	Rarely, Gram-negative bacilli
Older than 40 y	
Without rheumatoid arthritis	*N. Gonorrhoeae*
	S. aureus
With rheumatoid arthritis	*S. aureus*
	Streptococci
	Gram-negative bacilli

Toxic Synovitis

Toxic Synovitis is a disorder of children in which an inflammatory process affects the large joints of the lower extremity (i.e., the hip or knee). Allergic reactions, viral infection, trauma, and distant bacterial infection have all been suggested as possible causes, but none has been firmly proved.

Diagnosis

The child with toxic synovitis frequently presents with a limp associated with a painful hip or knee. Some limitation of active and passive range of motion is noted on examination accompanied by local tenderness with palpation and an effusion. A slight leukocytosis and a modestly elevated erythrocyte sedimentation rate may be noted on laboratory examination. Diligence to rule out septic arthritis is essential if clinical suspicion for an infectious source exists.

Treatment

Bed rest and analgesics for several days lead to complete symptomatic recovery. A small percentage of children with synovitis of the hip will eventually develop Legg-Calvé-Perthes disease, and for this reason, orthopaedic follow-up is advised.

Ruptured Baker Cyst

Cysts of the popliteal space or Baker cysts may cause sudden calf or knee pain. The lesion consists of a synovial cyst in the popliteal fossa that frequently communicates with the joint space. Such cysts are frequently associated with osteoarthritis and with rheumatoid arthritis, but their exact cause or developmental evolution is unknown. Unruptured cysts produce mild chronic discomfort in the popliteal space with slight joint pain. Cyst rupture produces an acutely painful calf often associated with swelling and erythema. Patients often give a history of the sudden onset of a "tearing" or "popping" sensation in the back of the leg on standing, after which pain and swelling of the calf develop.

Diagnosis

The clinical presentation and physical findings in patients with ruptured Baker cysts are often difficult to differentiate from deep venous thrombophlebitis, with which the former is occasionally associated. For this reason, when the diagnosis is unclear, a venous ultrasound or venogram should be performed and, if negative, the diagnosis of a ruptured Baker cyst (unassociated with deep venous thrombosis), if not suggested by the ultrasound findings, can be made electively by arthrography.

Treatment

Treatment consists of activity limitations, crutches, and the use of analgesics and anti-inflammatory agents for 10 to 14 days.

Osteochondroses

The osteochondroses are a group of atraumatic orthopaedic disorders of unknown cause in which the ossification centers of involved bones manifest abnormalities identical to those of avascular or aseptic necrosis. Legg-Calvé-Perthes disease, Osgood-Schlatter disease, and Köhler disease are the most common of these conditions.

Legg-Calvé-Perthes Disease

Legg-Calvé-Perthes disease is a self-limited disease of the proximal femoral epiphysis of unknown cause in which the epiphysis has undergone changes similar to those of avascular necrosis. It is most commonly found in boys between the ages of 5 and 8 years in whom the presenting symptoms are pain in the knee or hip, a limp, and limitation of joint motion. Treatment includes minimal weight-bearing status and analgesia with careful orthopaedic follow-up to assess the occasional need for surgical intervention.

Osgood-Schlatter Disease

Osgood-Schlatter disease is seen most often in adolescents, most of whom are athletic, and presumably results from a traction-type injury to the tibial tubercle at the site of insertion of the patellar tendon. Chronic symptoms are common; however, an acute presentation is often associated with minor trauma to the area. Point tenderness is noted over the tibial tubercle, which may be inflamed as evidenced by local swelling, erythema, and increased warmth. Radiologically, a lateral view of the proximal tibia may be normal, may demonstrate irregularity or prominence of the tibial tuberosity, or, in some patients, may demonstrate an avulsion of the tuberosity.

Treatment is determined by the patient's symptoms. Initially, in most patients, activities requiring repetitive knee extension, such as running and jumping, should be prohibited for 3 to 4 weeks. Salicylates or other nonsteroidal, anti-inflammatory agents are useful and should be instituted along with crutches for patients with significant symptoms or evidence of inflammation. Ice may be applied initially to the area and may be helpful. Immobilization of the knee and surgical repair are additional options for patients with persistent symptoms; orthopaedic referral in 5 to 7 days is appropriate.

Köhler Disease

Köhler disease has been defined to include either an osteochondral lesion of the tarsal navicular or the second metatarsal typically seen in boys of age 4 to 5 years. Tarsal navicular involvement is self-limited with a good prognosis after revascularization and reconstruction, whereas metatarsal disease requires a metatarsal bar or pad and close follow-up.

Hemarthroses

Hemophilia A is a sex-linked, recessive disorder resulting in defective coagulation factor VIII. The severity of hemophilia A is quantified on the basis of the level of factor VIII coagulant (VIII:C) activity. Cases with 1% or less activity are considered severe and are subject to spontaneous bleeding; 1% to 5% activity represents moderate severity, with major bleeding primarily associated with trauma or surgery, whereas cases with greater than 10% activity are considered mild, although bleeding after trauma and surgery similarly is noted. Bleeding may occur at multiple sites; however, recurrent hemarthroses with progressive joint destruction and intracranial bleeding remain the major causes of morbidity and mortality, respectively. Trauma remains a common and important precipitant of bleeding in all groups of patients.

Abrasions, Avulsions, Lacerations, and Puncture Wounds

EXTENSIVE INJURIES

After evaluation and stabilization in the emergency department (ED), many patients with multiple or extensive injuries are best managed in the operating room. This is especially true in young children, particularly those with extensive facial injuries; in patients with extensive abrasions; or in patients with such widespread injuries that the acceptable maximum limits of local anesthesia will be exceeded.

INJURIES IN THE UNCOOPERATIVE PATIENT

Most patients classified as "uncooperative" will be either intoxicated or very young. Most children may be treated satisfactorily after proper reassurance and manual or mechanical restraint, if required. Procedural sedation may be necessary to facilitate suturing children, especially with significant facial or perioral injuries. For pediatric sedation, see Chapter 60, pp. 544–549.

In the intoxicated patient, a period of observation, either in the ED or in the hospital, depending on the presence of other injuries, will generally facilitate primary closure after 2 to 4 hours.

INSTRUCTIONS REGARDING WOUND CARE AND FOLLOW-UP

Written instructions regarding the daily care of any wounds, the signs and symptoms of infection, and a specific referral at an appropriate interval for suture removal or other care should be provided to all patients (see Table 48-1).

ANESTHESIA

Allergy

There are two major classes of locally active anesthetic agents that may be used for infiltration, field, or block anesthesia. *Esters*, of which there are two principal types, procaine (Novocain) and chloroprocaine (Nesacaine), are chemically and antigenically distinct from the *amides*, which include lidocaine (Xylocaine), bupivacaine (Marcaine), and mepivacaine (Carbocaine). Patients who report an allergic reaction to one class of agents may safely be treated with a member of the other group without fear of crossreactivity. Most reported allergies are actually caused by preservatives contained in the solution (usually methylparaben). The use of solutions without preservatives (pure cardiac lidocaine) further reduces the incidence of allergic reactions. In some patients, it will not be possible to determine with certainty to which class of

Table 48-1	Recommended Suture Materials and Duration of Use According to Site		
Location	**Type**	**Size**	**Duration(d)**
Scalp	Nylon	3-0 to 5-0	7
Eyelid	Prolene or silk	6-0 or 7-0	3–5
Conjunctiva	Plain gut	7-0 or 8-0	—
Face	Nylon	5-0 to 7-0	3–5
Mucous membranes	Plain or chromic gut[a]	3-0 to 5-0	—
Near joints	Nylon	4-0 to 6-0	10–14
Chest, abdomen, arm, and leg	Nylon	3-0 to 5-0	7–10
Fingertip	Nylon	5-0 or 6-0	10–12
Foot/toe	Nylon	4-0 or 5-0	12–14
Subcutaneous tissue	Dexon or Vicryl	3-0 to 5-0	—
Muscle	Dexon or Vicryl	3-0 to 5-0	—
Back	Nylon	3-0 to 5-0	12–14

[a]See "Common Suture Materials."

agents an allergy actually exists; these patients can be given, by instillation, diphenhydramine, which should not produce an allergic reaction.

Maximum Safe Dose

The maximum total adult doses for the various anesthetic agents are listed below. These doses assume that local infiltration is the method of administration and that epinephrine is contained in the solution. In patients not treated with a solution containing epinephrine, local vasoconstriction is not provided, and systemic absorption of the anesthetic agent is rapid; topical application to abraded skin surfaces similarly results in accelerated absorption; therefore, under either of these conditions, dosage reduction is indicated.

When administered by local infiltration, and when epinephrine *is* present in the solution, the upper limits of safe dosage for the various agents are as follows: procaine (9 mg/kg), lidocaine (7 mg/kg), and bupivacaine (3 mg/kg); when epinephrine is *not* present in the solution, maximal safe doses are as follows: procaine (7 mg/kg), lidocaine (4.5 mg/kg), and bupivacaine (2 mg/kg). In adults, no more than 150 to 200 mg topical lidocaine and no more than 50 mg of tetracaine (Pontocaine) should be administered.

Duration of Action

The expected duration of action for the various agents when epinephrine is *not* present in the solution is as follows: procaine (15–45 minutes), lidocaine (1–2 hours), and bupivacaine (4–8 hours). When epinephrine is present in the solution, the duration of action for all these agents is approximately doubled.

Route of Administration

Topical

Topical agents are useful for providing local anesthesia for laceration repair without the pain associated with needle infiltration; these agents provide reasonable hemostasis and do not cause infiltration-related distortion of wound edges.

Topical solutions containing lidocaine, epinephrine, and tetracaine (**LET**) or *t*etracaine, *a*drenaline (or epinephrine), and *c*ocaine (**TAC**) have been shown to be quite effective in providing anesthesia before suturing. Typically, several drops of the agent are dripped into the wound using a syringe; alternatively, a piece of gauze is cut to approximately correspond to the size of the laceration, after which the gauze is applied over the laceration, and the solution, using a syringe, is dripped onto the pad, which when saturated is gently taped down; the gauze is resaturated in approximately 5 minutes. Blanching of tissue surrounding the laceration usually indicates that sufficient anesthesia has been provided.

For a variety of reasons, LET is the preferred topical agent; this is related to differences in cost, as well as to the status of cocaine as a controlled substance (which may limit availability of the agent). In addition, LET can often be used in locations where TAC is not recommended. Caution must be exercised when TAC is used in areas in proximity to the mucous membranes of the nose and mouth, because seizures, respiratory arrest, and a fatality have been reported in children, presumably resulting from the rapid absorption of cocaine from these sites. One must therefore carefully avoid any contact of the TAC solution with oral or nasal mucous membranes. Because of the particular vascular supply to the acral areas (nose, ear, fingers, toes, penis), the use of these solutions is contraindicated.

Topically active ophthalmic agents include proparacaine (Ophthaine) and tetracaine. These agents should be used routinely to facilitate fluorescein staining of the cornea, foreign body removal, irrigation, tonometry, and so on. They are also effective in the repair of conjunctival disruptions. Applying two or three drops, waiting approximately 1 minute, and then readministering a similar dose, will generally provide complete and sufficient anesthesia for most purposes. Topical ophthalmic anesthetic agents should not be provided to or prescribed for patients with ocular symptoms, because patient-initiated use, either currently or in association with subsequent injuries, may mask symptoms and thereby delay treatment. Indiscriminant use and therefore overdosage may also contribute to poor or delayed wound-healing and may cause toxicity.

The nose and throat may also be anesthetized topically with 0.5% or 2% tetracaine. When nasal procedures are contemplated that would benefit from local vasoconstriction, epinephrine may be added to the anesthetic solution. Viscous lidocaine (2%) or a combination of tetracaine and benzocaine (Cetacaine spray) is an additionally useful topical agent.

Topical lidocaine and tetracaine are also useful agents for anesthetizing abraded skin before cleansing or scrubbing for the removal of embedded foreign material.

Local Infiltration

In patients with lacerations that require cleansing, irrigation, debridement, or closure, needle instillation directly through and into the wound edges with 1% lidocaine is routine and most effective; when injuries are extensive, 0.5% lidocaine, usually without epinephrine, should be used to limit the total administered dose. Epinephrine is available commercially in many of these preparations and may be used to limit local bleeding; when injuries are extensive or involve the very young or elderly, however, the use of epinephrine should be limited. In addition and importantly, solutions containing epinephrine should not be used in patients with finger, toe, or penile lacerations, in digital blocks, or in patients with vascularly compromised avulsions or flaps; the use of epinephrine in these patients may precipitate or worsen ischemic injury via vasoconstriction of end arteries.

The usual discomfort associated with instillation of anesthetic may be limited by injecting first proximally with a 27- or 30-gauge needle and injecting very slowly.

Moderate mechanical pressure over the site before injection and cutaneous stimulation of the overlying skin during the injection may significantly reduce discomfort. Lidocaine solutions, using sodium bicarbonate and which are pH-balanced, significantly reduce discomfort associated with instillation anesthesia. These can be easily prepared in the hospital pharmacy or ED. Typically, nine parts of a 1% lidocaine solution is mixed with one part of an 8.4% solution of sodium bicarbonate.

Field and Nerve Blocks
Field blocks involve the instillation of anesthetic agents proximal to or surrounding the area to be anesthetized. Field blocks are often used to provide anesthesia for the cleansing of small abrasions, the repair of minor lacerations, and the draining of abscesses. A barrier of anesthetic agent is established proximal to or surrounding the area to be treated and provides appropriate anesthesia after 10 to 15 minutes.

Field blocks are most useful in the treatment of patients with distal finger or facial injuries. The use of a field block, particularly in these locations, circumvents the problem of distension or "ballooning" of tissue, which frequently interferes with wound edge apposition when anesthetic is injected directly.

Digital Blocks
Digital blocks are extremely useful for anesthetizing the digit, thereby facilitating the repair of lacerations, cleansing or debriding of wounds, paronychia drainage, nail removal, and so on. Each digit is supplied by two dorsal and two volar nerve branches, each of which courses along the four "edges" or "corners" of the digit adjacent to the phalanx. To obtain adequate anesthesia using a digital block, all four branches must be anesthetized with local instillation. A small-gauge needle (25- or 27-gauge) may be inserted dorsally, into the web space, and should touch the periosteum at the base of the proximal phalanx; after withdrawing the needle slightly, 1.0 to 1.5 mL of anesthetic agent, usually 1% lidocaine *without* epinephrine, is then injected. Without withdrawing the needle, it may then be redirected toward the volar "corner" and a similar volume of anesthetic agent injected. This procedure must be repeated on the opposite side of the digit and will produce total anesthesia within 10 to 15 minutes. "Failure" of digital block anesthesia often results from an insufficient waiting period after administering the agent.

Nitrous Oxide
Nitrous oxide is a nonflammable gas administered in combination with oxygen. A mixture of 50% nitrous oxide and 50% oxygen may safely be used in the ED to provide short-term analgesia without significant respiratory or cardiac depression. Onset of action is rapid, and duration of action after discontinuing inhalation is brief. Nitrous oxide may be used alone or as an adjunct to parenterally administered narcotics or sedatives or locally administered anesthetics.

Nitrous oxide should not be used in patients with head injury, with emotional or psychiatric disturbances, or when nausea or vomiting is present. In addition, because of the high concentrations of oxygen usually coadministered with nitrous oxide, patients with chronic obstructive pulmonary disease who retain carbon dioxide should not be treated with this regimen.

WOUND REVISION BY EXCISION

Primary repair of a variety of different injuries by excision of involved tissue continues to be a valuable technique both to eliminate crushed or devitalized tissue and to improve cosmetic results. Injuries amenable to this type of therapy in particular include multiple, closely spaced, parallel lacerations that would otherwise be difficult or impossible to close individually and wounds associated with central devitalization or crushing of tissue that will ultimately be nonviable.

Before excision, the amount of available tissue surrounding the area to be excised must be determined to be adequate. Excision to facilitate closure is typically not possible in the digit, for example, because of the paucity of available tissue in this area; too aggressive excision in these locations may result in irreparable defects that will ultimately require skin grafting. Frequently, adjacent tissue must be slightly undermined to permit adequate approximation of the wound margins. To optimize the final cosmetic result, the long axis of the excised tissue should be approximately 3.5 to 4 times the short axis. This dimensional consideration will ensure that puckering of the wound ends or "dog ears" are not produced. If present, these may be corrected by slightly extending the long axis of excision. After excision, which should include all nonstructural devitalized tissue, closure may proceed in the usual fashion.

ABRASIONS

- **Superficial abrasions** not associated with embedded foreign matter require only thorough cleansing with an appropriate antiseptic agent, removal of the agent by irrigation or cleansing of the wound with normal saline, application of an appropriate antibacterial ointment and a sterile dressing, recleansing and reapplication of antibacterial ointment at 24-hour intervals until healing is complete, and a wound check at 48 to 72 hours if indicated. Instructions regarding the signs and symptoms of infection should also be provided and antitetanus prophylaxis administered as discussed pp. 464 and 465.
- **Deeper abrasions** not associated with embedded material are treated similarly; however, an occasional patient with more significant injuries will require a wound check 'at 24 to 48 hours. If signs of infection have developed at that time, a wound culture should be obtained and antibiotics instituted. In addition to the administration of antitetanus prophylaxis as needed, analgesics may be required for 24 to 48 hours.
- When **embedded foreign material** is present, aggressive treatment is required to prevent permanent "tattooing" of the skin. The use of povidone–iodine-impregnated brushes and forceps will facilitate cleansing of the wound. Excision may occasionally be required in wounds with devitalized tissue or deeply embedded material not otherwise extractable. Locally applied or topical anesthetic agents are required for adequate cleansing of abrasions in these patients. In patients with relatively small abrasions, topically applied 2% lidocaine or tetracaine or locally instilled 0.5% to 1% lidocaine will be reasonably effective. Topically applied agents generally require 10 to 15 minutes to become maximally effective. It is important to note that topically active anesthetic agents are absorbed extremely rapidly from abraded skin; therefore, the total maximally acceptable dose should be reduced. In addition, in patients with large injuries, if local instillation of 0.5% to 1% lidocaine is elected, the use of solutions containing epinephrine should be avoided.
- When injuries are extensive, when the patient is uncooperative, or when the maximally safe dose of anesthetic is likely to be exceeded, early surgical consultation is recommended, because regional or general anesthesia may be required in the operating room.

AVULSIONS

Complete avulsions occur when tissue is torn away, exposing the underlying fat. Generally, when cosmetically or functionally significant areas are involved, that is, the face or finger, respectively, skin grafting will be required for primary repair.

- When the **fingertip** is involved, the general rule is that avulsions exposing more than 1 cm^2 of fat require grafting, whereas lesions smaller than this will heal completely without grafting. When the avulsed tissue is available, it should be thoroughly cleansed, defatted, and tacked in place with fine suture material. When grafting is not required, an antibacterial ointment, a nonadherent dressing next to the skin, and a bulky dressing should be provided. Most patients with fingertip injuries will require an analgesic for several days; patients should be instructed to strictly elevate the hand to reduce bleeding and discomfort. Patients should be seen in 48 to 72 hours for a dressing change, at which time, despite the use of a nonadherent dressing, hydrogen peroxide as a soak may be required to facilitate removal of the dressing without severe pain. A similar dressing should be applied, which can be changed at 24- to 48-hour intervals until healing is complete—usually within 2 weeks. Partial avulsions are defined as tangentially oriented lacerations that result in an undermined flap of tissue. Before considering the various treatment options for such injuries, the pathophysiology of the injury as it relates to vascular disruption and subsequently to scar formation and contracture should be noted.

- Clearly, when **tissue is undermined,** local vascular structures, including arteries, veins, and lymphatics, are disrupted. Because of venous and lymphatic compromise, swelling and edema of the flap evolve over several hours to several days. Such expansion of the flap places increasing traction on the wound edges that results in the spreading or widening of the scar as it forms. In addition, flaps tend to become "boggy" or edematous as intradermal scar tissue increases in density; this further aggravates the tendency of the scar to widen. Furthermore, as the peripheral skin scar contracts, a "heaping up" of the tissue that composed the original flap occurs. Last, particularly in patients with distally attached flaps, the blood supply may be inadequate to support the most proximal tissue, resulting in ischemic necrosis at or near the suture line. The combination of these processes in patients with injuries occurring in cosmetically significant areas often produces less than optimal results, unless special measures are taken to minimize their impact on the healing process. Flap-type avulsions of the nasal bridge and forehead often have such outcomes; for this reason, in selected patients, subspecialty consultation for repair is often appropriate.

- In patients with somewhat **larger flaps,** conservative excision of very thin or beveled edges of the flap to produce a more perpendicular union of tissue will reduce subsequent scar formation. In patients with extremely small flaps, excision of the flap and primary closure are acceptable therapeutic options and will often produce a cosmetically superior result.

- A special problem is the elderly patient with very **atrophic or thin skin** who presents with a superficial avulsing injury of the distal anterior tibial area, dorsal hand, or forearm. Such lesions are typically quite superficial and impossible to suture without further tearing of the skin. Occasionally, in patients with only superficial involvement, the application of a light pressure dressing or Steri-strips alone after routine cleansing will be sufficient. In other patients, the placement of one or two large, interrupted mattress sutures, the outermost pass of which should be placed at some distance from the wound edge, followed by the application of Steri-strips to complete the closure and a bulky dressing will produce optimal healing. Importantly, when an extremity is involved, the importance of strict elevation for 48 to 72 hours, along with a cool compress initially, should be clearly noted. A wound check at 72 hours is recommended.

LACERATIONS

Neurovascular Status

Motor, sensory, and vascular integrity must be carefully assessed in all patients with skin disruption, and all findings, including a normal examination, must be carefully recorded. Scalp, torso, and "tuft only" injuries of the finger or toe are the only exceptions to this important general principle. All patients with even minor lacerations will, if very carefully tested, demonstrate minor sensory deficits at the wound margin and distally. These patients should be reassured at the time of injury that sensory function should return over the subsequent several weeks to months. Patients presenting with abnormalities of motor function that result from nerve, tendon, or ligament disruption should be referred to the appropriate subspecialist. Patients with major sensory deficits should be similarly referred. Because long-term outpatient care will be required for such injuries, it is most appropriate that initial care be provided by the physician who will longitudinally follow the patient. Occasionally, depending on the nature and extent of the injury, the activity of the department, and the referral patterns of the hospital, extensor tendon repair may be undertaken by the emergency physician.

Patients with significant vascular disruption require emergency vascular surgical consultation after appropriate stabilization of the acute hemorrhagic event. The application of continuous pressure to the wound and, if an extremity is involved, elevation are the preferred maneuvers for controlling hemorrhage. If these prove unsuccessful, a sphygmomanometer cuff inflated above systolic pressure or a proximal tourniquet may be applied. When required, the cuff should be deflated or the tourniquet removed for 1 to 2 minutes every 15 to 20 minutes.

Treatment Implications of Delay in Presentation

Bacterial growth begins immediately after skin disruption occurs, with bacterial colony counts doubling by 12 hours after the injury. Although strict guidelines regarding "safe" postinjury intervals for the primary closure of lacerations have been proposed, these are frequently modified by individual practitioners based on personal experience and the details of the specific injury.

One approach to the patient presenting late after injury is simply to discuss the physician's dilemma, that is, the greater risk of infection with primary closure versus the potential cosmetic benefit and a shorter healing period. If closure is elected, close follow-up is essential, and patients should understand that if evidence of infection develops, removal of one, several, or all sutures may be necessary. The conversation with the patient or family should be documented.

The management of lacerations resulting from bites is specifically discussed in Chapter 57.

Guidelines regarding the treatment of older lacerations are as follows:

- Lacerations **less than 6 hours old** may be primarily closed, unless other contraindications exist.
- Lacerations **more than 24 hours old** should generally not be closed, with several exceptions.
  - It would appear that lacerations involving the scalp can be closed up to several days after the injury. Obviously, such lacerations should be thoroughly cleansed and irrigated, and a prophylactic antibiotic and a wound check in 48 hours are recommended.

- Lacerations should be closed in patients with a cosmetically insignificant but extensive injury that would require an extended period of healing and disability if left open. Such injuries not uncommonly involve large lacerations overlying or in close proximity to joints; these wounds should be cultured, their margins loosely approximated with nonabsorbable, interrupted, vertical mattress sutures at intervals of ½ to 1 inch, Penrose or gauze drains inserted between sutures, a prophylactic antistaphylococcal antibiotic instituted, and follow-up in 24 hours arranged. The interrupted, vertical mattress type of suture is effective at both establishing focal areas of healing and simultaneously allowing drainage of the wound. At follow-up in 24 to 48 hours, any drains may be removed or replaced and the results of wound cultures determined.
- Patients with cosmetically significant lacerations generally should be discussed with a surgeon, who may elect primary closure if appropriate.
- Patients presenting **between 6 and 24 hours** after the injury are evaluated in terms of the considerations that follow. Facial lacerations should be closed in most cases because of cosmetic considerations and the rich vascular supply of the face. After appropriate cleansing and irrigation, scalp and finger lacerations of similar age may also generally be closed, again because of the rich vascular supply to these areas. Conversely, lacerations that are infected, those considered more appropriately deep puncture wounds, those associated with nondebridable, crushed, or devitalized tissue, and small to moderately sized cosmetically insignificant lesions about which doubt exists as to the wisdom of primary closure should all be left open and should be treated initially as open wounds with consideration of delayed closure in 3 to 5 days. This includes obtaining an initial culture if possible, the use of an appropriate antistaphylococcal antibiotic such as amoxicillin clavulanate or cephalexin, soaks in warm water every 4 to 6 hours, elevation if an extremity is involved, and clear instructions for follow-up in 24 to 48 hours. As noted in section above, primary closure of lacerations overlying or in close proximity to joints may be preferable where continued movement, with subsequent and repetitive reopening of an unsutured laceration, would produce a protracted period of healing and often functionally significant scarring and contracture. Splinting of the involved joint is also helpful in limiting this complication.

Wound Cleansing and Exploration

All wounds must be carefully and meticulously cleansed and explored before closure to ensure that all foreign material and devitalized tissue are removed. Irrigation is felt by most authorities to be the most effective technique in wound preparation in terms of reducing contamination and infection rates; tap water has proven to be sufficient with no greater risk of infection than normal saline. To be optimally effective, high-pressure irrigation (with impact pressures between 5 and 8 lb/square inch) is considered the most effective technique. To achieve this, a 50-mL syringe with a 16- to 18-gauge needle (with a terminal plastic shield to prevent back splashing) is needed. Other solutions once commonly used, such as various dilutions of povidone-iodine, hydrogen peroxide, and various detergents or soaps, should not be used because of their tissue toxicity.

- **Grossly contaminated wounds, fragmented tissue, or multiple small foreign bodies** may be most easily removed with forceps followed by copious irrigation with normal saline. During irrigation, the wound should be manually explored to ensure that the irrigant floods all potentially contaminated areas and that occult foreign bodies are removed. An adequate volume for most patients is 250 to 500 mL of saline, whereas several liters are required for more extensive or more contaminated injuries.

- **Deeply embedded material or severely devitalized tissue** must often be excised and may require surgical consultation. The management of grossly infected wounds is discussed in "Management of Grossly Contaminated Wounds," p. 462
- As noted, **foreign bodies that have penetrated the skull, globe, thorax, or abdomen** are most appropriately removed in the operating room.
- **Lip lacerations** are often associated with trivial or unrecognized dental fractures and are notorious for incorporating such fragments into the margins of the laceration. If unrecognized, suppuration and cellulitis of the laceration will typically develop within 2 to 4 days; thus, careful exploration of such lacerations is imperative before primary closure. Lateral or "puckered" lip radiographs are useful in defining the presence and extent of any incorporated tooth fragments in these patients.

Closure

Many suture techniques are available for the closure of simple lacerations and are well described in a number of texts. One technique that is probably underused in most EDs and that is useful to minimize wound margin inversion and thereby optimizes wound edge apposition is the interrupted vertical mattress suture. Such sutures, when closely alternated with simple interrupted sutures, are additionally useful for stabilizing lacerations involving areas exposed to repetitive trauma or movement or overlying or in proximity to joints (Figs. 48-1 and 48-2).

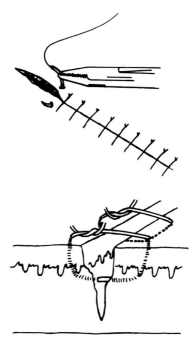

Figure 48-1. Simple interrupted suture. Individual simple sutures are placed and tied so that the width of each stitch equals the distance between the stitches. This helps to avoid inversion of the skin edges. (From Gomella Clinician's pocket reference, LG, ed. 6th ed. Norwalk, CT: Appleton and Lange; 1989, with permission.)

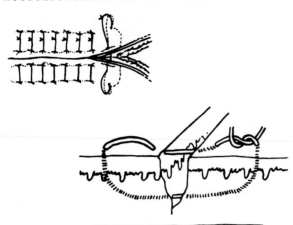

Figure 48-2. Vertical mattress suture. These sutures reduce tension of the skin and prevent inversion of the skin edges. (From Gomella Clinician's pocket reference, LG, ed. 6th ed. Norwalk, CT: Appleton and Lange; 1989, with permission.)

If simple interrupted sutures are used, optimal wound margin eversion and edge apposition may be achieved if the insertion and depth of needle penetration, the path of the needle through the laceration, and its exit from the adjacent side are carefully controlled. For example, if needle insertion into the skin occurs so that the path of the needle is initially directed away from the laceration, sufficient subcutaneous tissue will be grasped on the side of entry to result in wound-edge eversion when the knot is tied. The needle is then passed through the laceration at an equal depth and distance to ensure evenness of wound closure and then directed back toward the skin to exit at a distance equal to that of needle entry. To achieve maximum control of the wound edge and to minimize residual suture marks, sutures should be placed near the edge of the wound.

Avoidance of Skin Suture Marks

Permanent cross-hatching by suture material is unfortunately common and may be more cosmetically significant than if the original laceration had been left unsutured. Cross-hatching may be minimized if sutures are not tied too tightly and if they are placed near the wound margins to limit the amount of skin surface included in the knot. Appropriate and timely removal of sutures also minimizes such scarring, particularly in the face, where 4 to 5 days is the accepted limit. Many plastic surgeons prefer to remove alternate sutures from the face on the third day, apply Steri-strips, and remove the remaining sutures on the fifth day.

Common Suture Materials

- **Nonabsorbable** (such as nylon, prolene, or silk):
  - Used in general for skin. Nylon or prolene is preferred for closing most skin surfaces; however, in patients with lacerations involving tissue surfaces that are frequently apposed (such as the eyelid fold, tongue, or selected surfaces of the lip), fine prolene is often preferred because of its pliability.

- **Absorbable** (such as Dexon, Vicryl, or plain or chromic gut):
  - Used for subcutaneous tissue and mucosal surfaces. In the unreliable patient who, in the judgment of the physician, is unlikely to seek follow-up for suture removal, the placement of absorbable sutures, or the use of Steri-strips if the wound is superficial, is a reasonable alternative. Table 48-1 lists recommended suture materials in relation to the location of the injury.

Other Materials

Paper-Tape (Steri-Strips)

These have some, although limited, usefulness in the ED. Patients with relatively minor, superficial lacerations, not exposed to skin tension, moisture, or excessive movement can be treated with tape closure. Rates of infection are somewhat less than sutured wounds, and with the limitations noted regarding optimal candidates for tape closure, comparable cosmetic results are achieved, usually with less time required to close the wound. To ensure that tape remains in place for sufficient time for initial healing to occur, wound edges and surrounding tissue should first be treated with tincture of benzoin. Importantly, lacerations closed with tape must remain dry at all times, and one does not apply topical antibacterial agents. One situation that is amenable to tape closure is when a patient has very superficial, avulsion-type lacerations, typically involving the anterior tibial area or the arm or hand in elderly patients, particularly those using long-term steroid therapy. This tissue is often thin and friable, and suture material often further causes tears in these patients.

Stainless Steel Staples

These offer some advantages over traditional suture material (less reactivity, lower infection rate, and markedly less time to place) but cannot be used in locations where precise approximation of wound edges is important (cosmetically significant lacerations) or where skin traction forces or movement are significant (hands, fingers, etc.). Staples are most commonly used on the scalp and trunk where cosmetic results comparable to sutured wounds are achieved. Many patients also report pain associated with staple use, and obviously stapling cannot be used when the reliability of the patient in terms of staple removal is in question. Scalp sutures also interfere with computed tomography scanning of the head and should be avoided prior to scanning.

Tissue Adhesives

These are becoming more popular for wound closure as experience increases with this technique; adhesive (typically a cyanoacrylate) is applied to the wound edges (adhesive should not enter the wound) in several thin (three to five) layers, after the wound is irrigated or cleansed, effecting skin closure as the adhesive bonds to adhesive on either side of the laceration. To facilitate bonding, wound edges are gently pressed together after adhesive administration for 60 to 90 seconds. Wounds associated with excessive movement (over or around joints) or increased tension should not be closed with adhesives, nor should lacerations near the eye or those occurring on mucosal surfaces. Additionally, lacerations greater in length than 4 to 5 cm are prone to open when closed with adhesives and should generally be closed by suturing. Simple linear lacerations involving areas not exposed to repetitive movement or stress are the best candidates; cosmetic results are similar to closure with traditional sutures, time required for closure is generally less, and patient acceptance is better because the pain associated with anesthesia is usually eliminated. No topical antibacterial ointments should be used; a light topical dressing can be applied initially to protect the wound during activity, but if used, dressings must be changed frequently to prevent moisture from accumulating around the wound.

SPECIFIC LACERATIONS

Scalp

Most scalp lacerations can be primarily closed after thorough cleansing, irrigation, and removal of any foreign material or devitalized tissue. Shaving of the scalp has been shown to increase the rate of infection and should not be performed. Hair may be trimmed, if needed, with scissors or held away from the wound edges by applying an antibacterial ointment.

Foreign material embedded in the skull must be removed mechanically with forceps or rongeur. Interruptions of the galea may be closed separately with 4-0 Dexon, although some sources suggest that this may not be necessary.

Scalp lacerations in young children and infants can be closed with 5-0 chromic sutures; these do not increase the infection rate and do not require removal. Two final points involve cosmetic considerations in patients with scalp lacerations. One must remember that the normal hairline forms a smooth, uninterrupted curve, the misalignment of which causes distracting abnormalities of contour at conversational distance. Secondly, the hairline often recedes as one ages; this is true in both men and women and demands that lacerations involving the scalp be closed as carefully as possible, because these areas may subsequently become exposed. Patients may safely wash their hair on arriving home.

Eyelid

The improper repair of an eyelid laceration may produce disastrous and disabling consequences; for this reason, many such lacerations should be treated initially by a surgeon or ophthalmologist. Lacerations interrupting the lid margin or those involving the medial fifth of the lid should be referred for definitive repair, because the former may require longitudinal follow-up over several months and the latter may involve the lacrimal apparatus. Patients with full-thickness lacerations of the eyelid should generally be referred for definitive three-layered repair unless the emergency physician is skilled in this technique.

- **Simple lid lacerations** that do not cross the lid margin, do not involve the medial fifth of the lid, and do not involve muscle may be closed with a 6-0 or 7-0 nonabsorbable suture. Fine prolene or silk may be preferred in these patients because of their pliability. Sutures should be removed at 3 to 5 days because early removal will minimize scar formation. A topical ophthalmic antibacterial ointment should be provided or prescribed.
- If the emergency physician elects to close **deeper lacerations** of the eyelid, a layered closure is the preferred method. The eyelid must be thought of as consisting of three layers, two of which are anterior, the skin and orbicularis oculi muscle, and one posterior, the tarsus and palpebral conjunctivae. Each of these three layers must be separately closed. The tarsus and palpebral conjunctivae should be closed in a way that avoids contact of the suture material with the eye. Again, because of the time and potential technical difficulties associated with such injuries, consultation is often elected for repair.

Eyebrow

The eyebrow represents another important facial landmark, the misalignment of which produces noticeable and distracting abnormalities of facial contour. Eyebrows must *never be shaved* because in a small percentage of patients, regrowth may not occur. Even if regrowth does occur, disturbing asymmetries of texture may exist between the old and new brow. Obviously devitalized tissue should be debrided if necessary, but this must be performed with extreme caution. If debridement is considered necessary, one must remember that the orientation of hair follicles in the brow is not perpendicular but tangential to the skin surface. This fact suggests that when any tissue is excised, the orientation of the incision should correspond to the orientation of the follicles as they traverse the skin; this practice ensures that crosscutting of follicles does not occur with resultant bare areas.

Hairline

Lacerations crossing the hairline are of cosmetic significance because if improperly realigned, noticeable abnormalities of the normally smooth contour of the hairline are produced.

Nose

The nasal bridge is an important central facial landmark that is often difficult to repair. This is especially true when flap-type or avulsion injuries are present and transversely cross the nasal bridge. These injuries tend to spread or to become elevated or irregular on healing, often producing a significant deformity. For this reason, subspecialty consultation should be considered in selected patients with these injuries. Avulsions and partial or complete amputations of the nose should be referred promptly as well.

- **Closure.** Simple lacerations of the nose may be closed with a 6-0 nonabsorbable suture as usual. Through-and-through lacerations require a layered closure using a 5-0 or 6-0 absorbable suture in the deeper layers of mucosa and cartilage and a 6-0 nonabsorbable suture to close the skin. In all cases, alignment of the alar rim and columella is essential. Because of the relative avascularity of the nasal cartilage, irrigation of the mucosa and cartilage before their respective closure and local anesthetic *without* epinephrine are recommended.
- Unfortunately, local **infection** in the form of stitch abscesses or cellulitis is common with nasal lacerations and because of this, relatively early suture removal followed by the application of Steri-strips is often advised. In addition, many physicians prescribe an antistaphylococcal antibiotic for 3 to 5 days.
- In all nasal injuries, the presence of **septal hematoma** must be excluded by careful examination of the nasal septum; these appear as either unilateral or bilateral bulging of the septum that, if seen early, may be fluctuant. If present, these collections of blood must be incised or aspirated completely and the affected side or sides packed to tamponade the area and prevent reaccumulation. A short course of antibiotics is also indicated. If undiagnosed or insufficiently treated, permanent and cosmetically significant cartilaginous necrosis involving the nasal bridge may result.

Conjunctiva

Small conjunctival lacerations less than 1 cm may be treated conservatively with observation and a topical ophthalmic antibiotic. Lacerations 1 cm or larger require closure with 7-0 or 8-0 absorbable material such as plain gut; because of the possibility of associated intraocular damage, these cases should be evaluated by an ophthalmologist.

Cheek

Lacerations of the cheek may result in significant injury to the facial nerve, the parotid duct, or the parotid gland. Muscle function on the side of injury must be carefully assessed and, if abnormal, despite nonvisualization of the transected nerve, consultation should be obtained. Eyelid closure should specifically be assessed in patients with lacerations between the tragus of the ear and the lateral corner of the eye, because division of the temporal branch of the facial nerve may occur in this location and may produce an important functional deficit. Superficial injuries to the parotid gland are frequently left unrepaired, whereas interruptions of the duct require definitive correction.

Lip

Precise alignment of lip lacerations involving the vermilion border is most important to ensure an optimal cosmetic result. Misalignments of as little as 1 mm produce a noticeable deformity at conversational distance. Typically, the first suture is used to align the vermilion border precisely.

One must conscientiously explore lip lacerations because small, avulsed dental fragments may be present, may be asymptomatic, and, if unrecognized, may lead to significant infection. If dental fractures are present and foreign material cannot be excluded on the basis of simple inspection, a lateral "puckered" radiograph of the lip may be obtained to rule out such material. Although substantial loss of the lip can occur without producing a significant cosmetic defect, midline losses of greater than 20%, as well as peripheral defects of less than this percentage, require plastic repair by a surgeon with experience in this area. No tissue should be excised from the philtrum, which, if destroyed, requires extensive reconstruction. Deep lacerations require a layered closure with a 4-0, 5-0, or 6-0 absorbable suture in the deepest layers. Lacerations involving the apposing mucous membrane surfaces of the lip may be repaired with fine prolene or pliable silk, which will permit comfortable lip closure. Although the use of prophylactic antibiotics has not been shown to be of definite benefit in these injuries, they are generally recommended for a 3- to 5-day course to decrease the risk of infection given the presence of a foreign body (suture) in a cosmetically important area obviously exposed to oral bacteria. Penicillin is a common choice.

Tongue

Superficial lacerations of the tongue may be left unsutured; deeper lacerations, however, must be repaired to minimize the risk of infection and the entrapment of food particles therein. Lacerations less than 1 cm long generally do not require suturing. A 4-0 or 5-0 absorbable suture is generally recommended, and patients should be instructed to rinse their mouth with half-strength hydrogen peroxide after meals and at bedtime. Although prophylactic antibiotics have not been shown to prevent infection, the use of oral penicillin or erythromycin for 3 to 5 days is commonly recommended. When deep muscle involvement occurs, a layered closure is indicated.

Suturing the tongue may be difficult, particularly in the child or uncooperative patient; in these patients, an assistant or two, a mild sedative, or general anesthesia may be required. The head should be stabilized and the tongue must be adequately exposed; this can often be accomplished simply by having an assistant apply traction on the distal tongue with a dry gauze pad. In other patients, local anesthesia may be instilled into the distal tongue and a large suture placed through this area, on which traction may be applied for adequate exposure and control.

Ear

Several principles govern the management of patients with ear lacerations.

Debridement

Because the blood supply to the ear is excellent and because donor sites for transplantation of tissue are few and often unacceptable, debridement of tissue should be extremely conservative, and only tissue that is obviously nonviable should be removed.

Closure

Through-and-through lacerations require a layered closure, which may be performed by suturing the cartilage with 6-0 Dexon and the medial and lateral skin with 5-0 or 6-0 nylon or prolene. The dressing is as important as closure, because those producing unequal distributions of pressure may distort the contour of the ear. In most patients, the ear must be "splinted" in a normal or neutral position by carefully placing saline-moistened pledgets or cotton balls behind the auricle and in its recesses, followed by the circumferential application of a loose dressing. The final dressing is meant simply to cover the ear rather than to provide hemostasis. A wound check in 48 hours is often recommended, depending on the extent of injury.

Anesthesia

Anesthesia for the ear may conveniently be provided by infiltrating 1% or 2% lidocaine *without epinephrine* superficially around the base of the ear, which will anesthetize 80% to 90% of the external ear. Lacerations involving the canal, however, will require additional direct instillation of anesthetic agent.

Hematomas

Hematomas involving the ear, if left untreated, frequently result in significant deformity; these have been termed "cauliflower ear." Such hematomas must be evacuated in the usual sterile manner using either aspiration, which is most often successful, or incision followed by splinting the ear as previously outlined. One must take care to dress the ear so that slight pressure is applied to the area of the hematoma, which prevents reaccumulation. Most often, posterior and anterior splinting of the area of the hematoma will tamponade the ear without undue discomfort or deformity, but patients should be advised that reaccumulation may occur and reaspiration may then be required. ENT consultation is often sought initially to assist with drainage or at 1 to 2 days for follow-up.

Oral Cavity

Superficial lacerations of the oral mucosa less than 1 cm in size usually do not require closure. Adults should be advised to rinse their mouths with half-strength hydrogen peroxide after meals and at bedtime. In patients with lacerations greater than 1 cm, closure with a 4-0 or 5-0 absorbable suture is indicated after appropriate cleansing. In patients with through-and-through lacerations, a layered closure is indicated using a 4-0 or 5-0 absorbable suture for the mucosa and muscle layers and a 5-0 or 6-0 non-absorbable suture for the skin. Although the use of prophylactic antibiotics has not been shown to be of definite benefit in these injuries, they are generally recommended for a 3- to 5-day course.

PUNCTURE WOUNDS

Puncture wounds should be managed with the following guidelines.

- **Deep puncture wounds,** particularly those involving muscle, should not be closed; these are best treated with culture of any expressed material, appropriate cleansing with antiseptic solution, irrigation if possible, drain insertion to the depth of the puncture tract, and a wound check with drain removal or replacement in 24 hours. Prophylactic antibiotics should be initiated if wounds are deep or extensive, if they result from bites, or if evidence of infection is apparent at the time of presentation. Antitetanus prophylaxis is discussed in "Antitetanus Prophylaxis" on pp. 464 and 465.
  - If **infection-prone areas of the hand** are involved, aggressive initial therapy is imperative and should include an initial culture, irrigation if possible, the application of wet heat or soaks four to six times per day; the institution of an appropriate antibiotic, such as amoxicillin-clavulanate; a wound check in 24 hours; and elevation. In these patients, hospital admission should be considered for parenteral antibiotic therapy when evidence of infection is already present; when puncture wounds are extensive; when discomfort is increased by gentle, passive movement of the fingers; or when the wound is the result of a bite, particularly a cat or human bite. Regarding antibiotic therapy, ampicillin-sulbactam, cefoxitin, or ticarcillin/clavulanate is acceptable. Penicillin-allergic patients can be given clindamycin plus ciprofloxacin.
- Puncture wounds, in general, should not be closed; those associated **with an entry and exit site** should similarly not be closed unless the face is involved and the injury is cosmetically significant. These wounds are best treated by following the course of the wound with a sterile snap or probe, if possible, and pulling through an appropriate drain such as plain sterile gauze or sterile umbilical tape. When the offending instrument is still present in the wound, sterile gauze or umbilical tape may be tied to the smaller end of the object with suture material and pulled through the wound as the instrument is removed; this will provide excellent drainage over the subsequent 24 to 48 hours. In either case, a dry sterile dressing should then be applied.
  - Puncture wounds of the **distal foot**, particularly when the puncture occurs through tennis sneakers, are particularly prone to infection; *Pseudomonas* organisms are often responsible, and prophylactic antibiotics treatment should be considered, that is, ciprofloxacin, and 24-hour wound reassessment advised.
- **Superficial puncture wounds** may generally be left open; however, when cosmetically significant and not associated with infection or the result of bites, primary closure or excision and primary closure may be the most appropriate therapy. Other injuries may be treated with delayed excision and closure.

MANAGEMENT OF GROSSLY CONTAMINATED WOUNDS

Grossly contaminated wounds are distinguished from infected wounds in that contamination implies that significant numbers of bacteria have entered the wound at the time of and as a direct result of the mechanism of injury, whereas infection, which may result from such contamination, implies that local cellulitis or abscess formation has occurred.

- **Closure.** Many grossly contaminated wounds may be closed primarily after proper cleansing, irrigation, and debridement, while infected lacerations must always be treated with delayed closure.

- **Cleansing and irrigation.** Grossly contaminated wounds should be cultured and copiously lavaged. Normal saline or tap water may be used with gravity flow or a variety of high-pressure methods, the latter being most effective at dislodging foreign material and reducing in-wound bacterial counts. Mechanical exploration of the wound and its recesses during irrigation will further facilitate the removal of foreign material and is recommended. Material that is embedded may be mechanically removed with forceps if possible or excised along with any devitalized, nonstructural tissue.
- Patients with **grossly contaminated, cosmetically significant facial wounds** require extremely aggressive management to optimize the final cosmetic result. A wound culture should be obtained, which should be followed by copious irrigation and manual or mechanical debridement; very small wounds are often best managed by primary excision and repair. Larger wounds may be managed by closure in the usual manner, the institution of prophylactic antibiotics, a wound check in 24 hours, and a warning to the patient that one or more stitches may require removal should infection develop.
- **Grossly contaminated, cosmetically insignificant injuries** require that a decision be made as to whether the laceration should be closed definitively, closed loosely, closed loosely with drain placement, or not closed at all. This decision must be based on the physician's personal experience, the size and location of the wound, the degree of contamination, the adequacy of cleansing, the postinjury interval, and the reliability of the patient.

WOUNDS PARTICULARLY PRONE TO INFECTION

A variety of wounds are considered by most authorities as particularly prone to infection. Although these injuries are discussed in detail elsewhere, they are recounted here to emphasize the higher probability of infection associated with them. Conservative treatment of these injuries often involves delay of primary closure, initial bacterial cultures, vigorous irrigation and debridement, drain insertion, the use of prophylactic antibiotics, and early referral (24 hours) for a wound check. The following are particularly prone to infection:

- Wounds resulting from **bites,** particularly when the hand is involved, are especially infection prone. In general, unless the face is involved, primary closure of bites is not recommended. It should also be noted that many human bites are unintentional, such as those resulting from sports collisions or altercations involving hand-mouth or hand-teeth contact; these must be recognized as human bites and treated accordingly.
- Wounds, particularly deep puncture wounds, that involve the distal foot (see previous) and the "**closed spaces**" **of the hand;** these include the midpalmar space, the thenar and hypothenar eminences, and the web spaces
- Wounds that are **grossly contaminated** with soil or other substances with high bacterial counts
- Wounds **left untreated** for 12 to 24 hours, depending on location
- Wounds associated with **significant crushing or devitalization of tissue** that cannot be adequately debrided

MANAGEMENT OF INFECTED WOUNDS

Patients who present with evidence of wound infection after suturing may have simple cellulitis, local abscess, or both. Patients may be divided into those with injuries that involve the face and those with injuries that do not.

- Patients with **cosmetically significant facial lacerations** unassociated with fluctuance, but with moderate erythema within the first 48 hours after suturing, should have every other suture removed, be treated with an antistaphylococcal antibiotic such as dicloxacillin, should have any expressed material sent for culture and sensitivity testing, and should receive instructions to apply heat to the area four to six times per day. A wound check is advised in 24 hours, and patients should be instructed to return if signs of systemic infection develop sooner. Patients presenting after 48 to 72 hours, again without fluctuance, should have all sutures removed and Steri-strips applied. If the patient appears systemically ill on presentation, hospital admission and parenteral antibiotic administration are required. Occult abscess must be suspected in such patients and drained if detected. When local fluctuance is appreciated, one or two adjacent sutures should be removed, the wound opened, drainage established, and a sterile rubber band or small Penrose or gauze drain inserted. A wound culture should be obtained and, in most patients, antibiotics instituted. A wound check is advised at 24 hours, with drain removal or reinsertion and determination of preliminary bacterial sensitivities; warm soaks are advised every 4 to 6 hours during this initial period.

- Patients with **cosmetically insignificant lacerations** associated with either significant erythema or fluctuance require adequate suture removal to exclude local abscess formation. Small lacerations unassociated with abscess can be treated by simply removing all sutures, applying Steri-strips to the wound if necessary, instituting an appropriate antibiotic, and applying heat four to six times per day; a wound check at 48 hours is appropriate. Patients with local abscess require removal of sufficient sutures to ensure drainage, drain insertion, a wound culture, and the institution of soaks four to six times per day; a wound check at 24 to 48 hours is also advised. Larger lacerations are treated similarly; however, when local abscess is noted, sutures overlying the area of fluctuance or alternate sutures should be removed and the wound opened at these sites to ensure drainage. Drains can then be inserted centrally or between sutures. The application of heat, a wound culture, the institution of antibiotics if appropriate (see previous), and a wound check at 24 to 48 hours are recommended.

ANTITETANUS PROPHYLAXIS

Tetanus is a completely preventable disease, and antitetanus prophylaxis must be provided to all patients when indicated.

Hypersensitivity

Hypersensitivity to antitetanus preparations may occur, although it is rare. Hypersensitivity to "horse serum" is the most common explanation for previous reactions to antitetanus immunization and is not a contraindication to the administration of currently available preparations, all of which are human derived.

Criteria

The administration of antitetanus prophylaxis is determined by the patient's age, previous immunization status, and the physician's assessment of the likelihood of *Clostridium tetani* contamination. Criteria have been established to define a particular wound as very tetanus prone or not tetanus prone. Wounds considered very tetanus prone are those seen later than 12 to 24 hours after the injury, those of a stellate configuration, avulsions, wounds greater than 1 cm deep, and those caused by missiles, burns, frostbite, or crushing injuries associated with devitalized tissue. Relatively clean wounds seen within the first 24 hours are considered not tetanus prone.

Treatment

Patients are placed into three categories based on their history of antitetanus immunization (Table 48-2):

- A history of complete immunization with a tetanus booster within the past 5 years; no treatment is required regardless of the type of injury.
- A history of complete immunization is present, but the most recent tetanus booster was received more than 10 years ago; all patients require Td (tetanus and diphtheria toxoids) only. Note that the CDC now recommends use of Tdap (tetanus, diphtheria and acellular pertussis toxoids) in lieu of Td for any adult ages 19 to 64, and for any adolescent ages 11 to 18 not already given the booster.
- A history regarding antitetanus immunization unavailable or incomplete; very tetanus-prone injuries require treatment with Tdap in adults, DPT (diphtheria and tetanus toxoids with pertussis vaccine) in children younger than 7 years of age, and 250 units of TIG-H (tetanus immune globulin-human) in adults, 125 U in children 5 to 10 years of age, and 75 U in children younger than 5 years of age. Injuries not considered tetanus prone require treatment with Tdap in adults and DPT in children younger than 7 years of age. Patients with an incomplete immunization history should be referred for the completion of immunization as follows:
  - In children 7 years of age and older and for all adults, immunization consists of three doses of tetanus toxoid (Td may be used), the first of which should be administered at the time of injury and the second and third at 1 and 7 months thereafter, respectively.

Table 48-2	Tetanus Immunization Regimen			
Tetanus Immunization	**Tetanus-Prone Wound**[a]		**Not Tetanus-Prone Wound**	
	Td[b]	**TIG**	**Td**[c]	**TIG**
Unknown or fewer than three immunizations	Yes	Yes	Yes	No
Three or more immunizations	No (yes if over 5 y since last booster)	No	No (yes if over 10 y since last booster)	No

[a]Tetanus-prone wounds include those that are 6–24 h old, are stellate or avulsions, are more than 1 cm deep, are contaminated by dirt, foreign material, or saliva, have devitalized tissue, or are caused by burns, frostbite, missiles, or crush injuries.

[b]Td is for children younger than age 7 y. Td is for adults and has one-tenth the amount of diphtheria toxoid as Td.

[c]Tdap (tetanus, diptheria, and acellular pertussis toxoids) now used in lieu of Td for adults ages 19–65, and adolescents ages 11–18 who have not already received the scheduled booster.

- In unimmunized children between the ages of 6 weeks and 7 years, immunization consists of four doses of tetanus toxoid given as DPT, the first administered at the time of injury and the second, third, and fourth given at 1, 2, and 12 months after the injury, respectively.
- Separate injection sites should be used in all patients receiving Td, Tdap, or DPT and TIG-H.
- In children older than 10 years of age and for adults, Tdap (tetanus, diphtheria, and pertussis toxoids) is the preferred treatment, rather than tetanus alone. Td should be used for children ages 7 to 10.
- As noted previously, in children younger than the age of 7 years, DPT should be given as a booster.
- If an allergy to human-derived tetanus toxoid is present, TIG-H may be given without hazard.
- Pregnancy is not a contraindication to the use of antitetanus prophylaxis. Tdap is not yet recommended for routine use in pregnancy (Td is acceptable).

PART 10

Environmental Emergencies

Diving Accidents

CLASSIFICATION

Diving injuries continue to increase as the popularity of underwater diving increases. Injuries related to diving are best classified into those associated with descent, those associated with ascent, and those related to prolonged exposure to significant depths.

DESCENT

During descent, not only is the pressure exerted on the diver great, but it also increases quickly; at a relatively shallow depth of 33 ft, atmospheric pressure has doubled. The air-filled spaces of the body (primarily the middle ear, sinuses, lungs, and bowel) become compressed on descent (as pressure increases) and expand on ascent.

Middle Ear Barotrauma

Probably the commonest syndrome associated with diving occurs during descent, when problems related to middle ear equilibration are noticed. The middle ear is an air-filled bony cavity communicating with the external environment via the eustachian tube. It is via the eustachian tube that air enters and exits the middle ear to maintain an equal pressure as ambient pressure changes. As the diver descends, increasing pressure is exerted against the tympanic membrane; this is countered as the diver voluntarily forces air through the eustachian tube into the middle ear resulting in equalization of pressures. Failure to achieve equilibration results in a "squeeze" manifest as pain in the affected ear; this is usually reversible by a small ascent and additional efforts to reequilibrate. If descent is uncontrolled and equilibration does not occur, pressure differences result in closure or collapse of the proximal eustachian, subsequent to which air flow through the eustachian tube ceases. Rupture of the tympanic membrane occurs with further descent, allowing water into the middle ear, which typically produces nausea and vertigo; this occurs in relatively shallow depths (5–15 ft) if equilibration has not occurred. Diagnosis is based on history (failure of the diver to notice "clicks" or "pops" associated with equilibration during descent, sharp pain in the ear, or a sound reported with tympanic membrane rupture, followed by vertigo) and physical examination (the tympanic membrane may demonstrate capillary engorgement, edema, or hemorrhage, or rupture may be noted). In some patients, signs of a seventh nerve palsy are noted; this is usually self-limited. Treatment includes avoidance of diving for several weeks until complete healing of the tympanic membrane occurs, oral and topical (spray) decongestants, and exercises to force fluid from the middle ear through the eustachian tube (Frenzel maneuvers); this is performed by repeated swallowing with a closed glottis, pursed lips, and pinched nose. Oral antibiotics should be prescribed if tympanic membrane rupture has occurred, and oral steroids may hasten improvement in seventh nerve palsy. Prevention includes avoidance of diving when upper airway congestion is present and recognizing early in descent that signs of middle ear equilibration are failing to occur; the prophylactic use of pseudoephedrine, typically 60 mg taken 30 minutes to 1 hour before diving, is sometimes recommended, although controversial.

External and Inner Ear Barotrauma

Barotrauma may also involve the external auditory canal (external ear squeeze) and the inner ear; these injuries are far less common than middle ear barotrauma. External ear squeeze occurs during descent when the external ear canal is occluded, thereby preventing equilibration of pressure during descent. Obstruction can occur if obstructing cerumen or earplugs are present. Pain is noted, often with blood reported in the canal. On examination, the canal is typically hemorrhagic; tympanic membrane rupture may also be noted. Inner ear barotrauma results when significant differences in pressure between the middle and inner ear develop suddenly (with very rapid or uncontrolled descents); patients report severe nausea, diaphoresis, lightheadedness, confusion, and disorientation. The "classic" symptoms of inner ear barotrauma are tinnitus, vertigo, and hearing loss. Symptoms may be delayed. Treatment includes bed rest with the head elevated, avoidance of diving until full resolution occurs, and otherwise supportive measures.

Facial Barotrauma

Facial barotrauma is infrequently seen in divers when negative pressure developing in one's mask during descent fails to equilibrate ("mask squeeze"); this can produce dramatic facial and conjunctival petechiae and edema, which typically resolve without sequelae. Visual acuity should be assessed, and diving should be proscribed until resolution of symptoms.

Barotrauma Involving the Sinuses

Barotrauma involving the sinuses ("sinus squeeze") is sometimes seen when equilibration of pressure via the nasal chambers is limited because of congestion or sinus obstruction; pain over the affected sinus is reported, and treatment is symptomatic with decongestants and elevation of the head of the bed. Symptoms most commonly involve the maxillary and frontal sinuses. When infection is suspected, a course of antibiotics should be instituted. ENT referral is appropriate in that a small group of patients may require surgical treatment.

ASCENT

General Considerations

Individuals exposed to environments of inert gases at partial pressures higher than that of the normal environment incorporate these gases into tissues; the rate and extent of incorporation occur as a function of the partial pressure of the gas and the rate of entry or solubility of the specific gas in the constituents of cells (i.e., water, lipid).

Individuals using a self-contained underwater breathing apparatus (SCUBA) are routinely exposed to environments in which the partial pressure of nitrogen gas becomes unusually high; therefore, nitrogen becomes incorporated into the body's tissues as a function of the depth reached and the time involved. Once nitrogen dissolves in the tissues, if environmental pressures fall for whatever reason, nitrogen comes out of solution forming bubbles. The rate and extent of pressure change determine the rate and extent to which nitrogen bubble formation occurs. Two major clinical syndromes occur as a result of this phenomenon; they are discussed later and include the pulmonary overpressurization syndrome (POPS) and decompression sickness or the "bends."

Pulmonary Overpressurization Syndromes

The volume occupied by an inhaled gas increases as the diver ascends (i.e., at the surface, a given volume of gas occupies four times the volume it occupied at 99 ft). Clearly, then, as the diver ascends, this volume of gas, as it expands, must be gradually and continuously expelled from the chest; too rapid of an ascent associated with breath holding or laryngospasm may rupture both pulmonary veins and alveoli as large pressure gradients are generated. Depending on their location within the chest, rupture of alveoli may result in pneumothorax, pneumopericardium, pneumomediastinum, subcutaneous emphysema, or a combination of these disorders. Symptoms may be noted at the surface or may be delayed. Mediastinal and subcutaneous emphysema are most commonly noted, present with neck pressure, hoarseness, and chest tightness, and if unaccompanied by other more serious abnormalities (pneumothorax), are usually self-limited and require no specific treatment, aside from rest, and in some patients supplemental oxygen. An upright, end-expiratory, PA chest film should be obtained to exclude pneumothorax, which may require specific therapy. **Air embolus** occurs as a result of rupture of pulmonary veins which allows bubble-laden blood to return to the heart, the arterial circulation, and commonly the carotid vessels; this is not unexpected, because ascent occurs with the head up. Free air entering the cerebral circulation may result in cessation of blood flow.

Symptoms typically appear within seconds or minutes of embolization and include headache, dizziness, subtle changes in personality, confusion, focal neurologic deficits including aphasia, apraxia, blindness, and hemiplegia, as well as loss of consciousness, seizures, coma, and death. These symptoms are usually noted immediately at the surface or within several minutes. A variety of chest symptoms related to free air within the chest, pericardium, and mediastinum are also noted; these include dyspnea, chest pain, and hemoptysis. The treatment of arterial gas embolization is immediate recompression; this is discussed in "Treatment."

Decompression Sickness

As a diver descends, as described in "Descent," ambient pressures rise and nitrogen gas dissolves in the body's tissues; too rapid ascent, associated with falling ambient pressures, results in the formation of nitrogen bubbles as the gas expands and comes out of solution. Because the central nervous system and the bone marrow are preferential sites for nitrogen deposition, it is in these locations, as well as within the intravascular space, that nitrogen expansion and bubble formation produce symptoms.

Symptoms usually occur within the first hour of surfacing but may be delayed by as much as 24 hours and may be both nonspecific and vague. Divers should be carefully questioned regarding their adherence to required decompression time stops. The closer the onset of symptoms to the end of the dive, the more severe the illness is expected to be. Severe muscular aching described as "deep" by most patients is common and reflects nitrogen decompression occurring within bones and around joints; this pain is referred to as the "bends." Divers presenting with muscular aching should be assumed to have the bends until proved otherwise.

Symptoms referable to the skin may also occur and are manifest as mottling, pain, pruritus, and paresthesias. Nitrogen decompression within the pulmonary vascular space results in substernal aching, cough, a feeling of impending suffocation, dyspnea, and in some patients cyanosis and shock; these early symptoms have been referred to as the "chokes." Cardiac involvement may also occur, and approximately 25% of patients present with neurologic abnormalities, including paraplegia, paraparesis, urinary retention, and a variety of peripheral deficits. Venous air may also enter the arterial circulation (paradoxical embolization) via right to left shunting in the heart (presumably from occult patent foramen ovale) and pulmonary circulations. Spinal cord injury results from retrograde venous thrombosis producing patchy necrosis of the cord; the lower thoracic and upper lumbar areas are most commonly involved.

NITROGEN NARCOSIS

Nitrogen narcosis or "rapture of the deep" is the result of CNS exposure to increased concentrations of nitrogen gas for an extended period of time; symptoms include confusion, disorientation, lack of coordination, and a sense of euphoria. These symptoms are usually seen at depths more than 75 ft but can occur in shallower water if prolonged exposure has occurred. Generally, symptoms are not severe and gradually resolve with ascent, although as a result of confusion and disorientation, failure to recognize falling oxygen reserves and distance from shore/rescue can result in severe secondary injury.

TREATMENT

The basic techniques of cardiopulmonary resuscitation are undertaken in the usual manner. When the possibility of air embolus is present, the patient should be placed in a supine position. Placement in Trendelenburg position is not recommended; 100% oxygen should be administered with a tightly fitting mask. Plans for transfer to a recompression facility should then be formulated. Seizures should be treated with intravenous diazepam in the usual manner; hypotension is initially managed with lactated Ringer solution and plasma. Patients presenting to the emergency department stating that they have miscalculated their required decompression time stops, even though currently asymptomatic, may require transfer to a hyperbaric facility for recompression therapy. Similarly, patients with symptoms attributable to air embolus or decompression sickness require emergent transfer; the accepting facility will also provide information as to how best to transfer the patient (i.e., using aircraft capable of generating high cabin pressures or those able to fly at low altitudes). Recompression is advised and effective even when several days have elapsed between the injury and presentation, although it is most effective if instituted early; 24-hour information regarding treatment may be obtained by calling the National Diving Accident Network (919-684-4326), the Medical Laboratory Experimental Diving Unit, U.S. Navy, Panama City, Florida (904-234-4351), or the U.S. Air Force School of Aerospace Medicine, Decompression Management Team, San Antonio, Texas (512-536-3281).

50 Near Drowning

GENERAL CONSIDERATIONS

Near drowning occurs when patients survive at least temporarily after water immersion. Near drownings are relatively common, usually involve children younger than age 4 years or young adults, and present dramatically to the emergency department.

Traditionally, major emphasis has been placed on whether immersion in fresh or salt water occurred; the incidence of hemolysis, electrolyte disturbances, intravascular volume changes, and prognosis were said to be determined by the osmotic nature of the aspirated fluid. Although experimentally valid, these considerations have more recently been deemphasized.

When immersion occurs, a period of breath holding is followed by involuntary inspiration; aspiration of water, which may be contaminated with bacteria and other particulate matter, usually follows. Interestingly, however, approximately 15% of patients who die as a result of drowning do not aspirate. In these patients, intense and immediate laryngospasm prevents aspiration; death occurs as a result of asphyxia ("dry-drowning").

PULMONARY INJURIES

A variety of **pulmonary injuries** are seen in patients who aspirate during immersion; these include varying degrees of interstitial and alveolar edema, injury to the alveolar capillary membrane, loss of surfactant resulting in alveolar collapse, obstruction of airways secondary to any variety of particulate matter, and a number of delayed complications resulting from bacterial deposition within the lung. If significant, singularly or collectively, these abnormalities produce hypoxemia, which in approximately 20% of near-drowning victims causes profound neurologic damage despite adequate resuscitative efforts.

CLINICAL PRESENTATION

Clinically, patients may present totally without symptoms; with cough and slight dyspnea; or with apnea, hypothermia, and coma. In patients with cerebral anoxia, the prognosis for recovery of normal neurologic function is not well understood. Important **prognostic factors** include
- The duration of submersion
- The extent and duration of hypoxemia
- Water temperature
- The extent of hypothermia
- Age
- The presence of aspiration

- The adequacy of initial resuscitative efforts
- Coexistent medical problems
  Two clinical points should be emphasized:
- Initially, many patients with evolving pulmonary compromise will have normal arterial blood gases and chest x-rays; these criteria therefore must not be used to exclude aspiration or evolving pulmonary injury.
- Trauma is frequently the initial event that precipitates submersion; cervical and thoracic injuries frequently coexist and are occasionally unappreciated, leading to disastrous consequences. Patients with abnormalities of consciousness or cognitive function or those with trauma to the head or neck should be considered to have possible spinal cord injuries until proven otherwise.

TREATMENT

- All patients with submersion-type injuries should be promptly evaluated in the hospital. Asymptomatic patients should remain under observation for 2 to 6 hours, and if they remain completely asymptomatic during this interval and have adequate oxygen saturation demonstrated, they may be discharged. Patients with very mild symptoms and normal oxygen saturation, and who become asymptomatic over a period of several hours, may be discharged if the social situation lends itself to careful reliable observation. Patients with reduced oxygenation, even if normalized by oxygen administration, and persistent or progressive symptoms, should be admitted for a period of observation.
- Injuries to the cervical and thoracic spine must be considered in all seriously injured near-drowning patients. This is particularly true when trauma preceded immersion or when a history of diving is elicited or suspected; patients with evidence of trauma to the head or neck must be considered to have spinal cord injuries until proven otherwise.
- At the scene, the patient should be removed from the water (bearing in mind the possibility of cervical spine injury), and ventilation, preferably with supplemental oxygen, initiated, along with other standard protocols.
- Maneuvers to "drain fluid from the lungs" are ineffective and potentially dangerous; these should be abandoned and emphasis placed on early aggressive CPR.
- One hundred percent oxygen should be administered at the scene as soon as possible.
- Transport to an appropriate facility in a manner that protects the cervical spine and minimizes the possibility of aspiration is essential. Patients who are vomiting or nauseated may be placed in the lateral decubitus or prone position with the neck supported and protected as much as possible.
- On arrival in the emergency department, the usual criteria for resuscitation and intubation are followed. Injuries to the cervical and thoracic spine must be considered. Oxygen, 100% by mask or 40% by endotracheal tube, should initially be administered; a chest x-ray, oxygen saturation, and other routine studies are obtained, and intravenous access established in all patients.
- Patients who are hypoxemic despite being given 100% oxygen by mask should be intubated and receive 40% to 50% oxygen. Persisting hypoxemia (<60 mm Hg) despite maximal oxygen may be corrected by PEEP (positive end-expiratory pressure) or CPAP. Correction of hypoxemia is an absolute priority that may necessitate increasing the FIO_2 beyond 40% to 50%.

- Hypothermia frequently complicates the management of patients with submersion injuries, although low temperatures may be neurologically protective. Hypothermia must be treated in the usual manner (see , "Hypothermia," in Chapter 56). A rectal temperature taken with a low-reading or hypothermia thermometer is mandatory. Severe hypothermia may mimic the clinical state of death, and survival with normal neurologic function may follow prolonged submersion; on the basis of these considerations, resuscitative efforts should be aggressive, often protracted, and continue until such time as the temperature reaches 30°C to 32.5°C or 86°F to 90.5°F.
- There is no evidence that prophylactic antibiotics or steroids are helpful in the management of near-drowning patients. Appropriate antibiotics should be administered if evidence of pulmonary infection develops.

51

Electrical and Lightning Injuries

ELECTRICAL INJURIES

A variety of discrete injuries may result from exposure to electricity.

Thermal Injuries

Thermal injuries secondary to electrical flashing occur when radiant energy is released because of the rapid passage of current from an electrical source to a ground outside the body. These are true burns, which may be of any extent and severity and are treated as such. (The treatment of burns is discussed in Chapter 55.) Importantly, actual transmission of electrical current through the body does not occur in these patients.

Conductive Injuries

Conductive injuries are the most common of the electricity-related injuries seen in the emergency department. Several points about diagnosis and pathophysiology should be made.

- **Heat-Generated Tissue Injury:** When electrical current travels through the body, tissue injury occurs along the path of travel as a result of the generation of heat. Interposed tissues provide varying degrees of resistance to current, and as a consequence, heat is generated. Injuries to nerves, muscles, and the vasculature (resulting in thrombosis) are the most significant types of injury. The extent of tissue damage is directly related to a number of factors:
  - The intensity of the current (measured in amperes, which is increased at higher voltages)
  - Duration of contact
  - Resistance and general diameter of interposed tissue
  - The current's specific path through the body
  - The specific type of current (AC or DC)
- High voltage (generally considered that in excess of 600–1,000 V) is associated with a higher incidence of death and serious injuries. Most household appliances operate at 110 V (dryers and house power lines are at 220 V), with residential feeding or trunk lines carrying 7,620 V. Commercially available "stun guns" or Tazers produce generalized, intense muscle contraction and result in the collapse of the victim; although the voltage produced with these weapons is high (50,000 V with the Tazer), serious injuries are unusual.
- Direct contact burns are typically, but not always, seen at the point of current entry and exit from the body; these are characterized by a charred or dark center, with a surrounding area of pale or necrotic tissue. Electrical current may also produce injury via arcing; this is the phenomenon whereby current travels to the victim, through interposed air, from and between areas of high and differing electrical

potential. Arcing may occur across significant distances (approximately 1 ft for each 100,000 V of differing potential), may ignite the victim's clothing, and, because of intense muscular contraction at the time of contact, produce falls and other injuries.

- It is not possible to predict or define the extent or type of damage along the suspected course of current transmission, even when entry and exit wounds are found.

- **Tissue necrosis**, which can be dramatic, extensive, and rapidly evolving, is classically delayed for several hours to days and may complicate injuries originally assessed as trivial in the emergency department. Compartment syndromes related to vascular injury and extensive muscular injury must also be suspected and treated aggressively.

- **Cardiac arrest** caused by ventricular fibrillation is the most common cause of death in electrocuted patients; a variety of other cardiac arrhythmias, which may not be present initially, are also seen. Monitoring is therefore appropriate.

- **Extensive muscle necrosis** may produce significant hyperkalemia, hypocalcemia, and renal failure caused by myoglobinuria.

- **Neurologic abnormalities** are common in patients exposed to high voltage; a variety of mental status changes are reported and include loss of consciousness, restlessness, depersonalization, anxiety, and mild confusion. Most of these changes are transient. Coma, which may be prolonged, is also seen occasionally. Spinal cord damage, usually reported in association with hand-to-hand or head-to-hand transmission, is occasionally noted and may not be fully manifest when the patient is first seen. Interventricular hemorrhage can occur when high voltage passes through the brain.

- As a result of intense muscular contraction at the time of contact, or as a result of a "blast," patients may be thrown from ladders, etc., and significant **musculoskeletal and other injuries** may be sustained; these include vertebral compression and long-bone fractures and dislocations (typically posterior dislocations of the shoulder). Similarly, loss of consciousness at the time of contact may also occur and result in injury. Fractures involving long bones frequently coexist, and occult injuries to the cervical and thoracic spine are common; these injuries are often not initially suspected.

- **"Kissing" or arc burns** involving contact areas of the flexor surfaces of the upper extremity are common, occur when electricity-induced muscular contraction occurs, and are diagnostic of conductive-type injuries. These burns frequently involve the axilla, flexor creases of the palm and wrist, and the antecubital fossa; when they are present, a significant underlying injury should be suspected.

- In pregnant patients, although uncommon, **fetal death** has been reported, often in the absence of significant injury to the mother; amniotic fluid is an excellent conductor. When exposed to household or higher current, pregnant patients should be observed for a period of time, along with obstetrical consultation. Fetal monitoring will be recommended for patients with gestational ages more than 24 weeks; auscultation of fetal heart sounds and an ultrasound are appropriate for gestational ages less than this.

- **Electrical injury to the mouth** and oral mucosa, typically occurring in infants who chew through household electrical wire, presents a unique problem. Unfortunately, occult injury to the labial artery (which is unrecognized because of arterial spasm and local tissue injury) can result in delayed and significant hemorrhage (as the overlying eschar separates from the underlying tissue). This typically occurs approximately 5 days after the injury.

- **Disposition Recommendations**
  - Asymptomatic adults exposed to high voltage (>600 V) should be admitted for observation; telemetry is not required unless the patient's EKG is abnormal or an arrhythmia is suspected or identified. Patients with any evidence of significant complications of electrical injury (vascular, muscular injury, cardiac, neurologic) should be observed in a burn unit. Adults exposed to less than 600 V, with any complications, similarly require admission and observation.
  - Asymptomatic adults with no physical findings who are exposed to household (110 V) current can be safely discharged provided their EKG is normal and the risk of cardiac exposure is minimal (no projected cardiac path implied, no tetany, wet skin, or immersion). Exposure to 220 V probably carries little additional risk of delayed cardiac arrhythmias, although there are fewer data supporting this.
  - Most children exposed to household current (110 V) have isolated hand or oral injuries; the risk of serious local or delayed cardiac complications are small; children with tetany, loss of consciousness or other neurologic symptoms, wet skin at the time of exposure, or vertically transmitted current should be admitted for a period of observation, including cardiac monitoring.
  - Children with oral injuries from electrical cords can be safely discharged provided there was no loss of consciousness, the EKG is normal, the child can tolerate oral fluids, and other complications are absent. The postdischarge environment must also be safe and the parents/caretaker must be reliable; the patient should return for a wound check in 24 hours. If bleeding occurs, direct pressure should be applied and the head should be elevated; if continuing, the patient should be promptly evaluated in the ED. Prolonged splinting is usually needed to limit wound contracture and the need for subsequent commissuroplasty. Patients discharged should be discussed with the pediatrician and plastic or oral surgeon to whom the patient would be referred for follow-up.
- **Specific Treatment Considerations**
  - Because of the unique nature of electrical injuries, the physician must maintain a high degree of suspicion regarding the presence of musculoskeletal injuries, particularly injuries to the spine, long-bone fractures, and specific dislocations.
  - Cutaneous burns are treated in the usual fashion.
  - Additionally, in patients with significant injuries to muscle, rhabdomyolysis must be considered and treated aggressively if myoglobinuria is present (with early and aggressive fluid replacement and urinary alkalization). The latter is achieved via the infusion of alkalinized normal saline or Ringer lactate solution (44–50 mEq of sodium bicarbonate is added to each liter); optimal urinary output is approximately 1.5 to 2.0 mL/kg/h with an optimal blood pH greater than 7.45. Mannitol may hasten the urinary clearing of myoglobin but is contraindicated in hypovolemic patients and when thermal burns are present (because of the risk of hypovolemia). Standard formulae regarding the rate of fluid replacement in burn patients based on percentage and type of burn present are not applicable to patients with electrical injuries; fluid requirements are high and always underestimated by such formulae. An initial fluid challenge with Ringer lactate or normal saline (20–40 mL/kg over the first hour) is usually indicated; further assessment of volume replacement may require guidance via central venous or pulmonary artery wedge pressure measurements. Tetanus prophylaxis should be confirmed or provided.

LIGHTNING INJURIES

Exposure to lightning involves a variety of pathophysiologic mechanisms:

- An initial exploding or blast-type injury, often followed by a decelerating injury or a fall
- Exposure to artificially generated electricity (which is alternating current), usually produces a prolonged exposure, resulting in extensive damage to deep tissues
- Exposure to lightning (which is direct current) is extremely brief, with most of the current actually passing over (the "flashover") or across the body.
- Burns involving the skin are mild and usually superficial
- Deep or internal damage caused by conductive injury is less commonly seen
- Death is most common in "direct strikes" (when lighting directly strikes the victim) and results from asystole and/or respiratory arrest

It is estimated that lightning strikes the earth more than 100 times each second; additionally, at any one time, more than 1,500 to 2,000 thunderstorms are active in the earth's atmosphere. Lightning occurs when a "circuit" is completed between the bottom of a storm cloud and the surface of the earth. There is contact between downward- and upward-moving electrical currents, thereby essentially making a "complete circuit." Temperatures reached instantaneously exceed those on the surface of the sun. Energy levels have been calculated to be as high as 30 million volts and 50,000 A. The actual diameter of the lightning "bolt" is unknown, but estimates based on strike sites through metallic structures range from approximately 4 inches to extremely small. When air is heated to this extent and this quickly, rapid expansion or exploding occurs. Rapidly moving air, with its related turbulence, is heard as thunder. Because of the differences in velocity between light and sound, one can calculate the distance from lightning's impact to one's current location; the distance in miles can be calculated by determining the interval in seconds between seeing the flash and hearing thunder and by dividing this number by 5.

Diagnosis

Although asystole and respiratory arrest are reported after lightning exposure, most victims survive. Although the mortality rate associated with lightning exposure is unknown, it is estimated to be between 15% and 20%. In survivors, long-term and serious sequelae are common. Other cardiac abnormalities include transient alterations in conduction and rate as well as delayed myocardial infarction, because of coronary artery endothelial damage. Elevation of creatine kinase isoenzymes, as well as other markers of cardiac injury, is common. Actual myocardial infarction occurs in only approximately 10% of patients. Neurologic abnormalities include a variety of acute and late complications:

- Acute mental status changes include loss of consciousness, amnesia, lethargy, confusion, and coma.
- Intracerebral hemorrhage and infarction are also reported.
- Spinal and peripheral nerve deficits, which may be transient, and direct injuries resulting from falls or other trauma after the initial blast also occur.
- A wide variety of late neurologic sequelae may be seen.
  Other injuries include the following:
- Direct injury to the liver, spleen, or bowel may occur, and ileus is common.
- Pulmonary complications include contusion, pneumothorax, and adult respiratory disease syndrome, all secondary to the blast injury.

- Hematuria may be noted, in which case computed tomography or ultrasound should be obtained to exclude a structural injury to the kidney. The urine should also be evaluated for myoglobin.
- Retinal detachment and optic nerve degeneration or atrophy may follow lightning exposure; the development of cataracts is also reported, and many authorities recommend an initial or baseline slit-lamp examination.
- Occult fractures of long bones and the spine are common; radiologic evaluation of the cervical spine is recommended in all patients, particularly those with abnormalities of mental status.
- Injury to the tympanic membrane is present in approximately 50% of patients.
- Because of overwhelming vasospasm and sympathetic nervous system dysfunction, many patients present with cold, pulseless, often blue extremities. These findings are usually transient with gradual clearing over several hours.
- Characteristic Lichtenberg markings are noted on the skin (fern-like or lace-like, red or brown areas) and represent first-degree thermal injuries associated with a large entry site; smaller entry sites produce second-degree or third-degree burns.

Disposition Considerations

Most patients exposed to lightning should be admitted for a period of in-hospital observation; this is particularly true for patients with
- Suspected or documented loss of consciousness
- Scalp, facial, or leg burns
- Evidence of evolving complications (myoglobinuria, EKG changes, including any arrhythmias, neurologic abnormalities)

   If admitted, central cardiac monitoring is recommended for the first 48 to 72 hours. Initially occult conductive injuries, although uncommon, may be associated with extensive damage to deep tissues and may be identified early in admitted patients. Pregnant patients should be admitted for observation, ultrasound, and fetal monitoring.

Treatment

- The treatment of **cardiac and respiratory arrest** is undertaken in the usual fashion. Resuscitative efforts should be aggressive. The usual criteria for termination of resuscitative efforts are less applicable in patients with electrical injuries because a number of reports describe recovery of neurologic function despite a prolonged resuscitative effort.
- Patients with **abnormalities of mental status**, loss of consciousness, symptoms referable to the spine, or significant facial or cervical trauma must be considered to have vertebral or spinal cord injuries until proved otherwise. Stabilization of the neck and appropriate transport of the patient until such time as stability of the spine is demonstrated radiologically are indicated in all such patients. Direct injury to the central nervous system as a result of a fall after the initial injury is common.
- **Thermal injuries** are managed as discussed in Chapter 55. It is important for the physician to realize that severe thermal injury may mask significant conductive insults. Because of this, in patients with important thermal injuries, transfer to definitive burn services is appropriate. In patients with minor thermal injuries, the possibility of occult conductive injury is still present, and we generally recommend a period of in-hospital observation is generally recommended.

- Patients with **true conductive injuries** must be admitted and closely followed clinically for evidence of evolving or progressive tissue injury. Twelve to twenty-four hours of central monitoring, serial electrocardiograms, and measurement of cardiac isoenzymes are indicated.
- In selected patients, the adequacy of **intravascular volume and urinary flow** should be ensured by central venous pressure or Swan-Ganz line and Foley catheter placement, respectively; a urinary flow of 1.0 to 1.5 mL/kg/h is reasonable in adults.
- **Myoglobin,** released from damaged muscle, if present in significant quantity may cause acute renal failure. Baseline initial urinary myoglobin determinations should be made, along with sequential studies. Many authorities recommend forced alkaline diuresis to decrease the possibility of renal injury when urinary myoglobin is detected (discussed previously). The presence of hematuria indicates the need for imaging to exclude structural injury to the kidney.
- As noted, **pregnant patients** should be admitted for a period of observation, determination of fetal heart sounds, ultrasound, and obstetric consultation.

52

High-Altitude Illness

GENERAL CONSIDERATIONS

Acute high-altitude illness consists of a spectrum of clinical syndromes occurring in nonacclimatized individuals traveling to altitudes greater than 8,000 ft and ranges from a mild, almost flulike, systemic illness (acute mountain sickness or AMS) to life-threatening high-altitude pulmonary edema (HAPE), to high-altitude cerebral edema (HACE), to death. In general, the incidence and severity of illness increase with higher altitudes and rapid rates of ascent. All age groups may be affected, including otherwise healthy young persons and persons currently living in and adapted to high altitude who travel to a lower elevation and then reascend.

Acute high-altitude illness typically has an onset within 2 to 8 hours of ascent; this is important in our increasingly mobile society, in which a sea level resident may fly to a high-altitude destination within a few hours. Commercial airlines cruising at altitudes of 29,000 to 37,000 ft have cabin pressures equivalent of an altitude of approximately 6,000 to 8,000 ft (1,800–2,400 m) (FIO_2 of 15.2%–17.6%); thus, the airline passenger may be briefly exposed to conditions otherwise associated with the development of mild high-altitude illness.

Acute hypoxia is the syndrome resulting from severe and sudden exposure to extremely low levels of oxygen. This is typically seen during accidental decompression of commercial aircraft or associated with sudden failure of supplemental oxygen in individuals at very high altitudes. Less dramatic situations resulting in arterial desaturation include massive pulmonary embolus and flash pulmonary edema. Symptoms are related to the degree and time course of desaturation and include light-headedness, weakness, dizziness, changes in vision, and lethargy.

PATHOPHYSIOLOGY

Although the ill effects resulting from rapid ascent to high altitudes have been known for years, much of the pathophysiology remains poorly understood. When a nonacclimatized person reaches a high altitude, the decreased ambient oxygen partial pressure results in immediate hypobaric hypoxemia; compensating for hypoxemia, the carotid artery and aortic body chemoreceptors and the brainstem induce an increased respiratory rate, resulting in hypocapnia and respiratory alkalosis. Unfortunately, alkalemia depresses the ventilatory drive, thus operating to increase hypoxemia further during this initial period of alkalosis, usually in the first 24 to 36 hours after ascent.

Physiologic Changes

Numerous physiologic changes occur during high-altitude exposure:
- The heart rate increases with ascent to high altitude, and although the cardiac output may be initially increased, it is eventually reduced as a result of a decrease in stroke volume.
- Electrocardiographic monitoring of healthy Mount Everest climbers revealed sinus tachycardia, marked sinus arrhythmia, right axis shift, T-wave flattening or inversion, premature atrial and ventricular depolarizations, and, rarely, right bundle branch conduction disturbances. These changes reverted to normal on descent from high altitude.
- An increased pulmonary, splanchnic, and skeletal muscle vascular resistance is observed in travelers to high altitude—this is because of vasoconstriction induced by hypoxemia.
- The effects of high altitude on the cerebral vasculature are more complex. Hypoxia produces vasodilation, whereas hypocarbia induces vasoconstriction. The overall effect of these changes is believed to cause an increased cerebral blood volume and a variable increase in cerebral blood flow, depending on the amount of hypocarbia present.
- Exercise tolerance is reduced at high altitude, and vigorous exercise clearly worsens resting hypoxemia.

Acclimatization

Acclimatization begins when a reduced arterial oxygen saturation is first detected.
- Hypoxia results in a compensatory increase in minute ventilation, which produces a respiratory alkalosis.
- After approximately 24 to 36 hours, renal compensation for respiratory alkalosis causes a bicarbonate diuresis.
- Restoration of a more physiologic pH reverses the blunting effect of alkalemia on the respiratory drive, the respiratory rate increases, and hypoxemia improves.
- Improved oxygenation at this time signals acclimatization, and symptoms resolve.
- Any further incremental ascent will again expose the person to a further decrease in ambient oxygen levels, after which the acclimatization process must begin anew.

In addition, a person who has only mild symptoms at an altitude of 10,000 ft (3,050 m) cannot be predicted to acclimatize well at 12,000 ft (3,660 m); in fact, a serious high-altitude illness may result. Acclimatization of individuals chronically exposed to high altitudes occurs gradually, with hypoxia stimulating the release of erythropoietin. Hypoxia also results in increased 2,3-diphosphoglycerate, which produces a favorable rightward shift in the oxygen-hemoglobin dissociation curve.

ACUTE MOUNTAIN SICKNESS

History

Symptoms of AMS usually occur within the first several hours of ascent, peak at approximately 36 hours, and then gradually resolve over the next 1 to 2 days. Some patients will have mild symptoms for 1 week; symptoms usually occur at more than 8,000 to 10,000 ft or 2,440 to 3,050 m and correspond to the initial period of uncompensated respiratory alkalosis. Symptoms may include
- Fatigue
- Light-headedness

- Dizziness
- Irritability
- Difficulty concentrating
- Headaches
- Nausea, vomiting
- Dyspnea on mild exertion
- Palpitations
- Insomnia and poor sleep quality

Dyspnea at rest is not part of this syndrome and should raise suspicion regarding the development of HAPE; similarly, evidence of central nervous system dysfunction, which may include any impairment in cognitive function or ataxia, raises concern regarding the development of HACE. If this is noted, descent should be undertaken. Of patients with AMS at elevations of approximately 14,000 ft, approximately 1 in 10 will have HAPE or HACE with further ascent. Most patients with AMS note resolution of symptoms within 12 to 16 hours of onset; however, some patients will continue to experience symptoms for 3 to 4 days.

Physical Examination and Diagnostic Tests

The results of the physical examination, chest x-ray, and laboratory data are usually normal, except for possible evidence of mild dehydration secondary to increased pulmonary water loss, anorexia, and, if acclimatization has begun, the bicarbonate diuresis. During sleep, periodic breathing may be observed with alternate episodes of apnea and hyperpnea.

Treatment

The treatment of mild high-altitude illness consists of the following:
- Encourage bed rest and fluid intake until acclimatization is complete.
- Any additional ascent is contraindicated.
- Despite headache and poor sleep quality, narcotic analgesics and sedatives are best avoided because they may depress respiration and thereby accentuate hypoxemia.
- The administration of oxygen (1–2 L/min) usually relieves mild symptoms, as will acetaminophen.
- The efficacy of acetazolamide in reducing symptoms in AMS, as well as preventing the development of symptoms, is relatively clear; this agent is most effective if given early (250 mg given orally at the first symptom and 125–250 mg twice daily thereafter). Acetazolamide is a carbonic anhydrase inhibitor, which reduces reabsorption of bicarbonate by the kidney, resulting in a metabolic acidosis; this stimulates ventilation, correcting hypoxemia; treatment should continue until symptoms resolve. Acetazolamide belongs to the sulfa family and should not be given to patients with sulfa hypersensitivity.
- Nausea and vomiting may be treated with prochlorperazine, 5 to 10 mg intramuscularly.
- Patients presenting with more serious or progressing symptoms or whose symptoms persist beyond 72 hours despite treatment will require the administration of supplemental oxygen and evacuation to a lower altitude for relief of symptoms. Evacuation to sea level is not typically necessary in patients with mild symptoms; fortunately, relatively small changes in altitude (1,500–2,500 ft) can result in prompt resolution of symptoms.
- Dexamethasone, 4 mg every 6 hours (orally, intramuscular, or intravenous), has been shown to reduce the symptoms of AMS and should be given to patients with moderate AMS.

- Portable, hyperbaric bags, in which the patient is exposed to approximately 2 psi of pressure, are now available in some areas and effectively simulate a descent of approximately 5,000 ft. These may be very useful when descent to lower altitudes is impossible or delayed.

HIGH-ALTITUDE PULMONARY EDEMA

HAPE may occur when ascents more than 8,000 ft or 2,400 m are made. HAPE is a type of noncardiogenic pulmonary edema and is usually observed approximately 48 to 96 hours after ascent.

History

In addition to the symptoms of AMS, which may coexist, patients with HAPE typically complain initially of
- Dry cough
- Low-grade fever
- Weakness
- Dyspnea with exertion
    Moderate illness is characterized by
- Fatigue
- Increased weakness
- Anorexia
- Headache
- Increasing cough (which may now be productive)
- Progressive dyspnea
    Severe HAPE is associated with
- Dyspnea at rest
- Productive cough
- Overwhelming fatigue and weakness
- Lethargy
- Stupor
- Eventually, coma and death

Physical Examination

Physical examination reveals the findings characterizing progressive hypoxemia.
- Increased heart and respiratory rates
- Crepitant rales
- Cyanosis
- Progressive neurologic findings
- Temperatures up to 38.5°C
- Signs of elevated right- or left-sided filling pressures are not present (jugular venous distention, S_3 gallop, cardiac enlargement); a prominent P2 is often noted.

Diagnostic Tests

- The chest x-ray confirms a normal cardiac silhouette but is remarkable for typical interstitial or patchy alveolar infiltrates, followed by generalized alveolar infiltrates. A unilateral pulmonary infiltrate may suggest unilateral pulmonary artery atresia, and a ventilation-perfusion lung scan should be performed to assess this possibility.

- Arterial blood gases will show hypoxemia and a respiratory alkalosis, unless respiratory failure has evolved.
- The electrocardiogram typically shows a sinus tachycardia and occasionally evidence of right atrial and ventricular strain.
- Studies have shown that patients with HAPE have elevated pulmonary artery but normal left-sided filling pressures.

Treatment

The treatment of patients with HAPE is determined by the availability of oxygen and hyperbaric units, and the specific options regarding descent.

- If descent to lower altitudes is an option (even by 2,000–2,500 ft), then this is the optimal treatment, although in mild and some moderate cases, it is not always necessary. If descent is elected, physical activity must be minimized and supplemental high-flow oxygen (as noted), if available, should be provided. During descent, oxygen is helpful, but if unavailable, descent should proceed.
- If the patient can be carefully observed, bed rest and supplemental oxygen may provide adequate treatment, provided evacuation to lower altitudes, if symptoms worsen, is immediately available.
- The immediate availability of a portable hyperbaric device provides additional safety in the patient being observed.
- Oxygen should be administered via an expiratory positive airway pressure mask, if available, which improves oxygenation.
- If patients are unable to descend, oxygen should be administered as noted and may be lifesaving; similarly, if a portable hyperbaric device is available, it may be lifesaving as well; if unavailable, all efforts must be directed toward having oxygen and a portable chamber airlifted in.
- Patients with severe HAPE may require intubation, mechanical ventilation, and positive end-expiratory pressure; supplemental oxygen and emergent evacuation to low altitudes remain the mainstays of treatment.
- Treatment of HAPE with medications used for cardiogenic pulmonary edema is often successful. Furosemide and small doses of morphine improve pulmonary congestion and reduce symptoms. Intravascular volume is typically reduced in these patients, and caution with these agents must therefore be exercised to avoid hypotension. Nifedipine, a pulmonary vasodilator, is sometimes helpful, particularly if other treatment options are unavailable, and is given orally via the 10-mg capsule or the 30-mg sustained-release preparation.
- In treated patients, symptoms usually improve or resolve over 36 to 48 hours.

HIGH-ALTITUDE CEREBRAL EDEMA

HACE, defined as a progressive neurologic syndrome occurring in patients with AMS or HAPE, may occur during the first 24 to 48 hours of ascent to elevations more than 12,000 to 15,000 ft or 3,660 to 4,570 m.

Diagnosis

Initial signs and symptoms
- Nausea, vomiting
- Lethargy or confusion
- Difficulty with coordination and concentration
- Headache

- Papilledema
- Cerebellar dysfunction and a variety of focal neurologic deficits (as a result of increased sensitivity of the cerebellum to hypoxia, ataxia, which is initially often mild, should alert the physician that HACE is developing; ataxia alone represents an indication for immediate descent.)
- Retinal hemorrhages may be noted as well but may also be seen in patients without cerebral edema.
- As intracranial pressure increases, patients have increasing impairment of neurologic function, eventually progressing to coma and death.

Autopsy demonstrates endothelial vascular damage with thrombosis and hemorrhage; evidence of pulmonary and cerebral edema is detected as well.

Treatment

The treatment of patients with HACE includes the administration of high-flow oxygen, steroids, and immediate evacuation to lower altitudes. Dexamethasone, 8 mg given orally, intravenously, or intramuscularly, followed by 4 mg repeated at 6-hour intervals, is helpful and should be administered. If descent is not possible, supplemental oxygen, steroids (if available), and hyperbaric treatment may be lifesaving. The role of mannitol, hypertonic saline, and diuretics, if any, is unclear at present.

PREVENTION

- Patients with medical conditions in whom decreased ambient oxygen concentrations could be deleterious (chronic obstructive pulmonary disease, cyanotic congenital heart disease, congestive heart failure, pulmonary hypertension) should receive supplemental oxygen when traveling to areas of high altitude, if possible.
- The American Lung Association recommends that patients with arterial Po_2 less than 80 mm Hg, but with normal or low Pco_2 and normal minute ventilation, may travel by conventional air traffic without difficulty. However, those patients with Po_2 less than 60 mm Hg at sea level will need continuous supplemental oxygen in flight.
- In all patients, slow ascents to areas of high altitude may prevent or lessen the severity of symptoms.
- Vigorous or strenuous activity should be avoided during the first 24 to 48 hours of ascent, during which time acclimatization occurs.
- Patients with sickle cell disease are at substantially increased risk for a vasoocclusive crisis with ascent (this may occur at altitudes simulated by travel in pressurized commercial planes). Patients with sickle trait do not appear to be at risk. All patients with hemoglobin SC and sickle thalassemia require supplemental oxygen during air travel.
- The incidence and severity of AMS and HAPE have been shown to be decreased by the prophylactic administration of **acetazolamide**; doses of 125 mg twice daily started 1 full day before ascent and continued for 2 to 3 days are recommended. Patients with a previous history of AMS or HAPE should receive prophylactic treatment with acetazolamide, as should individuals required to ascend rapidly without adequate acclimatization.
- Patients allergic to sulfa may be given dexamethasone, 4 mg orally every 12 hours, starting 24 hours before ascent and continuing for 48 hours after ascent.
- The avoidance alcohol and overexertion is also recommended.
- **The most important preventive measure is gradual acclimatization with ascent.**

53

Radiation Injury

INTRODUCTION

The widespread use of radiation and radioactive materials in medicine, research, and industry, the transport of radioactive materials throughout all parts of the country, and the unfortunate looming threat of radioactive materials used in acts of terrorism (so-called "dirty bombs") mandate that every emergency department (ED) develops protocols for the treatment of victims of radiation injury. Emergency physicians should be familiar with recognition of exposure and treatment protocols. Telephone numbers for regional Department of Energy Assistance Offices by state are listed in Table 53-1.

There are two mechanisms of radiation injury that must be recognized and treated: actual **contamination** with radioactive, particulate matter, which may be external or internal, and **exposure** to particulate or electromagnetic radiation. This chapter discusses some of the physical aspects of radiation, the common nuclides involved, ED planning with respect to radiation injury, and the nature and initial treatment of radiation illness.

PHYSICAL PROPERTIES

Particulate Radiation

Particulate radiation includes alpha and beta particles, neutrons, protons, and positrons.

Alpha Particles

Alpha particles are composed of two protons and have an atomic mass of 4 and a +2 charge. The decay of certain heavy elements, such as uranium, radium, and plutonium, results in the emission of alpha particles, each with its own discrete energy. Alpha particles, because of their charge, have significant ionizing ability but virtually no penetrating ability; they are stopped by paper and keratin and cause injury by internal contamination only. Alpha particles cannot be measured by most radiation survey meters.

Beta Particles

Beta particles is composed of electrons, each carrying a −1 charge, and is often produced during the decay of lighter elements (such as tritium), usually resulting from the conversion of a neutron to a proton in the atom's nucleus. Beta rays have a continuous spectrum of energy from 0 to a maximum value characteristic of each beta emitter. Although beta radiation may travel several meters in the air, it penetrates only a few millimeters of skin tissue and is stopped by clothing.

Table 53-1	United States Department of Energy Regional Coordinating Offices for Radiologic Assistance[a]		
Region	**State**	**Regional Office**	**Address**	**Telephone**
1	Maine, New Hampshire, Vermont, New York, Massachusetts, Connecticut, Rhode Island, New Jersey, Pennsylvania, Maryland, Delaware	Brookhaven area office	Upton Long Island, New York 11973	516-344-2200
2	Virginia, West Virginia, Kentucky, Arkansas, Tennessee, Mississippi, Louisiana, Missouri, Puerto Rico, Virgin Islands	Oak Ridge operations office	P.O. Box E, Oak Ridge, Tennessee 37830	423-576-1005
3	North Carolina, South Carolina, Georgia, Alabama, Florida	Canal Zone Savannah River operations office	P.O. Box A, Aiken, South Carolina 29801	803-725-3333
4	Kansas, Oklahoma, Texas, New Mexico, Arizona	Albuquerque operations office	P.O. Box 5400, Albuquerque, New Mexico 87185	505-845-4667
5	Ohio, Indiana, Michigan, Illinois, Wisconsin, Iowa, Minnesota, Nebraska, South Dakota, North Dakota	Chicago operations office	9800 S. Cass Ave, Argonne, Illinois 60439	630-252-4800
6	Montana, Idaho, Wyoming, Utah, Colorado	Idaho operations office	785 DOE Place, Idaho Falls, Idaho 83402	208-526-1515
7	California, Nevada, Hawaii	San Francisco operations office	1301 Clay Street MS 700 North Oakland, California 94612	510-637-1794
8	Washington, Alaska	Richland operations office	P.O. Box 550, Richland, Washington 99352	509-373-3800

[a]The Radiation Emergency Assistance Center and Training Site (REAC/TS) at Oak Ridge, Tennessee, is a part of the Department of Energy and provides 24-h medical consultation assistance. Telephone: 423-576-313 (during the day); 24-h line: 423-481-1000.

Positrons

Positrons have the same mass and energy characteristics as the electron but have a charge of +1; they result from conversion of a proton to a neutron in the nucleus or by electron capture.

Neutrons

Neutrons, resulting from elements decaying by spontaneous fission, have a mass of 1 and are uncharged; free neutron particles are unstable and decay with a half-life of approximately 13 minutes into a proton, electron, and a neutrino. Neutron particles readily penetrate all human tissues and may cause widespread ionization by collision or neutron capture. Protons produced within tissues by neutron radiation are potent ionizers.

Protons

Protons are the same as hydrogen nuclei, having a mass of 1 and a charge of +1.

Electromagnetic Radiation

Electromagnetic radiation is composed of *gamma* and *x-rays*. Gamma radiation originates from the decay of unstable atomic nuclei, often accompanies the emission of alpha and beta particles, and has discrete energy levels related to the nuclide from which it is emitted. Gamma rays easily penetrate tissues and are detected by Geiger-Müller counters. X-rays originate outside the atomic nucleus and have a penetrating power related to the energy of the particular photon from which they are emitted. X-ray machines produce x-rays by applying a high positive voltage between the source of electrons and a collecting terminal in a vacuum tube. The electrons produced strike a target, such as tungsten, and their energy is converted into x-ray photons. X-rays and gamma radiation produce ionization in tissues by a variety of indirect mechanisms that involve the ejection of a high-speed electron.

DOSE UNITS

The curie (Ci) is the basic unit used to describe the quantity of radioactivity in a sample of material. One curie equals 3.7×10^{10} disintegrations per second (dps), the approximate rate of decay of 1 g of radium. The roentgen is the unit of exposure related to the amount of ionization caused in air by gamma or x-radiation. The rad is the unit of measure of *r*adiation *a*bsorbed *d*ose and represents the actual amount of radiation energy deposited in any material; 1 rad equals 0.01 J/kg in any medium. The rem (*r*oentgen-*e*quivalent-*m*an) is equal to the absorbed dose (rad) multiplied by a specific quality factor (QF) derived for each source of radiation. The QF is based on the linear energy transfer of the radiation—the rate at which charged particles transfer energy to the medium. Generally, the higher the linear energy transfer, the greater the tissue injury for a given absorbed dose. The QF for electrons, positrons, and x-rays equals 1. Although the QF for alpha particles and neutrons is currently under discussion, the International Committee on Radiation Protection recommends the use of a QF of 10 to 20 for these particles.

The International Committee on Radiation Units and Measurements recommends that the aforementioned units, which continue to be used, be replaced with the International System of Units. These are as follows and are being increasingly used.

- 1 Becquerel (Bq) = 1 dps = 2.703×10^{-11} Ci
- 1 Gray (Gy) = 100 rad = 1 J/kg; 1 rad = 1 cGy
- 1 Sieverty (Sv) = 100 rem = 1 J/kg × QF; 1 rem = 1 cSv
- Roentgen is to be expressed as coulomb/kg (C/kg).

RADIATION SOURCES

Ambient sources of radiation include cosmic rays and naturally occurring nuclides (65–235 mrem/y); medical diagnostic and therapeutic radiation (77 mrem/y); medical radiopharmaceuticals (4 mrem/y); nuclear power reactors and weapons testing (4 mrem/y); and miscellaneous industrial, research, and consumer sources (4 mrem/y). An airplane trip from Boston to London will expose a traveler to 5 mrem, whereas a chest x-ray gives a skin dose of approximately 20 to 30 mrem. Generally, the yearly amount of radiation to which a person is exposed depends on occupation, geographic location, and the number of diagnostic medical or other tests using radioactive materials to which he or she is exposed.

MECHANISM OF INJURY

Ionizing radiation reacts with molecules in two ways:
- **Ionization,** in which an orbital electron is ejected from the molecule resulting in the formation of an ion pair
- **Excitation,** in which an orbital electron is raised to a higher energy level
- In both cases, reactive free radicals are produced that may then react with biologically important molecules. These reactions have been shown to involve proteins, enzymes, nucleic acids, lipids, and carbohydrates. Cytopathologically, such reactions may result in cell death, temporary cellular injury, or genetic mutation.

SPECIFIC RADIONUCLIDES

Familiarity with the more common radionuclides used in medicine, research, and industry is useful when developing treatment protocols. Efforts should be made to determine which, if any, nuclides are being used in the hospital and local area; this information should be included with the radiation treatment protocol. Medical centers may use ^{131}I, ^{99m}Tc, ^{67}Ga, ^{32}P, ^{133}Xe, ^{201}Tl, and ^{60}Co. Laboratories may use ^{3}H, ^{14}C, ^{125}I, ^{60}Co, and ^{238}U. Industrial processes may use ^{60}Co, ^{137}Cs, ^{192}Ir, and enriched or depleted uranium. Nuclear power facilities produce ^{3}H, ^{131}I, ^{137}Cs, ^{60}Co, ^{90}Sr, ^{144}Ce, ^{239}Pu, and numerous other radionuclides.

Radium

Radium is a metabolic analog of calcium and after exposure becomes deposited in bone. It is a source of alpha, beta, and gamma radiation with a physical half-life of 1,622 years. Inhalation or ingestion is associated with an increased incidence of bone sarcoma and carcinomas of the head and neck. Radium, a disintegration product of uranium, is used in medicine, industry, and research.

Strontium

Strontium-90 is a metabolic analog of calcium and is deposited in bone. Strontium is a beta emitter with a half-life of 28 years. It is abundant in the fission products of nuclear weapons and power plants. It is readily absorbed and produces an increased incidence of bone and bone-related sarcomas. Long-term ingestion is associated with a high incidence of myeloproliferative disease and overt leukemia.

Iodine

Iodine-131 is absorbed rapidly and is nonuniformly deposited in thyroid tissue. It is a low-energy beta and gamma emitter with a half-life of approximately 8 days.

It is widely used in medicine and found in nuclear weapons and power plants. An increased risk of thyroid carcinoma is associated with exposure to [131]I. [125]I has a half-life of 60 days and otherwise has similar properties to [131]I.

Cesium

Cesium-137 is a metabolic analog of potassium that is rapidly absorbed and distributed throughout all tissues of the body. It is an energetic beta and gamma emitter with a half-life of 30 years. Symptoms of acute toxicity are similar to those of whole-body radiation exposure; death is caused by bone marrow failure. Chronic low-level contamination may be associated with a variety of neoplasia; ^{137}Cs is an abundant product of nuclear detonation and power plants, is present in nuclear fallout, and is used in certain industrial applications.

Cerium

Cerium-144 is an abundant nuclide found in association with the processing of uranium, nuclear reactors, and nuclear weapons. It is an energetic beta emitter with a half-life of 285 days. It is poorly absorbed from the gastrointestinal tract. Most toxicity is caused by inhalation. The effective half-life of cerium in the lung is measured in days to weeks, and most of the element is translocated to the liver (47%) and the skeleton (37%). Both moderate- and high-level exposure may be fatal because of radiation pneumonitis, hepatic necrosis, and ultimately bone marrow aplasia. Lower level exposure may be associated with the development of bone and liver neoplasia and leukemia.

Uranium

Uranium, including [238]U, [235]U, and [234]U, is abundant and is used in nuclear power plants, nuclear weapons, and research. It is an energetic alpha and gamma emitter with a half-life between 2.5 million and 4.5 billion years, depending on the specific isotope involved. In addition to systemic damage associated with radiation toxicity, soluble forms are also thought to be directly nephrotoxic. Insoluble inhaled forms have been shown to cause severe pulmonary fibrosis, metaplasia, and neoplasia in animals.

Plutonium

Plutonium-239 and its 15 known isotopes occur naturally in small amounts but are usually produced from neutron bombardment of uranium. It is an extremely energetic alpha emitter with a half-life up to 82 million years. Plutonium is used as nuclear fuel, in weapons and breeder reactors, and for the generation of electric power in space. When inhaled, soluble forms are translocated and tenaciously retained in the liver and the skeleton. Animal studies have shown that death is caused by pulmonary and hepatic injury and a variety of cancers.

Radon

Radon is a gaseous product of the disintegration of radium and thus uranium; this is of particular concern to uranium miners and persons exposed to uranium mine tailings. It is a potent alpha emitter, with slight gamma radiation, and has a half-life of 3.8 days. Radon and its disintegration products are inhaled and have been associated with an increased incidence of small cell carcinoma of the lung.

Tritium

Tritium or ^{3}H is formed in large quantities in nuclear fusion and fission power plants and is present in their effluent. It is also found in nuclear weapons and the reaction of cosmic rays with atmospheric gases. Tritium is a beta emitter with an approximate half-life of 12 years. As tritiated water, it is readily absorbed into the bloodstream from skin, pulmonary, or gastrointestinal tract contamination and is then widely distributed in total body water; radiation effects are thus similar to those of whole-body irradiation. It is, however, a minimal health hazard.

Iridium

Iridium-192 is a member of the platinum family of metals. It is a potent gamma emitter with a half-life of 74 days and is widely used in industrial radiography.

Cobalt

Cobalt-60 is distributed throughout the body when internalized; it has widespread use in industrial radiography, medical therapy, and metallurgy and is present in nuclear power plant coolants. It is a potent gamma emitter with a half-life of approximately 5 years.

Technetium

Technetium-99 is a metallic element that has 14 isotopes; ^{99m}Tc has widespread medical uses and is a gamma emitter with a half-life of 6 hours. ^{95m}Tc is used in the laboratory and industry and has a half-life of 60 days.

Phosphorus

Phosphorus-32 is used by the medical community as a sealed source for intracavitary radiation therapy and for treatment of polycythemia vera. It is a high-energy beta emitter with a half-life of 14 days.

Polonium

Polonium-210, commonly used in devices that eliminate static charges and dust in textile mills and photographic plates, emits alpha particles with a half-life of approximately 50 days. It came into public awareness in 2006 when it was implicated in the assassination of a former Russian spy.

ACUTE EXTERNAL RADIATION ILLNESS

The effect of external radiation is modified by several factors. The amount of radiation received over a given period of time is called the dose rate, usually measured in mrem/y for low-level exposure and rad/h or rem/h for high-level exposures. In general, the lower the dose rate at which exposure occurs, the less likely the injury will result. For example, a total body dose of 600 rad occurring over a few hours is likely to be fatal, whereas the same dose spread over several months is not expected to be. The effect of radiation exposure is also somewhat dependent on age; a dose of 100 rad, for example, received by a fetus or embryo may cause a number of developmental abnormalities. The distance from the source of radiation also affects the dose received. The dose decreases as a function of the square of the distance. Finally, the presence of shielding may decrease the amount of radiation received, depending of course on the type of radiation involved and the specific shielding used.

The late effects of external radiation are significant and include an increased incidence of certain cancers, genetic mutation, and gross chromosomal aberrations. Radiation exposure has been linked to increased risks for the development of leukemia and thyroid, lung, and breast cancers. The minimum dose and dose rate of radiation required to produce these effects are not clear; however, many scientists believe that any increase in ambient radiation results in an increased rate of carcinogenesis, whereas others argue that a "threshold" dose and dose rate must be exceeded before the rate of carcinogenesis is enhanced. Much more uncertain is the cumulative genetic impact of radiation exposure because clearly such mutations become hidden within the genetic material of families, are variably and unpredictably manifest, and are difficult to measure. In experimental animals, the most frequent aberration resulting from radiation exposure is reciprocal translocation, which results in embryonic death or physical and mental abnormalities in the live-born. Other chromosomal lesions seen are inversion, rings, dicentrics, and tricentrics with fragments.

Acute External Whole-Body Exposure

Acute external whole-body exposure may produce four frequently overlapping syndromes of radiation illness. Whole-body exposure of less than 75 rad is generally not associated with any symptoms.

- Patients exposed to doses between 75 and 240 rad have **prodromal syndrome** characterized by a constellation of symptoms including anorexia, nausea, vomiting, diarrhea, apathy, tachycardia, fever, and headache. The pathogenesis is unclear.
- The **hematopoietic syndrome** may result after exposure to between 50 and 1,000 rad. These patients typically have lymphopenia within 48 hours, and a lymphocyte count less than $300/\mu L$ at this time is indicative of a poor prognosis. Lymphocyte counts greater than $1,200/\mu L$ at 48 hours are associated with a good chance of survival with proper medical treatment. In most patients, neutropenia and thrombocytopenia become evident 15 to 30 days after exposure; the return of counts into the normal range may be quite slow and counts may, in some patients, be decreased for months to years.
- The **gastrointestinal syndrome** occurs after exposure to 400 to 5,000 rad, reaches a peak symptomatically at 3 to 5 days, and is associated with severe vomiting, diarrhea, fluid and electrolyte loss and imbalance, and shock. Pathophysiologically, death of radiosensitive crypt cells in the gut is noted, leading to ulceration and hemorrhage within the bowel. The gastrointestinal epithelium may regenerate within 2 weeks if the patient can be supported during this period.
- The **cerebral syndrome** is caused by exposure to doses greater than 5,000 rad. This syndrome is associated with the rapid onset of vomiting and drowsiness, followed by tremors, ataxia, convulsions, and death within 24 to 72 hours. The syndrome is caused by widespread vasculitis, meningoencephalitis, and cerebral edema.
- As previously noted, the various syndromes widely overlap. In addition, the presence of other trauma, for a variety of reasons, dramatically increases morbidity and mortality. Without medical treatment, it has been calculated that the median lethal dose (LD_{50}) for humans is approximately 450 rad of whole-body radiation. Acute exposures greater than 1,000 rad are lethal despite treatment.

Acute External Partial-Body Exposure

Acute external partial-body exposure, although dependent on the amount and type of tissue exposed, is less likely to result in an acute radiation illness syndrome. Such exposures, however, account for the majority of radiation injuries.

- Radiation burns to the **skin** are usually the result of direct contact or exposure to a high-dose radiation source. Patients may report localized burning pain, usually without erythema, or they may be asymptomatic. Importantly, when patients are seen early, physical findings may be deceptively minor because radiation burns may take 2 weeks or longer to fully develop. At doses up to 500 rad, the skin typically becomes erythematous and brawny, followed by dry desquamation, vesiculation, loss of hair (which may not regrow), and persistent dryness. Higher doses may produce ulceration, gangrene, and full-thickness destruction of the skin caused by damage to the underlying vasculature. After initial healing, skin damaged by irradiation continues to exhibit poor healing even after otherwise minor trauma.

• Exposure of the **testes** to doses greater than 10 rad will cause a dose-related depression of spermatogenesis manifested 45 to 60 days after exposure. Doses greater than 500 rad are associated with permanent sterility. Exposures to lower doses are usually associated with gradual recovery of testicular function. In women, this dose causes destruction of oocytes and the germinal epithelium.

• Radiation exposure to the **eye** may result in cataracts, the formation of which appears to be dose related. A latency period of 5 years after exposure is often reported. Cataracts in humans have been observed with doses of 200 rem of x-ray or gamma radiation and with 20 rem of neutron exposure.

INTERNAL RADIATION EXPOSURE

Internal radiation exposure may occur if radioactive material is ingested, inhaled, or deposited in or on open wounds.

• **Ingestion** of contaminated food or water and the absorption of inhaled nuclides are common mechanisms resulting in internal exposure. In these patients, the radiation dose received is a function of the "effective retention time," which is a combination of the physical and biologic half-lives of the specific nuclide. Toxic effects of internal exposure may be related to systemic absorption of the nuclide, local irradiation of the gastrointestinal tract or lung, or both. Importantly, however, the actual amount of radionuclide absorbed is variable and depends on the specific nuclide ingested and the physical and chemical form of the nuclide.

• **Inhalation** of radioactive material is an important route of internal radiation. Clearance from the lung of such nuclides is a complex function of systemic absorption and ciliary, macrophage, and lymphatic clearance rates. Currently, nuclides are classified into three groups depending on their overall clearance rates from the lung.

  • **Class D**: Maximal clearance occurs in less than 24 hours and is seen with cesium chloride, for example.

  • **Class W**: Moderate clearance rates from a few days to less than 6 months; calcium sulfate and cerium carbonate are examples.

  • **Class Y**: Poor clearance rates with retention from more than 6 months to years, which is typical of cerium, uranium, and plutonium oxides.

• Radioactive contamination of **open wounds** can cause local injury and, if significant absorption occurs, systemic toxicity as well.

DIAGNOSIS

An estimation of the potential severity of radiation exposure may be determined if the following are known:

• Time and duration of exposure
• Radiation type and source
• Mechanism of contamination
• Dose readings at the site of exposure

In most patients, this specific information will be unknown, incomplete, or inaccurate; however, the likelihood of systemic illness can be estimated based on the interval between exposure and the onset of any prodromal symptoms, the lymphocyte count at 48 hours, and lymphocyte karyotyping.

The following are some guidelines to estimate the amount of radiation exposure and prognosis:

- Symptoms developing less than 2 hours after exposure suggest that a dose greater than 400 rem was received, whereas a symptom-free interval of more than 2 hours is seen in patients receiving less than 200 rem.
- Onset of symptoms after 6 hours correlates with a dose less than 50 rem.
- Lymphocyte counts at 48 hours, as previously stated, can be helpful in that normal counts are observed in patients with whole-body exposures of less than 25 rad.
- A mild decrease in the lymphocyte count occurs in whole-body doses between 50 and 125 rad.
- A 50% decrease in the lymphocyte count occurs at doses of 125 to 200 rad.
- A 75% decrease or greater in the lymphocyte count is seen in patients exposed to doses exceeding 240 rad and correlates with at least 50% mortality if not aggressively treated.
- In general, lymphocyte counts at 48 hours of more than 1,200/mL are indicative of a good prognosis.
- Lymphocyte counts between 300 and 1,200/mL indicate a guarded prognosis.
- Lymphocyte counts of less than 300/mL are associated with a poor prognosis.
- Additionally, lymphocyte karyotyping provides another measure to estimate the amount of radiation received, because the number of abnormal chromosomal forms (e.g., rings, dicentrics) increases in a nearly linear relationship to the dose of radiation received more than 15 rem.

TREATMENT PLANNING

Although all nuclear power–generating plants must have identified medical treatment referral facilities, every ED should develop a protocol for the treatment of radiation accident victims. The current widespread transportation and use of nuclides and radiation in industry, research, and medicine mandate such a posture.

Patients who are not contaminated but who have received whole-body or partial-body exposure to gamma or x-radiation are not radioactive and may be treated in the usual manner in the ED. Conversely, accident victims who are known or suspected to be contaminated or who have been exposed to neutron particle beams, which may induce radioactivity, must be treated in a special manner as outlined on pages 495 to 498.

Contaminated patients should be treated utilizing the following techniques:

- Patients should be treated in specifically designated areas away from other patient treatment areas.
- A separate securable entrance to this area should be identified in the radiation plan and used.
- The floors of the entry, passages, and treatment areas should be covered with plastic sheeting or heavy paper, secured by tape to the floor, during the treatment of accident victims.
- Areas through which contaminated patients will pass and the treatment room should be cordoned off and appropriate cautionary signs affixed.

- A "buffer" zone or area between the contaminated treatment area and clean areas is highly recommended to ensure that contaminated materials do not leave the treatment area before decontamination.
- This area is ideally staffed with a nurse or aide who will obtain and transfer any needed supplies to the treatment personnel.
- The ventilation system in the designated treatment area should be able to be turned off. Contamination of the hospital through the ventilation system, although unlikely, is thereby prevented.
- In the absence of a separate radiation treatment area, the autopsy suite frequently provides an adequate treatment area because stainless steel drainage tables, a separate shower facility, an independent ventilation system, and a mechanism for collecting effluent are usually present.
- Properly labeled bags and receptacles for the collection of contaminated materials, including liquids, must be available.
- Surgical scrub suits, caps, eye protection, masks, water-repellent gowns, gloves, and foot covers should be readily available for use by treatment personnel.
- During the treatment of any patients, all nonessential equipment should be removed from the treatment area.
- Electrical and nondisposable equipment to be used during treatment should be covered with clear disposable plastic bags to minimize contamination.
- Because patients and personnel will be frequently checked with radiation survey meters for contamination, the location of the nearest meter should be noted in the treatment protocol.
- If a situation in the community increases the likelihood of significant alpha-particle contamination, then the protocol should state the location of the nearest alpha-particle survey meter because the common Geiger-Müller counter will not detect alpha contamination. Members of the treatment team should be familiar with the operation and calibration of these counters.
- In addition, personal dosimeters and film badges must be available for all members of the treatment team.
- Treatment team personnel should not include pregnant women.
- Other persons may accumulate up to 100 rem in a single isolated event rendering lifesaving treatment.
- In less urgent situations, the National Council on Radiation Protection and Measurements emergency dose limit is 25 rem; however, in general, treatment team personnel should be rotated after exposure to doses between 100 and 125 milliroentgen (mR).
- Health physicists for consultation and appropriate referral facilities should be identified and clearly noted in the protocol. Regional Department of Energy Assistance Offices are noted in Table 53-1 and may provide useful information.

TREATMENT

On notification that the ED will be receiving casualties from an accident involving radiation, the radiation treatment area should be prepared to receive the patient or patients. Assistance regarding treatment may be obtained from the Department of Energy, and these offices are noted by state in Table 53-1. Treatment protocols should include the following:

- The nature of the accident, types of radiation or radionuclides involved, and all measures to treat the patient at the scene and en route should be carefully documented.

- On arrival, if the patient is critically injured and requires emergent measures, treatment should proceed in the usual manner, followed by decontamination.
  - If possible, before entering the department, the patient should be placed on clean linen and a clean stretcher.
- The treatment team should wear full surgical attire, including cap, mask, eye protection, scrub suit, gown, and gloves.
  - All seams and the cuffs of the suit and gown should be sealed with tape and the shoe covers tucked inside the pants and similarly taped.
  - A second pair of gloves is always worn over the first taped pair; these should be removed whenever contamination occurs.
  - In addition, a second gown may be worn over the first and similarly removed.
- Persons using liquid for decontamination should also wear waterproof coveralls or aprons.
- Dosimeters should be worn at the neck and over the gown at the chest or hip.
- With respect to specific treatment, patients may be divided into those uncontaminated but irradiated, those externally contaminated, and those internally contaminated.

Irradiated

Patients exposed to significant doses of whole-body, penetrating radiation have signs and symptoms referred to as the **acute radiation syndrome**, with a severity and a postexposure interval depending on the total dose received, the mechanism of exposure, and the time interval of exposure. Most whole-body exposures resulting in the syndrome occur over a brief (<24 hours) period of time and exceed 1 to 2 Gy or 100 to 200 rad. Prodromal symptoms occur within 48 hours at this dose, within several hours at doses exceeding 6 Gy or 600 rad, and within several minutes at doses more than 30 Gy or 3,000 rad. Prodromal symptoms include nausea and vomiting, diaphoresis, fever, fatigue, myalgias, and headache. Diarrhea is associated with higher doses. After the prodrome, a latent period occurs, typically lasting between 1 and 3 weeks in lower dose exposures (2 Gy or 200 rad), several days in exposures involving more than 6 Gy or 600 rad, and a few hours in doses greater than 15 Gy. No latent period is seen in exposures exceeding 30 Gy. After the latent period, if any, injury to tissues and end organs becomes apparent: hematopoietic sensitivity to injury is greatest and occurs first, followed by GI (>600 rad) and cardiovascular and neurologic (>2,000–2,500 rad) involvement. Lower dose exposures are anticipated to produce hematologic toxicity with pancytopenia, followed by infectious or bleeding complications. Toxicity to the gastrointestinal system occurs in exposures greater than 6 Gy and is manifest as GI bleeding, electrolyte abnormalities, and enterocolitis, followed by generalized cardiovascular and CNS dysfunction at doses more than 20 to 25 Gy.

After acute exposure, the irradiated patient must be carefully assessed. History from the patient, co-workers, and others should be detailed and dosimeters (if any) obtained for processing. Metallic articles such as coins and belt buckles should be analyzed for induced activity if neutron radiation was involved or suspected.

Baseline blood work should be performed and a sample of blood retained for cell and HLA typing and for measurement of ^{24}Na if neutron radiation exposure is suspected. A health physicist should be consulted and a preliminary absorbed dose estimated. If whole-body exposure is more than 1 Gy or 100 to 200 rad, the patient should be transferred to a hospital equipped to treat the sequelae of severe radiation injury (e.g., bone marrow transplant). If the absorbed dose is less than 100 rad, close outpatient follow-up is usual, although consultation from an expert in radiation exposure is advised to guide individual therapy.

Externally Contaminated

If the patient is externally contaminated or suspected of being contaminated, all articles of clothing should be removed and separately placed in plastic bags and labeled. The patient is then wrapped in clean blankets and transferred to the treatment area on a clean litter. The ambulance equipment and personnel should remain with the vehicle until surveyed and decontaminated if necessary. Before the patient's arrival in the treatment area, a background count should be obtained and recorded with the survey meter.

When the patient arrives in the treatment area, a careful survey is made over all body surfaces for contamination. If survey equipment is not available, then routine decontamination should proceed; when available, the survey meter's probe should be covered with plastic wrap to avoid contamination and slowly moved to 3 to 5 cm above the skin surfaces. The survey meter's readings should carefully be noted on an anatomic chart. Devices with audible clicking and alarms should be avoided if possible. Before decontamination, specimens should be obtained with saline swabs from both ears, both external nares, the mouth, and all wounds. Skin surface wipes measuring an area of 10 cm × 10 cm should be taken from all contaminated skin surfaces using filter paper or a 4 × 4. All samples should be placed in separate containers and carefully labeled. Urine samples should be obtained as soon as practical. Blood samples should be obtained for routine admission studies and type and cross-matching. Venipuncture sites should be chosen in an uncontaminated area and covered or deferred until decontamination has been performed, if possible. If roentgenogram studies are needed before decontamination, the x-ray cassettes should be wrapped in plastic bags to avoid contamination.

Decontamination proceeds from open wounds first. All visible fragments and debris are first carefully removed with forceps and placed in suitable containers. If the debris is radioactive, it should be stored in lead containers or in a remote area away from personnel. Wounds are then copiously irrigated with normal saline until resurvey shows the area to be free of contamination or at a steady-state level. Once decontaminated, wounds should be covered with a waterproof material such as surgical plastic adherent skin drapes (Steri-Drape, Op-Site). Decontamination then proceeds from the highest to the lowest areas of contamination. Skin areas can be decontaminated with lukewarm water and disposable surgical sponges, resurveying every 3 minutes until background or stable counts are obtained. It is important to avoid abrading the skin or causing erythema. The face and hair are cleansed with particular care taken so that the solution does not enter the mouth, nose, ears, or eyes and become internalized. The hair may be clipped if washing is insufficient. Showers should be avoided unless cutaneous contamination is widespread.

The patient, when free of external contamination, is then dried; clean flooring should be placed along the exit path and a clean stretcher or wheelchair brought into the room by attendants not involved in the decontamination process. The patient is then taken to the ED for further care.

All equipment must be surveyed for contamination before being removed from the treatment area. Personnel exiting the treatment area must remove their caps, gowns, shoe covers, masks, and gloves and be carefully surveyed for contamination before leaving the area. Dosimeters are collected and labeled as to name and location, and liquid and solid wastes are disposed of specifically as the health physicist or radiation safety officer directs.

Internally Contaminated

If internal contamination is suspected or has occurred, treatment must be initiated as early as possible. Internal contamination may occur as a result of ingestion, inhalation, or absorption of material via mucous membranes, wounds, or abrasions. Treatment is generally aimed at preventing uptake and absorption or enhancing the excretion of the nuclide and is facilitated if the specific radionuclide is known. When unknown, assistance in identification may be obtained from sources noted at the end of the chapter. Nuclides likely to be responsible for internal contamination should be determined, if possible, from the site of the accident or nature of the work. For ingestions, gut decontamination should be attempted; emesis, lavage, and cathartics have been used with success. Common radionuclides associated with internal contamination are products of iodine-131, cesium-137, plutonium-239, and hydrogen-3. Although previously not described as such, polonium-210 was found to be responsible for the death of a Russian spy in a presumed assassination in 2006.

Patients exposed to **radioactive iodine (I-131)**, either via inhalation or ingestion, should receive potassium iodide (KI), 390 mg, daily for 7 to 14 days. Blockage of I-131 uptake by the thyroid is the goal of therapy. Treatment is optimal if given within 1 hour of exposure, with little benefit seen after 12 hours. In these patients, treatment with propylthiouracil or methimazole should be considered. A clue to I-131 exposure, in the absence of specific identification, is early urinary excretion and enhanced activity over the patient's thyroid.

Patients with internal contamination caused by the transuranic elements such as **Plutonium-239**, which result in alpha radiation, may be treated with chelating agents (calcium or zinc diethylenetriamine pentaacetic acid [Ca-DTPA and Zn-DTPA]); Ca-DTPA is typically used in the first few (1–2) days of treatment, and both agents are most effective if given within 2 hours of exposure. Zn-DTPA is used in pregnant patients. In inhalation injuries, aerosolization of the chelating agent has been used successfully.

Exposure to **cesium-137** is typically treated with ferric ferrocyanide, 1 g orally, in 100 to 200 mL water three times per day for several days. In addition, isotopic dilution or displacement therapy may decrease the concentration of the radionuclide and thereby reduce the effective half-life. Water diuresis is helpful for hydrogen-3 or ^{99m}Tc, and calcium is a competitor of strontium at uptake sites. Gaviscon, ten tablets or 40 mL orally every 2 hours, may be given as mobilizing agents for certain radionuclides, such as strontium and cesium.

Hydrogen-3 exposure is treated via water dilution and enhanced excretion. Urine, vomitus, and feces should be retained for radioassay.

Polonium-210 emits alpha particles and may therefore benefit from treatment with chelating agents such as dimercaprol.

Whole-body gamma cameras can localize and measure most types of internal contamination and may be useful in this regard. After decontamination, initial assessment, and treatment for internal contamination, patients should be referred to appropriate facilities for definitive care. Such facilities must have sophisticated capabilities in hematology (bone marrow transplants), infectious disease, and plastic and general surgery.

54 Smoke Inhalation

GENERAL PRINCIPLES

Inhalation of smoke represents exposure to a complex mixture of toxic gases and suspended particulate matter. Although the major cause of death in patients with smoke inhalation is cerebral hypoxia related to carbon monoxide exposure, a number of other toxic substances formed during combustion may produce significant pulmonary, cutaneous, and conjunctival injury. These substances include ammonia, hydrochloric acid, sulfur dioxide, hydrogen cyanide, and nitrous dioxide. In addition, when contact is made with lung or skin water, several substances form extremely toxic, corrosive alkalies or acids. These include ammonium hydroxide and nitric, sulfurous, and sulfuric acids. Phosgene, an extremely toxic gas, may be liberated when carbon tetrachloride—containing fire extinguishers are used to treat fires involving chlorinated hydrocarbons.

Clinically, carbon monoxide exposure must always be considered in any patient exposed to excessive smoke because this represents a potentially treatable disorder that if unrecognized may produce serious neurologic sequelae or death.

Clinical Presentation

Patients suffering smoke inhalation may present to the emergency department in a variety of ways. It is important to note that many patients in whom severe pulmonary injury will develop over the next 12 to 24 hours may initially have normal laboratory and radiologic studies and may be completely asymptomatic; therefore, a very conservative approach to therapy is warranted.

Patients' symptoms include:
- Sore throat, hoarseness, dyspnea, cough, and substernal discomfort typically accentuated by inspiration
- Headache, dizziness, nausea, and vomiting
    Physical signs include:
- Tachycardia, tachypnea, stridor, and retractions
- The skin color may be normal, cyanotic, or "cherry red" (when carbon monoxide exposure has occurred concurrently).

The possibility of serious pulmonary or inhalation injury is strongly suggested by the following:
- A history of containment in a closed space
- Situations associated with a reduced level of consciousness (associated with drug or alcohol abuse, seizure, head injury)
- Full-thickness facial, perioral, or perinasal burns
- Hoarseness, singeing of nasal hair, and burns of the oral mucosa
- Carbonaceous sputum
- When wheezing is noted initially, a serious and evolving respiratory injury should be suspected.

Laboratory Tests

Arterial blood gases, a carboxyhemoglobin (COHb) level, and a chest x-ray should be obtained initially and will serve as baseline studies. Importantly, even in patients with evolving severe pulmonary injury, these studies may initially be normal and cannot be relied on to exclude or make less likely the diagnosis of inhalation injury.

Criteria for Admission

The initial criteria for admission therefore are clinical in most patients:
- Patients likely to have had a respiratory injury based on the history
- Patients with a history of loss of consciousness or seizure, amnesia, or other abnormalities of mental status that are otherwise unexplained
- Patients with significant CO intoxication

Treatment

Treatment should begin based on the patient's history.
- The administration of humidified, cooled 100% oxygen by a nonrebreathing mask is recommended in all patients.
- Bronchodilators are useful if evidence of bronchospasm is present.
- The patient should be encouraged to cough frequently and breath deeply, as secretions can be copious, and frequent suctioning may be necessary.
- A specimen of sputum should be sent for routine culture and sensitivity.
- Antibiotics are not administered prophylactically, and the role of steroids in this setting has not clearly been defined.
- Indications for intubation include
  - A reduced or falling Po_2 despite maximal supplemental oxygen
  - Hypercarbia due to respiratory or CNS depression
  - Full-thickness burns of the face or perioral area
  - Acute respiratory distress or air hunger
  - Pulmonary secretions not effectively cleared with suction
  - Evidence of rapidly increasing upper airway obstruction (progressive hoarseness or direct visualization of supraglottic edema via bronchoscopy)

CARBON MONOXIDE EXPOSURE

Carbon monoxide is a colorless and odorless gas released when virtually any carbonaceous material is incompletely combusted. Automobile and other similar engines typically produce an exhaust with approximately 5% carbon monoxide; other important sources include exhaust from flame-type heating units (excluding natural gas) and charcoal fires (Table 54-1).

Carbon monoxide binds preferentially and with great affinity to the hemoglobin molecule, thereby limiting its oxygen-binding capacity. The need and urgency of treatment are determined by the patient's clinical evaluation; COHb concentrations, although used in the past to guide therapy, can be misleading in a large percent of patients and are not reliably predictive of subsequent, long-term morbidity or mortality. Nonetheless, certain symptoms may be seen in relation to general COHb levels and are briefly reviewed here:
- Patients with less than 10% COHb typically have no symptoms or signs.
- Patients with levels of 10% to 20% produce mild headache and irritability.
- Patients with levels between 20% and 40% develop light-headedness, confusion, dizziness, agitation, nausea, vomiting, and dyscoordination.

TABLE 54-1	Effects of Carbon Monoxide Exposure

Concentration of CO in Air (ppm)	Approximate Inhalation Time and Symptoms Developed
50	This is the maximum allowable concentration for continuous exposure for healthy adults in any 8-h period.
200	After 2–3 h, slight headache, dizziness, nausea
400	After 1–2 h, frontal headaches
	After 3 h, life-threatening CO levels develop.
800	After 45 min, dizziness, nausea, and convulsions
	After 2 h, unconsciousness
	After 2–3 h, death
1,600	Within 20 min, headaches, dizziness, and nausea
	Within 1 h, death
3,200	Within 5–10 min, headache, dizziness, and nausea
	Within 25–30 min, death
6,400	Within 1–2 min, headaches, dizziness, and nausea
	Within 10–15 min, death
12,800	Within 1–3 min, death

- Patients with concentrations of 40% to 60% are associated with syncope, dyspnea, lethargy, and coma.
- Patients with concentrations that exceed 60% may develop respiratory and cardiac arrest.

Diagnosis

The diagnosis of carbon monoxide exposure should be made on the basis of history and, if present, the characteristic cherry red color of the optic fundus, skin, mucous membranes, and fingernails. COHb levels should be obtained in order to confirm CO exposure. One must remember that the determination of oxygen saturation by pulse oximetry, in the setting of CO exposure, routinely overestimates the percent of oxygen saturation; this is because this methodology fails to differentiate COHb and oxyhemoglobin. Co-oximetry is required to obtain accurate levels of oxygen saturation. Non-invasive co-oximetry units with CO detection capability similar to oxygen pulse oximeters are now widely available.

Treatment

Treatment decisions are based on the patient's history and clinical presentation:
- Patients with mild symptoms (headache, fatigue, dizziness, nausea, and weakness) require treatment with continuous, 100%, high-flow oxygen via a nonrebreather mask and a period of observation in the emergency department; 100% oxygen therapy alone reduces the half-life of CO in the blood from 320 to 60 minutes. In patients with mild toxicity, symptoms will usually gradually subside over 3 to 4 hours and patients can be safely discharged. Patients should be instructed to return

if symptoms recur and have a repeat evaluation in 24 to 48 hours. If mild symptoms persist despite treatment, an additional 4-hour period of 100% oxygen therapy is advised; patients with worsening symptoms should be considered candidates for hyperbaric oxygen (HBO) treatment.

- Patients presenting with signs of significant CO toxicity (including loss of consciousness, syncope, reduced levels of consciousness, confusion, focal neurologic abnormalities, cardiac ischemia, and persisting acidosis) should be considered candidates for HBO treatment. In terms of HBO treatment, the half-life of COHb, which is approximately 60 minutes while breathing 100% oxygen, falls to 23 minutes by exposure to HBO (chambers typically exert 2.8 atm of pressure, with a typical treatment lasting 90 minutes). In addition, the threshold for initiating treatment with HBO should be reduced in elderly patients, particularly those with significant comorbidities. There is also some evidence that exposures associated with loss of consciousness (or syncope) are more often associated with the development of late neurologic and/or psychiatric abnormalities and that treatment with HBO may reduce the severity of these conditions; further studies are needed to clarify the exact indications and benefits related to HBO treatment in this setting. The relative lack of HBO treatment facilities (and thus often long transport times); the inherent difficulty in treating seriously ill, intubated patients in HBO chambers; and the time-sensitive nature of HBO therapy further complicate treatment; HBO is most effective if initiated within 6 to 8 hours of exposure.

The closest HBO chamber may be determined by calling the Divers Alert Network (DAN), at Duke University, Durham, North Carolina, at 919-684-4326. High-flow oxygen (100%) and continuous observation/monitoring are appropriate interval measures.

Patients with possible coexposure to other irritant gases, the symptoms of which are often delayed in onset, require more aggressive management, including expectant observation for developing pulmonary distress.

Lastly, in **pregnant patients**, it is important to remember that fetal hemoglobin has a much higher affinity for CO than adult hemoglobin; this means that potentially serious fetal hypoxia can persist long after maternal serum COHb levels have normalized. For this reason, and because HBO therapy is safe in pregnancy, HBO therapy can be used in pregnant patients with COHb levels greater than 15%.

Burns

INITIAL ASSESSMENT

As with all seriously injured patients, one must first insure that a functional airway is present, that air exchange is occurring within the chest, and that intravascular volume is adequate. An additional priority in patients with ongoing thermal injury is to stop the process of burning; this includes removing any metallic objects (which retain heat) and any clothing, particularly synthetics, which may continue to smolder for prolonged periods after the fire has otherwise been extinguished.

In the field, oxygen (100%) by mask should be given, burned areas should be covered with clean sheets, and the airway must be carefully reassessed; depending somewhat on transport time, prophylactic intubation should be considered in patients likely to have had a significant respiratory injury (severe respiratory symptoms, progressive bronchospasm or hoarseness, confinement in a closed, burning space, facial, perioral, or intraoral burns, etc.). Isotonic solution should then be infused and transport initiated.

Estimation of Extent and Depth of Injury

The entire skin surface should be examined for evidence of thermal and other injury and estimation as to the extent and depth of injury made.

- **"Rule of nines":** The "rule of nines" provides a reasonable initial approximation of the percent of total body surface area (BSA) involved.
  - In adults, the head (including the neck) and each upper extremity are assigned 9% of total BSA, with the back–buttocks, chest–anterior abdomen, and each lower extremity assigned 18%; the genitalia are assigned 1%.
  - In the newborn, the head is relatively larger and together with the neck represents 19% of the total BSA, with the lower extremities each assigned a percentage of 12.5. For each year of life up to age 10, 1% is subtracted from the head and neck and added to the lower extremities; at age 10, adult proportions are reached. Lund and Browder charts, which are age-specific, provide a more accurate measure of the area of burn in children.
- An additional, simple method to estimate percent of involvement is to assign a value of 1% to the *patient's* palm and then use this as a way of estimating total percent. Importantly, first-degree burns are not included in the extent of burn injury, unless they account for more than 25% to 30% of the BSA (Table 55-1 and Fig. 55-1).

Classically, the depth of burn injury has been described as first-, second-, or third-degree. More recently, the terms superficial, partial-thickness, and deep, partial-thickness have been used to more fully describe "second-degree" burns; third-degree burns are described as full-thickness burns. This terminology is common and well understood and is thus appropriate and interchangeable.

- **First-degree burns** involve only the epidermis, are characterized by simple erythema that blanches with pressure, are painful, and are not associated with evidence of skin

Table 55-1	American Burn Association Grading System	
Minor Burns (Outpatient)	**Moderate Burns (Inpatient)**	**Major Burns (Burn Center)**
First-degree <15% TBSA	Second-degree 15%–25%	Second-degree >25%
Second-degree <15% TBSA	Third-degree <10%	Third-degree >10%
Third-degree <2% TBSA		Burns of hands, face, eyes, ears, feet, or perineum; inhalation burns; electrical burns; those associated with major trauma and in poor-risk patients (previous medical illness, head injury, cerebrovascular accident, psychiatric illness, closed space injury)

TBSA, total body surface area.
From Harwood-Nuss A, Wolfson A, Linden C. *The clinical practice of emergency medicine.*
Philadelphia: Lippincott-Raven; 1996, with permission.

disruption or blister formation. First-degree burns typically heal within 3 to 7 days, do not scar, and require only symptomatic treatment.
- **Superficial, partial-thickness burns** result in destruction of the epidermis and extend into the outer portion or papillary layer of the dermis; extension into the inner dermal layer (the reticular layer) does not occur. As a result of this, hair follicles and sweat and sebaceous glands are spared. Any visible dermis is red and moist and appears viable; blisters are typically present, and adequate capillary refill is noted. These burns are very painful, and resolve over a 2- to 3-week period, typically without scarring.
- **Deep, partial-thickness burns** involve the inner portion of the dermis (the reticular dermis), do not blanch with pressure, are not painful, and are usually characterized by the presence of blisters. Any underlying or visible dermal tissue typically has a white appearance. Capillary refill is absent, and these injuries are sometimes difficult to differentiate from full-thickness burns. In fact, deep, partial-thickness and full-thickness burns commonly alternate in any given area. These burns require 1 to 2 months to heal and produce significant scarring.
- **Fourth-degree** burns extend into the underlying subcutaneous tissue and may progress further into muscle and bone. These burns may resemble deep, partial-thickness burns and typically require surgical intervention.

Airway Involvement
Thermal injury involving the upper airway may produce few if any signs at presentation; however, rapid airway obstruction may occur as swelling progresses. Both the history and the physical examination are useful in determining those patients at risk for upper airway or pulmonary injury. The following suggest the possibility of airway injury and the risk for the development of airway complications:
- Patients who were burned within an enclosed space
- The very young or elderly

BURN SHEET

Name_____ Age_____ Number_____

Burn Record. Ages—Birth-7½   Date of Observation_____

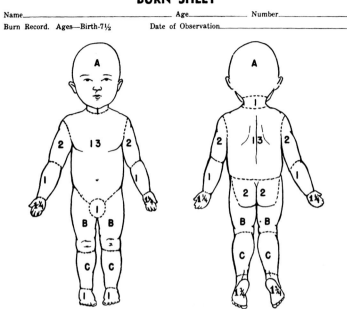

RELATIVE PERCENTAGES OF AREAS AFFECTED BY GROWTH

Area	Age 0	1	5
A = ½ of Head	9½	8½	6½
B = ½ of One Thigh	2¾	3¼	4
C = ½ of One Leg	2½	2½	2¾

% BURN BY AREAS

Probable   { Head_____ Neck_____ Body_____ Up. Arm_____ Forearm_____ Hands_____
3rd' Burn   { Genitals_____ Buttocks_____ Thighs_____ Legs_____ Feet_____

Total Burn { Head_____ Neck_____ Body_____ Up. Arm_____ Forearm_____ Hands_____
            { Genitals_____ Buttocks_____ Thighs_____ Legs_____ Feet_____

Sum of All Areas_____ Probably 3rd' _____ Total Burn_____

Figure 55-1. Modified Lund and Browder chart for estimation of BSA burn involvement in infants and children. (From Harwood-Nuss A, Wolfson A, Linden C. *The clinical practice of emergency medicine.* Philadelphia: Lippincott-Raven; 1996:1207, with permission.)

- Patients with abnormalities of mental status, or reported loss of consciousness in the fire
- Physical evidence of facial burns
- Loss of facial hair including the eyebrows and nasal hair
- Pharyngeal burns, hoarseness, or change in voice
- Cough, wheezing, or carbonaceous sputum
- Carboxyhemoglobin level greater than 15% to 20%

Baseline arterial blood gases, a chest x-ray, and a carboxyhemoglobin level should be obtained and humidified and 100%, high-flow oxygen administered by mask to all patients in whom respiratory injury is suspected; smoke inhalation injuries are discussed in Chapter 54. Patients with possible airway injury require admission along with serial reassessments of oxygen saturation, physical examination, and chest x-ray to detect early those patients who will require intubation or assisted ventilation. The chest x-ray is initially insensitive as an indication of the severity or extent of pulmonary thermal injury.

Fluid Resuscitation

Fluid replacement will be required when second- or third-degree burns involve 20% or greater of the total BSA. Ringer lactate solution is the preferred replacement fluid by many, but isotonic saline is acceptable. In general, the upper extremities are preferred sites for intravenous line placement given the high incidence of simple and suppurative thrombophlebitis in association with lower extremity lines; upper extremity burns do not necessarily contraindicate intravenous line placement. A 16-gauge line or larger is appropriate in most adult patients.

The **Parkland formula** may be used to calculate initial fluid requirements in children and adults; 50% of the total calculated 24-hour fluid requirement should be given over the first 8 hours and the remainder over the next 16 hours. The Parkland formula is as follows:

4 mL × body weight (kg) × percent of second-degree and third-degree burn/24 hours

An alternative formula in children is to calculate the child's 24-hour maintenance fluid requirement, to which is added the product of 3 mL multiplied by the child's weight in kg multiplied by the percent BSA; one half is given in the first 8 hours and the remainder over the next 16 hours. It is important to keep in mind that all formulae represent only an initial estimation and may require adjustment based on close clinical observation of the patient. Urine output is a useful indicator of the adequacy of fluid replacement; this is expected to be approximately 0.5 to 1.0 mL/kg/h adults and 1 mL/kg/h in children. In some patients, invasive monitoring of intravascular volume will be needed to guide fluid replacement.

Other Treatment Considerations

- **Inhalation injury and CO toxicity** should always be considered in burn victims, particularly if the patient was confined within the burning area; a **carboxyhemoglobin level** should be obtained, and treatment is discussed in Chapter 54.
- **Prophylactic intubation** may be required for transport.
- There is no role for prophylactic **antibiotics**.
- **Tetanus status** should be determined and brought current.
- If the patient requires **transfer to a burn center**, burned areas should be covered with saline-moistened, sterile dressings; topical agents should not be used, because the receiving facility must reassess the patient's injuries.
  - Debridement should similarly be deferred to the receiving facility.
  - The decision regarding transfer to a burn center should be made early.
  - If available, sterile linen or large, sterile, surgical drapes should be placed under and used to cover the patient before and during transfer.
- **Pain** will usually require parenteral narcotic analgesics, which can be titrated as needed.
- Patients with significant burns should have a **Foley catheter and nasogastric tube** inserted. In general, the stomach should be emptied to prevent aspiration; antacids and H_2-receptor antagonists are given to prevent stress ulceration of the stomach.

- If the patient requires transfer, all administered fluids, medications, and laboratory data, including a copy of the original chest x-ray, if obtained, should be transmitted to the receiving facility; a copy of the patient's flowchart is most useful. Information regarding drug allergies, tetanus status, family members to contact, religious contraindications to usual treatment, and so on should be ascertained initially and recorded.

Whether to Admit and to Where

In general, the following types of injury require treatment in a burn center:
- All patients with second- or third-degree burns of greater than 20% of the BSA
- Patients older than age 50 years and younger than age 10 years, with second- and third-degree burns over more than 10% of BSA
- Patients with second- and third-degree burns involving the face, hands, feet, genitalia, major joints, or perineum
- Burns associated with a significant inhalation injury
- Burns occurring in immunologically compromised patients

Patients who are unable to care for themselves at home will require regular hospital admission; children with suspicious burn injuries, even if minor, should be hospitalized until the home situation is clear.

CIRCUMFERENTIAL CHEST, NECK, AND EXTREMITY BURNS

Restriction of chest wall movement and ischemia of the extremity secondary to circumferential burns and eschar formation must be recognized and require aggressive treatment. These conditions must occasionally be treated in the emergency department (ED) and should be undertaken by physicians skilled in the technique of escharotomy.
- In patients with chest constriction, as manifested by reduced respiratory excursions or respiratory failure, bilateral incisions are required and should be made in such a way that the edges of the eschar are seen to separate clearly and thereafter move with each respiratory effort. Anesthesia is not required, because the area of eschar generally is in the area of deep, partial-thickness or third-degree burns. To mobilize the chest wall, bilateral axillary incisions (along the anterior axillary line from approximately the level of the rib 2 through rib 12) should be made; these are connected anteriorly by two transverse, spaced incisions. Incisions should extend slightly beyond the eschar.
- Distal extremity ischemia, manifest by the usual clinical signs of peripheral underperfusion or demonstrated by Doppler analysis of distal pulses, is an indication for medial and/or lateral escharotomy along the long axes of the extremity.

OUTPATIENT TREATMENT

Patients not requiring admission or transfer may be treated as outpatients. An initial assessment of the depth and percent of total body involvement is made and tetanus prophylaxis administered as usual. Patients presenting acutely with significant pain can be improved symptomatically by the application of sterile gauze saturated with sterile, cooled saline; this may also reduce ongoing tissue injury in borderline areas.

First Degree Burns

- Patients with simple first-degree burns generally do not require additional treatment, although some patients will benefit from a mild analgesic.
- If the extremities are involved, elevation is helpful to reduce swelling.
- In addition, simply covering the skin for 24 hours will prevent the elicitation of discomfort related to air movement or clothing touching the injured area.

Second- and/or Third-Degree Burns

- After cooling as described above, the injured area should be cleansed with mild soap or antiseptic solution (dilute)
- Blisters that have broken should be sterilely debrided.
- Intact blisters should similarly be debrided if large, tense such that bursting is imminent, if occurring in locations exposed to repetitive movement or pressure (i.e., fingers, toes, feet, hands), or if the patient is unlikely to be compliant with postdischarge recommendations.
- After debridement, apply a topical antibacterial preparation; 1% silver sulfadiazine is a common choice, after the application of which (one applies a very thin coating), a *nonadherent gauze* dressing is applied, followed by a bulky dressing.
  - Sulfadiazine cannot be used in patients allergic to sulfa compounds and should be avoided on the face and in patients with glucose-6-phosphate dehydrogenase deficiency.
  - Patients with burns in proximity to the eye should be treated with a topical, ophthalmologic, antibacterial preparation.
  - Bacitracin and any of the available triple-antibiotic topical preparations are also acceptable alternatives; these tend to be used in smaller burns.
- If an extremity is involved, rings, bracelets, watches, etc. should be removed by cutting, if necessary. Advise the patient to elevate the extremity to prevent swelling.
- In general, patients should be reevaluated in 24 hours for evidence of infection, a dressing change, and further instructions regarding wound care.
- Dressings should be changed twice daily thereafter if the burned area is weeping, and changed daily otherwise, until resolution is complete.
- Small areas involving the face may be treated with an appropriate antibacterial ointment; these may then be left open with instructions to reapply the ointment every 12 hours until healing is complete.
- Another option in patients with partial-thickness burns is the application of one of the newer, occlusive dressings (Tegaderm, Biobrane); these are applied after cleaning and wound debridement and are reevaluated in 24 to 48 hours, at which time one hopes that the dressing has become adherent to the underlying tissue. If so, the dressing is left in place and will separate from the tissue as healing occurs. This type of dressing is most useful for burns occurring on flat areas of the body and away from joints or other areas associated with movement.

It is appropriate to recommend that all patients have a reevaluation after discharge from the ED in 24 hours, at which time the presence of infection is determined and a more accurate estimate of the extent of the burn can be made. Discharged patients should be provided with appropriate analgesics; discharge instructions should recommend a reevaluation in the event of suspected infection and should describe in detail how the patient should attend to the wound at home. Burned extremities should be elevated to minimize swelling; patients with significant injuries (typically deep, partial-thickness and full-thickness burns) should be referred to a plastic surgeon because surgical restoration or skin grafting may be required.

CHEMICAL BURNS OF THE SKIN

Chemical burns of the skin may result from a variety of substances. In all patients, copious tap water irrigation or normal saline should be used initially. In all injuries, if pH paper is immediately available, it is very useful to determine the pH of the offending agent; clearly, alkaline agents require more prolonged periods (sometimes hours) of irrigation to be thoroughly removed. Any solid material present on the skin should be removed by brushing before irrigation, followed by debridement if needed. After irrigation, a topical antibiotic preparation and a nonadherent dressing are applied; tetanus prophylaxis should be provided as needed. Follow-up in 24 hours in the ED is appropriate as noted; referral to a physician skilled in the management of burns at 2 to 4 days is appropriate. A few specific types of exposure are somewhat unique and are discussed.

- The initial treatment of patients exposed to any of the various lacrimators or tear gas–like substances (***p*-chloroacetophenone [Mace], chlorobenzlidenemalonitrile, and dibenzoxapine**) is essentially as for other chemical burns (copious irrigation); tetracaine administration should precede ocular irrigation. Clothing exposed to such substances should immediately be removed and taken outside the hospital, which will prevent distribution of the material throughout the hospital through the ventilation system. These agents produce ocular, skin, and mucous membrane irrigation. An additional agent is pepper-gas or **pepper-spray** (trichloronitromethane), which causes similar symptoms, along with upper respiratory irritation and wheezing. After irrigation, patients with ocular exposure should undergo fluorescein staining to demonstrate or exclude cornea injury.

- Exposure of the skin to some of the **cyanoacrylate glues** may provide a special problem, particularly when the eye, eyelashes, or mucous membranes are involved. In these locations, gently swabbing the involved area with vegetable oil will eventually soften the material; in other locations, acetone is effective.

- Exposure of the skin to **hydrofluoric acid** represents another relatively special problem in that extensive damage to skin and underlying tissues may occur and a specific antidote exists as calcium gluconate (the calcium ion binds to fluoride rendering it nontoxic). Copious irrigation of exposed areas for 15 to 30 minutes may be sufficient treatment, without the need for calcium gluconate administration, if a mild exposure has occurred (brief exposure to the acid, concentration <20%, and prompt [at the scene] irrigation). Persistent pain after irrigation requires that additional, specific treatment be provided; sterile gauze saturated with 10% calcium gluconate should be applied to the area of involvement and preparations made for local (subcutaneous and intradermal) or intraarterial administration of calcium gluconate. There are no clear data indicating which approach is superior at this point. In the former, a 5% to 10% calcium gluconate solution is injected into the subcutaneous and dermal tissues via a 27- to 30-gauge needle at the rate of 0.5 mL of solution per square centimeter of skin. Many patients report rapid pain relief, which if persistent, implies that sufficient solution has been administered and that toxicity has been neutralized. Conversely, persistent or increasing pain is noted when acid remains active in the skin, and further therapy is then indicated. Intra-arterial infusions of calcium gluconate have been successfully used to neutralize acid; after placement of the intra-arterial catheter in an artery proximal to and supplying the area to be treated, calcium gluconate can be infused. It is recommended that the arterial line be connected to a three-way stopcock, to which is attached (1) a 50 mL syringe containing 10 mL of a 10% calcium gluconate solution and 40 mL of 5% dextrose and (2) an arterial pressure monitor. The latter insures that the infusion catheter remains in the artery (extravasation of calcium into the tissues will result in additional damage to the tissues). This can be infused over a 2- to 4-hour period and repeated if pain persists or recurs within a 4-hour period. In patients with **intraocular exposure**, irrigation with, or injection of, calcium carbonate into the subconjunctival tissues is not recommended; 1% calcium carbonate eyedrops has in one case been helpful in limiting corneal injury. Systemic absorption of HF acid may be fatal; absorption produces an acidosis, along with a variety of electrolyte abnormalities (including hypocalcemia, hyperkalemia, and hypomagnesemia). Death is caused by ventricular irritability.

SUNBURN

Patients frequently present to the ED with varying degrees of skin damage secondary to sun exposure. Mild sunburn associated with erythema only and mild symptoms require no treatment other than recommending aspirin or ibuprofen for discomfort and avoiding further exposure. More severe burns, which are often associated with blistering, require elevation if an extremity is involved, cool compresses, and the institution of aspirin or ibuprofen as an anti-inflammatory agent. Emollients, such as Eucerin®, Lubriderm®, or Nivea®, may soothe the skin and relieve dryness and local discomfort after cool compresses are discontinued. Some practitioners recommend that patients with severe sunburn, in addition to the previous measures, be treated with a 5- to 7-day rapidly tapering schedule of prednisone, beginning with 40 mg/day (unless contraindicated).

In all patients, over-the-counter preparations containing topical anesthetics, which may sensitize the patient, should be avoided.

Heat Illness and Cold Exposure

HEAT ILLNESS

Heat illness represents a spectrum of disorders, including mild and moderate forms in which the thermoregulatory mechanisms of the body remain intact (heat cramps, heat exhaustion) to life-threatening heat stroke, in which the body's thermoregulatory mechanisms fail. The factors that predispose patients to develop heat illness include:

- An increased wet-bulb globe temperature (WBGT) found when there is a high ambient heat and humidity
- Lack of acclimatization or physical conditioning
- Obesity
- Strenuous exertion and fatigue
- Cardiovascular disease
- Alcohol consumption
- Anticholinergic drug ingestion
- Old age
- A history of heat illness.

Environmental factors play an extremely important role in the development of heat illness; the WBGT is the most accurate measure of the environmental heat load and reflects the impact of humidity and radiant heat on dry air temperature. It has been estimated that 90% of cases of heat stroke occur when the WBGT is 30°C (85°F) or more.

Heat Cramps

Heat cramps typically occur in hot weather when heavily exercising muscles (most often the legs) contract without reflex inhibition from antagonist muscles. The shoulders may also be affected. Cramping may occur during exercise or may be delayed by several hours. Although the cause of heat cramps is poorly understood, loss of salt during exertion and replacement with free water seem implicated. Patients usually have a history of profuse sweating during strenuous exertion with inadequate or inappropriate fluid replacement. Treatment consists of rest in a cool environment and water and salt replacement either orally with a 0.1% salt solution (made by adding one-quarter teaspoon of salt to each quart of water) or intravenously with normal saline, 1 L intravenously over 1 to 3 hours. A variety of commercially available replacement drinks can also be used. Plain salt tablets are not recommended, because their dissolution in the stomach produces a hypertonic solution often causing gastric irritation, nausea, and vomiting. Enteric-coated salt tablets are poorly absorbed and not recommended.

Heat Exhaustion

Heat exhaustion is also caused by salt and water loss; heat exhaustion caused by predominant water loss typically develops rapidly over a few hours, whereas that caused by predominant salt loss may have a more insidious onset over several days.

Diagnosis
- Symptoms include headache, light-headedness, giddiness, anorexia, nausea, vomiting, malaise, excessive thirst, and muscle cramping.
- The examination usually reveals the patient to be flushed and sweating profusely; the rectal temperature is usually less than 38°C to 39°C (102°F) but can be as high as 40°C (104°F); evidence of dehydration, including tachycardia and orthostatic hypotension, is often noted as well. The mental status examination, except as noted, should be normal; patients with abnormalities of mental status should be considered to have heat stroke (see "Heat Stroke").
- Laboratory data may reveal evidence of dehydration (a mildly elevated BUN and concentrated urine and hematocrit); the serum sodium may be mildly elevated (if no rehydration has occurred) or normal (if fluids have been ingested). Mild to moderate rises in creatinine kinase and hepatic enzymes may be found as well; hypoglycemia is also occasionally noted.

Treatment
Treatment includes rest in a cool environment and intravenous replacement of salt and water initially with 5% dextrose in normal saline, adjusted subsequently based on the patient's electrolytes. Patients with significant hyperthermia should be treated with cooling in the usual manner. Young, physically fit patients may require up to 3 to 4 L of fluid over 4 to 8 hours and generally become completely asymptomatic and well within approximately 6 to 12 hours. Patients with little improvement after 6 to 8 hours of treatment in the emergency department (ED) should be admitted to the hospital for further therapy; similarly, patients with persisting orthostatic hypotension or cardiovascular compromise, as well as elderly patients, require admission for more gradual intravenous fluid replacement.

Heat Stroke

Heat stroke develops when the body's thermoregulatory mechanisms fail or are overwhelmed; the body temperature then rises to levels that produce widespread cellular damage. The diagnosis is based on a core temperature above 40.5°C (104.9°F) and evidence of CNS dysfunction; anhidrosis (lack of sweating) may or may not be present (see later).

History
Although temperatures above 42°C (107.6°F) are universally associated with heat stroke, symptoms may occur at lower temperatures, but always, however, above 40.5°C (104.9°F). Two types of heat stroke have been described: nonexertional (or classic) and exertional.
- **Nonexertional** or classic heat stroke occurs in infants and ill or elderly patients and usually develops over a period of several days, often during a period of excessive ambient temperatures. Patients with classic heat stroke may be severely dehydrated; therefore, sweating may not be seen.
- In contrast, the patient with **exertional** heat stroke may be a healthy young person, often unacclimatized, with symptoms that develop in a matter of hours and that

are most often caused by an unusually heavy heat load associated with exercise or exertion. The patient with exertional heat stroke may not be severely dehydrated and is most often sweating. Symptoms may include chills, headache, nausea, unsteadiness, light-headedness, piloerection involving the arms and chest, paresthesias of the hands and feet, bizarre behavior, syncope, seizures, and coma.

The Physical Examination

The physical examination in patients with heat stroke reveals the rectal temperature to be above 40.5°C (104.9°F), although it may be lower if prehospital treatment has been initiated. The skin may be red and flushed, or ashen gray and dry, or patients may be sweating profusely. The respiratory and heart rates are usually elevated; hypotension may occur as a result of high-output or low-output cardiac failure as well as severe dehydration. Seizures and coma are the most frequent serious central nervous system findings in the ED, although a wide variety of other disturbances are described. These include oculogyric crises, tremors, dystonia, muscle rigidity, decerebrate or transient hemiplegia, dilated and fixed pupils, and a flatline electroencephalogram (EEG).

Diagnostic Tests

A variety of abnormal laboratory studies are noted.
- ABG: Arterial blood gases usually reveal an acidosis, particularly in exertional heat stroke, caused by elevated lactate levels.
- Complete blood count (CBC): A leukocytosis is common and may be as high as 30,000 to 50,000.
- LFTs: The AST, ALT, and lactate dehydrogenase enzymes are markedly elevated. The AST levels in the first 24 hours are said to be prognostic. If the level is less than 1,000 IU/L, the prognosis is generally good with serious injury to the brain, liver, and kidneys unlikely; if levels are above 1,000 IU/L, the prognosis is generally poor, with damage to all three organs likely.
- CPK: Creatinine kinase levels are markedly elevated because of muscle fiber damage. Rhabdomyolysis is especially common in exertional heat stroke, and myoglobinuria, hyperuricemia, and a creatinine elevated out of proportion to the BUN are seen.
- BMP/electrolytes: The sodium, BUN, and osmolality will vary depending on the state of hydration. Hyperkalemia caused by muscle cell damage may be noted after 12 to 24 hours, in addition to hypocalcemia as a result of its deposition in injured muscle. Serum glucose levels may be normal or low; the latter is common in the hypotensive, preterminal state. Hypophosphatemia as low as 1 mg/dL has been described.
- Coagulation studies: Evidence of coagulopathy is common, with disseminated intravascular coagulopathy seen in severe cases.
- ECG: The electrocardiogram (ECG) may show nonspecific ST-segment and T-wave abnormalities, evidence of injury, and a variety of arrhythmias and bundle branch blocks; most of these are reversible with cooling.
- A toxic screen should be ordered as well.

Treatment

Treatment of this lethal disease must be prompt and aggressive.
- **Cooling**. The first priority is immediate cooling of the patient. The means by which this is undertaken is controversial, and no controlled studies comparing one method with another exist at this time. Antipyretics are ineffective.
  - **The evaporative technique** is simple to implement and unlike immersion, minimally impairs the ability of the staff to monitor and/or treat the patient. The evaporative

technique results in cooling rates of up to 0.33°C/min and is undertaken by removing all of the patient's clothing, wetting the skin with a spray of lukewarm water, and circulating cool, dry air rapidly over the patient's body with fans; the patient is kept wet with the use of a tepid or lukewarm water spray bottle. Cold water should not be used because shivering, which is counterproductive, may be provoked.

- **Ice packs** can be used as well; they should be placed in areas of maximal heat transfer: the groin, axillae, and neck. Cooling rates of 0.1°C/min have been reported with this technique.

- **Ice-water immersion** requires that patients be placed in a container of ice water, sufficiently deep to cover the abdomen and chest and the proximal extremities; ice-water immersion results in a cooling rate of 0.11°C/min but is technically difficult when patients are ill, is not feasible in most EDs, and probably should not be used.

- Ice-water gastric lavage may be useful in refractory cases; however, the patient must be intubated.

- Ice-water peritoneal lavage can also be used in refractory cases but is recommended neither in pregnant patients nor in patients with previous abdominal surgery.

- Covering the extremities with ice packs may induce vasoconstriction and thereby reduce the cooling rate; it is not generally advised. Cold water enemas and the inhalation of cooled air are not useful.

- If all other measures to reduce temperature have failed, **cardiopulmonary bypass**, if available, will be effective. To avoid overcooling, the rectal temperature should be continuously monitored with a rectal thermistor probe and the cooling process stopped immediately when the rectal or core temperature reaches 40°C or 104°F.

- **Other therapeutic measures** include
  - Maintenance of an adequate airway and oxygenation; comatose patients should be intubated and intravenous glucose should be given to all patients after blood is drawn for laboratory studies.
  - Peripheral intravenous fluids such as 5% dextrose in one-half normal saline or Ringer lactate solution should be administered; however, fluid balance must be carefully monitored and a Swan-Ganz line may be necessary in selected patients.
  - A Foley catheter should be inserted and hourly measurements of urine output made.
  - Violent shivering should be suppressed, since this will interfere with efforts to cool the patient by generating heat. Benzodiazepines or phenothiazines (chlorpromazine, 25–50 mg intravenously) will effectively suppress shivering in most patients; benzodiazepines should be tried initially because phenothiazines lower the seizure threshold.
  - Seizures should be treated with intravenous diazepam or phenobarbital, because phenytoin is reported to be ineffective in this clinical setting.
  - Acidosis should be treated with intravenous bicarbonate only if the pH is less than 7.2.
  - Hypocalcemia should be treated only if ECG abnormalities consistent with hypocalcemia are noted and then only judiciously, considering the incidence of subsequent renal dysfunction (see p. 390).
  - Hypotension is common and generally responds to measures used to cool the patient. If the patient is clinically dehydrated, a fluid challenge with 200 to 400 mL of normal saline should be given; if blood pressure improves, additional saline may be infused. Vasopressors should be used cautiously when hypotension persists despite adequate intravascular volume replacement.

• Dantrolene, used in treating malignant hyperthermia or neuroleptic malignant syndrome induced by antipsychotic medications, is *not* recommended for use in heat stroke.

Importantly, *rebound hyperthermia,* which may recur 3 to 6 hours later, must be recognized early and treated in the above manner. In addition, patients may show evidence of thermoregulatory instability for several weeks after the acute episode and will always be predisposed to heat stroke in the future. Despite thorough attention to the details of management, the mortality of this illness remains high, particularly among the elderly.

COLD EXPOSURE

Hypothermia

Hypothermia is defined as a core temperature less than 35°C, or 95°F. Predisposing factors include
• Increased age
• Abnormalities of mental status or mobility
• Intoxication with ethanol, barbiturates, or phenothiazines
• Endocrine abnormalities, including hypoglycemia, hypothyroidism, adrenal insufficiency, and hypopituitarism
• Malnutrition
• Uremia
• Overwhelming sepsis
• Exposure, particularly that associated with high wind chill, improper or inadequate clothing, and immersion in cold water

Hypothermia is classified as mild (rectal temperature above 32°C or 89.6°F), moderate (rectal temperature above 26°C or 78.8°F), or severe (rectal temperature below 26°C or 78.8°F). Hypothermia clearly occurs in warm environments and must always be suspected.

Clinical Assessment
Patients with mild hypothermia manifest shivering, which is maximal at 35°C (95°F), and disappears at temperatures below 32°C (89.6°F), mild confusion, poor judgment, dysarthria, and ataxia. Moderate hypothermia is associated with progressive deterioration in mental status; atrial and ventricular arrhythmias, including ventricular fibrillation; a falling pulse and respiratory rate; dilated and nonreactive pupils; absent voluntary motor function; and loss of reflexes are noted. Severe hypothermia is characterized by coma and hypotension; at a temperature of 19°C (66.2°F) the EEG becomes flat, and at 15°C (59°F) asystole occurs. Patients appear cold and pale and have rigid extremities; opisthotonus may be seen in some patients. The mental status may range from confusion to coma, as a function of the degree of hypothermia. Evidence of dehydration is usually present. Body temperature should be followed with the use of a rectal thermistor probe; the esophageal temperature, which may be followed in intubated patients, is more reflective of core temperature but is technically more difficult to obtain. Foley catheters are now manufactured with bladder (core) temperature measurement capability.

Diagnostic Tests
All patients presenting with hypothermia should have blood drawn for a CBC and measurement of BUN, glucose, electrolytes, calcium, creatinine, amylase, liver function studies, and ABG (corrected for hypothermia). A toxic screen, thyroid function studies, and a serum cortisol should be requested in selected patients.

Laboratory studies confirm dehydration with an elevated hematocrit and BUN. The serum glucose is usually high (unless hypothermia is secondary to hypoglycemia) and is caused by impaired insulin secretion, reduced cellular uptake, and reduced insulin effectiveness at low temperatures. Acidosis is typically found and is metabolic (because of increased lactate production and reduced hepatic clearance) and respiratory. ABG must be corrected to reflect the patient's temperature; uncorrected gases typically demonstrate a factitiously high Po_2 and Pco_2 and a low pH. To correct the pH, 0.015 should be added to the measured pH for each degree less than 37°C. For changes above and below 37°C:

	>1°C	<1°C
pH	minus 0.015	plus 0.015
Pco_2	plus 4.4%	minus 4.4%
Po_2	plus 7.2%	minus 7.2%

The effect of hypothermia on the serum potassium and chloride is variable; however, the serum amylase is often elevated as a result of hypothermia-related pancreatitis. The ECG may show tachycardia, bradycardia, atrioventricular block, and a variety of atrial and ventricular arrhythmias; Osborn (or J) waves are occasionally noted at temperatures from 25°C to 30°C and are manifest as a shoulder or "hump" between the QRS and ST segments.

Treatment
Hypoglycemia should be excluded by a bedside glucose determination; if present, hypoglycemia should be treated in the usual manner, followed by the judicious administration of 5% dextrose in one-half normal saline. Ringer lactate solution should be avoided because of the lactate load. The bladder should be catheterized in patients with moderate and severe hypothermia to assess renal perfusion via urine output. In unconscious patients, the cervical spine should be immobilized until it is cleared. The precipitation of ventricular fibrillation by movement or excessive manipulation of the patient with hypothermia is well known; effects should be made to minimize this. This is important in the prehospital setting, in that patients with severe hypothermia (temperatures <28°C [82.4°F]) may have undetectable vital signs if assessed in the usual manner. CPR undoubtedly can precipitate ventricular fibrillation in this setting; therefore, some authorities recommend withholding CPR until the patient's rhythm can be determined. This is a reasonable approach, provided that the time required to determine this is brief. Initial efforts to palpate a pulse in these patients require an entire minute of careful observation; this exercise may still provide inaccurate data as to the presence or absence of a pulse.

Patients with a history of **hypothyroidism**, other characteristics suggestive of myxedema coma, or evidence of a previous thyroidectomy can be given intravenous levothyroxine, 500 μg, and hydrocortisone, 100 mg. Similarly, patients with a history of **adrenal suppression** should be given hydrocortisone, 100 mg as noted. Admission for 24 hours of observation and cardiac monitoring is typically advised.
• Patients with **mild hypothermia** (rectal temperature above 30°C–32°C or 86°F–89.6°F) are capable of endogenous thermogenesis and generally require treatment

with **passive external rewarming** only; this simply involves covering the patient with an insulating material, such as warm, dry blankets, in a warm environment. During rewarming, the rectal temperature should increase approximately 1°C/h. When this is not the case, specific precipitating causes should be considered. Passive rewarming is unlikely to be effective alone in patients with specific (and presumably ongoing) precipitants of hypothermia (e.g., sepsis); active rewarming should be considered in these patients.

- Although somewhat controversial with respect to the method of rewarming, several points regarding the therapy of patients with **moderate and severe hypothermia** are accepted by most authorities. First, because patients with temperatures below 30°C are unable to generate heat, active rewarming is essential. Second, attempts at resuscitation should be aggressive, often prolonged, and continued until the body temperature is 35°C (95°F) or greater, at which time the usual criteria for termination of resuscitation are valid; below this temperature they are not. In addition, in the hypothermic patient, the usual neurologic indicators of central nervous system function, and therefore prognosis for recovery, are inapplicable.

- A number of **metabolic derangements** are commonly observed in patients with hypothermia, the correction of which must be cautious and conservative. Extreme hyperglycemia may be treated with small intravenous doses of regular insulin. With respect to ventilatory support, the rate of ventilation should be reduced by approximately one-half, given that carbon dioxide production is dramatically reduced. One should attempt to maintain the P_{CO_2} at approximately 40 mm Hg; in patients with hypoxia, this may require the addition of carbon dioxide to the inspired mixture. Rapid fluctuations in the pH or P_{CO_2} must be carefully avoided.

- As noted, **cardiovascular complications** are common. Ventricular fibrillation should be treated initially with a 2 Watt-sec/kg defibrillation, after which, if unsuccessful, cardiac compressions at approximately one-half the normal rate should be provided while active rewarming proceeds. A variety of factors have been suggested as precipitants of ventricular fibrillation in the hypothermic patient; these include rapid fluctuations in pH or P_{CO_2}, endotracheal intubation and other procedures undertaken without adequate preoxygenation, and patient movement. Importantly, lidocaine (as well as propranolol) has been shown to be minimally effective at low temperatures, and procainamide may actually increase ventricular irritability. In addition, electrical defibrillation is unlikely to be effective at temperatures below 28°C. Atrial arrhythmias, ventricular premature contractions, and atrioventricular block when unassociated with significant hemodynamic compromise should not be treated; pharmacologic therapy is unlikely to be effective and may precipitate or worsen irritability or block, and these rhythm disturbances typically resolve with rewarming without specific treatment. The role of cardiac pacing in the treatment of bradyarrhythmias is controversial.

- **Hypotension** should be treated initially with isotonic fluid replacement (normal saline, not Ringer lactate), which should be administered cautiously; central venous pressure or Swan-Ganz catheter guidance is often helpful in avoiding volume overload. Vasopressors may be used in patients with refractory hypotension.

- In patients with **moderate and severe hypothermia,** authorities agree that **active rewarming measures** are essential. Two types of active rewarming are available and include active external rewarming and active core rewarming.

  - **Active external rewarming** uses heated or electric blankets, heated water bottles, or warm water immersion. It is generally recommended that measures to achieve active external rewarming be applied initially primarily to the trunk, followed by rewarming of the extremities. The reasons for this are partly historical and partly anecdotal; it was thought that rewarming of the extremities, which produces vasodilation of peripheral vessels, might thereby result in loss of heat from the core to the periphery as peripheral blood flow improves and relatively colder blood returns to the core (explaining the phenomenon of core temperature afterdrop). This was also felt to explain some aspects of the phenomenon referred to as rewarming shock (a transient fall in blood pressure after rewarming); this was also attributed to heat-induced, peripheral vasodilatation. Both phenomena probably result simply from redistribution of heat from the core to the periphery as peripheral perfusion improves. Both phenomena are transient.

- The aforementioned techniques are appropriate for patients with hypothermia and normal hemodynamic function; the best candidates are young, otherwise healthy patients who have become acutely hypothermic.
- **Active core rewarming**, which is indicated in patients with hemodynamic instability, includes inhalation rewarming (the administration of heated oxygen by mask or endotracheal tube), the intravenous infusion of heated crystalloid, peritoneal lavage using an isotonic, heated dialysate with 1.5% dextrose, pleural lavage, gastrointestinal lavage, bladder lavage, and extracorporeal blood rewarming. Mediastinal irrigation by chest tubes or open thoracotomy has been used anecdotally in severely ill patients, but the indications for this modality are unclear. The more invasive techniques are reserved for patients with asystole or refractory ventricular fibrillation.
- **Inhalation rewarming** is noninvasive and although providing only a minimal net heat gain, does reduce pulmonary heat loss (which is significant), and should be considered in all patients.
- Similarly, **the heating of intravenously administered fluids** is simple, noninvasive, and recommended in all patients.
- **Peritoneal lavage**, by which two catheters are placed (one for infusion and the other for removal of fluid) is another technique which can be instituted rapidly and is relatively noninvasive. Dialysis solutions (without potassium) are warmed between 40°C and 45°C (104°F–113°F) and are extremely effective.
- Circulation of warmed fluids in the pleural cavities via chest tubes, in the stomach via a nasogastric tube, and the bladder via a Foley catheter are additional effective core rewarming techniques.
- Extracorporeal rewarming is generally reserved for those patients who do not respond to less invasive techniques.

Local Injuries

Local injuries resulting from cold exposure include chilblain, trench or immersion foot, frostnip, and frostbite.

Chilblain

Chilblain (pernio) is caused by repetitive exposure to dry, cold (but not freezing) environments and manifests clinically as patches of erythema and swelling, often mildly painful, usually occurring on the face, dorsal surface of the hands and feet, and pretibial areas; these can appear up to 24 hours after cold exposure. Blue nodules, plaques, and small ulcerations or vesicles may also develop. Most patients are female; itching and burning may also be reported. Individuals appear to be predisposed to develop chilblain on the basis of increased vascular tone; it appears that the collagen vascular diseases, hyperviscosity, and Raynaud disease increase one's risk for chilblain. Pathophysiologically, persisting vasoconstriction resulting in edema of the dermis and a mild vasculitis involving the dermal vessels are noted. Lesions may persist throughout the cold months, resolve with warm weather, and recur annually. Treatment is largely preventive and symptomatic (with warming and elevation); however, nifedipine has been shown effective in some patients.

Immersion or Trench Foot

Immersion or trench foot results from exposure to cold (not freezing) temperatures and dampness, occurring over a relatively prolonged period (several days). The syndrome appears likely to develop in patients wearing socks that remain damp or wet, or socks or boots that prevent the escape of moisture. The typical evolution of injury includes an initial vasospastic or ischemic period associated clinically with swelling, decreased pulses, local pallor, and reduced or absent sensation; a hyperemic or vasodilatory phase follows that may last 5 to 10 days, during which time pulses may be bounding. The extremity is usually described as warm or hot and erythematous, with edema, blistering, and ulceration; gangrene is noted in severe cases. A recovery phase follows. Pathologically, edema and injury to small vessels and nerves are noted. Importantly, it may not be possible to estimate the depth or extent of injury at presentation; treatment is conservative, with elevation, avoidance of pressure, and meticulous attention to asepsis. Loss of feeling in the foot may be permanent; hyperhidrosis, pain with weight bearing, and cold intolerance may be noted as well and can result in severe, long-term disability. During exposure, the syndrome is preventable by frequently insuring that the feet are dry.

Frostnip and Frostbite

Frostnip represents a mild, superficial freezing injury that is reversible and produces mild discomfort; the extremity appears pale. Symptoms resolve with rewarming and there are no sequelae. **Frostbite** occurs as a result of exposure to freezing temperatures; cell death reflects both the effects of actual freezing of tissues as well as ischemic necrosis caused by vasoconstriction, vessel injury, and stasis. Frostbite may be classified as superficial or deep.

- **Superficial frostbite** (also known as first- and second-degree injury) involves only the skin and subcutaneous tissues, which are described as white, without blanching or evidence of capillary filling after mild pressure. Diagnostically, when compared with deep frostbite, superficially injured tissues are somewhat soft or rubbery to palpation; prognosis for recovery is good.
- **Deep frostbite** (also known as third- and fourth-degree injury) involves the skin, subcutaneous tissues, muscle, blood vessels, nerves, tendons, and often bone and produces a hard or wooden-like extremity. Patients may report mild burning or stinging of the involved extremity, which may be described as clumsy; numbness is also commonly noted. The prognosis is poor. Most patients with frostbite should be admitted to the hospital for a period of observation; this is particularly true when treating patients unable to care for themselves properly.

Treatment involves transportation of the patient to a facility where rapid warming in water may be undertaken without any risk of refreezing or the need for ambulation on the thawed extremity. Dry heat, rubbing snow on the injured tissue, and gradual warming are all to be avoided. Frostbitten nasal and facial tissue (including ears) can be appropriately thawed by applying gauze compresses soaked in warm water. If an extremity is involved, it should be rapidly warmed in a circulating (if possible) water bath at 40°C to 42°C (104°F–107.6°F) for 10 to 30 minutes (until the thawed extremity feels somewhat soft). Hot water directly from the tap must not be used because temperatures are typically too high and will further injure tissue. Most patients will experience severe pain with warming and will require parenteral narcotics for relief. Clear blisters should be incised and debrided, whereas hemorrhagic blisters should be left intact; topical treatment with aloe vera (Dermaide Aloe Cream) should be started and reapplied every 6 hours. Affected digits are treated as noted but should then be separated by placing dry gauze between them. Extremities should be elevated to minimize swelling. Tetanus prophylaxis should be brought current. Although controversy surrounds the use of prophylactic antibiotics, treatment with penicillin G, 500,000 U intravenously every 6 hours, for 2 to 3 days, may be considered. Ibuprofen, in a dose equal to 12 mg/kg/day, in divided doses, is recommended in addition to other analgesics, in that they are helpful in interrupting the arachidonic acid cascade (which locally produces prostaglandins and thromboxane, both severely detrimental to tissue preservation).

Patients frequently present to the ED after a period of treatment (or neglect) at home, often with a partially thawed extremity; warming should proceed in these patients as noted.

Many other treatment modalities exist, the efficacy of which is unproven or anecdotal at present; these include heparin, oral anticoagulants, low molecular weight dextran, hyperbaric oxygen therapy, tissue plasminogen activator, and prostaglandin E analogs. MRI with magnetic resonance angiography (which has replaced technetium-99m scanning), is helpful to delineate viable tissue and estimate the extent of injury. In the past, it is acknowledged that surgical intervention in the treatment of frostbite has occurred too early; surgical treatment is now delayed until approximately the third week after the injury, at which time the demarcation between viable and nonviable tissue has usually become clear.

57 Bites and Stings

HYMENOPTERA STINGS

Hymenoptera (honeybees, bumblebees, wasps, hornets, fire ants, harvester ants, and yellow jackets) stings may produce local toxic reactions, local allergic reactions, local cellulitis, abscess formation, generalized urticaria, angioedema, serum sickness, and anaphylaxis, the last causing approximately 40 deaths each year in the United States. The order Hymenoptera is distinguished by the successful adaptation of the ovipositor (a tubular structure protruding from the abdomen, used for depositing eggs) such that the organ is additionally used to inject the insect's venom.

Most Hymenoptera stings produce immediate pain followed by local itching, erythema, and edema, all of which generally resolve over 2 to 3 hours. Stings that occur directly into peripheral nerves may be associated with a local temporary paralysis.

Discussion of treatment is divided into that for acute (first 2 hours) and delayed presentations.

Acute Presentations

Local Reactions

Patients presenting acutely after a presumed Hymenoptera sting with only localized symptoms and signs should be questioned as to whether reactions have occurred in the past. Patients with no history of angioedema, bronchospasm, urticaria, or anaphylaxis should be observed for 1 to 2 hours and carefully monitored for evidence of evolving anaphylaxis; importantly, most patients with anaphylaxis have no history of significant reactions, and many deny any previous exposure. Patients with documented anaphylaxis caused by Hymenoptera envenomations in the past should receive prophylactic treatment as discussed in "Systemic Reactions." The wound should be carefully examined for a stinger, which should be removed by gentle scraping to prevent further envenomation. Mouth parts or other foreign material should similarly be removed. The wound should be thoroughly cleansed, tetanus prophylaxis administered if appropriate, and ice applied. Patients who remain asymptomatic 2 hours after the injury may be discharged with instructions to return immediately if shortness of breath, wheezing, generalized pruritus, oropharyngeal swelling, or rash occurs. Instructions regarding local wound care and the possibility of local reactions should be provided as well.

Systemic Reactions

- Adult patients who present with or develop **generalized pruritus, urticaria, bronchospasm, or angioedema** should immediately be treated with aqueous 1:1,000 epinephrine in a dose equal to 0.3 to 0.5 mg (0.3–0.5 mL); the pediatric dose is 0.01 mg/kg up to a maximum of 0.3 mg (0.3 mL); epinephrine in this setting should be administered subcutaneously. Caution should be used when weighing the risks and benefits of epinephrine administration in patients with preexisting cardiovascular disease. Intravenous access should then be established and plans made for at least 2 to 4 hours, and up to 8 to 12 hours, of observation. Patients will also benefit from intravenous or intramuscular diphenhydramine, 50 mg in adults and 0.5 to 1.0 mg/kg in children. Ranitidine, 50 mg intravenous, or an analogous H_2-blocker can also be administered, though the benefit is controversial. Steroids, although having little effect on the immediate reaction, should generally be given and may limit the course of urticaria and/or edema. Local wound care should be undertaken as in "Local Reactions" and a cool compress applied to the sting site to induce local vasoconstriction. Patients requiring treatment with epinephrine should be closely observed for evidence of recurring reactions.

- Adults with **significant bronchospasm** should receive standard bronchodilatory therapy by nebulization. An early intravenous dose of methylprednisolone, 100 to 125 mg, or hydrocortisone, 500 mg, may be indicated and may prevent or lessen recurrences over the next 24 hours.

- Patients who have minimal symptoms, who rapidly respond to therapy, and who remain asymptomatic after several hours of observation may be discharged; oral antihistamines may be helpful in reducing symptoms after discharge. Patients must be instructed to return immediately if symptoms recur.

- Adult patients who present with **anaphylaxis** manifest as hypotension, shock, life-threatening or irreversible bronchospasm, or impending airway obstruction caused by laryngeal edema should immediately receive subcutaneous aqueous 1:1,000 epinephrine in a dose equal to 0.5 mg (0.5 mL); the pediatric dose is 0.01 mg/kg up to a maximum of 0.3 mg (0.3 mL), followed by intravenous diphenhydramine, 50 mg in adults and 0.5 to 1.0 mg/kg in children (up to 50 mg); intravenous ranitidine, 50 mg, can also be administered. In severe reactions, subcutaneous epinephrine may need to be readministered in 5-minute intervals for several doses. Importantly, adults presenting with anaphylaxis who are taking β-blockers should receive glucagon, 1 mg intravenous, which may need to be repeated at 5-minute intervals. In all patients, intravenous access should be established immediately, concurrent with the administration of subcutaneous epinephrine, and preparations for possible intubation, cricothyrotomy, or tracheostomy made. Normal saline should be rapidly infused to assist with blood pressure support. In patients **not responding** to the initial dose of epinephrine or with persisting and severe symptoms, aqueous **1:10,000** epinephrine, 1 to 2 mL, should be administered intravenously. This dose is equivalent to 0.1 to 0.2 mL of a 1:1,000 dilution and may be repeated if no response is observed or if significant symptoms persist. Cardiac monitoring should be initiated and maintained. The dose of intravenously administered epinephrine must be determined by the patient's clinical condition, whether any response has occurred to the subcutaneous injection, and the possibility of precipitating cardiovascular complications. In addition, **oxygen** should be administered, and ice should be applied to the site.

- Patients with **inadequate ventilation** or persistent cyanosis despite therapy require emergent intubation; patients with progressive respiratory obstruction or patients who are unable to be intubated because of local swelling require needle or surgical cricothyrotomy or tracheostomy. In the child younger than 12 years old, needle cricothyrotomy with a 14- or 16-gauge needle followed by pressure insufflation with 100% oxygen is indicated; adequate oxygenation may also be maintained in adults in this manner.

Prevention

Patients with reactions to Hymenoptera stings should be provided with and instructed in the use of any of the commercially available "bee sting" kits; kits contain a tourniquet and injectable epinephrine. An EpiPen (epinephrine autoinjector) is commonly prescribed and will deliver 0.3 mg of epinephrine automatically; EpiPen Jr. is also available and delivers 0.15 mg of epinephrine. The Ana-Kit contains a syringe with two individually injectable 0.5 mL (0.5 mg) doses of epinephrine. Patients should also be advised to obtain an appropriate identification bracelet indicating their Hymenoptera allergy. Further measures to prevent subsequent envenomations involve avoiding scented toiletries and brightly colored clothing while outdoors and using an insect repellent containing diethyltoluamide when possible. Patients with systemic reactions should strongly consider Hymenoptera hyposensitization after discharge; therefore, referral to an allergist may be appropriate.

Delayed Presentations

Delayed reactions to stings are relatively common and result from four different mechanisms:
• Local toxic reactions to venom
• Local allergic reactions
• Local infection
• Systemic allergic reactions
    Clear differentiation of the first three of these entities is extremely difficult clinically because all patients present with the signs and symptoms of local inflammation (redness, heat, swelling, and pain), and many patients with toxic and allergic reactions will have low-grade fevers. Infection is said to be somewhat more common after wasp, hornet, or yellow jacket stings than after bee stings; however, this is often not helpful in the individual patient. Infection is, however, unusual in the first 12 to 24 hours after injury. A practical approach to the treatment of patients with delayed presentations involves the use of both an antihistamine and an oral antibiotic. Diphenhydramine, 25 to 50 mg four times daily for 3 to 5 days, and a first-generation cephalosporin, for 5 to 7 days, are a reasonable treatment regimen. The wound should be thoroughly cleansed, examined for foreign material, and tetanus prophylaxis administered if needed. Elevation is advised if swelling is present; wounds that are fluctuant may require incision and drainage (see Chapter 44).
    One should note the specific delayed or "toxic" reaction produced by the "killer bee." These bees were imported into Brazil from Africa in 1956 and have now migrated into the southern United States via northern Mexico. Although the venom of the killer bee is similar to that of other bees, fatal and severe toxic reactions have been seen, primarily because of the bee's aggressiveness and the large number of stings. As a result of the large amount of venom injected, direct toxic effects of the venom are produced; these typically evolve over 2 to 3 hours, as distinguished from anaphylactic reactions, and include fever, drowsiness, light-headedness, abdominal cramping, vomiting, diarrhea, and, in severe cases, seizures, coagulopathy, cardiovascular collapse, and death. Although less common, other delayed presentations include serum sickness, vasculitis, hemolysis, renal failure, and Henoch-Schönlein and thrombotic thrombocytopenic purpura.

HUMAN BITES

Human bites may occur intentionally or may be inadvertent; these inadvertent bites are often unrecognized, and therefore, therapy is inadequate or inappropriate. Inadvertent or accidental bites most frequently involve the hand when the face and mouth are struck during an altercation (closed fist injury or CFI) or as a result of a "head-on" collision in sports. The human mouth contains a number of both aerobic and anaerobic organisms that may produce an extremely aggressive, necrotizing infection, particularly when the so-called closed spaces of the distal extremities are involved. Patients with CFIs require a careful evaluation of the wound along with plain films; integrity of tendons must be determined and foreign material (teeth) and/or fractures identified. One must remember that when striking an object, making a fist requires that the fingers are flexed; injuries will occur in this position. When evaluating such a wound, typically with the fingers extended, tendon injuries will therefore be missed, because they will now be proximal to the site of skin injury.

Antibiotic Therapy

Preferred oral antibiotic therapy is recommended for 5 days and includes amoxicillin-clavulanate (Augmentin), 875 mg twice daily, dicloxacillin plus penicillin, a first-generation cephalosporin plus penicillin, or a fluoroquinolone (Ciprofloxacin, 500–750 mg every 12 hours). Children may be treated with Augmentin, 40 mg/kg/day in three equally divided doses. When parenteral treatment is required, ampicillin-sulbactam (Unasyn), 1.5 to 3.0 g every 6 hours; cefoxitin, 1 to 2 g intravenous every 6 hours (pediatric dose is 80–160 mg/kg/day intravenous divided every 6 hours); or ticarcillin/clavulanate (Timentin), 3.1 g intravenous every 6 hours, is recommended. Penicillin-allergic patients can be given clindamycin plus ciprofloxacin.

Hospitalization

Given the difficulty in treating infection associated with human bites, a markedly reduced threshold for recommending hospital admission for parenteral antibiotic therapy is appropriate.

Superficial Abrasions or Minor Scrapes

Superficial abrasions or minor scrapes are occasionally produced, and these may be treated with thorough cleansing and the application of an appropriate antibacterial ointment. Tetanus prophylaxis should be administered as usual, and the patient should be instructed to recleanse the area in 24 hours, reapply an antibacterial ointment, and return for a wound check in 48 hours if evidence of infection occurs.

More Significant Injuries

The treatment of **more significant injuries** depends on location.

Face

Cosmetically significant lacerations involving the face occurring as a result of human bites should be thoroughly cleansed, copiously irrigated, and debrided if necessary and will thereafter usually be primarily closed; plastic surgical consultation is often sought in these injuries. Antitetanus prophylaxis should be administered as needed, and antibiotic coverage initiated as outlined in Table 57.1. A wound check in 24 to 48 hours is recommended. Puncture wounds are best treated with thorough cleansing, irrigation, if possible, and a prophylactic antibiotic; patients should be instructed to open the lesion four to six times per day for the first few days, express any purulent or bloody material, and apply a warm, moist compress for 20 to 30 minutes.

Distal Extremity and Tendon

Lacerations involving the distal extremity, particularly the hand or fingers, resulting from human bites should not be closed; subspecialty consultation and treatment are often recommended. This is particularly important when injuries are extensive or occur in close proximity to joints, where delayed closure may result in prolonged disability and contracture related to scar formation. In other less serious injuries, a thorough cleansing, copious irrigation, debridement if needed, the institution of antibiotic therapy as outlined in "Antibiotic Therapy," p. 524, and a wound check in 12 to 24 hours will be elected; delayed closure by the plastic or hand surgeon is typically elected. Tendon lacerations resulting from human bites will typically also be repaired by the consulting subspecialist, often after evaluation of the wound in the OR; this is also the case in patients with foreign material (teeth) and/or fractures involving the hand. Puncture wounds should not be closed.

Other
Lacerations or deep puncture wounds resulting from human bites that are not cosmetically significant and do not involve the distal extremity or tendons should be cleansed, irrigated, debrided as necessary, and reexamined in 24 to 48 hours; primary closure is not recommended. Antibiotic coverage should be provided as noted in "Antibiotic Therapy." Consideration can be given to delayed primary closure after the initiation of antibiotics and appropriate wound care.

NONHUMAN MAMMALIAN BITES

General Considerations
Injuries occurring as a result of nonhuman mammalian bites may cause abrasions, puncture wounds, major lacerations and avulsions, or occasionally crushing injuries. Rabies prophylaxis should be a consideration in all such injuries and is discussed in "Rabies," p. 526; antibiotic therapy is discussed in "Antibiotic Therapy," p. 526. See Table 57-1 for animals and organisms.

- **Superficial abrasions** should be treated routinely with thorough cleansing and the application of an appropriate antibiotic ointment. Antitetanus prophylaxis should be administered if needed.
- **Significant puncture wounds** that involve the distal extremity, enter joint spaces, or involve tendons must be treated aggressively. Aerobic and anaerobic cultures, thorough cleansing, copious irrigation and debridement, if needed, and subspecialty consultation should all be undertaken with consideration given to hospital admission for parenteral antibiotic therapy. Puncture wounds in other locations, depending on their extent, may generally be treated with cleansing, irrigation if possible, a prophylactic antibiotic, and early reexamination. Puncture wounds resulting from some canine species (pit bulls, etc.) should be x-rayed, because bony injuries may be present and require specific treatment.
- Patients with **facial and neck wounds that are cosmetically significant** can generally be closed primarily after appropriate local care; this includes thorough cleansing, copious irrigation, judicious debridement, if needed, and 24-hour follow-up. Cultures should be obtained, tetanus prophylaxis administered if appropriate, and prophylactic antibiotics instituted.
- **Lacerations that are not cosmetically significant** should generally be left open and allowed to heal by secondary intention. Injuries to the hands and fingers are typically left open and treated with delayed closure in 3 to 6 days. A possible exception would be injuries that are extensive, particularly in areas associated with movement, where a period of prolonged healing and disability could be expected; subspecialty consultation is recommended in these cases.

TABLE 57-1	Prophylactic Treatment of Animal Bites[a]	
Animal	**Organism**	**Prophylactic Antibiotics**
Bat, raccoon, skunk	Undefined	Amoxicillin/clavulanate (Augmentin)
Cat (80% become infected)	*Pasteurella multocida*[b]	Amoxicillin/clavulanate or cefuroxime or doxycycline
	Staphylococcus aureus	
Dog (5% become infected)	*Streptococcus viridans* *Pasteurella multocida* *Staph. aureus* *E. corrodens* *Bacteroides* sp. *Fusobacterium* *Capnocytophaga*	Amoxicillin/clavulanate or clindamycin plus a fluoroquinolone (for adults) or clindamycin plus sulfamethoxazole/ trimethoprim (for children)
Pig	Polymicrobial	Amoxicillin/clavulanate or a third-generation cephalosporin
Rat	*Streptobacillus moniliformis*	Amoxicillin/clavulanate or doxycycline
Pit viper	*Pseudomonas* sp. Enterobacteriaceae *Staphylococcus epidermidis* *Clostridium* sp.	Ceftriaxone

[a]Given within 12 h of bite or empirically if the wound is infected.
[b]*Pasteurella multocida* is resistant to dicloxacillin, cephalexin, clindamycin, and, for some strains, erythromycin.

Rabies

Rabies is an acute viral illness affecting the central nervous system transmitted to human beings by infected saliva or other secretions; these must be inoculated through the skin by a bite or a scratch, deposited on mucous membranes, or inhaled as aerosolized virus (i.e., from infected bats). The causative organism, an RNA rhabdovirus, can survive for 24 hours in carcasses at 20°C and longer at lower temperatures. Saliva is infectious for 24 hours at 4°C. The asymptomatic incubation period varies from 10 days to 1 year and depends on the size and site of the inoculation and age of the victim. Shorter incubation periods are seen in large wounds, in wounds closer to the brain, and in young victims. Bites resulting from livestock, rabbits, squirrels, chipmunks, guinea pigs, gerbils, rats, mice, other rodents, and hamsters rarely require antirabies prophylaxis.

Diagnosis
Patients present with a typical viral prodrome (sore throat, fever, cough, fatigue, headache, and myalgias), at which time approximately 70% of patients report paresthesias, fasciculations, or both at the site of the original injury or inoculation. Neuromuscular hyperexcitability, agitation, hallucinations, confusion, muscle spasms, "posturing,"

localized paralysis, and evidence of autonomic and brainstem dysfunction follow. The diagnosis is based on demonstration of virus in saliva or cerebrospinal fluid or serologic evidence of evolving infection.

Treatment

Recovery from rabies after symptoms appear is extremely rare and has been reported in only three patients; prevention must therefore be a primary concern. Treatment includes aggressive cleansing of the wound with soap and water, followed by saline and 0.1% benzalkonium chloride, 50% to 70% alcohol, or tincture of aqueous iodine irrigation. Postexposure rabies prophylaxis in unimmunized (unvaccinated) individuals is outlined in Table 57-2. Patients with a demonstrated antibody response to prior immunization, either via preexposure or via postexposure prophylaxis, do not need rabies immune globulin (RIG) but should receive a 1-mL intramuscular (deltoid) dose of human diploid cell rabies vaccine (HDCV), rabies vaccine adsorbed (RVA), or purified chick embryo cell (PCEC) vaccine on days 0 and 3. Day 0 is the first day of vaccine administration. Importantly, rabies does not occur in birds, reptiles, fish, or other nonmammals.

When **treatment** is indicated, **HDCV** (or RVA or PCEC) and **RIG** should be given. **HDCV** (or RVA or PCEC), 1 mL, is given intramuscularly (in the deltoid) on days 0, 3, 7, 14, and 28. Day 0 is the first day of vaccine administration. The deltoid area is preferred in adults and older children; younger children can be given the vaccine in the outer aspect of the thigh. The vaccine should not be given in the gluteal area. RIG is administered once on day 0; it should never be given in the same syringe as the vaccine. The dose is 20 IU/kg of body weight, which, if possible, should be infiltrated around the bite or bites; any remaining medication should be administered intramuscularly at a site distant from vaccine administration. The recommended dose of RIG should not be exceeded, because active antibody production by the patient can be suppressed. RIG can be given up to 7 days after initial vaccination, but administration on day 0 is preferred. Importantly, because of the potentially long incubation period in rabies, postexposure prophylaxis should be given to anyone with an exposure provided that symptoms of rabies have not developed; incubation periods in excess of a year have been reported in humans.

SNAKEBITE

Diagnosis

Bites resulting from poisonous snakes in the United States may produce no injury, local injury, or local injury and systemic manifestations; these latter phenomena include fever, widespread hemolysis, shock, and death. The role of the emergency physician in the evaluation of the patient with snakebite involves the following issues: Was the snake poisonous? If so, did envenomation occur and, if so, to what extent?

- **History.** In all patients, it is important to determine the exact time of the bite, what initial first aid was provided, and whether local or systemic symptoms have progressed. Specifically, the presence, degree, and progression of pain and/or numbness at the bite site should be determined. Systemic symptoms should also be noted if present; these can include nausea, dizziness, shortness of breath, cramping, paresthesias, perioral tingling or numbness, and a metallic taste.
  - Patients should also be questioned regarding any prior allergic reaction to horses, any previous treatment with horse serum, and any history of asthma or urticaria.

TABLE 57-2	Postexposure Rabies Prophylaxis Recommendations	
Animal Species	**Condition of Animal at Time of Attack**	**Treatment**
Domestic dog, ferret, or cat	Healthy and available for 10 d of observation	No treatment is indicated unless animal develops signs of rabies during the observation period; if so, treatment with HDCV or RVA and RIG is initiated, the animal is killed, and the diagnosis confirmed or excluded.
	Rabid or suspected to be rabid	Begin treatment with HDCV or R VA and RIG, sacrifice animal, and confirm or exclude diagnosis.
	Animal not available for observation or examination	Consult public health officials with details of attack, whether provoked, etc.
Bat, coyote, bobcat, raccoon, fox, skunk, other carnivores (including wild dogs and cats)	Not relevant	Regard as rabid unless proved otherwise by state laboratory examination; initiate treatment with HDCV or RVA and RIG.
Livestock, rabbits, squirrels, chipmunks, guinea pigs, gerbils, rats, mice, hamsters	Not relevant	Treatment usually not indicated; however, state public health officials should be consulted with specific details and recommendations followed for specific attack.

- **Was the snake poisonous?** Although not applicable to coral snakes, a variety of morphologic criteria for designating a snake as poisonous are useful:
  - **Poisonous**: a vertically elliptic pupil, well-developed hinged fangs, and a single row of posterior ventral plates or scales.
  - **Nonpoisonous:** Snakes generally have round pupils, several rows of small teeth, and a double row of posterior, ventral plates.
  - As noted, these criteria do not apply to the coral snake, a colorful reptile with alternating black, yellow, and red bands; a round pupil; and very short fangs. The yellow bands are narrow and separate the broader red and black bands (the red and black bands do not touch each other in the coral snake). The phrase "red on yellow may kill a fellow; red on black—venom lack" may help differentiate the coral from other striped, nonpoisonous snakes. Coral snakes account for only approximately 1% of poisonous bites per year; the other 99% result from bites of the family Crotalidae, which includes the rattlesnake, copperhead, and water moccasin or cottonmouth. This family may be identified by the criteria noted for poisonous snakes.
- **Did envenomization occur?** Deciding whether envenomation has occurred is straightforward except when the coral snake is believed to be the culprit. Up to 50% of venomous snakebites result in little or no envenomation ("dry bites"). Crotalidae snakebites resulting in envenomation are accompanied by immediate and severe pain at the site, often rapidly developing swelling and ecchymoses, and one to four adjacent fang marks. Necrosis of the surrounding area may develop, often rapidly, depending on the extent of envenomation. Systemic signs and symptoms are related to deranged hemostasis and neurotoxicity (manifest as muscle weakness, paresthesias, fasciculations, dysphagia, abnormalities of behavior, paralysis, and seizures). Nausea, vomiting, and diarrhea are also commonly noted. Conversely and importantly, coral snakes produce no typical bite marks and little or no local reaction. Because systemic toxicity, including death, may occur in these patients without evidence of significant local injury, patients with a coral snakebite should be admitted for antivenom administration, as discussed in the section "Treatment" in "Snake Bite," and warrant careful observation in the hospital for 18 to 24 hours. Evidence of evolving neurotoxicity, manifest as slurred speech, dysphagia, ptosis, pupillary dilatation, and respiratory paralysis, should be carefully monitored, because these may be the first signs of toxicity.

Treatment

- Patients with wounds resulting from bites by snakes judged **nonpoisonous** should be treated with antitetanus prophylaxis, cleansing, a period of observation (~6 hours) in the emergency department (ED), and a wound check in 24 to 48 hours. After this interval, patients without evidence of local or systemic toxicity can be discharged. Snakes do not transmit rabies.
- **Poisonous undetermined.** Patients in whom a judgment as to the poisonous status of a particular snake cannot be made should be observed in the ED, as discussed, for evidence of evolving local or systemic envenomization.
- All patients with bites from snakes judged to be **poisonous** should be treated as follows:
  - **Prehospital**. In the field, efforts are taken to calm the victim and ensure that a second bite does not occur. If an extremity is involved, it should be placed in neutral position below the heart; intravenous access should not be established in the bitten extremity. Wounds should not be incised and oral suction is not recommended.

The Sawyer Extractor is a suction device that, when placed over snake bites (no incision is made), produces sufficient suction to remove some venom in animal models; whether the device is helpful in humans is unknown. It probably does no harm, provided that transport to a hospital is not delayed using it; intuitively, the device must be used within minutes of the bite to be effective. The placement of an arterial interrupting tourniquet (to slow or prevent venom absorption) is not advised; alternatively, "compression or constriction bands," which are placed proximally around the bitten extremity and interrupt venous and lymphatic flow, may be helpful (in limiting systemic absorption of the venom), particularly if transport time to a hospital is long. The band is placed so that a finger slips under the band and distal arterial pulses are easily palpated. Bands may be made from clothing, rope, rubber gloves, etc. Oxygen should be administered and the patient transported as soon as possible.

- **In the ED**, blood is obtained for complete blood count, electrolytes, BUN, blood sugar, creatinine, prothrombin time, partial thromboplastin time fibrinogen, fibrin split products, creatine phosphokinase, and type and cross match, and request a urinalysis should be obtained. Patients with significant envenomization should have 2 to 4 U of packed RBCs available. Poison center consultation is useful at this time.

- Intravenous access should be established in an unbitten extremity. A careful baseline should be established regarding the appearance of the local site. Peripheral pulses should be noted, marked, and documented. The circumference of any bitten extremity should be determined and documented at, and approximately 4 to 5 inches proximal to, the bite. The distance from the bite of any surrounding edema should be marked and documented. These measurements should be rechecked at approximately 15-minute intervals to help determine the extent of envenomation.

- If an extremity is bitten, it should be kept slightly dependent and slightly cooled.

- **Tetanus toxoid** or human tetanus immune globulin (or both) should be administered if indicated. Evolving **compartment syndromes** must be excluded by frequent reassessment of the extremity, and therefore any dressing should be loosely applied and not cover the most distal extremity.

- The patient should be kept **quiet and calm** to avoid tachycardia and vasodilation-induced augmentation of absorption.

- Obtain appropriate **antivenom** for possible use. Two types of antivenom are commercially available. Crotalidae polyvalent antivenom is effective against bites caused by rattlesnakes, copperheads, and water moccasins or cottonmouths; coral snake antivenom is effective against bites resulting from this snake.

  ○ In all suspected **Eastern and Texas coral snakebites,** most authorities recommend the administration of three vials of North American coral snake antivenom intravenous, after dilution in 300 to 500 mL of normal saline, and skin testing. Additional antivenom should be administered to patients with signs or symptoms of a bite.

  ○ In **Crotalidae** envenomations, antivenom is the mainstay of treatment, but it is not administered prophylactically. **Rattlesnake** bites are the most serious, followed by **water moccasin** bites. In general, **copperhead** envenomations do not require treatment with antivenom; this is true unless the victim is a small child or a debilitated person, the snake was extremely large, or multiple bites are involved. Patients with no systemic symptoms, only mild to moderate pain (which is stable), and minimal local reaction (<1–2 inches of edema and erythema surrounding the bite) may be cautiously observed; if evidence of increasing toxicity is noted, locally (increased pain, swelling, and advancing erythema), systemically (hypotension, alterations in mental status, and respiratory distress), or serologically (reduced platelets, markedly prolonged clotting parameters [PT, PTT, and fibrinogen]), then antivenom should be administered.

- The introduction of polyvalent immune Fab of ovine origin (FabAV or CroFab) has improved the efficacy and safety profile of treatment for crotalidae envenomations. Nevertheless, antivenom should be given in a critical care setting with epinephrine and antihistamines prepared for the possibility of anaphylaxis. Four to six vials of FabAV, given intravenously, is the recommended initial dose in children and adults; this dose is repeated if no clinical or laboratory improvement has occurred or systemic toxicity is rapidly progressive or severe. Recurrence of local or systemic symptoms is common; after initial control is established, three maintenance doses of FabAV, two vials each 6 hours apart, are recommended to reduce the incidence of this recurrence. All patients must be carefully observed for evidence of increasing toxicity.

- **Other measures.** The role of steroids, if any, in the treatment of snakebites has not been defined. In patients with the possibility of a compartment syndrome, a pressure monitor should be inserted; a pressure of 30 mm Hg or greater requires that the limb be elevated and additional Crotalidae antivenom be administered. Additionally, some authorities suggest the concurrent administration of mannitol, 1 to 2 g/kg intravenously over 30 to 40 minutes. Surgical consultation for fasciotomy is indicated if pressure remains elevated or increases.

- **Disposition.** Patients bitten by a coral snake, exotic snake, or the Mojave rattlesnake, because of the possibility of delayed symptoms, should be admitted to the hospital for observation. Patients with pit viper bites presenting with only minor local evidence of envenomation, which is improving, can generally be discharged from the ED after approximately 12 hours of observation. Prophylactic antibiotics are not generally recommended. Information relevant to treatment may be obtained from the regional poison control center or your local zoo.

SPIDER BITES

Most significant spider bites in the United States involve two species: the black widow (*Latrodectus mactans* and *hesperus*) and the brown recluse spider (*Loxosceles reclusa*). Treatment differs depending on the species involved; thus, accurate identification of the spider is helpful.

Most significant spider bites in the United States result from the female black widow, the most characteristic marking of which is a red or yellow-orange hourglass on the ventral abdomen, which may be subtle or absent in young spiders. This is said to stand out brightly against the shiny black body of the adult spider. The brown recluse spider, as well, has a characteristic marking: a dark violin pointing backward on the dorsal cephalothorax. Both spiders are approximately 1 cm in diameter with a leg span of approximately 5 to 6 cm. Members of the genus *Latrodectus* currently inhabit the entire United States; however, more than 50% of bites occur in California. The brown recluse spider is found primarily in the south central and southeastern portions of the United States.

Although the black widow frequently produces substantially more systemic toxicity, bites that result from the brown recluse spider are accompanied by extensive local tissue injury. Treatment strategies recognize this difference and are discussed.

Black Widow Bites

Diagnosis

Bites from the black widow are accompanied by an initial pinprick sensation (caused by the spider's two fangs), followed by a dull ache; this is followed rapidly by mild erythema and swelling. The tissue immediately around the puncture may become pale, producing a target-type lesion. Some bites are not associated with any physical findings. In significant envenomations, a variety of constitutional symptoms follow within 20 to 30 minutes, the most striking of which are widespread muscle spasms. These may involve all muscle groups, occur in waves, and are said to be intolerable. The abdominal muscles may be involved producing a "board-like" abdomen, although examination reveals that actual abdominal tenderness is absent. In some patients, the interval between the bite and the onset of symptoms is prolonged; muscle spasms are usually followed by headache, nausea, vomiting, tremor, hypersalivation, generalized rash, and periorbital edema; hypertensive crisis has also been reported. Symptoms generally subside over 4 to 6 hours, but minor recurrences are reported for up to 72 hours and total recovery usually requires 3 to 7 days. Death from cardiac or respiratory failure is rare and occurs primarily in the debilitated, elderly patient and in small children. Some patients will experience residual symptoms for several months following the bite; these include fatigue, weakness, headache, insomnia, and paresthesias.

Treatment

The **treatment** of black widow bites involves the limitation of symptoms and the administration of *Latrodectus* antivenom to selected patients.

- Local discomfort and muscle cramping are most effectively treated with a combination of intravenous narcotic analgesics and benzodiazepines, titrated carefully to reduce symptoms.
- Intravenous calcium gluconate, 10 to 20 mL of a 10% solution given intravenously over 20 minutes, may also help relieve symptoms and may be repeated every 4 to 6 hours as needed.
- Hypertensive crisis should be treated with nitroprusside, or other titratable intravenous anti-hypertensive. Less severe elevations in blood pressure usually respond to treatment for muscle cramping and pain, as outlined above.
- Antivenom should be administered when envenomation appears severe or life threatening (respiratory distress, severe hypertension, refractory, and severe muscle spasms); antivenom is derived from horse serum and can be administered after skin testing for horse serum sensitivity (a testing kit accompanies the antivenom).
  - Symptomatic pregnant patients should receive antivenom and a markedly lowered threshold for the administration of antivenom should be maintained in children younger than 16 years of age, patients with significant chronic illnesses, and the elderly debilitated patient.
  - Antivenom is currently administered as follows: one vial (2.5 mL) is added to 50 to 100 mL of normal saline and intravenously infused over 15 to 20 minutes; clinical improvement is usually noted within 1 to 3 hours and is often dramatic, and repeat doses are rarely needed.
- Symptomatic patients should be admitted to the hospital; asymptomatic patients who have a documented black widow bite should be observed for 6 to 8 hours after which, if they remain asymptomatic, they may be discharged. Patients

with undocumented bites should generally be observed for 2 to 3 hours before discharge.

Brown Recluse Spider Bites

Diagnosis
L. reclusa bites are accompanied by an initial stinging sensation followed by a progressively severe ache. Bleb or vesicle formation, intense local ischemia, and underlying necrosis evolve over the subsequent 48 to 72 hours. Systemic reactions may occur but are rare, usually begin 24 to 72 hours after the bite, and include fever, chills, mild nausea, vomiting, diarrhea, and arthralgias. DIC and thrombocytopenia, both of which may be severe, have been reported as has severe hypotension.

Treatment
The treatment of brown recluse spider bites is very controversial.
- Many patients with minor bites can be treated with analgesics, antihistamines, and local wound care.
- Early excision had been recommended in the past; however, it is now recommended to be delayed 6 to 8 weeks after the bite.
- The administration of steroids has been suggested and may limit local injury, although no conclusive trials have documented their efficacy; if used, methylprednisolone, 125 mg intravenous initially, followed by 5 to 7 days of oral prednisone (50 mg daily), is appropriate.
- Antitetanus prophylaxis should be administered as needed; prophylactic antibiotic therapy is not advised unless infection is present.
- There is no effective antivenom available in the United States.
- In adults, an escalating dosage of oral dapsone has been used in this setting to limit local injury; clinical experience is limited, however, and no clear guidelines exist to direct treatment; this is also the case with hyperbaric oxygen therapy. Before initiating treatment with dapsone, screening for G6PD deficiency is recommended; complications of treatment include hemolysis and methemoglobinemia.

SCORPION STINGS

Scorpions are present in most states in the United States, and envenomations are relatively common. With the exception of one potentially lethal species confined to Arizona and small sections of adjoining states, most stings involve relatively minor local reactions and may be treated as such. Prudent treatment includes cleansing, examining the wound for any foreign material, cooling the area of the wound slightly, administering tetanus prophylaxis as needed, observation for systemic symptoms, and advising elevation for 24 to 48 hours. Scorpion venom is extremely rapidly absorbed, and thus incision and suction are not recommended.

Importantly, *Centruroides exilicauda*, which is geographically limited to the southwestern United States, may occasionally produce lethal stings, particularly in the elderly, debilitated patient and in the very young child. In such stings, very little local evidence of tissue injury can be found, but local, advancing paresthesias and numbness follow. In significant envenomations, systemic symptoms include hyperexcitability, restlessness, agitation, hypersalivation, lacrimation, rhinorrhea, nausea, vomiting, and seizures. Coma, respiratory arrest, and death may follow. The use of narcotic analgesics should be avoided in these patients because of drug–venom interactions. Treatment consists of slight cooling, general supportive measures, and the administration of specific antivenom when symptoms suggesting severe envenomation appear; antivenom is not currently FDA approved. The dose is one to two vials administered intravenously after dilution in 50 mL of normal saline; skin testing should precede antivenom administration, since the antivenom is derived from goat serum. Antivenom is available from the Antivenom Production Laboratory at Arizona State University. The Central Arizona Regional Poison Management Team can be called with specific questions regarding management (602-253-3334). Hypotension, disturbances in cardiac rhythm, and allergic reactions, including anaphylaxis, are treated in the usual fashion; tachycardia and hypertension respond to β-blockers or calcium channel blockers. Intravenous diazepam can be administered for muscle cramping/spasm. Patients should generally be observed for 18 to 24 hours in the hospital. As noted, children are at greatest risk for the development of severe reactions and require cautious in-hospital observation.

MARINE ENVENOMATIONS

Marine envenomations may result from a wide variety of both vertebrate and invertebrate organisms.

Invertebrates

Invertebrates include coelenterates (anemones, jellyfish, Portuguese man-of-war, soft corals), corals, cone shells, octopuses, sea urchins, sea cucumbers, and sponges. The sea wasp or box jellyfish, *Chironex fleckeri,* a coelenterate, produces the most lethal marine venom (it is deactivated topically by 5% acetic acid [vinegar]). Local problems related to envenomation or exposure include
• Lacerations (corals)
• Irritant and allergic dermatitis (coelenterates, octopuses, sea cucumbers, sponges)
• Local toxic injury (coelenterates, cone shells, octopuses, sea urchins, sponges)
• Infection (most commonly corals and sponges)
• Retained or occult foreign body (corals, coelenterates, sea urchins, sponges)
• Severe corneal irritation (after exposure to the excreted venom of the sea cucumber)
   Systemic reactions include anaphylaxis (sponges, coelenterates) and, in severe envenomations, paralysis, dysphagia, dysphonia, muscle cramping, cardiac arrhythmias, respiratory failure, coma, and death (coelenterates, cone shells, and octopuses).
   Local treatment includes foreign body removal, aggressive irrigation of any open wounds with normal saline, and antitetanus prophylaxis if needed; spicules resulting from sponge exposure can often be removed with adhesive tape and forceps. A wound culture may be helpful in patients with lacerations or deep abrasions. Patients with coelenterate or sponge envenomation benefit from an initial application or soaking of the involved area in 5% acetic acid (household vinegar) or isopropyl alcohol; this may be repeated as needed during the healing process. Hot water immersion of the site (up to 112°F) for 60 to 90 minutes may be symptomatically and therapeutically helpful in patients with cone shell, sea urchin, sea cucumbers, starfish, and octopus envenomations; this may be related to heat inactivation of the venom. Any visible spines should be immediately removed. Conjunctival irritation caused by sea cucumber venom is treated with normal saline irrigation. Local infection, which may be difficult to differentiate from local toxic reactions, should be treated with tetracycline or

trimethoprim-sulfamethoxazole; patients with extensive infections require admission and parenteral antibiotic therapy. Allergic or urticarial reactions are treated in the usual manner depending on the extent and severity of symptoms. Patients not requiring admission should be seen in 24 to 48 hours for a wound check.

Vertebrates

Vertebrates responsible for envenomations include the family Scorpaenidae (scorpionfish, lionfish, and stonefish) and the catfish, stingray, weeverfish, and the sea snakes. Local problems related to envenomation or exposure include lacerations or puncture wounds (catfish, stingray, and weeverfish); severe, local, toxic reactions (scorpionfish, lionfish, stonefish, and weeverfish); and infection. Stingray envenomations are usually associated with increasing discomfort, which may last for 48 hours; systemic symptoms result from envenomation and include fatigue, weakness, nausea, vomiting, diaphoresis, headache, vertigo, muscle cramping, seizures, hypotension, and death. Serious complications are also reported after scorpionfish envenomations; these include the lionfish (mild symptoms), the camouflaged scorpionfish (moderate to severe), and the stonefish (severe); symptoms are similar to stingray envenomation. The weeverfish occupies the Mediterranean Sea, the eastern Atlantic Ocean, and the European coast; stings occur when the fish is stepped on. Other venomous, stinging fish include the catfish (fresh and saltwater varieties), surgeonfish, toadfish, ratfish, and leatherbacks. Local treatment recognizes the heat-labile nature of most venom and includes immediate immersion in hot water (up to 112°F) for 60 to 90 minutes, which is followed by foreign body removal, antitetanus prophylaxis if needed, and copious irrigation with normal saline and povidone-iodine. Prophylactic antibiotics are not advised, but elevation and a reexamination in 24 to 48 hours should be recommended. Patients with fish stings, unless the species has been positively identified and is known to produce only local toxicity, should be considered for hospitalization for 24 hours; delayed symptoms, including respiratory, cardiac, and central nervous system depression, can occur. No antivenom is available for patients with weeverfish envenomations; treatment is supportive. Although infrequently required, stonefish antivenom is available for patients with severe symptoms; it may be obtained from the Health Services Department, Sea World, San Diego, California, (619-222-6363, extension 2201) or Sea World, Aurora, Ohio (216-562-8101, extension 2151).

Venomous sea snakes are found in Southeast Asia, the northern coast of Australia, and the Persian Gulf; one species is found in Hawaii. Most bites do not result in envenomation; diagnosis is based on the description of the snake, multiple "fang" wounds at the bite site, and the absence of an immediate local reaction. Systemic symptoms begin 30 minutes to 1 hour after envenomation and evolve over 8 to 12 hours. Signs and symptoms include muscle aching and stiffness, restlessness, difficulty speaking, ascending paralysis, myoglobinuric renal failure, seizures, respiratory distress, and coma. An 8-hour symptom-free period after the bite means that sea snake envenomation did not occur. The treatment for sea snake envenomation is pressure immobilization of the affected extremity (to prevent systemic absorption of the venom) and administration of polyvalent, sea snake antivenom. Antivenom is given after skin testing and can be given up to 36 hours after envenomation. All patients with sea snake envenomations should be hospitalized; antivenom is available from Commonwealth Laboratories, Melbourne, Australia. Tiger snake antivenom is an option if sea snake antivenom is unavailable.

PART 11

Selected Pediatric Emergencies

Child Abuse

INTRODUCTION

- Legally, the term *child abuse* has many definitions; it includes physical, sexual, mental, or emotional abuse and neglect. Practically, child abuse is diagnosed when the person responsible for the care or supervision of the child has injured the child or has failed to demonstrate a reasonable level of care or protection.

- In the hospital emergency department, it is estimated that approximately 10% of children younger than 5 years of age present with trauma as a result of abuse. Approximately, one third of abused children are younger than 6 months of age, and these children must be identified early if serious, permanent physical and emotional injuries are to be prevented.

- Laws currently exist in all states that mandate the reporting of **suspected cases of child abuse** to the appropriate protective state agency or local police department. Furthermore, these laws protect the healthcare professional from personal liability arising out of cases subsequently litigated and found not to involve abuse. This protection is present to ensure that a low threshold for reporting suspected abuse is maintained by all personnel and that abused children are therefore identified before further physical or emotional damage can occur.

- The causes of child abuse are multiple and involve factors related to the personalities of the parent and child, the family situation, and the emotional climate within the home at the time of the incident. Ninety percent of cases of child abuse involve parents who are neither psychotic nor sociopathic. Abused children are often unplanned and unwanted and may be perceived to misbehave consistently. The life of the parent or parents is often described as regularly punctuated by crises, usually involving lack of emotional support, economic difficulties, or failing relationships.

DIAGNOSIS

Physical Abuse

History
- The diagnosis of child abuse is often difficult and subtle and may come to one's attention as the family or patient reports the history of the injury.
- An undue delay in seeking care for a significant injury should raise suspicion of abuse.
- Explanations that are not compatible with the injury should raise concern of abuse.
- History of similar episodes or a reluctance to give a sufficient history may suggest abuse.

Physical Examination
- Certain physical injury patterns should raise the concern of possible abuse:
  - "Dunking" or scalding burns involving the buttocks and genitalia or the hands
  - Circular, pencil–eraser-sized burns usually occurring on the palms or soles or torso, resulting from cigarettes
  - Geographic, loop or circular, right-angled, or otherwise complex patterns of erythema or petechiae resulting from being slapped or struck with some object, such as a coat hanger or belt
  - Bruising confined to the back or buttocks
- Evidence of neglect as manifested by malnutrition or an unusual lack of care for the child's hygiene or disinterest in the child's medical care or needs
- The presence of multiple, healed fractures or bony deformities should raise the suspicion of abuse.
- Subdural hematoma, which often results from violent shaking, may be suggested by the presence of associated retinal hemorrhages. These children most often present with a reduced level of consciousness, seizures, or coma.
- Intra-abdominal injuries are also common, because small children do not know how to or cannot protectively flex the abdominal muscles before trauma (see Table 58-1).

Diagnostic Tests
- The laboratory serves to demonstrate normal hemostatic function in children with reported "easy bruising." A bleeding time, a complete blood count with platelet count, and prothrombin and partial thromboplastin times are appropriate and will confirm or exclude abnormalities of hemostasis.
- Children who appear calorically deprived or chronically ill require a CBC, erythrocyte sedimentation rate, urinalysis, chest roentgenogram, and measurement of blood sugar, BUN, electrolytes, calcium, and creatinine.
- Multiple fractures present in the child at varying stages of healing are a strong reason to suspect child abuse. In young children suspected of being abused, a complete skeletal survey should be obtained to address this question. Rib fractures are particularly suspicious in children; this is true because of the extreme resiliency of the child's rib cage and consequently the tremendous force necessary to fracture a rib or ribs. The Salter type 2 fracture, or the so-called bucket-handle fracture, is a relatively uncommon injury that results from major torsion or rotational force applied across a joint; abuse should be considered when this injury is noted—most often at the wrist.

Table 58-1	Signs of Potential Child Abuse

1. Emotional status
   a. Passivity of child, depression, and/or apathy
   b. Child has excessive fears
   c. Child frightened in presence of parent
2. Bruising, especially of
   a. Genitals (toilet training)
   b. Thighs (toilet training)
   c. Earlobes
   d. Cheeks (slapping)
   e. Neck (choking)
   f. Upper lip, frenulum, floor of mouth (forced feeding)
   g. Upper arms, trunk (grab marks)
3. Human bites
4. Strap marks (look for eyelet impressions and buckle marks)
5. Loop-shaped marks or scars (doubled-cord beatings)
6. Marks of gags (on mouth) or binding (wrists or ankles)
7. Burns
   a. Uniform circular burns (from cigarettes)
   b. Hot plate or radiator burns
   c. Scalding of buttocks
   d. Stocking or glove distribution burns
8. Multiple fractures in different stages of healing
9. Epiphyseal separations, metaphyseal chip fractures, corner fractures
10. Joint dislocations (other than "nursemaid's" elbow)
11. Posterior rib fractures
12. Hyperflexion/extension injuries of the spine
13. Signs of intracranial injury
14. Skull fractures
15. Retinal hemorrhage
16. Subconjunctival hemorrhage
17. Developmental delay

Mental or Emotional Abuse and Neglect

• Mental or emotional abuse and neglect may be suggested by the interaction between the parent and child or by the parent's description of the details of the accident. Neglect may be manifest as caloric deprivation, evidence of gross inattention to the child's medical or hygienic needs, or withdrawal or depressive features in the child's personality.

Sexual Abuse

• Sexual abuse is similarly difficult to establish because the actual episode may have involved fondling or oral contact, may have been remote, and would not be expected to have produced any physical evidence of abuse. Children capable of describing or demonstrating sexual abuses against them should generally be believed or taken seriously; this is true to the extent that the average child does not possess the intellectual or sexual experience required to fabricate such a history. Perpetrators often have close legitimate access to the child.

MANAGEMENT

- All children of suspected abuse must be reported to the child protective agency or the police.
- The child's pediatrician should be contacted and the details of the case discussed, and the intention to report the case formally as possible child abuse specifically noted.
- The emergency physician should then report the suspicion of child abuse by telephone to the appropriate state agency responsible for investigating such cases. The details of this interaction must be recorded on the patient's record.
- If the child is not thought to be at immediate risk of further abuse (i.e., suspected perpetrator is a teacher, neighbor, etc.) and the parents can provide a safe environment, the child may be discharged after appropriate contact with and input from child protective services.
- All children suspected of being abused and deemed at further risk of injury should be admitted to the hospital for further clarification of the extent of injury, for observation, and for the treatment of any injuries or nutritional abnormalities.
- The suspicion of child abuse should be raised with the parents. This should be performed in the hospital in conjunction with the child's pediatrician.
- Although no personal liability exists on the part of the physician or nurse who reports a case of suspected child abuse regardless of the outcome, the law is not clear with respect to physically preventing a parent from removing a child from the emergency department. The suggested approach, which initially avoids some of these issues, is to recommend admission, after which time the pediatrician, the emergency physician, a representative of the social service department, and the parents may then jointly discuss the injury, the formal suspicion of child abuse, and the absolute legal obligation of the physician to report those injuries not clearly explained by the details provided. Furthermore, hospital admission allows the parents to focus on the problem as it is perceived, and any counseling or emotional support required by the patient or the family may be initiated at this time.
- If hospital admission is refused by the parents and ongoing abuse is an immediate concern, the hospital administration, child protective services agency, and local police should immediately be contacted and a request made for emergency custody for protective admission.

59 Fever

INTRODUCTION

- Fever is defined as an elevation of basal body temperature above 38°C (100.4°F), when measured rectally, and has a multitude of causes. Infection is recognized as the major cause of fever in the pediatric patient. In addition, drug reactions, collagen vascular diseases, neoplastic processes, recent immunization, allergic reactions, heat illness, and tissue infarction all produce fever and must be considered in the differential diagnosis.
- The evaluation of the febrile child is dependent upon the child's age. Newborns and infants are less likely to have focal findings and are unable to relate associated symptoms. Older children will often have focal finding to guide therapy, and clinical impression is more reliable.

COMMON CAUSE OF FEVER

- Infection

OTHER CAUSES OF FEVER

- Collagen vascular diseases
- Drug fever
- Tissue injury or infarction
- Immunization reactions
- Inflammatory disorders
- Malignancy
- Heat illness
- Allergic reactions
- Thyrotoxicosis
- Hypothalamic injury
- Hyperactivity
- Factitious fever
- Malignant hyperthermia

ETIOLOGY

- Aside from the common causes of fever routinely handled in emergency practice and discussed at length in other parts of this text, several causes of fever produce no striking physical findings or laboratory abnormalities. Sepsis, bacteremia, and UTI are common bacteria infections that may cause fever without localizing findings.

- A young infant (<8 weeks) may have serious bacterial illness without any specific findings. Decreased feeding, irritability, excessive crying, or lethargy may be the only signs of sepsis. The infant may be pale and lethargic and have mottled skin or grunting respirations. Physical exam may not reveal any focal abnormalities.
- As the child ages, history and exam become more reliable. Changes in behavior, nuchal rigidity, and localizing signs become more apparent.
- In the non–toxic-appearing child 3 months to 3 years old, occult bacteremia has historically been a concern. The pneumococcal vaccine has lowered the risk of serious bacterial infection in this age group to less than 1%.

DIAGNOSIS

- The emergency evaluation of patients with fever includes a thorough physical examination, carefully noting the commonly overlooked sites of infection that include the gingiva and dentition, sinuses, perirectal tissues, and lower extremities.
- Basic diagnostic studies, including a complete blood count, ESR, and blood cultures, should be obtained in patients who appear systemically ill or who are immunocompromised.
- A catherized urine specimen should be obtained on all uncircumcised men less than 1 year of age and women less than 2 years of age without an obvious source of fever.
- A chest x-ray should be obtained when there are pulmonary signs or symptoms.
- If diarrhea is a prominent symptom, a stool smear for WBC and test for occult blood should be completed.
- Infants and young children present a special diagnostic problem in that meningitis must be considered in all such patients with fever, especially because of its often subtle manifestations in this age group: irritability, lethargy, poor feeding, and weakness. For this reason, one's threshold for performing a lumbar puncture in these young patients should be quite low.
- It should also be noted that discovering a clear source for a patient's fever never warrants neglecting the remainder of the evaluation of the patient; children with otitis media may also have meningitis, for example.

TREATMENT

- Specific causes of infection should be treated as indicated.
- Newborns and infants less than 4 weeks should be admitted to the hospital and treated with broad-spectrum antibiotics until sepsis or meningitis is excluded.
- Infants 4 to 8 weeks may be discharged after a complete sepsis evaluation if the workup is negative and the child appears well, and daily reevaluation can be assured.
- Infants 8 weeks to 6 months may be discharged if they are well appearing. Localized infections should be treated. Follow-up must be assured. Urinary tract infection must be excluded. Ill-appearing children must be admitted.
- Children 6 to 36 months may be discharged if they are well appearing and follow-up can be assured. Risk of occult bacteremia and serious bacterial infection is low. Ill appearance or excessive fever, persistent vomiting, or respiratory retractions require further workup.
- Acetaminophen 15 mg/kg or ibuprofen 10 mg/kg should be given every 4 to 6 hours to relieve the patient's suffering and minimize insensible water losses. Acetaminophen and ibuprofen may be alternated every 4 hours to treat persistent fevers.

Table 59-1	Dehydration in Children		
Signs and Symptoms	Mild (<5%)	Moderate (5%–10%)	Severe (>10%)
Tachycardia	Variable	Present	Present
Dry mucous membranes	Present	Present	Present
Depressed fontanelle	Absent	Present	Present
Sunken eyes	Absent	Present	Present
Abnormal skin turgor	Absent	Present	Present
Decreased urine output	Variable	Present	Present
Prolonged capillary refill	Absent	Variable	Present
Weak peripheral pulses	Absent	Absent	Present
Hypotension	Absent	Absent	Present
Hyperpnea	Absent	Absent	Present
Altered mental status	Absent	Variable	Present
Serum acidosis	Absent	Variable	Present
Urine specific gravity	Normal to high	Normal to high	High

- To decrease the possible risk of Reye syndrome, aspirin should not be given to children with viral illnesses.
- Fever-related dehydration may, in certain cases, become severe enough to require hospitalization and intravenous fluid replacement (Table 59-1).
- In children younger than 3 or 4 years of age, febrile convulsions may be of sufficient concern to warrant vigorous suppression of fever; this is particularly true when a history of febrile seizures is obtained or when temperatures exceed 40°C (104°F).
- When sponging is elected, tepid (rather than cold) water should be used, thereby decreasing the tendency for peripheral vasoconstriction to occur.
- Cooling blankets may also be used, which work by enhancing conductive heat loss. The physician must carefully monitor the rectal temperature so as to avoid producing hypothermia; use of the cooling blanket should be discontinued when the body temperature reaches 37.7°C to 38.3°C (100°F–101°F).

Pediatric Sedation

GENERAL CONSIDERATIONS

- The evaluation and treatment of patients in the emergency department often involve performing procedures that may be painful and/or frightening to the patient. Although older patients may be able to tolerate a certain degree of discomfort once given an understanding of the need for the procedure, pediatric patients, particularly in the preschool age group, may lack the ability to comprehend what is being performed. This may result in a lack of cooperation, fear of healthcare providers, and a sense of being betrayed by parents or other adults.
- The emergency physician should make every effort to allay the patient's fears and minimize any discomfort. Providing a soothing environment and reassuring, honest explanations of procedures can greatly reduce fear, even in younger children. In some patients, however, pharmacologic means may be necessary to provide sedation during a procedure. Anxiolysis, analgesia, and amnesia may all be goals of sedation. The agent, route, and dosing should be carefully chosen to meet the needs of the particular patient, procedure, and estimated time involved. Although some additional time may be taken in sedating and recovering a patient, improved efficiency and quality in performing the procedure can offset the additional time.
- **Minimal (Light) sedation** describes a drug-induced state during which patients respond normally to verbal commands. Although cognitive function and coordination may be impaired, ventilatory and cardiovascular functions are unaffected. **Moderate ("Conscious Sedation") sedation/analgesia** describes a drug-induced depression of consciousness during which patients respond purposefully to verbal commands, either alone or accompanied by light tactile stimulation. No interventions are required to maintain a patent airway, and spontaneous ventilation is adequate. Cardiovascular function is maintained. **Deep sedation/analgesia** describes a drug-induced depression of consciousness during which patients cannot be easily aroused, but respond purposefully following repeated or painful stimulation. The ability to independently maintain ventilatory function may be impaired. Patients may require assistance in maintaining a patent airway and spontaneous ventilation. Cardiovascular function is usually maintained.
- **The appropriate level of sedation/analgesia should be determined by the procedure being performed**

INDICATIONS

Consider using sedating agents for any pediatric patient who will be undergoing painful or frightening procedures during which nonpharmacologic means will not be adequate to relieve anxiety and discomfort.

- Young children and mentally handicapped or psychologically disturbed older children may not be able to comprehend the need for a procedure. Some patients capable of understanding may still be unwilling to cooperate for lengthy or particularly painful procedures. Even among those patients who can understand and are willing to cooperate, providing adequate analgesia and anxiolysis may still require sedation.

- Sedating agents should not be used in patients with altered levels of consciousness or in whom local anesthetics or oral analgesics can provide adequate relief of discomfort.

- Any procedure in the emergency department that causes moderate or severe levels of pain or anxiety may be an indication for sedation of the patient. Examples include burn management, wound debridement and repair, fracture/dislocation reduction, incision and drainage, foreign body removal, thoracostomies, and sexual assault examinations.

- Nonpharmacologic measures aimed at reducing anxiety and pain perception can be successful in young children and have the benefit of having few side effects. Procedures should be performed away from the normal background sounds and scenes of an emergency department, in an area containing pleasant images familiar to the child. A calm reassuring manner in which the physician explains the procedure in simple language with carefully chosen words can remove much of the fear of the unknown. Children generally have rich imaginations, and this can be used to suggest diversions, fantasies, or illusions that the child can control to reduce negative perceptions during the procedure. The presence of parents or familiar adults is reassuring, particularly to the small child, and should be encouraged even if it increases the anxiety of the healthcare provider in some cases.

TYPES OF AGENTS

- There are a variety of types of medications available that provide sedation. Primary sedatives reduce the patient's perception of stimuli or awareness of surroundings. They may also reduce anxiety, although that feature is not inherent in all sedatives. Primary analgesics reduce the patient's perception of pain but may secondarily cause sedation.

- It is important to select the appropriate agent for the patient and procedure. Pure sedating agents offer no pain relief, so analgesics or anesthetics must still be used for performing painful procedures even though the patient is sedated. If a single agent does not meet the needs for a given situation, combinations of agents may be used. However, side effects may be additive or synergistic in combination as well.

Sedatives

Benzodiazepines

Benzodiazepines are the most commonly used pure sedatives in the emergency department. They are also anticonvulsive and anxiolytic and cause skeletal muscle relaxation. Their primary untoward side effect is respiratory depression. Benzodiazepines can be reversed by giving the **competitive antagonist flumazenil** (0.002–0.02 mg/kg intravenous).

Midazolam

Midazolam (0.01–0.1 mg/kg intravenous, 0.2–0.7 mg/kg orally, intranasal) has a duration of action of 20 to 60 minutes, making it an ideal sedating agent for many emergency department procedures. The intravenous route is preferable for rapid onset and titration of sedation. Oral and intranasal routes for single-dose administration have longer time of onset and duration of action. The intranasal route can be associated with a burning sensation on administration. Midazolam also regularly causes amnesia aside from its sedating effects, which may be beneficial for children undergoing future procedures.

Lorazepam

Lorazepam (0.02–0.05 mg/kg intravenous) has a half-life of 3 to 24 hours and is not as effective for moderate sedation as midazolam or diazepam.

Diazepam

Diazepam (0.1–0.2 mg/kg intravenous, 0.3–0.5 mg/kg orally or rectally) has a duration of action of 1 to 3 hours intravenously and 2 to 4 hours orally, making it suitable for intermediate-length procedures.

Barbiturates

Barbiturates are sedative hypnotics. They also have anticonvulsant properties. They can cause significant respiratory depression and deep sedation, leading to loss of protective reflexes. There is no reversing agent currently available for these agents.

Pentobarbital

Pentobarbital (2–5 mg/kg intravenous) has a 30- to 60-minute duration of action. Sedation can be induced within 30 seconds by the intravenous route.

Methohexital

Methohexital (1 mg/kg intravenous, 18–25 mg/kg rectally) is an ultrashort-acting sedating agent with an onset of action within seconds when given intravenously and a duration of action of 10 minutes. Respiratory depression, deep sedation, and apnea can occur with this agent, and there are scant data reported on its use in the emergency department.

Other Sedative Agents

Chloral Hydrate

Chloral hydrate (50–100 mg/kg orally or rectally) has a duration of action of 2 to 3 hours and an onset of action of 20 to 30 minutes. It is used more commonly for scheduled procedures. It cannot be used in patients with hepatic failure.

Propofol

Propofol (0.5–2.0 mg/kg intravenous bolus followed by 0.025–0.13 mg/kg/min intravenous drip) has a very rapid onset and short duration of action such that it must be administered as an intravenous drip. It causes significant respiratory depression but also has antiemetic effects. Atropine can be used as a premedication to reduce secretions with this agent. Propofol has become a commonly used sedating agent in the ED for procedures lasting more than a few minutes.

Etomidate

Etomidate (0.1 mg/kg intravenous.) has an onset of action less than 1 minute and a duration of action of less than 5 minutes. It also acts as a respiratory depressant and may cause myoclonic jerking. Etomidate is widely used in the ED for both rapid sequence induction and for brief procedures lasting a few minutes or less.

Sedating Analgesics

Many nonsedating oral analgesics are available for treating mild to moderate pain. Narcotic agents should be used for moderate to severe pain relief either alone or along with sedation. These medications can be reversed with the **narcotic antagonist naloxone** (0.1 mg/kg intravenous). Naloxone has a duration of action of approximately 30 minutes, and this may be shorter than the clinical effect of the agonist agent it is reversing.

Morphine

Morphine (0.1–0.2 mg/kg intravenous, intramuscular, subcutaneous) has an onset of action of 20 to 60 minutes depending on the route of administration and a duration of 2 to 4 hours. Rapid intravenous administration can cause hypotension. Nausea and vomiting can occur as well, and antiemetics are frequently administered concurrently.

Fentanyl

Fentanyl (0.001–0.002 mg/kg intravenous) has a very rapid onset of action and duration of 30 to 60 minutes. Rapid intravenous administration may cause chest rigidity, requiring active respiratory support. Because of its short duration of action, **fentanyl used alone or in combination with midazolam** seems to be safe and effective for emergency department procedures when administered with proper monitoring and careful titration. Oral preparations have been developed and used in the preoperative setting.

Combination Sedative-Analgesic Agents

Ketamine

Ketamine (1–2 mg/kg intravenous, 3–5 mg/kg intramuscular, and 6–10 mg/kg orally) has an onset of action of 2 to 5 minutes by the intravenous route and duration of 30 to 60 minutes. It has analgesic, sedative, and amnestic properties. Ketamine induces a dissociative state in which the patient's eyes may remain open and staring, and there may be random nonpurposeful movements of the extremities. Protective airway reflexes remain intact, and bronchodilation occurs, making it a useful sedating agent for asthmatic patients. Another side effect, however, is hypersalivation, and atropine can be given as a premedication. Patients may have dysphoric emergence reactions with this agent. The incidence of this increases with age; therefore, the use of ketamine should be avoided in patients older than age 7. Low-dose benzodiazepines reduce the occurrence of emergence reactions. Ketamine may cause mild tachycardia, hypertension, and increases in intracranial pressure. Its use should be avoided in children with head injury, respiratory infections, congestive heart failure, or psychiatric conditions.

Nitrous Oxide

Nitrous oxide (30%–50% mixture with oxygen as an inhalation agent) has a rapid onset of action and short duration, lasting 3 to 5 minutes after cessation of administration. It can be administered safely with a demand valve mask held by the patient. It has analgesic, sedating, and anxiolytic effects. Nitrous oxide has minimal effects on the cardiovascular or respiratory systems. Side effects include light-headedness, nausea, vomiting, and excitement. Contraindications include altered mental status, pneumothorax, bowel obstruction, lung diseases, head injury, or facial anatomic abnormalities that preclude mask administration. Supplemental oxygen should be administered during the recovery period. Nitrous oxide use in children is well documented with few reports of problems. Use is limited in very young children who cannot self-administer the agent.

ROUTES OF ADMINISTRATION

Oral, intramuscular, intravenous, intranasal, inhalational, and rectal routes of administration can all be used for pediatric sedation administration, depending on the agent used.

Intravenous Administration

Intravenous administration allows careful titration of the agent, repeated dosing, and the most rapid onset and shortest duration of action. Obtaining intravenous access may be difficult, time consuming, and painful for the patient.

Intramuscular Administration

Intramuscular administration is used commonly but is more painful than intravenous dosing, causes more erratic absorption, and does not allow repeated dosing. For a single dose, it does allow more rapid administration than establishing intravenous access.

Oral Administration

Oral administration is probably the least uncomfortable route for the child. Not all sedating agents are available in oral form, however. This route requires the cooperation of the patient. Onset and duration of action are generally longer than by parenteral routes.

Intranasal Administration

Intranasal administration has primarily been described for midazolam. It does not require patient cooperation. Onset and duration are also longer than by parenteral routes but tend to be shorter and more predictable than by oral dosing.

Inhalation

Inhalation is only applicable to nitrous oxide for emergency department use. The demand valve mask allows the patient to self-administer the agent. Oversedation is avoided because the patient will not be able to continue using the mask. A scavenging unit must be a part of the system to avoid exposure of medical personnel to exhaled nitrous oxide.

Rectal Administration

Rectal administration is most applicable to very small children. Most agents have similar pharmacokinetics to oral dosing with the rectal route. Patient cooperation is not required.

MONITORING

Before Sedation

Children who are candidates for conscious sedation should be screened with a brief history and physical examination. Past medical history, allergies, current medications, last meal, current vital signs, and mental status must all be considered.

During the Procedure

Pediatric resuscitation equipment including sizes and doses for the age groups being treated must be immediately available in the emergency department. **Flumazenil and naloxone** should be present in the department if benzodiazepines or narcotics are being used. Physicians sedating children should be fully competent to conduct pediatric resuscitation including airway management. Monitoring of the patient throughout the procedure and during recovery is mandatory. Continuous pulse oximetry and either frequent vital signs or cardiac monitoring are needed. In addition to the physician performing the procedure, one other healthcare professional competent to observe monitors, vital signs, and mental status should be present throughout the procedure.

RECOVERY

Patients should continue to be observed after sedation until they return to baseline function. Objective parameters recommended include ability to follow commands, resumption of baseline verbal skills, ability to walk unassisted (in infants, sit unassisted), and return to baseline level of orientation. Patients should be discharged with a competent adult who has been given clear discharge instructions. Patients with prolonged recovery or complications should be considered for admission.

Foreign Bodies

GENERAL CONSIDERATIONS

Patients frequently present to the emergency department complaining of a foreign body or a foreign body sensation. Several general guidelines should be noted before discussing particular areas of involvement and the various methods of removal.

- Impaled foreign bodies, most often knives or other tools, that may have penetrated the chest or abdominal cavity, the eye, or the skull and are in place on initial evaluation of the patient should be removed only in the operating room. This recommendation is based on the probable tamponade or compression of severed vessels by the impaled object and associated hemorrhage upon removal.

- A foreign body incorporated into a laceration or puncture wound can be a vexing problem for the emergency physician. If undetected, such a foreign body can cause local infectious complications within 24 to 72 hours. Wood and glass are typical foreign bodies. Glass generally can be detected by radiography, but wood, unless it is painted with leaded paint, cannot. Ultrasound will frequently detect wood-based foreign bodies.

- Most patients who report a foreign body sensation localized to the soft tissues of the foot, hand, or fingers are correct in their suspicion; this is true even when the physical examination and radiographic studies fail to reveal a specific agent. In this setting, the physician should explain to such patients that blind dissection of the area without the ability to localize the foreign body accurately is rarely successful and may produce complications. These foreign bodies may require surgical extraction. Tetanus prophylaxis, if needed, a prophylactic antibiotic, crutches if a weight-bearing portion of the foot is involved, and consultation with general surgical or surgical subspecialty are all appropriate.

  - In contrast, foreign body sensations involving the cornea or throat are often misleading or inaccurate. Minor scratches or abrasions involving these areas are frequently responsible for the symptom, rather than a retained foreign body. After a simple corneal abrasion is demonstrated by fluorescein staining and any airway foreign body ruled out by radiologic and physical examination, reassurance and follow-up in 24 hours may be recommended.

- Occult foreign bodies must always be considered in patients presenting with unusual or infectious complications related to previous trauma. Children presenting with a foul-smelling discharge from the nose or the external auditory canal or with a recurrent or refractory pneumonia in the same anatomic location are prime suspects for an occult foreign body. Vaginal or urethral discharge or bleeding in the child should also suggest this possibility.
  - Similarly, patients presenting with local infection several days after suturing must always be questioned as to the nature of the original injury. If an occult foreign body is possible based on the history or if fluctuance is present, partial or complete suture removal, drainage, radiologic evaluation, and manual inspection of the wound may be indicated. Oral trauma with occult dental fractures may result in embedded dental fragments that may be diagnosed by lateral lip radiographs.
- The actual removal of foreign bodies that have penetrated the skin surface may require subspecialty consultation. What often appears to be a simple procedure, such as removing an embedded pin from the sole of the foot, may be both extremely difficult and time consuming. When removal is not straightforward or easily accomplished, early referral is appropriate.
  - Importantly, when infection is not present, removal is not urgently necessary. Consultation with the general surgeon and clear instructions for follow-up in 12 to 24 hours are recommended. If infection is suspected, however, removal should be undertaken as soon as possible.
- When foreign material is suspected, AP and lateral, soft-tissue films should be requested. Additional imaging with CT or US may be indicated.

SPECIFIC DISORDERS

Airway Foreign Bodies

History

- Patients with a foreign body sensation in the airway may report cough, pleuritic chest pain, dyspnea, or stridor or may be frankly moribund with severe hypoxia, cyanosis, and reduced or absent ventilatory efforts. Most alert adult patients who are able to speak will report that "something is caught" in the throat. Persons who are unable to speak will usually point to or grasp their throats. Airway aspiration is particularly common in children. This diagnosis must be considered in all children presenting with respiratory insufficiency or respiratory or cardiac arrest.

Physical Examination

In comparison to patients with esophageal foreign bodies, those with airway obstruction present with predominant respiratory symptoms and are able to swallow normally. Some diagnostic confusion may arise in children in whom relatively large esophageal foreign bodies may become impacted, producing tracheal compression and a presentation that often includes prominent respiratory symptoms, such as stridor, which typically began suddenly.

Diagnostic Tests

A lateral roentgenogram of the neck in such patients, if time permits, should demonstrate the foreign body lodged posteriorly in the neck. Compression of the tracheal air shadow posteriorly is noted and is an important diagnostic finding. Fluoroscopy, if available and if time permits, is similarly useful.

Treatment

Patients with suspected foreign bodies of the airway must be quickly triaged into either those with incomplete obstruction and adequate ventilatory function, or those without adequate ventilatory function. This latter group must be rapidly evaluated and managed in the following manner:

- A rapid Heimlich maneuver (abdominothoracic thrust) should be attempted and repeated once if unsuccessful; this may also be accomplished with the patient supine by exerting a similar abdominothoracic thrust. The pharynx should then be quickly visualized, and any foreign material that is freely movable should be manually extracted.

- The posterior pharynx should then be "swept" with the examining finger; material palpated deep in the posterior pharynx should not be removed without direct visualization unless its expulsion appears imminent. It is generally much wiser to use the laryngoscope gently, visualize the foreign body, and then proceed with forceps-aided removal. This approach will limit the tendency of such material to fragment or become further impacted in the airway. When foreign material is noted below the level of the cords, it may be possible, using forceps, to grasp and remove the material during expiration or cough, if the patient is alert, or during abdominal chest compression.

- If a foreign body is successfully removed, the upper airway should be inspected quickly unless normal and spontaneous respirations have been immediately and completely restored.

- When removal of a foreign body does not immediately restore normal ventilatory function, further resuscitative measures must be immediately undertaken.

- Material that completely occludes the airway, is distal to the level of the cricothyroid membrane, and is not accessible despite attempts to remove it must be displaced distally so that oxygenation may proceed; this is accomplished by placement of the endotracheal tube. In this uncommon setting, it is necessary in patients with life-threatening hypoxia to impact the material forcibly into one bronchus to the extent that the other lung may be ventilated; patients with more proximal obstructions that remain refractory to removal or displacement should undergo immediate cricothyrotomy by either needle or incision. In children younger than 12 years of age, needle cricothyrotomy is the treatment of choice and may be performed with a 14-gauge needle followed by pressure insufflation.

- In adults, when cricothyrotomy is unsuccessful, a 14-gauge angiocath may be rapidly inserted through the cricothyroid membrane and may provide adequate ventilation by pressure insufflation until a definitive airway is established. Patients without inspiratory effort obviously require mechanical ventilation. Surgical or incision cricothyrotomy is relatively contraindicated in children younger than 12 years of age, and needle cricothyrotomy should be undertaken when an airway is otherwise unavailable.

- In patients with adequate ventilatory function, oxygen should be administered, and the mouth, posterior pharynx, and chest quickly examined and radiologic assessment of the neck and chest undertaken. Foreign material identified by one of these maneuvers that does not significantly compromise ventilatory function may be removed laryngoscopically if present in the proximal airway. If the foreign material is localized more distally, subspecialty consultation is required for removal.

Foreign Bodies of the Ear and Nose

A variety of objects have been recovered from the auditory and nasal canals. Children may present with purulent drainage and pain in the nose or external auditory canal caused by the presence of a foreign body. Several points should be emphasized. When attempting foreign body removal from a child's ear or nose, two assistants are virtually always required except in the most trivial of cases. Procedural sedation may be required. Appropriate lighting and instruments are essential if removal is to be successful; a head lamp, a suction catheter, foreign body forceps, a pointed right-angle probe, right-angle forceps, and curved Kelly forceps are indispensable. The use of a nasal speculum to expand the visual field or the combination of an otic speculum and posterior-superior traction on the pinna in patients with aural foreign bodies facilitates both visualization of any foreign material and its removal.

- Many objects may simply be grasped with forceps or curved Kelly forceps and removed. Nonstinging insects may similarly be removed if adequately visualized. Stinging insects in the ear, however, should first be immobilized by instilling mineral oil or viscous lidocaine, after which removal is straightforward. The patient lies with the involved ear up, and several milliliters of fluid are instilled into the canal until it is filled. Several minutes later, the fluid and insect may be removed either manually or with the suction catheter. Objects within the ear that cannot be grasped because of their contour or location may occasionally be "floated" out of the canal with gentle irrigation provided the tympanic membrane is intact. This is accomplished by directing the stream of water above or to the side of the object so as to create a flow of water moving away from the tympanic membrane.

- Many small objects that are not otherwise retrievable from either the auditory or nasal canal may frequently be removed with a large-bore, rigid suction catheter connected to wall suction; the Frazier catheter works particularly well for this purpose.

- With nasal foreign bodies, care must be taken to avoid posterior displacement of these objects. Posterior movement of such objects associated with attempts at removal remains an indication for consultation. The pointed, right-angle probe may be very useful. Often, when the probe can be slipped either behind or to the side of the object, it can be gently nudged exteriorly. Furthermore, when the probe can be inserted beside the object and when the object can be penetrated, the point probe can be inserted into it and thus removed. An additional technique can be effective without instrumentation. Here, the physician gently occludes the unobstructed nare (without the foreign body), and a parent can then give the child a quick "puff" of air, orally, somewhat in "mouth-to-mouth" fashion. Although often requiring some "vigor" on the part of the parent, again while the unobstructed nare is closed by the physician, positive pressure generated in the nasopharynx often propels the foreign body exteriorly.

- Be cognizant of the possibility of multiple foreign bodies, particularly in children; a careful postremoval examination is indicated. Mucosal disruption may be noted, and a topical antibacterial ointment for 3 to 4 days is indicated.

Gastrointestinal Foreign Bodies

Pharynx

Fish or poultry bones are the most common pharyngeal foreign bodies.

Diagnosis

Sharp pain, often accentuated or changed in character with swallowing, is typical. The physical examination is usually normal unless the foreign body partially occludes the airway, in which case stridor or dyspnea may be noted.

Treatment

Patients presenting with symptoms compatible with pharyngeal foreign body should be triaged immediately and be seen as soon as possible.

- With the patient sitting at 75 to 90 degrees, the oral cavity and posterior pharynx should be carefully examined.
- Small, sharp objects may insinuate themselves into the recesses surrounding the tonsillar area and may easily be overlooked unless the examination is thorough and directed.
- Discomfort produced by objects located in the tonsillar recesses is often referred exteriorly just below the angle of the jaw.
- Foreign body forceps or a hemostat may be used to remove foreign bodies localized to this area. The deeper pharyngeal structures may be examined after topically anesthetizing the posterior pharynx, after which the tongue may be grasped with a dry sponge and pulled forward.
- Fiberoptic nasopharyngoscopy may then be used to examine the base of the tongue, the valleculae, the epiglottic area, and the pyriform sinuses.
- Once identified and well visualized, foreign bodies found in these areas may be removed.
- Often, otolaryngologic consultation is required for definitive removal.
- Minor scratches or abrasions involving these areas are important to note, because such injuries may be responsible for the patient's symptom.
- If radiographic studies are normal and significant symptoms persist, arrangements should be made for direct laryngoscopy by an otolaryngologist.
- Patients with improving or minimal symptoms in whom no evidence of foreign body is found and in whom no respiratory symptoms exist should be discussed with the otolaryngologist and arrangements made for direct laryngoscopy within 6 to 12 hours if symptoms persist.
- The patient should be instructed to return immediately if symptoms worsen or if respiratory symptoms occur.

Esophagus

Diagnosis

Esophageal foreign bodies produce localized discomfort that is relatively accurate with respect to localization; only foreign bodies lodged at the gastroesophageal junction fail to produce symptoms in that area and, instead, produce referred pain to the suprasternal notch.

- Fish or poultry bones or large, poorly chewed pieces of meat are the most common offenders. Patients with complete esophageal obstruction report drooling or immediate vomiting of ingested liquids or solids; substernal chest "tightness" or discomfort often occurs.
- Gastroenterology consultation for foreign body removal should be obtained before the administration of contrast agents, which may hinder later endoscopic removal. Cardiac ischemic pain must always be considered and excluded.
- If the diagnosis is less clear (drooling may not be present and patients may be able to tolerate liquids without immediate vomiting), anterior and lateral films of the suspected area should be obtained. Esophageal foreign bodies, if radiopaque, will be seen lying posterior to the tracheal air column. If these studies are unrevealing, a contrast study of the esophagus is indicated and should first be performed with meglumine diatrizoate (Gastrografin).
- If a perforation is not found, better mucosal detail and minute foreign bodies may be defined with a standard barium study.

Treatment

Objects embedded in the wall of the esophagus (such as pins, needles, or sharp bones) should be removed using fiberoptic endoscopic guidance.

- Occasionally, distal, nonpenetrating foreign material may be displaced by relaxation of the lower esophageal sphincter using glucagon, 1 mg given intravenously or benzodiazepines. Passage of the material into the stomach is signaled by the disappearance of discomfort and the ability to ingest liquids normally; solid material should not be given.
- In patients responding to glucagon, a referral for endoscopy should be obtained to exclude the presence of any obstructing lesions or abnormalities of mucosal contour. Endoscopy may be used to withdraw or push forward any nonpenetrating, obstructing foreign material, after which the esophageal mucosa may also be evaluated.

Stomach and Bowel

Patients with a suspicion of ingesting a foreign body include children, mentally disturbed persons, prisoners who allege ingestion, or persons involved in illicit drug trafficking. Persons in this last group typically ingest balloons, condoms, or packets filled with any variety of controlled substance, including opiates, cocaine, amphetamines, and barbiturates.

Diagnosis

Plain radiographs of the abdomen may confirm the diagnosis if the swallowed substance is radiopaque. To prevent artifactual radiographic information, prisoners purported to have ingested a foreign body should be disrobed prior to the radiographic study, should remain in the company of their escort during the evaluation, and should be re-examined just before the roentgenogram is taken. Objects taped to the skin or inside clothing that are not removed will appear superimposed on the abdomen and may result in substantial and unnecessary intervention.

Treatment

Treatment is dependent on the type of ingested material, its location, and its size.

- Most small, **smooth foreign bodies** will pass uneventfully through the gastrointestinal tract and will require only outpatient observation. Patients who are discharged should be instructed to return immediately if vomiting, abdominal pain, or gastrointestinal bleeding occurs. These patients may also be asked to examine the stool and note the passage of the foreign object; follow-up is indicated in approximately 48 to 72 hours or sooner if symptoms occur. Daily, serial films of the abdomen may be obtained but in asymptomatic patients are not necessary.
- **Disk batteries** typically contain lithium, mercury, silver, cadmium, zinc, or silver. Potassium hydroxide in high concentration may be found. All disk batteries can leak, and those containing potassium hydroxide or mercury pose significant hazards. When noted in the esophagus, this type of foreign body should be removed. If more distal, some specialists prefer expectant management, with close radiologic documentation of the intact battery's progress through the gastrointestinal tract. If rupture of the battery is noted, sequential determinations of blood heavy metal levels are undertaken followed by chelation therapy if indicated. If a **sharp object** has been ingested, surgical or gastroenterologic consultation should be obtained because endoscopic removal is the procedure of choice.
- With **suspected drug ingestion,** no real difference exists with regard to treatment between these and other patients ingesting a potentially harmful substance. When

balloons or condoms have been ingested and when dissolution or rupture of the container would result in significant toxicity (substances such as opiates, barbiturates, and amphetamines), endoscopic retrieval or whole body irrigation is necessary. Obtunded patients require intubation and endoscopic removal of the intact container or irrigation.

Rectum
Digital rectal exam should be avoided to prevent injury to the examiner or patient with potentially injurious/sharp foreign bodies. Plain film or CT imaging is required to define to object and its location. Anoscopic or vaginal speculum-guided removal of a distal rectal foreign body is relatively straightforward. A long Kelly clamp or ring forceps will prove most useful and facilitate removal. After removal, sigmoidoscopy should be performed to rule out intestinal perforation.

Ocular Foreign Bodies
See "Corneal Abrasions and Foreign Bodies" in Chapter 5 (p. 61)

Soft-Tissue Foreign Bodies
Diagnosis
Foreign bodies that penetrate the deep tissues of the neck, chest, abdomen, eye, or skull should be left in place and removed only in the operating room. A careful neurovascular examination and its documentation should be performed in all patients. This is particularly important in patients with gunshot wounds, in whom substantial damage to tissues and structures not in the obvious trajectory of the missile may be noted; urgent diagnostic and therapeutic evaluation is required. Vascular or neural injury requires urgent subspecialty consultation.

Treatment
Treatment depends on the nature of the object and its location. Extractions that are anticipated to be straightforward should be undertaken by the emergency physician. Lengthy attempts at foreign body removal should be avoided. The threshold for subspecialty consultation should be low.

   When evidence of infection is not present, semielective removal in 12 to 24 hours may be advised. Give clear instructions for 12- to 24-hour follow-up with a surgeon, anti-tetanus prophylaxis, and a prophylactic antibiotic. When an extremity is involved, elevation should be advised and crutches provided when a weight-bearing portion of the foot is involved.

Through-and-Through Puncture Wounds
Through-and-through puncture wounds or other injuries that are particularly deep require measures to reduce the risk of infection.
- With a **retained foreign body and a through-and-through injury,** particularly in the hand or foot, a high risk of infection exists and thus aggressive local and often systemic treatment is warranted. If possible, sterile plain gauze or umbilical tape may be tied with suture material to the smaller end of the foreign body and essentially "pulled through" the wound along the tract of injury; this will facilitate drainage over the next 24 hours and thereby reduce the risk of infection. A prophylactic antibiotic should be instituted and a reevaluation scheduled for 12 to 24 hours. With particularly infection-prone injuries, an initial intravenous dose of antibiotic may be helpful.

Fish-Hook Removal

Prior to providing anesthesia, neurovascular function must be determined and documented. With finger or toe injuries, a digital block with 1% lidocaine without epinephrine provides excellent anesthesia; in other anatomical areas, proximal field anesthesia is appropriate. If the hook is relatively small and not structurally significant and interposed tissues are thought to be present, **advancement after** local anesthesia is a simple effective technique. If the imbedded hook is curved, the hook may be grasped with a needle holder and provided that no significant neurovascular structures or bone is present in the projected path of the needle, the hook may simply be directed through the skin, completing its trajectory. The barb, after it passes through the skin, may be cut with wire cutters and the remainder of the hook removed in a retrograde direction. The cosmetic defect resulting from the exit site is usually trivial.

Such injuries should not be sutured; soaks three times per day, tetanus prophylaxis, if indicated, and early follow-up are advised. Prophylactic antibiotics may be considered in patients with injuries considered infection prone.

Urethral Foreign Bodies

Urethral foreign bodies should be suspected in the child presenting with urethral discharge, pain, or periurethral bleeding. In addition, some adult psychiatric patients and prisoners have self-introduced urethral foreign bodies and will give this history. Radiologic assessment will usually disclose the foreign object, which if visible or externally palpable may be easily removed. Care must be taken not to injure the delicate mucosa of the urethra. If removal is unsuccessful or if a suspected foreign body is not clearly delineated, urologic consultation is recommended.

Vaginal Foreign Bodies

- The removal of vaginal foreign bodies in **adults** is usually relatively routine and may easily be accomplished with a vaginal speculum and ring forceps or a Kelly clamp. The vaginal mucosa should be carefully examined after removal to detect lacerations or evidence of infection. Gynecologic consultation is indicated for repair of lacerations. Foreign body-related vaginitis may be treated with antibacterial vaginal creams.
  - Occasionally, tampons become lodged in the posterior fourchette. These can usually be grasped with ring forceps and removed.
- **Children** presenting with vaginal bleeding or discharge should be considered to have a vaginal foreign body until proved otherwise. Although many vaginal foreign bodies in children may be palpated on rectal examination, a pelvic soft-tissue radiograph may also be useful. Gynecologic assistance is often indicated to remove such objects, depending on the child's age and cooperativeness. Careful inspection of the vaginal mucosa and, in particular, the urethral meatus should be performed after removal of the object because urethral foreign bodies may cause similar symptoms and may be indistinguishable radiologically from vaginal foreign bodies.

62

Oncologic Emergencies

At times, oncologic emergencies may be the presenting complaint in a patient with a previously undiagnosed malignancy. The emphasis is on rapid diagnosis and initial treatment. Many patients with the conditions discussed will benefit from hospital admission. Early contact with the appropriate consultant or primary physician is often helpful.

COMMON ONCOLOGIC EMERGENCIES

- Superior vena cava syndrome (SVCS)*
- Hypercalcemia*
- Acute tumor lysis syndrome (ATLS) and hyperuricemia*
- Hyperviscosity syndrome (HVS)*
- Spinal cord compression*
- Neoplastic cardiac tamponade*
- Fever
- Neutropenia
- Increased intracranial pressure
- Deep vein thrombosis
- Pulmonary embolism
- Hemorrhage

SUPERIOR VENA CAVA SYNDROME (SVCS)

Epidemiology

Up to 85% of cases of SVCS are caused by malignancy. It is especially common in association with bronchogenic carcinoma, which accounts for 75% of cases, and in lymphoma. Central intravenous lines are the second most common cause. Most patients respond rapidly to treatment, and early diagnosis is important.

Etiology

The SVCS results when tumor growth in the mediastinum compresses the superior vena cava. This leads to venous hypertension in the head, neck, and upper extremities. Signs and symptoms are promptly relieved when treatment decompresses the superior vena cava. If thrombosis of the vena cava occurs, there is a poor prognosis.

Clinical Presentation

The most common symptoms of the SVCS are dyspnea (50% of patients) and swelling of the face and upper extremities (40%). Less common symptoms are cough, dysphagia, headache, chest pain, blurred vision, and altered mental status. Early signs include

---

*Discussed in this chapter.

periorbital edema and conjunctival injection. Later, the full-blown syndrome including thoracic and neck vein distention, facial edema with plethora or cyanosis, and edema of the upper extremities may develop. If left untreated, extrinsic vena cava compression may lead to irreversible thrombosis. This occurs in 10% to 20% of cases. Death may occur from intracranial propagation of the thrombus or from tracheal compression.

Differential Diagnosis

The differential diagnosis is relatively short and includes nephrotic syndrome, pericardial tamponade, and congestive heart failure. These can be differentiated by physical examination and basic ancillary testing.

Diagnostic Tests

Useful diagnostic tests include the chest x-ray and computed tomography (CT) scan of the thorax. Chest x-ray reveals a mass in almost all cases. There is often associated adenopathy, pulmonary parenchymal lesions, or effusion. The CT scan can provide detailed anatomic information about the location and extent of the obstruction. Upper extremity venous access should be avoided. Venous hypertension and low flow rates predispose to bleeding and thrombotic complications. Contrast venography is therefore also contraindicated. If venous access is necessary, it may be obtained through the lower extremity.

Primary Treatment

The primary treatment of SVCS is radiation therapy to the mediastinum. Seventy to eighty percent of treated patients will have a good symptomatic response within a week. Patients with lymphoma have the best response. Poor responders often have thrombosis of the superior vena cava. Chemotherapy is also used as a primary treatment modality in selected cases. The simple measure of elevating the head and upper body may provide significant relief of symptoms.

Prognosis

The prognosis for patients with SVCS depends on the underlying malignancy. Patients with lymphoma have better survival than those with bronchogenic carcinoma. The overall survival for all patients with SVCS is 25% at 1 year. Despite this poor prognosis, not all patients with the diagnosis of SVCS in the emergency department require admission. When the signs and symptoms are not severe and the underlying malignancy is known, reliable patients with access to timely and appropriate follow-up may be discharged. Patients who lack these characteristics require admission.

HYPERCALCEMIA

Etiology

Hypercalcemia is the most common metabolic emergency associated with malignancy. It is reported in up to 25% of cancer patients. Most cases are related to solid tumors, with lung (especially squamous cell carcinoma) and breast cancer being the most common. Many other solid tumors as well as leukemia and lymphoma have also been associated with hypercalcemia. The mechanisms by which malignancy causes hypercalcemia may include increased bone resorption at the site of metastases or increased osteoclastic resorption at sites distant from the tumor. The latter effect is mediated by tumor-secreted hormone-like substances. Hypercalcemia may therefore occur in the absence of disseminated malignancy.

Diagnosis

The earliest and most common symptoms of hypercalcemia are related to the gastrointestinal, renal, and neurologic systems. Central nervous system (CNS) effects include weakness, lethargy, fatigue, confusion and coma. Coma is especially likely when serum calcium rises rapidly. Anorexia, nausea, constipation, and nonspecific abdominal pain are common gastrointestinal manifestations. Acute pancreatitis is uncommon but does occur. Polyuria and polydipsia are often present. Bone pain may occur.

Hypercalcemia is usually diagnosed when clinical suspicion leads to laboratory confirmation. It is also a common incidental diagnosis when serum calcium is included in a panel of laboratory tests used for screening patients with nonspecific symptoms. Although the differential diagnosis is lengthy, malignancy and hyperparathyroidism account for 95% of all cases.

Treatment

Although the ultimate success of **treatment** for hypercalcemia depends on treatment of the underlying cause, emergency treatment is not dependent on the specific cause. The pace and nature of the treatment is dictated by the severity of the symptoms and the degree of elevation of the serum calcium. Associated fluid and electrolyte abnormalities such as hypokalemia and dehydration are common and must also be sought and treated. The general principles of treatment rely on correcting dehydration, increasing calcium excretion, and decreasing renal resorption.

The cornerstone of the emergency treatment of hypercalcemia is the induction of a calcium and saline diuresis. In mild cases, oral hydration may be sufficient. In more severe cases, especially when serum calcium exceeds 14 mg/dL, intravenous hydration with 0.9% normal saline is indicated. Electrocardiographic monitoring should be considered, especially when there is coexisting hypokalemia. The goal of saline administration is induction of a 200 mL/h (3–4 mL/kg/h) diuresis. After any dehydration is corrected, a loop diuretic (intravenous furosemide, 40–100 mg) may be given to promote diuresis and enhance calcium excretion. Serum potassium should be monitored even if the initial level is normal, because hypokalemia may develop secondary to diuresis. Fluid overload and hypomagnesemia are other possible complications of treatment that can be avoided with appropriate monitoring.

Forced diuresis is usually effective in beginning to lower serum calcium over a period of hours. Pharmacologic treatments that inhibit bone resorption of calcium are also an important part of treatment but require several days to be effective. Agents used include calcitonin, mithramycin, and diphosphonates. Hemodialysis is effective but is reserved for life-threatening cases.

Most patients with significant hypercalcemia should be considered for hospital admission. If the serum calcium is less than 12 to 14 mg/dL, the symptoms are mild or the patient is asymptomatic, no other significant electrolyte abnormalities are present, and discharge with close follow-up may be appropriate. Such patients should be considered for a regimen that includes oral hydration pending initiation of other treatment.

THE ATLS AND HYPERURICEMIA

Etiology

When hyperuricemia occurs in the setting of malignancy, it is most commonly in the context of the ATLS. In this condition, rapid cellular dissolution occurs soon after the initiation of chemotherapy, releasing large amounts of uric acid precursors. If the production of uric acid exceeds the excretory capacity of the kidneys, serum uric acid levels may rise rapidly. Underlying intrinsic renal insufficiency or dehydration makes the development of significant hyperuricemia much more likely. The ATLS is associated with multiple other metabolic abnormalities, including hyperkalemia, hyperphosphatemia, and hypocalcemia. Hyperuricemia may also occur because of rapid cell turnover in rapidly growing malignancies such as multiple myeloma or disseminated adenocarcinoma.

Diagnosis and Pathophysiology

Hyperuricemia is often asymptomatic. When symptoms occur, they are most often referable to the urinary tract. In less acute elevations of the serum uric acid level, nephrolithiasis may occur and present as classic renal colic. Chronic renal insufficiency may occur because of renal damage from interstitial deposits of uric acid. In the setting of a malignancy, especially in the case of recent chemotherapy, a patient who presents with renal colic or evidence of renal dysfunction should be suspected of having hyperuricemia. Relatively rapid increases in uric acid production may precipitate acute hyperuricemic nephropathy and acute renal failure. This occurs when uric acid crystals precipitate in the distal renal tubule. The low pH of the urine at this point decreases uric acid solubility and favors crystal formation. The resulting intrarenal obstruction may cause acute renal failure.

Serum uric acid may be elevated in a number of conditions not associated with malignancy. These include hereditary gout, hyperparathyroidism, sarcoidosis, renal failure, or as a consequence of long-term treatment with a variety of medications. Whereas hyperuricemia in these conditions is unlikely to cause acute renal failure, chronic renal failure, gouty arthritis, and renal colic may all occur. In any case, the immediate therapy of hyperuricemia does not depend on the primary cause.

Treatment

The decision to institute acute **treatment** of hyperuricemia depends on the serum uric acid level and the clinical situation. Serum levels more than 7 mg/dL carry an increased risk of gouty arthritis and renal stones but are often asymptomatic for many years. Levels greater than 13 mg/dL are associated with a high risk of nephrolithiasis and nephropathy. In the setting of the ATLS, any elevation of the serum uric acid level should be considered for aggressive treatment, and other electrolyte abnormalities sought and treated. Acutely, the primary treatment of hyperuricemia is the induction of an alkaline diuresis. The solubility of uric acid is increased in an alkaline environment. The goal of treatment is a urine pH greater than 7 and urine output of at least 2 mg/kg/h. This can be achieved by intravenous administration of a mixture of 50 to 100 mEq of sodium bicarbonate per liter of 0.25 normal saline. A loop diuretic (furosemide) may be added to promote diuresis. Allopurinol may also be administered to decrease uric acid production. If there is coexisting renal failure, hemodialysis may be required. Patients with symptomatic hyperuricemia or the ATLS should be admitted for treatment.

HYPERVISCOSITY SYNDROME (HVS)

Etiology and Pathophysiology

Normal blood flow in the microcirculation is dependent on a normal serum viscosity. Marked leukocytosis or elevation of certain serum paraproteins can result in the constellation of findings known as the HVS. The HVS occurs most commonly in the dysproteinemias, including the myelomas, Waldenström macroglobulinemia, and cryoglobulinemia. Leukemias are another cause of the HVS, especially when the white blood cell count exceeds 100,000. When the HVS occurs, microvascular sludging with resultant hypoperfusion in the retinal, cardiopulmonary, renal, and peripheral vascular systems and CNS is responsible for the observed signs and symptoms. The abnormal hemoglobin of sickle cell anemia also causes increased blood viscosity, and the pathophysiologic mechanism of painful sickle cell crisis is similar. Rapid treatment of the HVS is necessary to prevent irreversible ischemic complications.

Clinical Presentation

The most common clinical findings in the HVS are visual disturbances including complete, painless loss of vision. Physical examination may reveal retinopathy with exudates, microhemorrhages, and "boxcar-like" venous segmentation. A variety of CNS disturbances have been reported. They include headache, seizures, depressed level of consciousness or coma, and auditory disturbances. Congestive heart failure and myocardial infarction have been reported, as have peripheral vascular insufficiency and renal failure.

Diagnostic Tests

Patients may present with HVS caused by undiagnosed dysproteinemias or acute leukemias. A clue to the diagnosis may be a laboratory report of rouleaux formation on the peripheral blood smear or difficulty processing serum in an automated analyzer caused by increased serum viscosity. The diagnosis of the HVS rests on the measurement of an increased serum viscosity as compared with water. Water is assigned a viscosity of 1.0. Normal values for serum viscosity relative to water are 1.4 to 1.8. Symptoms related to hyperviscosity are likely when the ratio exceeds 4.0.

Treatment

In the presence of consistent signs and symptoms, a relative viscosity greater than 4.0 is considered an indication for emergency treatment of the HVS. Plasmapheresis or leukapheresis is used, depending on the cause of the HVS. As a temporizing measure, 1- or 2-U phlebotomy with simultaneous normal saline volume replacement may be used.

NEOPLASTIC PERICARDIAL TAMPONADE

Frequency

Neoplastic pericardial disease has been reported in up to 25% of patients with metastatic cancer at autopsy. Despite this, symptomatic pericardial disease is uncommon in patients with cancer. Although uncommon, malignant pericardial effusion with tamponade is a treatable, life-threatening emergency. Consideration of this condition is therefore important for emergency physicians.

Etiology

Neoplastic cardiac tamponade usually occurs as a consequence of malignant pericardial effusion. Bronchogenic and breast carcinomas, leukemia, and lymphoma are the most common causes. Many other tumors can also cause pericardial effusion. Tamponade from effusion may also occur in postradiation pericarditis. Tamponade without effusion can result from constrictive pericarditis caused by radiation-induced fibrosis or, more rarely, direct tumor involvement of the pericardium.

Diagnosis

The signs and symptoms of neoplastic or radiation-induced pericardial disease are similar to those observed in pericardial disease of other causes. Pericarditis usually presents as nonspecific chest pain. The classic pericardial pain pattern of pleuritic pain exacerbated by the recumbent position and relieved by an upright, bent-over posture also occurs. A pericardial friction rub is sometimes observed but is often transient or difficult to elicit. Patients may also report dyspnea or cough. These patterns are also seen in pericarditis associated with malignancy, but pain is reported less often than in other types of pericarditis. Electrocardiographic (ECG) changes of ST elevation in two or three limb leads and the lateral chest leads are commonly observed.

Malignant pericardial effusion is often asymptomatic until cardiac tamponade occurs, though it may be suspected when an enlarged cardiac silhouette is seen on chest x-ray. Cardiac tamponade caused by effusion occurs when a sufficient amount of pericardial fluid accumulates to raise the intrapericardial pressure and interfere with ventricular filling. This can occur when relatively small amounts of fluid accumulate rapidly or when large amounts accumulate over a long period. When compensatory mechanisms fail to maintain cardiac output, left ventricular end-diastolic pressure rises and circulatory collapse occurs.

Patients with pericardial tamponade may present with chest pain, anxiety, and dyspnea. With the development of hemodynamic compromise, the classic signs of hypotension, distended neck veins, narrow pulse pressure, tachycardia, enlargement of the cardiac shadow on x-ray, pulsus paradoxus, and muffled heart sounds are observed singly or in combination. Pulsus paradoxus is an ominous sign in pericardial tamponade and presages complete circulatory collapse. Nonspecific ECG findings are often seen, and low voltage is often observed. Electrical alternans may occur but is relatively uncommon, although specific for massive pericardial effusion. The most sensitive and specific diagnostic procedure is echocardiography. In the setting of a large effusion, right atrial or ventricular diastolic collapse is pathognomonic for hemodynamically significant tamponade and is both a sensitive and specific finding. An enlarged heart is usually seen on x-ray, but this is a nonspecific finding.

Treatment

When the diagnosis of cardiac tamponade is considered, **treatment** consisting of standard supportive care including intravenous access, oxygen, and ECG monitoring should be initiated. Inotropes such as dopamine or norepinephrine may be used. Even in patients with hemodynamic compromise, vigorous resuscitation may allow for temporary stabilization. Removal of pericardial fluid is a lifesaving procedure in cardiac tamponade. Pericardiocentesis may be performed with an over-the-needle catheter, which should be left in place pending a definitive drainage procedure. Performance with ECG guidance and/or echocardiographic monitoring may decrease the chance of cardiac damage. Removal of only a small amount of fluid (50–100 mL) may provide hemodynamic improvement. Subxiphoid surgical drainage may be performed under local anesthesia by experienced personnel. Radiotherapy, chemotherapy, or surgical pericardiectomy may be used to definitively prevent recurrence of malignant pericardial effusion.

Patients who present with pericarditis should be evaluated for the presence of effusion and tamponade. In the absence of a large effusion, outpatient management may be elected. Nonsteroidal anti-inflammatory drugs may be prescribed for pain. When there are signs of tamponade or a large effusion, the patient should be admitted.

SPINAL CORD COMPRESSION

Etiology

Spinal cord compression is a common, serious, and treatable complication of malignancy. It occurs most commonly in carcinoma of the lung, breast, and prostate. Cord compression occurs when tumor metastasizes to the epidural space or a vertebral body, extends into the spinal canal, and compresses the spinal cord. Lymphoma may extend from paravertebral lymph nodes through the neural foramina and thus cause compression. The lower thoracic spine is the most common site of involvement, accounting for two thirds of cases, followed by the lumbar and cervical regions, respectively.

Clinical Presentation

The initial symptom of cord compression is pain at the site of bony metastases, occurring in more than 90% of patients. Signs include weakness on physical examination, which is noted in 75%. Autonomic dysfunction, manifested as alterations in the pattern of urination or defecation, is present in 50% of patients at presentation. Sensory changes are less common, occurring in less than 50% of patients. The spinal level at which symptoms are noted depends on the level of the compression. Lower extremity symptoms are therefore more common than upper.

Diagnostic Tests

When the diagnosis of vertebral metastatic disease with or without suspected cord compression is suspected, plain films of the involved area should be considered. Tumor involvement is seen on plain films in approximately 90% of patients. Immediate MRI or myelography is indicated when there are signs or symptoms of cord compression. MRI does not require a lumbar puncture and provides superior anatomic detail. Because of the prevalence of multiple lesions, the entire spine should be imaged.

Treatment

Spinal cord compression may progress rapidly. Treatment should therefore be initiated as soon as the diagnosis is suspected. High-dose corticosteroids are given to reduce cord edema. A reasonable regimen includes an initial dose of dexamethasone (Decadron), 10 mg intravenous. In most cases, immediate radiation therapy should follow confirmation of the diagnosis by MRI or myelography. Most patients respond to radiotherapy, but surgical therapy may be indicated in selected cases to provide a tissue diagnosis or when maximal radiation has already been given. Patients with signs or symptoms caused by cord compression usually require emergency admission for diagnosis and management.

63 Pain Management

INTRODUCTION

Pain is the most common complaint in the emergency department. Prolonged, untreated pain may exacerbate ongoing conditions, and can generally be treated without obscuring signs or symptoms of underlying processes. Perception of pain can be modified by culture, by previous experiences with pain and by underlying emotional state. One patient may react intensely to a painful stimulus that elicits only a minimal response in another.

PAIN EVALUATION AND DOCUMENTATION

No truly objective means of measuring pain exists. The use of visual analog scales has been accepted as a means to quantify pain. The use of pain scales prompts recognition of painful states that require early intervention (see Fig. 63-1).

EMERGENCY DEPARTMENT APPROACH TO ANALGESIA

Agents with a wide margin of safety should be preferentially used, and patients should be evaluated for both the effect and any side effects, to ensure that harm does not outweigh benefit in the treatment of pain. Optimal agents should have a rapid onset of action and be simple and painless to administer.

Parenteral Opioids

Opioid analgesics are the agents of choice for many patients. Opioids act by binding with specific receptors in the brain, spinal cord, and peripheral nervous system. **Morphine** has a duration of action of 3 to 4 hours when given parenterally, is metabolized by the liver, and undergoes renal excretion. It has minimal cardiovascular effects at therapeutic doses but can cause decreased cardiac contractility and histamine release, resulting in vasodilation (arterial and venous), urticaria, and bronchospasm. It also causes decreased gastrointestinal (GI) motility. **Meperidine** should be avoided due to its many side effects. Lethal interactions can occur when meperidine is given to patients taking monoamine oxidase inhibitors. **Fentanyl,** a synthetic opioid that causes no histamine release or decrease in cardiac contractility, has a short half-life, which makes it excellent for procedures and is lipid soluble for rapid onset of action. High or repeated doses can cause muscle rigidity. **Hydromorphone** is very soluble, allowing small volumes to be used in injection. It has a duration of 2 to 4 hours when given parenterally and is also available in oral and rectal forms.

Oral Opioids

Oral opioids are indicated for moderate pain states. These agents undergo first-pass metabolism, so the doses used are often greater than parenteral doses of the same

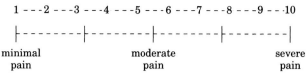

Figure 63-1. Visual analog scale for pain.

drug. They are often prescribed in combination with acetaminophen or a nonsteroidal anti-inflammatory drug (NSAID). **Codeine** has limited analgesic effect and is not a very potent analgesic. It often causes nausea and sedation but is an excellent antitussive. **Hydrocodone,** a synthetic analog of codeine, offers increased analgesia with decreased GI side effects. **Oxycodone** is a potent oral analgesic but causes more euphoria, increasing abuse potential. Oral preparations of morphine and hydromorphone are available. Morphine is available in long-acting preparations that are most commonly used in chronic pain states. **Methadone** has a long half-life and minimal euphoria and is most commonly used in treating opioid dependency. **Propoxyphene** has been removed from the market in the United States. However, toxic overdoses can cause seizures and respiratory depression.

Opioid Agonist-Antagonists

Opioid agonist-antagonists eliminate some of the negative effects of opioids but preserve their analgesic properties. This results in less respiratory depression, less euphoria, and less smooth muscle contraction but also limits the amount of analgesia. Agonist-antagonist agents should be prescribed with care in opioid-dependent patients because they can precipitate withdrawal. Specific agents include pentazocine (Talwin), nalbuphine (Nubain), butorphanol (Stadol), tramadol (Ultram), and buprenorphine (Buprenex).

Nonopioid Analgesics

Nonopioid analgesics include **NSAIDs** and **acetaminophen** (Table 63-1). They are most commonly used in the treatment of musculoskeletal pain. NSAIDS are anti-inflammatory as well as antipyretic agents that work through inhibition of prostaglandins and decreased production of leukotrienes. Adverse effects include gastrointestinal irritation, renal failure, anaphylaxis, and platelet dysfunction. Acetaminophen has the fewest adverse effects. Maximum daily dose is 1 g every 6 hours. Six hundred milligrams of ibuprofen provides the maximum analgesic effect. Doses of 800 mg provide

Table 63-1	Equianalgesic Doses of Common Nonopioid Analgesics
Drug	**Dose (mg)**
Aspirin	650
Acetaminophen	650
Ibuprofen	400–600
Naproxen (Aleve, Naprosyn)	250–500
Indomethacin (Indocin)	25–50

Table 63-2	Pediatric Doses of Common Analgesics	
Drug	**Route**	**Dose**
Codeine	PO	0.5–1.0 mg/kg
Morphine	PO	0.08–0.1 mg/kg
	SC	0.1–0.15 mg/kg
	IM	0.1–0.15 mg/kg
	IV	0.2–0.4 mg/kg
Fentanyl (in	IV	1.0–4.0 µg/kg
µg/kg)	PO[a]	10.0–15.0 µg/kg
Acetaminophen	PO	10.0–15.0 mg/kg
	PR	15.0–25.0 mg/kg
Ibuprofen	PO	5.0–10.0 mg/kg

[a]Fentanyl incorporated in a citrate matrix is available in candy form for ease of administration to children.
PO, orally; IV, intravenous; IM, intramuscular; SC, subcutaneous; PR, rectally.

increased anti-inflammatory activity without additional analgesic effect. **Ketrolac** (Toradol) is a parenteral NSAID. In chronic pain conditions, **tricyclic antidepressants** such as amitriptyline provide adjunctive relief. Gabapentin (Neurontin) is effective for neuropathic pain such as postherpetic neuralgia or diabetic neuropathy. Anxiolytics provide adjunctive relief when combined with analgesics.

Pediatric Doses

These are outlined in Table 63-2.

Miscellaneous Modalities of Analgesia

Acupuncture is used rarely for emergency department analgesia. Theories for its efficacy include inhibition of pain perception because of selective stimulation of other nerve fibers and stimulation of endogenous endorphin release. Hypnosis and distraction are two techniques that work by allowing the patient to focus attention on something other than pain. In hypnosis, a trancelike state is the goal, established by suggestion of pleasant images or thoughts. Distraction involves using media such as music, reading material, or biofeedback tapes to draw attention away from pain. Placebos are believed to inhibit descending pain channels and may stimulate endogenous endorphins as well.

Analgesics During Pregnancy

Acetaminophen is considered to be safe for minor pain. NSAIDs and salicylates are not recommended in pregnancy. Opiates may be used if benefits outweigh risks, for example, sickle cell pain crises.

64

Poisoning and Ingestions

GENERAL ASSESSMENT AND MANAGEMENT

Ensuring an adequate airway, appropriate gas exchange within the chest, and circulatory support as required is an initial priority.

Patients with a diminished level of consciousness or alteration of mental status should receive 50 mL of 50% dextrose in adults and 1 mL/kg for children intravenous (IV), naloxone, 0.8 to 2.0 mg IV, and thiamine, 100 mg IV. Naloxone may be repeated in 1 to 2 mg bolus every 2 to 3 minutes up to 8 to 10 mg, before narcotic intoxication is excluded.

In some ingestions, the administration of a specific antidote will be indicated. In others, decontamination of the skin or gastrointestinal (GI) tract, followed by specific measures to enhance excretion, should be undertaken if appropriate.

- History includes agent, time of ingestion, approximate amount of ingestion, route of exposure, and resulting symptoms. All sources of information should be sought (observers at the scene, EMS personnel, current and old prescription bottles from the scene, medical alert bracelets, prescriptions, hospital and clinic records, etc.). Patients with nonaccidental overdose may fail to reveal all of the agents ingested.
- **Physical examination** may be helpful in suggesting a particular agent or toxidrome. Blood pressure, temperature, pulse, respiratory pattern, skin (presence of needle marks, bullae, cyanosis, erythema, dermatographism, etc.), diaphoresis, respiratory and cardiovascular status, bowel sounds, the odor of the breath, and neurologic function should all be assessed. The neurologic examination should specifically assess mental status, pupillary size, focal deficits, deep tendon reflexes, the presence of nystagmus, and the gag reflex.
- **Routine laboratory assessment** in overdose patients generally includes pulse oximetry, a complete blood count (CBC), electrolytes, BUN, creatinine, blood sugar, anion gap, urinalysis, and electrocardiogram (ECG). History and clinical status guide further studies such as specific drug levels or toxicology screens.
- The regional Poison Control Center can assist in identifying particular agents, predict the anticipated toxic effects or severity of exposure, recommend further diagnostic evaluation, and help guide therapy. In most seriously ill patients, general and specific therapeutic measures must be undertaken before toxicologic confirmation of a particular substance. Toxicology screens vary by laboratory and detect limited types of ingestants.

  Qualitative determination of a substance may be sufficient to guide therapy. However, **quantitative levels** of some substances are required to treat specific overdoses (Table 64-1).
- **Skin decontamination** should be performed when percutaneous absorption of a substance may result in systemic toxicity or when the contaminating substance may produce local toxic effects.

Table 64-1	Intoxications in which Quantative Levels are Helpful

Acetaminophen
Arsenic
Carbamazepine
Carboxyhemoglobin
Depakote
Digoxin
Ethanol
Ethylene glycol
Iron
Lead
Lithium
Mercury
Methanol
Methemoglobin
Phenobarbital
Phenytoin
Salicylates
Theophylline
Valproic acid

Decontamination is necessary for corrosives, hydrocarbons, metals, salicylates, pesticides, cyanide, methanol, irritants (e.g., Mace), and radioactive isotopes (see Chapter 53).

Treating staff should take appropriate measures to prevent exposure, as directed by the agent. The patient's clothing should be removed and sealed in plastic bags. Involved surfaces of the skin should be washed at least twice with a mild soap and water. Particular attention should be paid to body folds, nails, and hair when appropriate.

- **Gastrointestinal decontamination**
  - **Emesis.** There is little evidence that the use of emetics (syrup of ipecac) improves the outcome of patients with toxic overdoses. In addition, the use of emetics can lead to adverse outcomes, particularly aspiration pneumonia. Hospital use of syrup of ipecac is not recommended.
  - **Gastric lavage.** If the patient presents within 1 to 2 hours of ingesting a significant toxic substance and is symptomatic (obtunded, comatose), orogastric lavage after endotracheal intubation, followed by activated charcoal with sorbitol added as a cathartic, is recommended. For an asymptomatic patient, emesis, lavage, catharsis, or activated charcoal is not recommended *unless* the patient is seen within 1 to 2 hours and there is evidence of the ingestion of large amounts of a toxic drug, in which situation activated charcoal is recommended.

    Contraindications for gastric lavage include the ingestion of caustics when perforation of the esophagus may have occurred or may be caused, the ingestion of hydrocarbons of low viscosity when aspiration may be caused, and the ingestion of glass or other sharp material.

    Small-diameter nasogastric tubes are not effective. Number 28- to 40-French Ewald tubes should be used in adults and number 16- to 26-French orogastric tubes used in children. After placement, the position of the tube is confirmed by passing air into the tube with a 50-mL syringe and listening over the stomach for "bubbling." If any doubt exists as to tube location and gastric contents cannot be aspirated, the position of the tube should be confirmed by x-ray before lavage.

For lavage, the patient is placed in the left lateral decubitus position, the stomach emptied as completely as possible by aspiration, and normal saline or tap water instilled into and then suctioned out of the stomach. Aliquots should be 200 to 300 mL in adults and 50 to 100 mL in children. Lavage is continued until the return is clear or, if the initial return is clear, after 2 L of solution has been used. The first 100 mL of lavage solution or gastric aspirate should be separately collected for toxicologic analysis.

- **Activated charcoal** should be considered unless specifically contraindicated. **Activated charcoal is relatively contraindicated when** an oral antidote or endoscopy will be used (e.g., ingestions of caustics). In adults, the dose of activated charcoal is 1 g/kg with a minimum dose of 30 g; the dose in children is 1 g/kg. The method of administration is to dilute the appropriate amount of activated charcoal in approximately four parts of water or sorbitol. The slurry is then instilled by the lavage tube or given to the awake patient orally. Patients with vomiting should be controlled with ondansetron prior to attempting charcoal administration. Activated charcoal is tasteless but has an unpleasant appearance and gritty texture. Toxic ingestions with drugs having an enterohepatic circulation, such as theophyllines, phenobarbital, the tricyclic antidepressants (TCAs), the phenothiazines, and digitalis, generally require that activated charcoal be readministered every 4 to 6 hours to limit reabsorption during recirculation. The administration of multiple doses of charcoal has also been reported to be effective in dapsone, digitoxin, salicylates, phenytoin, propoxyphene, carbamazepine, phenylbutazone, nadolol, and meprobamate overdoses. Activated charcoal does *not* adsorb simple alcohols such as ethanol or methanol; strong acids or bases; or simple ions such as iron, lithium, or cyanide (Table 64-2).
- **Cathartics** are **contraindicated** in infants, in patients receiving an oral antidote, and in patients with adynamic ileus, severe diarrhea, intestinal obstruction, abdominal trauma, or recent abdominal surgery. Magnesium-containing cathartics are contraindicated with renal failure or when the ingested substance is likely to be associated with renal injury. Sodium sulfate should not be given to patients with hypertension, significant left ventricular dysfunction, or congestive heart failure.

Laxatives should not be used for catharsis, because activated charcoal may bind these agents and render them ineffective. Adults may be given magnesium citrate, sorbitol (150 g maximum), or sodium phosphate, 15 to 30 mL diluted 1:4 with water. Children may be given magnesium citrate, 4 mL/kg. Sorbitol is also probably safe in children; however, sodium phosphate should not be given because of the probability of severe electrolyte imbalances.

- **Enhanced elimination.** Acceleration of elimination by diuresis, dialysis, or hemoperfusion may be useful therapeutic options in specific ingestions. An important measure of a particular drug's ability to be actively eliminated is its **volume of distribution** (V_d), which is conceptualized as the hypothetical volume of body water that *would be* required to contain the amount of drug ingested at the same concentration as that found in the blood. V_d is expressed in liter per kilogram and is defined for each particular substance. In general, V_d is a measure of whether a drug is highly

Table 64-2	Activated Charcoal Absorption of Commonly Encountered Drugs and Toxins

Well absorbed	*Moderately absorbed*
Amphetamines	Acetaminophen
Antidepressants	Benzene
Antiepileptics	DDT
Antihistamines	Disopyramide
Atropine	Kerosene
Barbiturates	Malathion
β-Blockers	Mexiletine
Cimetidine	Nonsteroidal anti-inflammatory drugs
Digitalis preparations	Phenol
Ergot alkaloids	Tolbutamide/chlorpropamide
Furosemide	*Poorly absorbed*
Glutethimide	Acids, strong
Indomethacin	Alkalis, strong
Meprobamate	Cyanide
Opioids	Ethanol
Phenothiazines	Ethylene glycol
Phenylbutazone	Iron
Phenylpropanolamine	Lithium
Quinidine	Methanol
Strychnine	
Tetracycline	
Theophylline	

tissue soluble (large V_d) or remains confined within the vascular compartment (small V_d). A substance with a large V_d, therefore widely distributed within tissues, is not very amenable to diuresis, dialysis, or hemoperfusion. Conversely, a substance with a small V_d, therefore relatively confined within the vascular space, may be amenable to enhanced elimination by one of these techniques.

• **Diuresis.** Forced diuresis may enhance elimination of a drug if excretion is primarily renal and if the substance is polar and has a relatively small V_d with little protein binding. Forced diuresis is accomplished by establishing a urinary flow rate of 5 to 7 mL/kg/h using IV supplemental solute, such as 0.45% normal saline and spaced boluses of furosemide (20 mg). Forced diuresis is contraindicated in patients with hypotension and pulmonary edema. Serum electrolytes must be monitored because both hyponatremia and hypokalemia may develop; in addition, mannitol may induce hyperosmolality. The total dose of mannitol, if this agent is chosen, should never exceed 300 g, and in most patients, 20 to 100 g is sufficient.

• **Alkaline diuresis.** Alkalinization of the urine promotes the ionization of weak acids, thereby preventing their reabsorption by the kidney and thus facilitating elimination. Alkaline diuresis is useful for toxic amounts of the long-acting barbiturates (phenobarbital, mephobarbital, primidone), salicylates, lithium, and isoniazid.

Alkaline diuresis is accomplished by giving adults 1 ampule of sodium bicarbonate ($NaHCO_3$) IV, followed by a constant infusion of 1 to 2 ampules of $NaHCO_3$ in 1 L of 0.25% to 0.45% normal saline to maintain the urine at the desired pH of approximately 7.3 to 8.5. Furosemide should be given concomitantly, along with supplemental solute such as 0.45% normal saline, to increase urine output to approximately 5 to 7 mL/kg/h. Complications of alkaline diuresis include metabolic alkalosis, hypernatremia, hyperosmolality, and fluid retention. In salicylate intoxication, which frequently is accompanied by dehydration, the patient must be rehydrated before the institution of forced alkaline diuresis, and dextrose should be included in the infusion.

- **Acid diuresis.** Acidification of the urine may enhance the elimination of weak bases by way of the mechanism noted in "Gastric Lavage" discussed under the section "General Assessment and Management." Substances optimally excreted should have a small V_d, little protein binding, and be excreted primarily by the kidney.

- **Dialysis.** Hemodialysis has an important but limited role in the active elimination of intoxicating substances. The ability of a particular substance to be dialyzed depends on a number of factors including its molecular weight, lipid solubility, Vd, extent of plasma protein binding, and the ability of a concentration gradient to be maintained in the dialysate.

  Immediate dialysis is indicated for patients ingesting toxic amounts of ethylene glycol, methanol, and paraquat. When other substances amenable to dialysis are involved (e.g., theophylline, lithium, the salicylates, the long-acting barbiturates, bromide, and ethanol), indications for dialysis include severe intoxication with progressive deterioration despite intensive supportive therapy or significant impairment of excretory function.

- **Hemoperfusion** is a technique in which anticoagulated blood is passed through a column containing activated charcoal or resin particles. Although many of the same physical limitations of hemodialysis apply to the ability of a substance to be successfully removed by hemoperfusion, such factors as lipid solubility and molecular weight are circumvented.

  Hemoperfusion should be considered for severe intoxications unresponsive to intensive supportive care with barbiturates, glutethimide, methaqualone, ethchlorvynol, meprobamate, chloral hydrate, and certain other agents.

  Complications of hemoperfusion include platelet depletion; reduction of plasma calcium, glucose, and fibrinogen; and transient leukopenia. Hemoperfusion cannot correct electrolyte abnormalities.

- **Exchange transfusions.** Exchange blood transfusions are used principally in the treatment of severe poisonings involving hemolysins and methemoglobinemia.

- **Immunotherapy.** The recent introduction of digoxin-specific antibody fragments has proved successful in treating patients with serious digoxin toxicity. Hyperimmune antisera are available for the treatment of certain snake and arthropod envenomations.

- **Antidotes** are important with specific ingestions. Very few substances have specific antidotes. Antidotes reverse the physiologic effects of specific substances through a variety of differing mechanisms. Although some antidotes are nontoxic, others can cause severe toxic effects if used improperly. Table 64-3 lists a variety of substances and their specific antidotes. Details regarding the use of each antidote are further discussed under the management of specific ingestions.

Table 64-3   Antidotes Used in the Emergency Department

Toxin	Antidote	Dose and Comments
Organophosphates and carbamates	Atropine	Test dose 1–2 mg IV in adults, 0.03 mg/kg in children; titrate to drying of pulmonary secretions.
Arsenic, mercury, and lead	BAL	3–5 mg/kg intramuscular only
Tricyclics	Bicarbonate	44–88 mEq in adults; 1–2 mEq/kg in children; best used by slow IV push.
Calcium channel blockers	Calcium	1 g calcium chloride IV in adults; 20–30 mg/kg per dose in children, over a few minutes with continuous monitoring.
Rattlesnake bite	*Crotalidae* antivenom	Five vials minimum dose, by infusion in normal saline, at increasing rate dependent on patient tolerance; may cause anaphylaxis.
Serotonin syndrome	Cyproheptadine	4 mg orally as needed; no parenteral form available; antidote may cause anticholinergic findings.
Iron	Deferoxamine	15 mg/kg/h IV; higher doses reported to be safe.
Digitalis glycosides	Digoxin-specific FAB fragments	10–20 vials if patient in ventricular fibrillation; otherwise, dose is based on serum digoxin concentration or amount ingested.
Lead	DMSA	Reported useful for arsenic as well; one 100 mg capsule per 10 kg body weight three times daily for 1 wk and then twice daily with chelation breaks.
Arsenic, lead, and mercury	D-Penicillamine	20–40 mg/kg/d; 500 mg three times daily in adults; may cross-react with penicillin in allergic patients.
Methanol and ethylene glycol	Ethanol	Loading dose 10mL/kg of 10%; maintenance dose of 0.15 mL/kg/h of 10%; double rate during dialysis.
	Fomepizole	15 mg/kg IV and then 10 mg/kg q12h.

Benzodiazepines	Flumazenil	0.2 mg, then 0.3 mg, and then 0.5 mg; not to be used if patient has signs of TCA toxicity; only if necessary to prevent need for intubation.
Methanol	Folate or leucovorin	50 mg intravenously every 4 h in adults with serious toxicity.
β-blockers and calcium channel blockers	Glucagon	5–10 mg in adults and then infusion of same dose per hour.
Black widow spider bite	Latrodectus antivenom	One vial, by slow IV infusion, usually curative; may cause anaphylaxis.
Methemoglobin-forming agents	Methylene blue	1–2 mg/kg IV; 1% solution (10 mg/mL) give 0.1–0.2 mL/kg. 100 mg is a common initial adult dose (100 kg).
Acetaminophen	N-acetylcysteine	140 mg/kg and then 70 mg/kg every 4 h; IV form available.
Opiates	Nalmefene	2 mg; much longer half-life than naloxone.
Opiates	Naloxone	2 mg; less to avoid narcotic withdrawal, more if inadequate response; same dose in children.
Anticholinergics	Physostigmine	1–2 mg IV in adults, 0.5 mg in children over 2 min for anticholinergic delirium, seizures or dysrhythmias.
Organophosphates and carbamates	Protopam	Loading dose 1–2 g IV in adults; 25–50 mg/kg in children; adult maintenance 500 mg/h or 1–2 g every 4–6 h.
Isoniazid, hydrazine, and monomethylhydrazine	Pyridoxine	5 g in adults, 1 g in children, if ingested dose unknown; antidote may cause neuropathy.
Ethylene glycol	Pyridoxine	100 mg IV daily
Cyanide, H_2S	Sodium nitrate (antidote kit)	10 mL of 3% (300 mg; 1 ampule) in adults; 0.33 mL/kg in children, slowly IV.
Cyanide	Sodium thiosulfate	50 mL of 25% (12.5 g; 1 ampule) in adults; 1.65 mL/kg in children, IV.
Ethylene glycol, chronic ethanol	Thiamine	100 mg IV

SPECIFIC AGENTS

Central Nervous System Depressants

Benzodiazepines

Numerous benzodiazepines (e.g., diazepam [Valium], oxazepam [Serax], chlordiazepoxide [Librium], clorazepate [Trauxene], lorazepam [Ativan], prazepam [Centrax]) are available and widely prescribed for anxiolytic, muscle relaxant, anticonvulsant, and hypnotic properties. Benzodiazepines have a wide therapeutic index, and death caused by an isolated oral ingestion of any benzodiazepine is rare if at all existent. The benzodiazepines are metabolized by demethylation or conjugation or both. Demethylation occurs slowly in the liver, and many of the resulting metabolites are active. Conjugation occurs rapidly and primarily leads to inactive metabolites. Individual differences among the benzodiazepines generally result from the type of biotransformation the drug undergoes and the presence, number, and biologic activity of metabolites. GI absorption is rapid and nearly complete, whereas absorption after intramuscular injection is erratic and incomplete; lorazepam is an exception to the latter.

Clinical Presentation

Symptoms and physical findings of intoxication include drowsiness, ataxia, nystagmus, dysarthria, coma, and occasionally paradoxical irritability, excitation, or delirium. Although oral overdoses rarely result in severe respiratory or cardiovascular depression, IV overdose is associated with a mortality of 2%; death occurs secondary to respiratory or cardiac arrest. Major ingestions of the benzodiazepines usually result in light coma; more profound depression in neurologic, cardiovascular, and respiratory function is virtually always the result of mixed ingestions most often including ethanol. Ingestions of triazolam (Halcion; 10-times the therapeutic dose) is an exception in that nonfatal apnea has been reported.

Laboratory Findings

Qualitative toxic screens usually reveal the presence of all the benzodiazepines except for clonazepam (Klonopin), which requires gas chromatography; quantitative levels are not useful in predicting clinical toxicity.

Treatment

Treatment consists of charcoal only if extremely large amounts have been ingested within 1 hour, and conservative support as needed. Hemodialysis, hemoperfusion, and diuresis are not effective.

Flumazenil is the antidote for unstable benzodiazepine overdoses. Flumazenil acts as a benzodiazepine receptor antagonist. In adults, give 0.2 mg by IV infusion over 30 seconds. If there is no response, give an additional 0.3 mg over 30 seconds. Thereafter, 0.5-mg doses can be given at 60-second intervals up to a total dose of 3 mg. The usual effective dose is 1 to 3 mg. The drug is not recommended in children and is contraindicated in mixed overdoses because seizures are likely.

Withdrawal

Withdrawal syndromes from chronic benzodiazepine use are similar to those associated with ethanol and the barbiturates but are less severe and less frequent. Seizures have been reported up to 12 days after abstinence, and neonatal withdrawal may produce seizures 2 to 6 days after delivery. Treatment consists of the reinstitution of the agent, intravenously if required, to terminate seizures, followed by its gradual withdrawal; phenobarbital may alternatively be used.

Meprobamate

Meprobamate (Equanil, Miltown) is a sedative hypnotic rarely prescribed or ingested. The reader is referred to the regional Poison Center.

Chloral Hydrate

Chloral hydrate, a halogenated hydrocarbon, is one of the oldest sedative-hypnotic agents still available. It is rapidly absorbed and quickly metabolized within the liver, kidney, and red blood cells. Its half-life is only a few minutes; however, an active metabolite, **trichloroethanol** (TCE), has a half-life of 4 to 14 hours, is highly lipid soluble, and is widely distributed. TCE is formed by the action of hepatic alcohol dehydrogenase on chloral hydrate. The concomitant ingestion of ethanol therefore markedly alters the metabolism of chloral hydrate, resulting in earlier and higher peaking of TCE levels. This combination of ethanol and chloral hydrate has been referred to as "knock-out drops" or a "Mickey Finn."

Laboratory Findings

Laboratory findings may include evidence of hepatic and renal injury. Toxicology specimens should be sent specifically to determine the presence of TCE, since chloral hydrate is not detected in blood. The lethal dose is quite variable (3–36 g); known lethal serum levels are 5 to 10 mg/dL.

Clinical Presentation

Symptoms of intoxication progress from mild sedation, incoordination, and ataxia, to stupor and coma. Respiratory depression, hypotension, and hypothermia occur in severe intoxications; the pupils are initially constricted, but later mydriasis is seen. Similar to other halogenated hydrocarbons, chloral hydrate depresses myocardial contractility and shortens the refractory period, producing cardiac arrhythmias and sudden cardiac arrest. The corrosive effects of chloral hydrate and TCE have produced esophagitis with stricture, hemorrhagic gastritis with necrosis, and enteritis.

Treatment

Treatment consists of the standard intensive support measures. Lavage is useful only if initiated soon after ingestion, activated charcoal may prevent absorption of any remaining drug, and oral demulcents (soothing agents) may be given to reduce GI tract irritation. Lidocaine will effectively suppress ventricular arrhythmias. Close observation for GI bleeding should be instituted initially. Hemodialysis and hemoperfusion are effective and may be indicated for patients with significant intoxications.

Dependence and Addiction

Dependence and addiction may occur in chronic users. A syndrome similar to ethanol withdrawal occurs with delirium and convulsions; mortality is high when the syndrome is unrecognized. Phenobarbital may be used to manage withdrawal symptoms.

Ethchlorvynol

Ethchlorvynol (Placidyl) is a hypnotic, rarely prescribed or presenting as a toxic ingestion. Refer to the regional Poison Center.

Methaqualone

Methaqualone, prescribed under the names Quaalude and Sopor, is not commercially available in the United States but occasionally appears on the black market. It was formerly a sedative hypnotic. It bears similarity to current "date-rape" drugs. Consult the regional Poison Center.

Hemoperfusion may be effective with severe intoxication (blood levels more than 10 mg/dL) unresponsive to conservative management.

Narcotic Analgesics

A tremendous variety of narcotic and non-pharmaceutical agents are available that may result in overdose. Overdoses are usually due to inadvertent excessive ingestion, not intentional overdose.

- **Clinical presentation.** Central nervous system (CNS) and respiratory depression (including coma and respiratory failure), noncardiogenic pulmonary edema, hypothermia, miosis, bradycardia, hypotension, and decreased GI tract motility are characteristic narcotic toxicity. These findings occur within minutes of an IV dose and within 20 to 30 minutes of oral ingestion. Typically, the respiratory depressant effects are longer lived than the analgesic effects of many of the narcotics and specific respiratory effects. Meiosis may be absent with meperidine overdose and may be absent hypoxemia. Death is due to respiratory depression.

- **Laboratory studies** should be guided by clinical status. Toxicology specimens may be sent for qualitative analysis.

- **Pentazocine, propoxyphene,** or **Lomotil** may present differently from other narcotics. Pentazocine is more likely to cause dysphoria, delusions, and hallucinations. Hypertension, tachycardia, flushing, chills, and diaphoresis are seen. Propoxyphene frequently causes seizures and cardiac rhythm dysrhythmias. Concomitant ethanol ingestion may greatly increase toxicity. Death is due to cardiac and respiratory arrest. Lomotil intoxication, especially in children, is characteristically biphasic. The first phase, due to anticholinergic effects of atropine, is marked by hyperpyrexia, flushing, hallucinations, lethargy, urinary retention, and tachycardia. After 3 hours, the characteristic findings of narcotic intoxication dominate the clinical picture.

- **Treatment** of narcotic overdose includes IV administration of naloxone, a specific opiate antagonist. There are no contraindications. A period of close in-hospital observation of respiratory status is also indicated. The IV administration of **naloxone** rapidly restores CNS and cardiopulmonary function in patients intoxicated with a narcotic agent; onset of action is 1 to 2 minutes when given intravenously with an effect lasting up to 60 to 90 minutes. Naloxone may be given subcutaneously, intramuscularly, sublingually, or by endotracheal tube if venous access cannot be established. In adults, the recommended dose is 0.8 to 2.0 mg every 5 minutes up to 10 mg, and 0.01 to 0.1 mg/kg in children. Patients ingesting toxic amounts of propoxyphene may initially require extremely large doses of naloxone. Importantly, when only a *partial response to naloxone occurs,* other coexisting factors such as a mixed overdose, hypoglycemia, head trauma, Wernicke encephalopathy, hypoxia, or posthypoxic encephalopathy should be considered.

Because the half-life of many narcotic agents is significantly longer than that of naloxone ($T_{1/2}$ = approximately 1 hour after IV or endotracheal tube administration), respiratory or cardiac depression may recur as blood levels of naloxone fall. Because most deaths in patients with narcotic intoxication are related to respiratory arrest, efforts to ensure adequate respiratory function are paramount. With severe ingestions or those associated with long-acting agents, a continuous IV naloxone infusion is required. Two mg of naloxone in 500 mL of normal saline is administered at 100 to 200 mL/h or titrated to the desired clinical response.

Noncardiogenic pulmonary edema may occur in patients with toxic amounts of narcotics and is managed with oxygen, positive pressure ventilation if required, and naloxone administration. Routine measures undertaken in patients with cardiogenic pulmonary edema are of no benefit. Seizures may occur and are treated with IV diazepam and phenytoin. Cardiac arrhythmias should be treated with an appropriate agent.

Lethargic or comatose patients require endotracheal intubation. Patients with prolonged symptoms may be admitted for observation. Naloxone infusion may be indicated for 12 to 48 hours, depending on the agent involved. Diuresis, dialysis, and hemoperfusion are not indicated.

- Symptoms and signs of **heroin withdrawal** are manifest after a latency period of approximately 12 hours; lacrimation, restlessness, rhinorrhea, "gooseflesh," insomnia, diaphoresis, muscle cramps, pupillary dilation, hot and cold flashes, vomiting, diarrhea, and fever are noted. Symptoms usually begin to subside after 72 to 96 hours of abstinence. Although most hospitals do not primarily manage detoxification from narcotics, admissions related to concomitant acute medical or surgical illness may be necessary. One approach is to administer methadone, 10 mg orally or intramuscularly when signs of opiate withdrawal appear, and to readminister additional 10-mg doses when objective signs of opiate withdrawal are noted. Further doses may be required every 8 to 12 hours; doses should be reduced approximately 50% every 2 days until detoxification is complete. Importantly, patient estimates of daily narcotic dose are generally inaccurate; the use of this estimate to calculate a starting dose of methadone is not appropriate.

Barbiturates

Barbiturates are weak acids, and are divided into classes based on their duration of action. Long-acting barbiturates (6–12 hours duration) include phenobarbital, barbital, mephobarbital, and primidone. Intermediate-acting compounds (3–6 hours duration) include amobarbital, butabarbital, and aprobarbital. Short-acting barbiturates (<3 hours duration) include hexobarbital, pentobarbital, and secobarbital. Ultrashort-acting agents (3 hours duration) include thiopental and methohexital. Agents with short durations of action are more lipid-soluble, are more rapid in onset of action, and cause more extensive CNS depressant effects than the longer-acting agents. Ingested barbiturates are absorbed in the small intestine and undergo hepatic metabolism primarily into inactive compounds.

- **Clinical presentation.** Early symptoms of barbiturate intoxication include drowsiness, slurred speech, or paradoxic excitement. More severe intoxication results in increasing sedation and progressive coma. Doses approximately three-times the hypnotic dose decrease the respiratory drive. Physical findings include initially reactive meiosis or, if CNS hypoxia secondary to respiratory depression has occurred, mydriasis. Respiratory depression may progress to apnea. Hypothermia and decreased GI motility are characteristic. Chronic users and acute overdoses show **bullous skin lesions** over pressure points on the hands and knees due to pressure stasis. Hypotension develops due to increases in venous capacitance and the direct myocardial depressant effects. Profound CNS depression associated with a flatline electroencephalogram (EEG) may be seen in severely intoxicated patients.
- **Laboratory data** may reveal acidosis and hypoxia. Qualitative identification of the specific barbiturate is much more important than quantitative levels, because

the clinical assessment of the severity of intoxication guides management and the phenomenon of tolerance is well recognized in patients chronically ingesting barbiturates.

- **Treatment** consists of intensive supportive therapy. Lavage should be performed up to 8 hours after ingestion because GI emptying is typically delayed; phenobarbital may form concretions necessitating endoscopic removal. Hypothermia is managed with the usual techniques. Hypotension is treated initially with fluid resuscitation followed by pressors. The long-acting drugs demonstrate an increased rate of elimination when **alkaline diuresis** is used; the urinary pH should be adjusted to between 7.5 and 8.0 with intravenously administered $NaHCO_3$. The details of alkalinization are discussed in "Gastric Lavage" discussed under the section "General Assessment and Management." Severe barbiturate intoxication that does not respond to intensive conservative therapy may respond to hemodialysis or hemoperfusion, particularly long-acting agents with hepatic or renal failure.
- Barbiturate **withdrawal** is manifest by insomnia, excitement, delirium, hallucinations, toxic psychoses, tremors (which may be dramatic), nausea, vomiting, orthostatic hypotension, and seizures. Treatment consists of phenobarbital, followed by its gradual withdrawal.

Central Nervous System Stimulants

Amphetamines

Amphetamines and its analogs have alpha- and beta-adrenergic CNS stimulant actions. Amphetamines may be taken orally, sniffed, or injected intravenously. They are generally metabolized in the liver by hydroxylation and deamination and excreted in the urine; the hydroxylated metabolites may be active. Amphetamines are weak bases, and urinary acidification results in increased excretion. Half-lives vary among the specific substances and excretion is enhanced with diuresis.

- **Clinical presentation.** Amphetamine intoxication ranges from restlessness and irritability to seizures and coma. Insomnia, tremor, diaphoresis, mydriasis, confusion, tachypnea, nausea, vomiting, nystagmus, tachycardia, hyperpyrexia, delirium, marked hypertension, and arrhythmias may occur. Amphetamine toxicity includes toxic psychoses, repetitive behaviors, renal failure, coagulopathy (caused by hyperthermia), and intracranial hemorrhage secondary to severe or accelerated hypertension. Because tolerance to the amphetamines occurs, quantitative serum levels do not reliably predict toxicity.
- The **treatment** of amphetamine toxicity is supportive; GI tract decontamination is undertaken if indicated, and seizures are treated with IV diazepam. Psychotic and behavioral disturbances should not be treated with chlorpromazine or haloperidol because these agents may potentiate seizures. Lorazepam 2 to 3 mg IV in an adult may control agitation. Hyperthermia must be aggressively treated with cooling blankets, and hypertensive crises may be treated with an alpha-blocking agent or nitroprusside. Beta-blockers alone should not be used to treat hypertension caused by amphetamines because they may raise the blood pressure due to unopposed alpha effects. Labetalol may be considered because it has alpha- and beta-adrenergic blocking effects.

Excretion of amphetamines is enhanced with acid diuresis using mannitol or furosemide and ammonium chloride (1–2 g orally or IV every 4–6 h) to achieve urinary flow rates of 5 to 7 mL/kg/h and a urine pH of less than 5.5. Acid diuresis is contraindicated in the presence of seizures and serious hyperthermia, because myoglobinuric renal failure may ensue. Both hemodialysis and hemoperfusion are effective in removing amphetamines but are not required except for progressive or prolonged toxicity despite supportive therapy and forced diuresis.

Cocaine

Cocaine is an alkaloid obtained from the plant *Erythroxylon coca*. It is absorbed after topical application to mucous membranes of the nose, smoked ("crack") or administered by IV injection; oral ingestion results in significant hydrolysis and poor absorption. Peak levels occur within minutes of IV injection and 60 minutes after topical application. Cocaine is metabolized within 2 hours by the liver and excreted in the urine; 20% of the drug is excreted unchanged. Cocaine interferes with the neuronal reuptake of norepinephrine and dopamine and interferes with serotonin activity.

- The **clinical presentation** is similar to amphetamine intoxication: CNS stimulation, tachycardia, chest pain, hypertension, hyperthermia, muscle twitching, seizures, nausea, vomiting and ventricular dysrhythmias, followed by CNS, cardiac, and respiratory depression. Patients may also have rhabdomyolysis and myoglobinuria. Death usually results from respiratory failure or cardiac infarction and arrest.
- **Treatment** is supportive; GI decontamination is not indicated. Ativan or diazepam should be used to control seizures, followed by phenobarbital if needed. Beta-blockers, when used alone, may cause an unopposed alpha-adrenergic reaction with further elevation of the blood pressure; therefore, phentolamine with esmolol can be used, or labetalol alone can be used, which itself has both alpha- and beta-adrenergic blocking activity. Hypotension in the depressive phases of intoxication should be treated with fluid expansion and vasopressors such as dopamine. Hyperthermia should be controlled with cooling blankets. Cocaine-induced psychosis has been successfully treated with neuroleptics. Forced diuresis, dialysis, and hemoperfusion are ineffective.

Strychnine

Strychnine is an alkaloid currently used only as a rodenticide; however, a variety of illicit drugs may be adulterated with strychnine because of its stimulatory effects. Strychnine causes diffuse stimulation of the CNS by depressing inhibitory pathways involving glycine receptors; it is rapidly absorbed and is quickly excreted in the urine (70% within 6 hours).

- **Clinical features** of strychnine toxicity include fever, muscle stiffness, hyperreactive reflexes, tetanic convulsions, opisthotonus, rhabdomyolysis, lactic acidosis, and death caused by respiratory failure.
- **Treatment** is supportive; airway control should be obtained and the gastric lavage initiated if within 1 hour of ingestion. Charcoal may bind some of the agents. Seizures are treated with diazepam, and a nonstimulating environment should be provided. Forced diuresis and dialysis are of little value because of the rapid urinary excretion of the agent.

Hallucinogens

Tryptamine Derivatives

Tryptamine derivatives produce hallucinatory effects. These substances include diphosphotryptamine (DPT), alphamethyltryptamine (AMT), dimethyltryptamine (DMT), diethyltryptamine (DET), psilocybin, psilocin, and serotonin. When ingested, sniffed, or smoked, onset of action occurs at 20 to 30 minutes. The duration of action varies, ranging from 1 hour (DMT) to 6 hours (psilocybin).

- **Clinical findings** include weakness, nausea, vomiting, abdominal pain, blurred vision, mydriasis, tachycardia, hyperpyrexia, and hyperreflexia. Visual hallucinations and perceptive distortions are also common.
- **Treatment** is supportive. The patient should be reassured as much as possible. If sedation is required, a benzodiazepine should be considered. **Phenothiazines should be avoided** (see below).

Phenethylamine Derivatives

Phenethylamine derivatives are hallucinogens **derived from amphetamine,** except for mescaline. After ingestion, these agents are rapidly absorbed, producing mild nausea and occasional vomiting within approximately 30 to 60 minutes; this is followed by a sensory phase lasting from 4 to 14 hours. During the sensory phase, visual distortion is common, whereas frank hallucinations are less often observed. The substituted amphetamines have been referred to as the hallucinatory "alphabet soup" and include 2, 5-dimethoxy-4-methylamphetamine (DOM; STP), 3,4-methylene-dioxyamphetamine (MDA), paramethoxyamphetamine (PMA), and 3,4,5-trimethoxyamphetamine (TMA).

- **Clinical presentation** is characterized by a variety of sympathomimetic effects, euphoria, and psychic effects similar to mescaline and the tryptamines at high doses. MDA has been associated with coma, seizures, and cardiovascular collapse when ingested in high doses.
- **Treatment** involves reassurance and conservative support as well as respiratory and circulatory assistance as needed. The patient should be placed in a monitored bed. The use of phenothiazines should be avoided because they lower the seizure threshold. Seizures should be treated with diazepam.

Phencyclidine

Phencyclidine (PCP) is a frequent adulterant of street drugs and remains an occasionally abused substance. It has onset of action 2 to 3 minutes after inhalation and 30 to 60 minutes after ingestion; effects last for approximately 6 hours. PCP is distributed widely in tissues; it is metabolized by the liver and excreted by the kidney. Substantial amounts of the drug are secreted into the stomach and undergo enterohepatic circulation and reabsorption.

- Distortions of time, space, and somatic sensation mark the **clinical presentation;** delusions, hostility, and bizarre and violent behavior are frequent. Vertical, rotatory, and horizontal nystagmus occurs, the pupil size is variable, and the corneal reflex may be decreased. Ataxia, dystonic posturing, muscle twitches, seizures, rhabdomyolysis, myoglobinuria, hyperthermia, and mild hypertension may also be noted. Respiratory stimulation is followed by depression and apnea in patients with severe intoxications.
- **Laboratory data** frequently demonstrate hypoglycemia and mild elevation of creatine kinase, AST, ALT, and myoglobin.
- The treatment of PCP intoxication should focus on reassuring the patient; diazepam or lorazepam may be used for sedation. Phenothiazines, such as haloperidol, should be used with caution because their use may result in hypotension and reduce the seizure threshold.

Activated charcoal should be administered initially and, because of enterohepatic recirculation, readministered at 4- to 6-hour intervals. Seizures are treated with IV diazepam and phenytoin if necessary.

Nonnarcotic Analgesics

Acetaminophen

Acetaminophen (*N*-acetyl-*p*-aminophenol) is an antipyretic-analgesic compound that may produce lethal hepatotoxic effects in untreated intoxications. Although accidental ingestion in children is the most frequent clinical scenario, intentional overdoses among adolescents and adults are responsible for most morbidity and mortality.

Acetaminophen is quickly absorbed from the GI tract, especially in liquid form. The half-life is 2 to 3 hours with normal doses in adults, slightly shorter in children, and slighter longer in neonates and in patients with hepatic dysfunction. Less than 5% is excreted unchanged in the urine, and the remainder is metabolized in the liver by three routes. The first two involve dose-dependent saturable pathways. These include glucuronidation and sulfation, which are responsible for greater than 90% of acetaminophen metabolism, and do not result in the formation of toxic metabolites. The metabolism of acetaminophen by the cytochrome P-450, mixed-function, oxidative enzyme system, however, results in the formation of a highly reactive, toxic, intermediate agent that under normal circumstances is rapidly detoxified by combining with endogenous hepatic glutathione and then metabolized to form an acetaminophenmercapturate conjugate. In patients ingesting large amounts of acetaminophen, the glucuronidation and sulfation pathways become saturated. This shunts increased amounts of acetaminophen into the glutathione pathway, resulting in the formation of excess amounts of the reactive intermediate and the relatively rapid depletion of available endogenous glutathione. When glutathione is no longer available to detoxify the intermediate, it combines with various hepatic macromolecules, for example, proteins and cell membranes, resulting in progressive hepatic damage.

It has been estimated that a 70% reduction in hepatic glutathione must occur before toxicity is noted. Although biochemically this percentage correlates with an ingestion of 15 g in the average adult, individual variability in glutathione stores is such that **7.5 g is conservatively used as the minimal potentially fatal dose.**

- **Clinical presentation.** During the initial 12 to 24 hours after ingestion (phase 1), signs and symptoms of severe acetaminophen overdose consist of mild nausea, vomiting, anorexia, diaphoresis, and pallor. Phase 2 is characterized by a relatively complete return to well being lasting as long as 4 days. During this period, laboratory data demonstrate a rising AST and other hepatic enzymes; mild right upper quadrant abdominal pain may be noted. In phase 3, which typically develops 3 to 5 days after ingestion in untreated patients, patients become symptomatic from hepatic injury. Symptoms include anorexia, nausea, malaise, abdominal pain, progressive evidence of hepatic failure, coma, and death. In those who survive, liver function tests return to normal within a few weeks; serious toxicity and death are rare in children for reasons that are not clear.

- **Laboratory studies. The level of plasma acetaminophen 4 hours or more after the ingestion** is critical; this test serves to predict the extent of potential toxicity and to guide specific management. The Rumack-Matthews nomogram or the regional poison center will assist in the interpretation of blood levels. It is very important that all reported levels, as well as the reported units, be double-checked. For example, some laboratories will report acetaminophen levels in micrograms/deciliter rather than micrograms/milliliter. If this is not recognized, the physician will make a major error and underestimate the actual level. In general, patients with **4-, 6-, 8-, or 12-hour levels greater than 150, 110, 75, or 40 μg/mL, respectively,** require specific treatment with *N*-**acetylcysteine** as outlined. Levels less than these parameters are not expected to be toxic, and specific treatment with *N*-acetylcysteine is not indicated. Similarly, if a calculated dose can be relied on (which it often cannot), ingestions of less than 7 g in the adult or less than 100 mg/kg in children are not expected to produce toxicity and, in general, patients ingesting these amounts or less do not require specific treatment. It is important to note that some patients, particularly the elderly or alcoholic patient, may sustain injury from ingestion of less than 7 g (i.e., even with acceptable daily doses of acetaminophen). Such patients may present with unexplained liver dysfunction. In general, however, adults with calculated doses greater than 7 g or children ingesting more than 100 to 150 mg/kg require treatment and a 4-hour or later plasma acetaminophen determination to guide specific therapy. Plasma acetaminophen levels drawn after the institution of treatment with *N*-acetylcysteine are unreliable as to toxicity and should not be used. Baseline liver function tests should be drawn in all patients.

- **Gastrointestinal decontamination.** Since acetaminophen is avidly bound by activated charcoal, the administration of this agent is recommended. Repeat doses are not recommended in acetaminophen ingestions alone, because absorption is rapid and a very limited enterohepatic circulation exists. Cathartic agents have a limited role in isolated acetaminophen ingestions.
- **Specific treatment with *N*-acetylcysteine.** *N*-acetylcysteine (Mucomyst) is given orally as 140 mg/kg, immediately followed by 70 mg/kg every 4 hours for an additional 17 doses. Most commonly 20% Mucomyst, containing 200 mg/mL of *N*-acetylcysteine, is diluted 1:3 with fruit juice or a soft drink (to mask its unpleasant taste). Five milliliters of 20% undiluted Mucomyst contains 1 g of *N*-acetylcysteine. If the dose is vomited within 1 hour of administration, it should be repeated, and in some patients, a nasogastric tube may be required to deliver the proper dose. *N*-acetylcysteine is most effective if given within 8 to 16 hours of ingestion but may exert beneficial effects if instituted within 24 hours. N-acetylcysteine may also be administered intravenously. Contact a regional poison control center for guidance. Seger and Murray have prepared a useful algorithm for the treatment of patients with acetaminophen ingestions (see Fig. 64-1). Patients presenting very early (within 1 hour of ingestion) can be given sorbitol along with activated charcoal; a 4-hour postingestion level of acetaminophen should be obtained and specific treatment with *N*-acetylcysteine initiated if the patient's level on the Rumack-Mathew nomogram (Fig. 64-2) exceeds that associated with hepatic toxicity. Patients presenting between 4 and 8 hours after ingestion should have an immediate acetaminophen level drawn; patients with levels exceeding those in the nomogram for hepatic toxicity should be treated with *N*-acetylcysteine. Patients presenting between 8 and 24 hours of ingestion should have an immediate acetaminophen level drawn and treatment with *N*-acetylcysteine initiated if the amount of ingestion is unknown or if the amount of acetaminophen ingested exceeds 140 mg/kg. Treatment can be discontinued if nontoxic levels are determined to be present. If the history is reliable, and the calculated amount of acetaminophen ingested is less than 140 mg/kg, treatment can be delayed pending the serum level; treatment with NAC should proceed based on levels exceeding those in the nomogram.

Patients presenting after 24 hours of ingestion require an acetaminophen level and liver function studies; the regional poison center should be consulted with these results, because delayed treatment with *N*-acetylcysteine may be appropriate in certain patients with acetaminophen detectable in the serum, particularly with laboratory evidence of hepatic injury. Consult the regional poison center when acetaminophen is ingested with other substances.

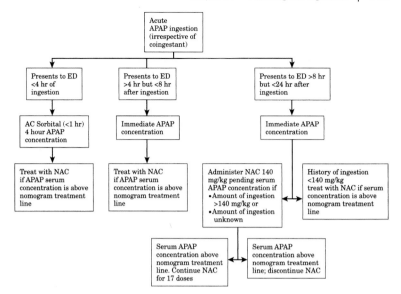

Figure 64-1. Treatment of acetaminophen ingestion. (APAP, acetaminophen; NAC, *N*-acetylcysteine; From Seger D, Murray L. Aspirin, acetaminophen, and nonsteroidal agents. In: Rosen P, et al., eds. *Emergency medicine, concepts and clinical practices,* 4th ed. St. Louis: CV Mosby; 1998:1257, with permission.)

Although children younger than 6 years old, in comparison with adults, have an increased sulfation capacity in relation to acetaminophen metabolism and a high turnover rate of glutathione, and therefore may be less susceptible to acetaminophen toxicity, this has not been clearly demonstrated. Treatment of children is therefore similar to that of adults. Treatment of pregnant patients is identical to that outlined. *N*-acetylcysteine does not appear to result in fetal injury. Although there are no clear guidelines for the management of patients with multiple-dose acetaminophen ingestions occurring over a period of time (the nomogram is intended for single acute ingestions only), some centers recommend consideration of *N*-acetylcysteine therapy when the total dose of acetaminophen over a 24-hour period exceeds 150 mg/kg or when laboratory evidence of hepatic injury is present. The regional poison center should be consulted in these cases. See Table 64-4 for some special considerations.

Salicylates
Acute and chronic salicylate toxicity remains a source of frequent morbidity and mortality in pediatric and adult populations. A tremendous variety of prescription and over-the-counter preparations contain salicylates in various forms for oral or topical use. Acute toxicity may occur from intentional overdose, accidental administration of a toxic dose (usually associated with the use of multiple preparations or chronic therapeutic administration of high doses, i.e., in the management of arthritis), or with normal doses in the setting of dehydration. Chronic and subacute salicylate poisoning is an increasingly important source of toxicity among both children and adults.

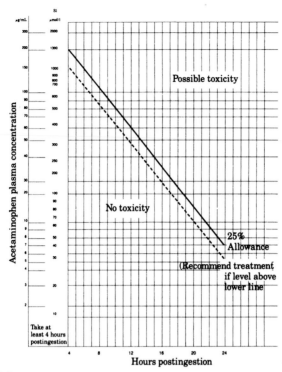

Figure 64-2. Acetaminophen toxicity. (From Rumack BH, Mathew H. Acetaminophen poisoning and toxicity. *Pediatrics* 1975;55:871, with permission.)

- **Acute toxicity.** The absorption of acetylsalicylic acid (ASA) is rapid and complete after the oral ingestion of normal doses; ingestion of toxic amounts may delay gastric emptying, and enteric-coated preparations are absorbed erratically and to a variable degree. ASA is rapidly biotransformed to salicylic acid; this is further metabolized in the liver to salicyluric acid, acyl and phenolic glucuronides, and to gentisic acid. Salicylates administered in therapeutic doses for the treatment of a variety of inflammatory conditions (4–6 g/day) result in a half-life of approximately 6 to 12 hours; in lower doses, used for the routine suppression of fever, a half-life of 2 to 3 hours is noted. In toxic ingestions, as a result of the saturation of metabolic pathways, the effective serum half-life may increase dramatically to more than 20 hours. Importantly, in toxic ingestions, 50% or more may be excreted unchanged in the urine.
- The **pathophysiology** of salicylate toxicity is complex. Salicylates directly stimulate the CNS (including the medullary respiratory center), resulting in the uncoupling of oxidative phosphorylation. Both the Krebs cycle dehydrogenase enzymes and amino acid metabolism are inhibited, which interferes with both platelet and vascular hemostatic mechanisms. These diverse effects combine to produce the various manifestations of toxicity.
  CNS stimulation may result in hallucinations, confusion, irritability, anxiety, seizures, cerebral edema, and coma. Stimulation of the medullary respiratory center

Table 64-4	Special Treatment Considerations for Acetaminophen (APAP)
Situation	**Treatment**
Vomiting after *N*-acetylcysteine (NAC) administration	Administer ondansetron 30 min before repeat administration of NAC.
APAP overdose in pregnant woman	Consult toxicologist. Consider IV NAC.
APAP overdose in chronic alcoholic	Treat with NAC at levels below nomogram treatment line.
APAP overdose in child	Use nomogram to determine treatment.
Chronic APAP ingestion	Treat with NAC if elevated liver function tests or any APAP present in serum.
Charcoal administration after overdose	Do not need to increase NAC dose

IV, intravenous.
From Seger D, Murray L. Aspirin, acetaminophen, and nonsteroidal agents. In: Rosen P, et al., eds. *Emergency medicine, concepts and clinical practice*, 4th ed. St. Louis: CV Mosby; 1998:1258, with permission.

produces hyperpnea and tachypnea, resulting in respiratory alkalosis. Respiratory alkalosis is compensated for by the exchange of intracellular hydrogen ions for extracellular cations and a renal bicarbonate diuresis. This contributes to metabolic acidosis and dehydration. The uncoupling of oxidative phosphorylation decreases the production of adenosine triphosphate, resulting in accelerated activity of the glycolytic and lipolytic pathways. Increased glycolysis and lipid metabolism result in production of lactic and pyruvic acids and acetone and acetoacetate, respectively. These organic acids also contribute to the development of metabolic acidosis, which is characterized by a *high anion gap;* their presence at the kidney, as an additional solute load, further enhances fluid loss. Furthermore, inhibition of amino acid metabolism results in an increase in serum amino acids, oxaloacetate, and α-ketoglutarate. These organic acids contribute further to the solute diuresis and the evolving anion gap. Dehydration is also caused by CNS-induced hyperventilation and from emesis, the latter resulting from the local irritant effects of the salicylates. Increased metabolic activity, particularly in children, may result in hyperthermia.

Glucose metabolism is uniformly deranged, but individual variability in blood sugar levels is common. Diabetics, for example, may present with and maintain severe hypoglycemia; the reasons for this are not clear. In other patients, the blood sugar is initially somewhat elevated, presumably as a result of increased mobilization and metabolism of lipids and hepatic glycogen; however, as toxicity increases or persists, blood sugar may fall. The impairment in glucose metabolism may also be manifest by delayed hyperglycemia; in all patients, blood glucose levels must be followed closely. It should be noted that CNS glucose concentrations might be decreased even with a normal plasma glucose concentration.

Disturbed hemostasis is common and results from decreases in prothrombin and factor VII production, decreased platelet adhesiveness, and increased capillary fragility and permeability. The latter may be the cause of pulmonary edema seen in some patients as well as a contributor to the facial petechiae and subconjunctival hemorrhages seen in others.

- **Clinical presentation.** Symptoms and physical findings include nausea, vomiting, abdominal and chest pain, tinnitus, hyperventilation, diaphoresis, hyperpyrexia, mental status abnormalities ranging from irritability and anxiety to coma, variable degrees of dehydration and oliguria, pulmonary edema, and signs of deficient hemostasis.

  Children are much more likely than adults to have hyperpyrexia, early acidosis, and CNS symptoms, whereas older children and adults usually present with alkalosis during the initial period of acute salicylate intoxication.

- **Laboratory data** should include a CBC, electrolytes, blood sugar, BUN, creatinine, arterial blood gases, liver function studies, prothrombin time, and partial thromboplastin time. A chest roentgenogram and ECG should also be obtained. Toxicology specimens should include **salicylate levels on presentation and 6 hours after ingestion;** additional levels drawn at 8 to 10 hours postingestion may be helpful to assess delayed salicylate absorption and elimination.

  The potential severity of acute salicylate intoxication may be estimated using either of the two methods. If a close approximation of the amount of salicylate ingested is known, the probability of toxicity may be estimated as follows: less than 150 mg/kg, none to mild; 150 to 300 mg/kg, mild to moderate; 300 to 500 mg/kg, serious; greater than 500 mg/kg, critical. Alternatively, the Done nomogram, based on measured serum salicylate levels, may be used for the same purpose (Fig. 64-3). Six-hour postingestion salicylate levels less than 40 mg/dL, for example, are typically seen in patients ingesting less than 150 mg/kg and are not associated with symptoms; patients with these levels may often be managed as outpatients.

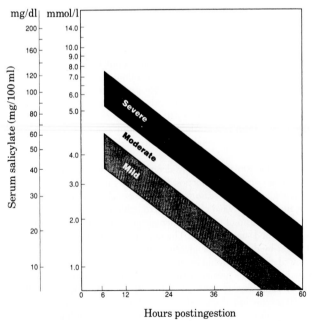

Figure 64-3. Salicylate toxicity. (From Done AK. Salicylate intoxication. *Pediatrics* 1960;26:805, with permission.)

Six-hour levels between 60 and 95 mg/dL are associated with moderate intoxication, and most patients demonstrate hyperpnea and CNS abnormalities including somnolence or excitability; admission and treatment are required. **Six-hour levels greater than 110 to 120 mg/dL are usually associated with severe toxicity,** and aggressive therapy is warranted.

- The **treatment** of acute salicylate intoxication involves the usual methods to stabilize respiratory and cardiac function as needed (Table 64-5). The patient's skin should be decontaminated if the salicylate was topically applied; this can be performed with simple soap and water. Emptying the stomach is not indicated if the ingestion occurred more than 2 hours before presentation or in patients with spontaneous emesis. Charcoal should be administered as indicated in Table 64-5. Because of oliguria and occasional renal failure, magnesium-containing cathartics should not be used, and dilution of gastric contents should be avoided, because this increases salicylate absorption. Vigorous fluid and electrolyte resuscitation should be undertaken to reverse dehydration and hypokalemia; acidemia should be treated with IV $NaHCO_3$. Dextrose and potassium chloride are routinely infused along with other fluids to replenish body stores; cerebrospinal fluid hypoglycemia may exist in these patients in association with relatively normal peripheral glucose concentrations. Sponge baths with tepid water or cooling blankets should be used to treat hyperpyrexia. Seizures are treated with IV diazepam. Pulmonary edema is treated by usual measures, except diuresis.

Table 64-5	Treatment of Acute Salicylate Poisoning

1. Gastrointestinal decontamination or activated charcoal (AC)
2. Repeat-dose AC
   50–100 g orally loading dose
   20–60 g orally every 2–3 h
   Change to aqueous charcoal when charcoal stool
3. Treat dehydration
   Maintain urine output at 2–3 mL/kg/h with D5LR or D5NS
4. Correct potassium depletion
5. Alkalinize urine
   Obtain baseline ABG values
   Administer 1–2 mEq/kg $NaHCO_3$ initially, then as needed (50 mL of $HaHCO_3$ increases serum pH 0.1)
   Intravenous fluid–D5 with 100 mEq $NaHCO_3$/L
   Monitor serum pH; do not cause systemic alkalosis
   Do not attempt forced diuresis
6. Dialysis indications
   Coma
   Renal, hepatic, or pulmonary failure
   Pulmonary edema
   Severe acid-base imbalance
   Deterioration in condition

From Seger D, Murray L. Aspirin, acetaminophen, and nonsteroidal agents. In: Rosen P, et al., eds. *Emergency medicine, concepts and clinical practice*, 4th ed. St. Louis: CV Mosby; 1998:1253, with permission.

Measures to eliminate the salicylates actively are effective and include both alkaline diuresis and hemodialysis; alkalinization is discussed in "Gastric Lavage" discussed under the section "General Assessment and Management," on p. 569. Salicylate excretion in the urine is enhanced when the urinary pH approaches 8.0. Thus, $NaHCO_3$ may be given intravenously to alkalinize the urine. Initial urinary pH may be quite low and difficult to increase; it is important to avoid severe alkalemia in an attempt to raise the urinary pH quickly. This treatment also causes a potassium diuresis, and serum K^+ levels should be monitored and potassium replaced if necessary. Because of the possibility of pulmonary edema, especially in older patients, alkaline diuresis may require central venous pressure monitoring. Acetazolamide is not indicated. Consider hemodialysis when the initial salicylate level is greater than 160 mL/dL; when the 6-hour level is greater than 130 mg/dL; when acidosis is profound (pH <7.1) and refractory to therapy; or when renal failure, severe persistent CNS dysfunction, or deterioration occurs despite maximum supportive and therapeutic intervention.

- **Chronic toxicity** is a frequently overlooked diagnosis is becoming increasingly common. Chronic salicylate intoxication usually results from high doses of salicylates given therapeutically for pain or control of inflammation in the adult or when normal doses are given to children who become dehydrated.
- **Clinical presentation.** Symptoms and physical findings are similar to those seen in acute intoxication but are typically more severe with prominent CNS symptoms, dehydration, and hyperventilation. Pulmonary edema is common in the elderly patient.
- **Laboratory data** establish the presence of an anion gap metabolic acidosis, and salicylate levels may be high or normal. The Done nomogram is not useful to predict morbidity in chronic intoxication.
- **Treatment** is similar to that of acute salicylate poisoning. Charcoal should always be considered and other treatment measures as for acute toxicity instituted aggressively.

Psychotropic Agents

Tricyclic Antidepressants

Tricyclic antidepressants (TCAs) are rapidly absorbed from the GI tract, whereas in large or toxic doses, gastric emptying may be delayed. The TCAs have large volumes of distribution (as reflected by their high tissue levels) and are therefore not amenable to accelerated elimination. These agents are up to 95% protein-bound; pharmacologically, protein-bound drug is inactive, and very small increases in systemic pH dramatically increase protein binding. Alkalinization therefore is a major therapeutic intervention. Metabolism occurs in the liver by demethylation, hydroxylation, and glucuronidation. In addition, the TCAs undergo an enterohepatic recirculation; half-lives vary from 24 to 72 hours with normal doses but are considerably prolonged in association with toxic ingestions. Although serum drug levels are not predictive of CNS or cardiac toxicity, a baseline **QRS duration greater than 0.10 seconds** predicts poor outcome.

- **Clinical presentation.** Signs and symptoms of TCA overdose are caused by anticholinergic, α-adrenergic, quinidine-like, and cardiac effects. Additionally, these agents block the reuptake of norepinephrine and serotonin, which is responsible for their therapeutic effect.

Anticholinergic effects in toxic ingestions result in the usual central and peripheral findings; CNS symptoms include confusion, anxiety, delirium, hallucinations, myoclonus, choreoathetosis, hyperactive deep tendon reflexes, positive Babinski signs, seizures, and coma. The time from ingestion to the onset of seizures and coma may be surprisingly short. Peripheral anticholinergic effects include mydriasis, peripheral vasodilatation, hyperpyrexia, tachycardia, urinary retention, decreased GI motility, and decreased secretions. The prevention of norepinephrine reuptake in adrenergic neurons may cause an initial sympathomimetic response that potentiates the anticholinergic peripheral effects; tachycardia, hypertension, and ventricular arrhythmias are noted.

The cardiac depressant effects of the TCAs are caused by sodium channel blockade. Myocardial conduction is delayed, and the **PR, QRS, and QT intervals become prolonged.** Progressive toxicity results in conduction delays with wide, bizarre QRS complexes. Ventricular tachycardia, fibrillation, torsades des pointes, and cardiac arrest are frequent. Pulmonary edema and cardiogenic shock result from decreased cardiac contractility. Although the earliest sign of TCA toxicity is sinus tachycardia, a QRS interval greater than 0.10 second is associated with severe toxicity.

- The **treatment** of TCA overdose should be aggressive. Patients should be continuously monitored. GI tract decontamination is warranted in all early ingestions because of decreased GI tract motility. Gastric lavage (particularly if performed within the first 2 hours after ingestion) is suggested in patients with severe overdoses, because seizures and coma may occur precipitously. After the stomach is emptied, activated charcoal (50–100 g in adults) should be given immediately and repeated every 4 hours. Sequential administration is intended to interrupt the enterohepatic recirculation. A nasogastric tube should be connected to continuous suction, because secretion into the stomach occurs. The administration of cathartics should follow.

- Ingestions associated with **serious cardiac toxicity** require treatment with *alkalinization,* and this should be undertaken at the first sign of significant toxicity. The goal of alkalinization is an arterial pH of 7.45 to 7.55 and is accomplished with $NaHCO_3$ given as 1 to 2 mEq/kg IV over several minutes, followed by an IV infusion of 2 ampules of $NaHCO_3$ in 1 L of 5% D/W running at 50 mL/h and adjusted as needed. Without a continuous infusion, a single bolus of $NaHCO_3$ (as noted) elevates the pH for only approximately 15 minutes. Normal saline should be avoided because of the potential for hypernatremia. If the patient requires intubation and mechanical ventilation, hyperventilation may also be used to raise the pH. Indications for alkalinization include significant or symptomatic bradycardia, ventricular or supraventricular arrhythmias, abnormalities of interventricular conduction (including QRS intervals more than 0.1 second or varying degrees of heart block), and hypotension.

- **CNS** manifestations of TCA toxicity may respond less well to alkalinization. With significant abnormalities of mental status or seizures, a trial of alkalinization is warranted. More aggressive treatment of minor abnormalities of mental status should not be pursued.

- If alkalinization is unsuccessful, **seizures** should be terminated with IV diazepam followed by phenytoin. Paralysis with neuromuscular blocking agents may be required when status epilepticus is present.

- **Symptomatic bradycardia** not corrected with alkalinization should be treated with temporary pacing. Atropine and physostigmine should not be used, and calcium is not effective.

- **Ventricular tachycardia** not responding to alkalinization should be treated with lidocaine. Phenytoin should **not** be used when second- or third-degree atrioventricular (AV) block is present. Electrical defibrillation may be tried but is usually not successful. Torsades de pointes may respond to 2 g $MgSO_4$ IV (adult dose).
- **Hypotension** refractory to alkalinization and saline administration should be treated with norepinephrine (Levophed).
- It is important to avoid quinidine, procainamide, and disopyramide (because of their sodium channel blocking properties), atropine and digoxin (because interventricular conduction may worsen), and pressors other than norepinephrine (because hypotension may worsen or be precipitated). Beta-blockers should also be avoided.

Neuroleptics

Neuroleptics include the phenothiazines, indoles, butyrophenones, thiothixene, and loxapine. These medications possess significant antidopaminergic, antiseritonergic, anti-α-adrenergic, and myocardial depressant effects and, as a result, substantially affect the central and autonomic nervous systems and the cardiovascular system.

The GI absorption of neuroleptic medications is nearly complete with peak plasma levels occurring 2 to 3 hours after ingestion. These agents have long half-lives (up to 30 hours) and, reflecting their high degree of protein and tissue binding, have high volumes of distribution (more than 20 L/kg). Metabolism occurs in the liver with excretion in urine and feces. Phenothiazines are radiopaque, and therefore tablets may be visualized with an abdominal roentgenogram.

- **Clinical presentation.** Large doses may produce respiratory depression, arrest, and coma. Children are more prone to profound sedation than adults in equivalent milligram per kilogram ingestions. Paradoxical excitation is seen in some patients, and the seizure threshold is reduced. Depression of the hypothalamic vasomotor and temperature homeostatic centers produces hypotension, and hypothermia or, less commonly, hyperthermia.

Extrapyramidal symptoms occur as a result of dopaminergic blockade within the basal ganglia; these reactions are commonly seen as acute dystonic reactions. Tardive dyskinesia and akasthisia are due to chronic ingestion.

The cardiovascular system is affected in a variety of ways; hypotension of CNS origin is compounded by myocardial depressant effects and peripheral α-adrenergic blockade with α-adrenergic blockade; when agents possessing both α- and β-stimulating properties are administered (e.g., epinephrine, isoproterenol, or dopamine), *paradoxical hypotension* may occur as a result of unopposed β-adrenergic stimulation producing vasodilation. Norepinephrine is appropriate for the treatment of hypotension.

Cardiac conduction abnormalities result from a quinidine-like effect on the myocardium; prolongation of the QT interval, convexity of the ST segment, blunting of the T wave, and the appearance of U waves may be noted. Other cardiac effects are similar to those of lidocaine; these include prolongation of the refractory period, QRS conduction delays, and varying degrees of heart block. Tachycardia is common and probably reflects a reflex sympathetic response to hypotension. Serious arrhythmias including ventricular fibrillation and asystole are seen as well. Autonomic nervous system dysfunction is primarily caused by the cholinergic blockade.

- **Treatment** of neuroleptic toxicity is supportive. Those ingesting phenothiazines should be given additional doses of charcoal (i.e., every 4–6 h for 24–48 h) to interrupt the enterohepatic recirculation characteristic of these compounds. Hypotension should be managed with isotonic fluids and norepinephrine specifically; epinephrine may produce paradoxical worsening of hypotension as a result of unopposed β-adrenergic stimulation. Cardiac arrhythmias may be treated with phenytoin or lidocaine. Seizures should be managed with diazepam. Hypothermia is treated with blankets and active rewarming if required; significant hyperthermia should be treated aggressively with the usual measures.

Acute dystonic reactions are managed with diphenhydramine IV or intramuscular (0.5–1.0 mg/kg in children and 50 mg in adults), or in adults, benztropine mesylate (Cogentin) 2 mg may be given intravenously over 2 minutes or intramuscularly or PO. Patients presenting with only extrapyramidal toxicity may be discharged if asymptomatic after treatment with a 3- to 4-day supply of diphenhydramine (25–50 mg four times daily) or benztropine mesylate (1–2 mg twice daily), because reactions commonly recur within the first 24 to 48 hours unless suppressed.

Lithium

Lithium is used in bipolar disorders. Lithium is rapidly and completely absorbed after oral administration; peak levels occur 1 to 2 hours after ingestion, but the half-life is approximately 29 hours because of slow tissue uptake and release. Lithium is freely soluble in water, is not protein-bound, and is excreted by the kidney (20%) or reabsorbed at the proximal renal tubule (80%). Factors increasing renal tubule reabsorption include hyponatremia, dehydration, ingestion of nonsteroidal antiinflammatory agents, and distal tubular diuretics.

Lithium has actions that affect a variety of organ systems. It competes for sodium, potassium, magnesium, and calcium at cellular sites; inhibits the release and augments the reuptake of norepinephrine at nerve endings; and inhibits adenyl cyclase. Most lithium toxicity is due to chronic ingestion.

- **Clinical presentation** of mild intoxication includes drowsiness, stupor, coarse tremor or muscle twitching, vomiting, diarrhea, excessive thirst, polyuria, and polydipsia. Serious intoxication produces coma, increased muscle tone and deep tendon reflexes, seizures, transient focal neurologic deficits, arrhythmias, hypotension, respiratory depression, hyperthermia, anuria, and renal abnormalities including tubular damage and necrosis, the nephrotic syndrome, and interstitial nephritis. Symptoms in general progress slowly; however, seizures may occur unexpectedly.

- **Laboratory data** reveal low or normal sodium and potassium levels; the ECG may be abnormal, demonstrating ST-segment depression and T-wave inversions. Hypokalemia is associated with a prolonged QT interval in lithium toxicity. Serum lithium levels are diagnostic and predictive of toxicity: Levels of 0.4 to 1.3 mEq/L are therapeutic, 1.5 to 2.4 mEq/L are mildly toxic, 2.5 to 3.5 mEq/L result in serious toxicity, and levels greater than 3.5 mEq/L imply critical toxicity.

- **Treatment** of lithium intoxication consists of supportive care. Activated charcoal does not bind lithium. Whole-bowel irrigation with Kayexalate may reduce intraluminal lithium amounts. Hypotension may reflect dehydration, and fluid and electrolyte replacement is often required. Hypotensive patients with normal intravascular volumes and patients not responding to fluid resuscitation should be managed with vasopressors. The administration of normal saline in patients with lithium-induced diabetes insipidus may worsen renal salt and water wasting; thus, patients with normal hydration should receive one fourth or one half normal saline. Seizures are managed with IV diazepam, phenytoin, or phenobarbital. Magnesium should be avoided due to potential renal failure and because hypermagnesemia potentiates the toxic effects of lithium. Previously prescribed thiazide and loop diuretics should be avoided because they may lead to renal lithium retention.

Hemodialysis is the treatment of choice in severe lithium intoxication and should be used in patients with renal failure, when serum lithium concentrations increase to more than 3.0 to 3.5 mEq/L, when prolonged coma or clinical deterioration occurs despite intensive supportive care, or when acute ingestions of life-threatening doses of lithium have occurred. Although serum lithium is quickly removed during dialysis, prolonged or repeated hemodialyses may be required because of the slow tissue release of stored lithium.

Corrosives

Corrosives imply that tissue contact results in direct chemically mediated damage. Corrosives include strong acids, alkalis, and certain oxidizing substances. These include hydrochloric acid (muriatic acid, some toilet bowl cleaners, swimming pool cleaners, and a variety of other products); sulfuric acid (battery acid, toilet bowl, and commercial drain cleaners); nitric acid; hydrofluoric acid, sodium or potassium hydroxides (various detergents, drain pipe and toilet bowl cleaners, lye, many paint removers, Clinitest tablets); ammonium, lithium, and calcium hydroxides; sodium hypochlorite (bleach); and potassium permanganate.

Acids

Numerous acids are used in household, laboratory, and industrial settings; exposure may result in severe burns or, rarely, death. Acids result in toxicity by direct contact, inhalation, or ingestion.

- Accidents in which acids are spilled onto the **skin** are the most common type of exposure. Although these usually result in first-degree burns, strong acids may quickly result in coagulation necrosis. Skin surfaces exposed to acids should be copiously irrigated with cool water; if only first-degree burns are apparent, mild soap-and-water cleansing is appropriate. Second- or third-degree burns necessitate prolonged and copious irrigation with cooled saline, gentle debridement, and early surgical consultation. Additional routine burn treatment should include tetanus prophylaxis. The treatment of chemical burns of the skin secondary to exposure to hydrofluoric acid is distinctive and is discussed in Chapter 55 (p. 509).
- Contamination of the **eye** with acid requires immediate and copious saline irrigation. When pH paper is readily available, an initial bilateral cul-de-sac determination of pH will be useful and should be documented. Redetermination of conjunctival cul-de-sac pH after irrigation with 1 L of normal saline and a resting period of 5 to 10 minutes may be used to guide the need for additional irrigation. These results indicate a normal pH or the need for additional irrigation. After irrigation, fluorescein staining of the cornea should be assessed. Ophthalmologic consultation, particularly when corneal staining with fluorescein is present, is advised at the time of injury along with ophthalmologic follow-up in 24 hours. In general, patching and ointments are not advised after acid exposure to the eye.
- **Inhalation** of acid fumes, such as chlorine, nitric acid, and hydrochloric acid, may affect the entire respiratory tract. The degree of injury depends on the concentration of the acid and the duration of exposure. Mild toxicity produces minor irritation that manifest as cough and mild burning pain of the pharynx and chest. More severe exposure may produce laryngeal swelling and obstruction, dyspnea, chest pain, hemoptysis, bronchospasm, pulmonary edema, and death caused by pulmonary consolidation and epithelial necrosis. The onset of pulmonary symptoms, including

pulmonary edema, may be delayed by several hours. Treatment is supportive and includes bronchodilators if evidence of bronchospasm is present; humidified oxygen, intubation, and mechanical ventilation as needed; and sequential chest roentgenograms and arterial blood gases to assess the extent of pulmonary injury. A low threshold for admission and observation is appropriate in patients with a history of exposure or pulmonary symptoms. Prophylactic antibiotics are not indicated, nor are diuretics; steroids may be beneficial.

- The **ingestion of strong acids** produces severe pain on contact with mucosal surfaces, and this often limits accidental ingestion. After ingestion, acids are rapidly transported through the esophagus and pool in the gastric antrum or pylorus. Mucosal surfaces contacting the acid rapidly develop coagulation necrosis; nitric acid turns mucosal surfaces yellow. Symptoms and signs include severe pain of the buccal, pharyngeal, and epigastric areas; dysphagia; nausea; vomiting; hematemesis; stridor from glottic edema; and shock. The ingestion of as little as 5 mL of mineral acid has been lethal. Perforation of the GI tract is rare but may occur. Late complications of acid ingestion include pyloric stenosis and less commonly gastric or esophageal stenosis. Initial treatment includes airway control and fluid resuscitation. When small amounts of **weak acid** have been ingested, moderate amounts of cold milk or water should be administered to dilute the gastric contents. In all patients, emesis is avoided, hospital admission is required for a period of observation, and surgical or gastroenterologic consultation is obtained early. Progression of local injury may occur over several days.

Alkalies

Alkalies with pHs greater than 11.5 are considered strongly alkaline and may result in rapid and substantial damage to the oral and esophageal mucosa caused by liquefaction necrosis. Products containing alkaline agents are widely available and are commonly ingested. Importantly, oral pain or burns may not necessarily be present in the context of severe and evolving esophageal injury; however, oral pain is a frequent clue to possible ingestion.

- **Skin and eye decontamination** should be performed immediately with copious irrigation. Cutaneous involvement is treated like other thermal injuries; surgical consultation should be obtained initially in patients with second- and third-degree burns. Copious irrigation of the eye with normal saline for at least 30 to 60 minutes must be performed repeatedly until such time as, after a waiting period of 10 to 20 minutes has elapsed, cul-de-sac pH remains normal. Prompt ophthalmologic consultation is indicated in all patients with alkaline ocular exposure. Fluorescein staining of the cornea should be performed after irrigation and any positive uptake discussed with the consultant. The use of antibacterial ointments and/or patching after exposure should also specifically be discussed with the consultant because their use is controversial and somewhat dependent on the extent of injury.

- **Ingestion** of a strong alkali requires emergent treatment. Emesis is contraindicated because this only serves to re-expose the esophagus to injury and increases the possibility of aspiration. Nasogastric tube passage followed by lavage is also *not* recommended; furthermore, the administration of charcoal is contraindicated because it is not ineffective and its administration makes endoscopic evaluation of the GI tract impossible. "Neutralization" with weak acids is *not* indicated because of the exothermic nature of the neutralization reaction. Most authorities recommend simple dilution as an initial treatment maneuver. This is accomplished by the administration of cold milk or tap water. Milk is preferred because of its tendency to agglutinate or precipitate around any solid particles. Steroids in high doses should be administered intravenously and early, and surgical and gastroenterologic consultation should be obtained. Antibiotics are indicated in patients with evidence of esophageal injury. Esophagoscopy should be undertaken within 12 to 24 hours of exposure to assess esophageal injury; upright films of the chest and abdomen along with baseline laboratory studies should be initially obtained to exclude mediastinal air or evidence of other visceral perforation. Oral intake is contraindicated.

Ingestion of "button" alkaline batteries is usually innocuous unless they fail to pass the esophagus or lodge in a Meckel diverticulum. A chest and abdominal roentgenogram should be obtained to document the presence and position of the battery, and gastroenterologic consultation and close follow-up should then be provided. The patient should be instructed to return immediately if abdominal pain, vomiting, or other symptoms occur or if the battery is not passed in the stool within 48 to 72 hours.

- **Inhalation** of alkaline fumes, such as industrial-strength ammonia solutions, may produce symptoms and signs of pulmonary damage similar to those of acid inhalation (see "Acids," p. 594); these are treated in a similar fashion.

Miscellaneous Agents

Digitalis

The digitalis preparations, which include digoxin and digitoxin, have a low toxic-to-therapeutic ratio.

- **Clinical presentation.** The signs and symptoms of toxicity typically progress in a somewhat predictable manner. Mild confusion (particularly in the elderly), anorexia, nausea, vomiting, and diarrhea commonly occur in that order and precede the ECG and hemodynamic manifestations of toxicity in most patients. Yellow vision and delirium also occur but are uncommon. Bradycardia, hypotension, and a host of ECG abnormalities, including nonspecific ST-T–wave abnormalities, first- and higher-degree heart block, ventricular premature depolarizations, sinus arrest, accelerated junctional rhythm, paroxysmal atrial tachycardia with AV nodal block, ventricular tachycardia (including bidirectional tachycardia), and ventricular fibrillation may all be seen. There is no good correlation between the serum digoxin level and the extent or severity of manifestations of toxicity. It is important to note that **hypokalemia** may accentuate the ECG and cardiac manifestations of digitalis toxicity as may hypercalcemia.
- **Treatment** is generally supportive and includes the usual measures to interfere with GI absorption; fluid and electrolyte repletion, particularly the administration of supplemental potassium as needed or dialysis if **hyperkalemia** predominates (usually only seen in patients with severe toxicity), and the control of arrhythmias. Ventricular ectopy and tachycardia may be treated with lidocaine or phenytoin; paroxysmal atrial tachycardia with block may respond to procainamide or phenytoin. Temporary artificial pacing or the administration of atropine may be required if bradycardia produces hemodynamic compromise. Digoxin-specific Fab antibody fragments (Digibind) are available for profound toxicity and have proved safe and efficacious. Indications for digoxin-specific Fab include VT, VF, high-degree AV block, and hyperkalemia (more than 5 mEq/L). Each Fab vial contains 40 mg Fab, which will bind 0.6 mg of digoxin. The total

body load (TBL) of an acute ingestion of digoxin is the dose ingested × 0.80. The number of vials needed to treat a patient is TBL/0.6 (mg per vial). The regional poison control center should be contacted.

Quinidine

- **Clinical presentation.** Quinidine toxicity may produce tinnitus, diarrhea, dizziness, hypotension, respiratory failure, and torsades de pointes, with the last being occasionally spontaneously reversible. ECG manifestations also include a prolonged PR interval, a lengthened QT interval, widening of the QRS complex, and ventricular premature depolarizations.
- **Treatment** is supportive and includes gastric decontamination as indicated, the administration of activated charcoal and a cathartic, and maintaining blood pressure with IV infusions and/or pressors as needed. Infusion of one sixth molar sodium lactate is said to reduce the toxic effects of the drug, and alkaline diuresis is effective in accelerating excretion; the latter must be undertaken with great caution in patients with left ventricular dysfunction (see "Alkaline Diuresis" discussed under the section "Enhanced Elimination" on p. 572).

β-Adrenergic Blocking Agents

Numerous β-adrenergic blocking agents are available. As the use of these agents has expanded, the number of clinically important overdoses has increased. Differences in the pharmacology of the individual agents determine the duration and to some extent the severity and specific clinical presentation. For example, propranolol is quite lipophilic, highly protein bound, and metabolized by the liver and has clinically important membrane depressant effects, whereas metoprolol, timolol, and pindolol are only moderately lipophilic and exhibit minimal to moderate protein binding. Metoprolol is metabolized in the liver, whereas timolol and pindolol are 20% and 40% excreted in the urine, respectively. Importantly, pindolol has membrane depressant effects and partial β-agonist properties, the latter of which become significant in major ingestions. Nadolol and atenolol are not lipophilic, are moderately protein bound, and are largely excreted in the urine. These pharmacologic differences are reflected in the differing treatment strategies that follow.

Importantly, in high or toxic doses, differences in the relative cardioselectivity or β_1-receptor specificity among the various agents disappear and are not clinically seen. β-blockers metabolized by the liver have half-lives of 3 to 6 hours, whereas those excreted by the kidney have longer half-lives (e.g., nadolol has a half-life of 14–24 hours).

- **Clinical presentation.** The signs and symptoms of toxicity are caused by β-adrenergic blockade and nonadrenergic effects such as membrane depression. These are usually manifest within the first 1 to 2 hours after ingestion. **Cardiovascular** manifestations include bradycardia and hypotension, pulmonary edema, AV block, widening of the QRS complex, sinus arrest, and asystole. Tachycardia and hypertension may be noted in patients ingesting pindolol because of its partial β-agonist properties; however, in general, these should not be treated. **CNS** manifestations include lethargy, delirium, hallucinations, coma, and recurrent, generalized, tonic-clonic seizures. **Bronchospasm, hyperkalemia,** and **hypoglycemia** may also be seen, the last especially in children and diabetics. Seizures, severe cardiac conduction abnormalities, and cardiovascular collapse are seen more frequently in patients ingesting agents possessing membrane depressant effects, such as propranolol, and these may occur suddenly.

- **Laboratory studies** should include routine admission blood studies, particularly noting serum potassium and glucose levels. A 12-lead ECG and continuous cardiac monitoring are indicated. A chest roentgenogram should be obtained and may demonstrate the presence of pulmonary edema. A toxic screen may help exclude the presence of other ingested drugs, but serum determinations of the various β-blocking agents are generally not useful in guiding therapy or in predicting toxicity.
- **Treatment** is specific and supportive and includes lavage (if less than 1 hour after ingestion) and the administration of charcoal; magnesium-containing cathartics should be withheld until adequate urine output is ensured, but non–magnesium-containing cathartics may be administered. Intravenous glucose should be administered as needed based on frequent and serial assessment of serum glucose levels; hyperkalemia is corrected in the usual manner. Seizures are managed with IV diazepam followed by phenytoin if the former is unsuccessful.

  Symptomatic bradycardia, conduction abnormalities, and hypotension may be treated initially with atropine, isoproterenol, and cautious fluid resuscitation, respectively. Although high doses of isoproterenol may be required to reverse these symptoms, its use may be limited by the induction of peripheral vasodilation and worsening hypotension. It is important to note that **glucagon**, 5 to 15 mg IV given over 1 minute, may dramatically reverse bradycardia and hypotension and should therefore be used early in the management of patients with hemodynamically significant β-blocker toxicity. Because the effects of glucagon may be delayed for 5 to 10 minutes, atropine, isoproterenol, and/or temporary pacing may be required, depending on the clinical situation. The effects of IV glucagon generally last approximately 20 to 30 minutes; if no response is seen after 10 minutes, a larger dose (up to 10 mg) should be administered. In patients responding to glucagon, the IV bolus should be followed by a maintenance infusion of 2 to 5 mg/h. It should be noted that the manufacturer distributes glucagon with a phenol diluent. Because large amounts of glucagon may be required in some patients, normal saline should be substituted for phenol as the diluent. Glucagon acts at sites distinct from the β-receptor and increases cyclic adenosine monophosphate levels in the myocardium, thereby increasing cardiac rate and contractility. Because glucagon may cause vomiting, ondansetron or nasogastric suction should be considered. **Calcium chloride** (0.2 ml/kg) intravenously may be helpful. High dose insulin euglycemia is another potential therapy. Intractable cardiogenic shock may necessitate an intra-aortic balloon; catecholamines with both α and β effects, such as dopamine and norepinephrine, may induce significant vasoconstriction before overcoming β-blockade; dobutamine, a more cardioselective catecholamine, may therefore theoretically have an advantage over these agents in this setting. Ventricular tachyarrhythmias may be treated with lidocaine, phenytoin or overdrive pacing; quinidine, disopyramide, and procainamide should be avoided because of their negative ionotropic properties. Hemoperfusion may be considered in patients with atenolol, sotalol, acebutolol, or nadolol poisoning unresponsive to conservative measures or associated with renal insufficiency.

Calcium Channel Blockers

Calcium channel blockers currently approved for use in the United States include verapamil, nimodipine, nifedipine, nicardipine, isradipine, felodipine, diltiazem, bepridil, and amlodipine. The usual onset of action and duration of action are approximately 30 minutes and 6 to 8 hours, respectively; however, in toxic ingestions, the duration of action may be prolonged. Additionally, some preparations are available in sustained-release formulations (diltiazem, felodipine, nicardipine, nifedipine, and verapamil) and may therefore not reach a peak serum level for 10 to 12 hours after ingestion.

- **Clinically, hypotension** and **bradyarrhythmias** are the most important findings; however, many patients report nausea and vomiting, with mild CNS depression, headache, dizziness, and seizures. Bradycardia in these patients may be sinus or a junctional rhythm, which is typically narrow complex. Serum drug levels are useful only for documenting a particular agent. **Hyperglycemia,** due to suppression of insulin release, may occur, although it is usually mild.

- **Treatment.** General measures include orogastric lavage when patients present within 1.5 hours of a potentially toxic ingestion. Activated charcoal should be administered to all patients with toxic ingestions; repeat dosing should be considered with long-acting or sustained-release preparations. Hypotension is treated with a cautiously administered fluid challenge (10–20 mL/kg of normal saline). Bradycardia often occurs with hypotension and should generally be corrected before the administration of a pressor. Most authorities recommend treating symptomatic bradycardia sequentially with calcium, atropine, glucagon, isoproterenol, epinephrine, and temporary pacing. Persistent hypotension, despite normalization of heart rate, should be treated with an inotropic agent; these include calcium, glucagon, dobutamine, and isoproterenol. If refractory, a pressor should be used. The dose of calcium in adults is 10 mL of a 10% calcium chloride solution intravenously; this dose may be repeated in 10 minutes. Additional doses require that the serum calcium be monitored. The dose in children is 0.2 to 0.25 mL/kg, up to 10 mL, of a 10% solution of calcium chloride. Glucagon is administered as a 1- to 5-mg IV dose initially, followed, if needed, by a 4-mg bolus; this latter dose may be repeated in 5 minutes. A maximum dose of 10 mg of glucagon is accepted initially. A continuous infusion may be indicated in patients responding to this agent (see "β-Adrenergic Blocking Agents," p. 598). The value of enhancing elimination is variable and depends on the particular agent, underlying renal function, and the degree of toxicity. A poison control center should be consulted in this regard.

Clonidine

Clonidine is an antihypertensive drug that acts centrally to stimulate α-receptors in the vasomotor centers of the medulla, producing inhibition of peripheral sympathetic activity. In addition, when clonidine is present in the serum in high concentration or administered intravenously, stimulation of α-adrenergic receptors of the peripheral vasculature occurs, resulting in vasoconstriction and hypertension. Sixty percent of absorbed drug is excreted unchanged in the urine, with a half-life of approximately 8.5 hours. Clonidine has numerous other potential side effects including sedation, hallucinations, dry mouth, postural hypotension, arrhythmias, impotence, hypothermia, and sodium and fluid retention. Clonidine is also used to treat migraine headache, narcotic withdrawal, and perimenopausal flushing.

- **Clinical presentation.** Clonidine overdoses may mimic the signs and symptoms found in narcotic overdose; patients exhibit bradycardia, hypertension followed by hypotension, respiratory depression, miosis, stupor or coma, and hypoactive deep tendon reflexes. Death occurs from respiratory or cardiac arrest.

- The **treatment** of clonidine overdose is supportive; the usual GI decontamination measures are indicated. Intubation and mechanical ventilation may be required. Hypotension should be managed with fluid resuscitation and the α-adrenergic antagonist **tolazoline,** given IV in a dose of 10 to 25 mg may be helpful. Vasopressors may be indicated in some patients. Bradycardia will usually respond to **atropine.** **Naloxone** may reverse hypotensive and respiratory depressant effects. Although clonidine is excreted unchanged in the urine, forced diuresis has not been shown to be of value.

The abrupt cessation of clonidine produces a **withdrawal syndrome** characterized by agitation, abdominal pain, nausea, vomiting, tachycardia, diaphoresis, mydriasis, and hypertensive crisis. The pathogenesis of the syndrome is unknown; however, high levels of circulating catecholamines are noted. Treatment of clonidine withdrawal involves the **use of both α- and β-adrenergic antagonists,** such as phentolamine and propranolol, respectively, or labetolal. The use of β-adrenergic blockers alone may exaggerate the hypertensive effect resulting from catecholamine excess and may precipitate or worsen hypertension; sodium nitroprusside, diazoxide, and trimethaphan may also be used to treat accelerated hypertension in these patients.

Nitrates and Nitrites

Nitrates and nitrites are found in a variety of settings including industry, agriculture, and medicine; the agents are abused as well. These compounds relax smooth muscle and oxidize hemoglobin to **methemoglobin,** which results in the most serious effects in severely poisoned patients.

- **Clinical presentation.** The signs and symptoms of nitrate or nitrite poisoning are caused by vasodilation resulting from smooth muscle relaxation and include orthostatic hypotension, syncope, tachycardia, and flushed and diaphoretic skin. The formation of methemoglobin results in hypoxia, the severity of which depends on the concentration of methemoglobin in the serum. Cyanosis occurs at concentrations between 10% and 20%; headache, dizziness, and tachypnea occur at concentrations between 20% and 30%; and at concentrations more than 50%, lethargy, stupor, coma, seizures, metabolic acidosis, and cardiovascular collapse occur.

- **Laboratory data** demonstrate metabolic acidosis and varying degrees of methemoglobinemia; blood is typically a chocolate brown color. Pulse oximetry is inaccurate and suggests a falsely high oxygen saturation. ABG measurement shows a falsely high pO_2 (because dissolved—not bound—oxygen is measured). Definitive diagnosis is by co-oximetry, a spectrophotometric method that differentiates various types of hemoglobin.

- **Treatment** includes the usual measures of GI and skin decontamination; the airway is controlled as usual, and oxygen is administered. Hypotension is managed by administering fluids and vasopressors. Patients with clinical signs of toxicity or methemoglobin levels greater than 40% should be given **methylene blue,** 1 to 2 mg/kg IV over 4 to 5 minutes (10 mL of a 1.0% solution or 100 mg is the usual adult dose). The methemoglobin level should be monitored and repeat doses given as needed approximately 1 hour after the initial dose. Methylene blue functions to reduce methemoglobin to hemoglobin through the action of a reduced form of nicotinamide-adenine di-nucleotide phosphate reductase. Patients with glucose-6-phosphate dehydrogenase deficiency will not respond to methylene blue.

Exchange transfusions may be used in patients with severe toxicity or those not responsive to methylene blue.

Cyanide

Cyanide is one of the most rapidly acting and deadly poisons known; inhalation of hydrogen cyanide may produce death within minutes. Compounds containing cyanide are widespread; they are used in numerous industrial processes; are found in rodenticides and in amygdalin in apple, apricot, peach, plum, cherry, and almond seeds;

and are produced during the treatment with nitroprusside. Cyanide is a protoplasmic poison that rapidly and reversibly inhibits the cytochrome oxidase enzymes involved in cellular respiration by combining with the ferric (3+) ion.

- **Clinical presentation** includes headache, dyspnea, occasional nausea and vomiting, ataxia, coma, seizures, and death; toxicity may be nearly instantaneous.
- **Treatment** must be instituted rapidly and is based on presumptive evidence of cyanide ingestion; a bitter almond odor may be detected on the breath of poisoned patients and should suggest the diagnosis. After airway control is established, the antidotes for cyanide ingestion are administered:
  - Amyl nitrite pearls are crushed and held under the patient's nose or the endotracheal tube for 15 to 30 seconds while an IV line is secured.
  - Three percent sodium nitrite is given intravenously over 3 to 5 minutes; the adult dose is 10 mL, and the pediatric dose is 0.33 mL/kg up to 10 mL. If blood pressure falls during the administration of sodium nitrite, fluids and vasopressors are administered.
  - Twenty-five percent sodium thiosulfate is given intravenously as a 50-mL dose in adults and 1.65 mL/kg in children up to 50 mL. If signs and symptoms of poisoning recur or persist, sodium nitrite and sodium thiosulfate may be readministered.

The mechanism of action of these cyanide antidotes results in the formation of methemoglobin, which competes with cytochrome oxidase for cyanide. Sodium thiosulfate is used to form thiocyanate, which is a harmless substance excreted in the urine. The goal of these measures is to produce 25% to 30% methemoglobin. If methemoglobin levels in excess of 30% are generated as a result of drug treatment, they may be reduced with methylene blue as described in "Nitrates and Nitrites," p. 600.

Isoniazid

Isoniazid (INH) poisoning is a potentially life-threatening overdose more common in populations with a high incidence of tuberculosis and suicide. Isoniazid is rapidly absorbed with peak levels occurring in 1 to 2 hours. Isoniazid is metabolized by acetylation, the rate dependent on whether an individual is a fast or slow acetylator. Plasma half-life averages 0.7 to 2.0 hours in fast acetylators and 2 to 4 hours in slow acetylators. The volume of distribution and renal clearance are not affected by acetylator status; protein binding is negligible.

INH toxicity is a result of its effects on brain gamma aminobutyric acid (GABA) metabolism. The synthesis and degradation of GABA are dependent on enzymes in which pyridoxal-5-phosphate, the active form of pyridoxine (vitamin B_6), is a necessary coenzyme. Isoniazid inhibits the action of pyridoxal-5-phosphate and also depletes body stores of pyridoxine by increasing its renal excretion. Isoniazid thus effectively decreases levels of GABA in the brain. GABA functions primarily as an inhibitor of synaptic transmission; doses of INH as low as 15 mg/kg reduce the seizure threshold. INH may also block the conversion of lactate to pyruvate in the Krebs cycle by competition with nicotinamide-adenine dinucleotide (NAD)—a required pyridine cofactor.

- **Clinical presentation.** Symptoms of INH overdose include nausea, vomiting, slurred speech, ataxia, blurred vision, and tachycardia. The patient may rapidly lapse into coma. Recurrent grand mal seizures are commonly seen, which are often refractory to the usual treatment modalities. Hypotension, hyperthermia, oliguria, and tachycardia are noted.

- **Laboratory data** reveal a severe lactic acidosis and often demonstrate hypoglycemia, mild hypokalemia, and a leukocytosis. Hyperglycemia, glycosuria, and ketonuria are sporadically reported. A toxicology screen may demonstrate the presence of INH and its metabolites in the urine by a simple dipstick method; quantitative serum levels are of no value in treating acute overdoses.
- The **treatment** of INH overdose involves lavage if performed early, activated charcoal, and a cathartic. The administration of IV pyridoxine has been found to prevent or hasten the resolution of INH-induced seizures, coma, and lactic acidosis if given on a gram-for-gram basis. Pyridoxine should be given early to patients suspected of ingesting toxic amounts; experimentally acute pyridoxine toxicity is not seen in doses less than 4 to 5 g/kg. *Pyridoxine hydrochloride,* 5 g in 50 mL of 5% D/W, is infused over 10 to 20 minutes and repeated as needed until the amount of INH ingested is exceeded or seizures stop and consciousness is regained. Alternatively, a gram-equivalent amount of pyridoxine hydrochloride equal to the amount of isoniazid ingested may be mixed as a 10% solution with 5% D/W and infused over 30 to 60 minutes. Seizures refractory to pyridoxine hydrochloride should be controlled with IV diazepam, which has been shown to act synergistically with pyridoxine to raise GABA levels. Bicarbonate may be given to correct significant acidosis based on the usual criteria (e.g., pH <7.15–7.20).

Hydrogen Sulfide

Hydrogen sulfide gas is formed in industrial processes, mines, and sewers and is associated with decomposing fish and manure treatment systems. It is colorless and smells like "rotten eggs." Toxicity is similar to that of cyanide (inhibiting cytochrome oxidase), but it is less toxic. The diagnosis is confirmed by the presence of sulf-Hgb on spectrophotometry. Levels of sulf-Hgb do not help with treatment decisions.

- **Clinical presentation** includes dermatitis, blepharospasm, ocular pain, conjunctival injection, blurred vision, headache, weakness, chest pain, bradycardia, dyspnea, confusion, stupor, cyanosis, coma, and respiratory arrest.
- **Treatment** is similar to that for cyanide poisoning (see "Cyanide," pages 600 and 601) except that sodium thiosulfate should not be administered.

Camphor

Camphor is used in many over-the-counter topical products primarily for its strongly medicinal odor. It is extremely toxic; as little as 5 mL of camphorated oil ingested by an infant may be lethal. Most ingestions involve the accidental substitution of camphorated oil for castor or cod liver oil. Camphor is a cyclic ketone, is lipid soluble, and is detoxified in the liver by hydroxylation and conjugation; excretion is renal.

- **Clinical presentation.** Symptoms of camphor poisoning include agitation, nausea, vomiting, confusion, lethargy, coma, and recurrent grand mal seizures. Symptoms occur 5 to 90 minutes after ingestion and are often abrupt in onset. The typical odor of camphor may be noted on the breath as well as in urine and gastric samples. Routine blood studies may reveal transient elevation of hepatic enzymes.
- **Treatment** includes gastric lavage and the use of activated charcoal. Cathartics containing oil should not be administered, as these may increase the absorption of camphor. Seizures are treated initially with IV diazepam followed by phenobarbital. Patients with recurrent seizures should be considered for hemoperfusion, which is effective in extracting the poison and thereby hastening the resolution of clinical toxicity.

Alcohols

Ethanol

Ethanol is the most common drug taken either alone or in combination in acutely overdoses. It is a sedative hypnotic that is also used as a solvent and antiseptic and is found in various cough syrups and mouthwashes. Ethanol is rapidly absorbed through the GI tract and is distributed throughout the total body water. One ounce of whiskey, a glass of wine, or a bottle of beer typically increases the blood alcohol level by approximately 25 mg/dL in the adult. Ethyl alcohol is largely metabolized by the NAD-dependent alcohol dehydrogenase present in hepatic cytosol. Tolerance to the effects of ethanol occurs in long-term users, making blood levels unreliable with respect to the prediction of toxicity. In persons not chronically exposed to ethanol, blood ethanol levels greater than 100 mg/dL are associated with the classic signs of intoxication, and levels greater than 400 mg/dL may be lethal.

- **Clinical presentation** includes CNS depression and gastric irritation. Other findings in acute intoxication include ataxia, dysarthria, visual impairment, nystagmus, stupor, hypothermia, nausea, vomiting, and postural hypotension. These may progress to coma, seizures, areflexia, and death due to respiratory depression. Laboratory studies may reveal hypoglycemia, which is common in children, ketosis, an elevated plasma osmolality (by the freezing-point method), and a variety of electrolyte disturbances. Calcium, phosphorus, and magnesium levels are typically low in the chronic user. A toxicology screen should be considered to determine whether other substances have been co-ingested.

- **Treatment** includes assurance of adequate ventilation and oxygen and the administration of thiamine and glucose. Importantly, the administration of glucose without the previous or simultaneous coadministration of thiamine may precipitate acute Wernicke encephalopathy in chronic users with severe thiamine deficiency. Ethanol is quickly absorbed through the gastric mucosa. GI decontamination may be considered if other coingestants are suspected. Hypothermia should be treated and may be associated with the degree of hypoglycemia present. Patients with a blood alcohol level greater than 400 mg/dL and who are unresponsive to conservative supportive therapy may be considered for hemodialysis, although this is rarely required.

- Chronic users of alcohol with malnutrition who become severely thiamine-deficient may present with Wernicke encephalopathy and/or Korsakoff psychosis. **Wernicke encephalopathy** is marked by **ataxia, confusion, and weakness or paralysis of ocular muscles,** particularly the lateral recti. Vertical and horizontal nystagmus may be noted. When this is suspected, IV thiamine, 100 to 500 mg, should be administered and may dramatically reverse the clinical signs; 100 mg should then be given PO or IM. Up to 1,000 mg thiamine may be required in the first 24 hours. Although the classic triad of signs may be noted, isolated ophthalmoplegia or confusion may dominate the early clinical picture and warrant prophylactic treatment. The hallmark of **Korsakoff psychosis** is a relatively clear sensorium with **confabulation,** which is due to a severe selective abnormality of recent memory formation resulting in amnesia. Both syndromes result from thiamine depletion, and other vitamin deficiencies commonly coexist. Korsakoff psychosis is generally not as responsive to thiamine repletion as is Wernicke encephalopathy. Patients with Wernicke encephalopathy require admission for further thiamine treatment.

- **Withdrawal.** Individuals chronically exposed to ethanol are at risk for several acute neurologic symptoms when ethanol is withdrawn. Early on, the patient startles easily, and anorexia, nausea, vomiting, and tremulousness develop ("the shakes").

The tremor is typically generalized and fluctuates widely in severity. In approximately one fourth of tremulous patients, disorders of perception are manifest, ranging from nightmares to visual or auditory hallucinations.

- "Rum fits," or **withdrawal seizures,** usually develop 12 to 48 hours after the cessation of ethanol ingestion, the majority within the first 12 hours. These seizures are typically grand mal. If a focus is expressed during the seizure, a structural abnormality should be considered.

- The most serious, and fortunately rarest, symptom of alcohol withdrawal is **delirium tremens.** Typically occurring 3 to 4 days (but up to 14 days) after cessation of ethanol intake, delirium tremens is characterized by profound confusion, delusions, hallucinations, tremor, agitation, and excessive sympathetic stimulation producing fever, tachycardia, hypertension, dilated pupils, and profuse diaphoresis. Approximately 15% of patients with delirium tremens die, so patients suspected of incipient delirium tremens require prompt diagnosis and treatment.

- **Therapy** of ethanol withdrawal symptoms depends on their major manifestations. Hallucinosis may be treated with antipsychotic agents such as haloperidol. Withdrawal seizures are not treated with anticonvulsants (unless the patient has a history of a chronic seizure disorder). There is no evidence to support the therapeutic or prophylactic benefit of these agents in this type of seizure disorder. Benzodiazepines in low doses are indicated temporarily. Delirium tremens is treated by suppressing the agitated, hypersympathetic state. The actual choice of sedative used is less important than using amounts sufficient to sedate the patient. Lorazepam or diazepam is titrated intravenously as needed to achieve adequate sedation. Treatment continues for several days, during which time the dose may be gradually decreased. Dehydration and electrolyte disorders are treated with thiamine, multivitamins, and folate replaced.

- Among the numerous interactions of alcohol with other drugs, the **ethanol-disulfiram (Antabuse) reaction** is common and varies from mild to life threatening; the precise mechanism producing these clinical effects is poorly understood. Signs and symptoms of a disulfiram reaction occur within minutes of the ingestion of alcohol and include a feeling of warmth, bright red skin, nausea, vomiting, diaphoresis, blurred vision, confusion, weakness, dizziness, dyspnea, and hypotension. Treatment is supportive and includes fluid administration, airway management, oxygen, and ventilatory support as needed. Vasopressors may be required if signs of fluid overload appear, while hypotension remains uncorrected. Correction of any electrolyte abnormalities and cardiac monitoring are indicated.

Methanol

Methanol has a wide variety of industrial and household uses including paint thinner, antifreeze, and fuel for food warmers (Sterno). Methanol, or wood alcohol, is extremely toxic in small doses (10 mL) and may be lethal when as little as 60 mL is ingested. Both by sight and smell, it resembles ethanol. Methanol is quickly absorbed from the GI tract and is distributed throughout the total body water. Thirty percent of an absorbed dose is slowly excreted unchanged through the lungs, and less than five percent through the kidneys; the remainder is metabolized by alcohol dehydrogenase at a zero-order kinetic rate one-seventh that of ethanol. Alcohol dehydrogenase will preferentially metabolize ethanol rather than methanol if both substances are present. The toxic effects are caused by its toxic metabolites, *formaldehyde* and formate.

- **Clinical presentation** is similar to ethanol intoxication except that drowsiness is more pronounced. These symptoms occur for a variable period, from 6 to 36 hours (depending on the rate at which toxic metabolites are produced), after which the major symptoms of methanol intoxication appear. These include severe vomiting and upper abdominal pain, diarrhea, dizziness, headache, restlessness, dyspnea, blurred vision, photophobia, hyperemic optic disks, papilledema, blindness, delirium, fixed and dilated pupils, coma, cerebral edema, cardiac and respiratory depression, opisthotonos, seizures, and death. **Blindness** in survivors is common and may result from as little as 5 mL of methanol; ocular damage results from retinal destruction and optic nerve degeneration due to the metabolite formic acid. The fatal dose of methanol is 0.5 to 3.0 mL/Kg.

- **Laboratory findings** include a **metabolic acidosis** characterized by an increased anion gap caused by the formation of formic and lactic acid. Hyperosmolality and hyperglycemia and hyperamylasemia may be noted.
- **Treatment** includes controlling the airway and gastric lavage with ingestions ≤1 hour. Charcoal is not effective. Acidosis is treated with IV **bicarbonate,** and large amounts are often required. **Intravenous ethanol** should be infused to provide a continuous ethanol level of between 100 and 150 mg/dL; this will effectively compete with methanol for metabolism and prevent the formation of toxic metabolites. A loading dose of 1 mL/kg of sterile absolute (95%–100%) ethanol should be diluted in 5% D/W and infused over 15 minutes, followed by a maintenance infusion of 0.1 mL/kg/h titrated to maintain the ethanol level more than 100 mg/dL. **Indications for Hemodialysis** are methanol level is greater than 20 mg/dL; pH < 7.15; and visual, CNS dysfunction or history of ingesting >30 mL. During hemodialysis, it is important to maintain the ethanol level above 100 mg/dL by increasing the maintenance infusion rate or adding ethanol to the dialysate. Patients who do not meet the criteria for hemodialysis may require ethanol infusions for 2 to 3 days. The administration of folic acid to enhance the metabolic degradation of formate at a dose of 1 mg/kg IV (maximum 50 mg) q4h and (4-methyl pyrazole) inhibits alcohol dehydrogenase. Fomepizole is given 15 mg/kg over 30 minutes and then 10 mg/kg q12h for four doses. Treatment with fomepizole does not alter the indications for dialysis.

Ethylene Glycol

Ethylene glycol is present in antifreeze as well as in a variety of industrial products and numerous cosmetic preparations. It is colorless, odorless, and has a somewhat sweet taste. As little as 100 mL may be fatal. Toxicity is caused by the formation of metabolites resulting in severe acidosis and tissue damage; these include lactic, glycolic, glyoxylic, formic, and oxalic acids.

- **The clinical presentation** occurs in three stages. The first stage occurs 0.5 to 12 hours after ingestion and is characterized by ataxia, nystagmus, nausea, vomiting, decreased deep tendon reflexes, and severe acidosis; more severe poisoning will result in hypocalcemic tetany and seizures, cerebral edema, coma, and death. The second stage, occurring 12 to 24 hours after ingestion, is marked by the onset of tachypnea, cyanosis, tachycardia, mild hypertension, pulmonary edema, and pneumonitis. This phase occurs as calcium oxalate crystals are deposited in the vasculature, myocardium, and pulmonary parenchyma. The third stage, occurring 24 to 72 hours after ingestion, is marked by flank pain, costovertebral angle tenderness, and oliguric **renal failure** due to interstitial nephritis and acute tubular necrosis.
  - **Laboratory data** reveal a severe metabolic acidosis associated with an increased anion gap. Hypocalcemia may be present, and the urine may demonstrate **calcium oxalate crystals** and microscopic hematuria.

- **Treatment** is similar to that of methanol intoxication (see "Methanol," p. 604–605) and includes the administration of **bicarbonate** to reverse acidosis, **ethanol** to block the metabolism of ethylene glycol, calcium, and early **hemodialysis.** Additionally, IV calcium gluconate should be given as needed to treat hypocalcemic tetany and seizures.

  Fomepizole (4-methylpyrazole), an inhibitor of alcohol dehydrogenase, demonstrates comparable efficacy without some of the hazards of ethanol (hypoglycemia, mental status changes) and can be used instead of IV ethanol with thiamine 100 mg IV plus pyridoxine 100 mg IV. Fomepizole is used in the same dosage as for methanol intoxication (see p. 605). Treatment continues until ethylene glycol concentration decreases below 20 mg/dL. Hemodialysis is indicated for (1) history, clinical presentation, and lab results consistent with ethylene glycol poisoning; (2) ethylene glycol levels >20 mg/dL; (3) nephrotoxicity; and (4) metabolic acidosis.

Isopropyl Alcohol

Isopropyl alcohol is often used as a home remedy for muscular aches and is rubbed into the skin; it is also commonly used as a solvent, a deicer and antifreeze, and a disinfectant. The lethal dose is approximately 2 to 4 mL/kg or approximately 150 to 250 mL in adults. Isopropyl alcohol is metabolized by alcohol dehydrogenase, after first-order kinetics, into acetone, carbon dioxide, and water.

- **Clinical presentation** is similar to ethanol intoxication, but a more severe hemorrhagic gastritis is noted. Increasing intoxication may be characterized by hypotension, hypothermia, areflexia, and stupor followed by deep coma, which precedes death secondary to respiratory arrest. Laboratory studies reveal the presence of an anion gap associated with acetonemia and acetonuria. Hyperglycemia is not seen, and acidosis, if present, is not caused by isopropyl alcohol or its metabolites but rather by other factors such as hypotension and hypoxemia.

Treatment is supportive and includes airway control and ventilatory support, and fluid resuscitation and vasopressors as required to correct hypotension. Lavage, if performed very early after ingestion, may be beneficial. Activated charcoal absorbs 1 mL of 70% isopropyl alcohol per gram of charcoal. Intravenous glucose should be given to treat hypoglycemia, and bicarbonate is used to treat acidosis. Early hemodialysis is indicated in patients with refractory hypotension. Patients who remain stable (normal vital signs and normal cognitive function) over a 6-hour period of observation may safely be discharged.

Hydrocarbons

Substances designated as hydrocarbons comprise a diverse group of substances, literally any organic compound containing carbon and hydrogen. Discussion here is limited to some of the petroleum distillates, turpentine, and chlorinated and aromatic hydrocarbons. The toxicity of hydrocarbons may arise from ingestion, inhalation, or percutaneous absorption, but it varies depending on the specific compound. Numerous hydrocarbons are used as solvents, and it should be noted that toxicity may result from either the solvent or the substances dissolved in the hydrocarbon (e.g., pesticides, heavy metals, camphor).

Petroleum Distillates and Turpentine

Petroleum distillates are products of crude oil and include petroleum ether, naphtha, mineral spirits, kerosene, gasoline, mineral seal oil, motor oils, tars, and petroleum jellies. Turpentine is distilled from pinewood oil. These substances are found in numerous household products including lighter fluids, paint thinners and other solvents, paint and laundry "spot" removers, and lubricating oils and jellies. Important routes of toxicity are inhalation and ingestion; toxicity from skin contact is generally limited to contact dermatitis and occasionally mild burns.

- **Ingestion** of a petroleum distillates or turpentine may be asymptomatic, but local irritation including a burning sensation of the mouth and throat, nausea, vomiting, diarrhea, and rarely hematemesis, glottic edema, and stridor may occur. The most severe toxicity is seen when the substance is aspirated either while swallowing or during emesis; aspiration produces a severe chemical pneumonitis. The hazard of aspiration increases as the viscosity of the substance decreases: mineral seal oil (red furniture polish) has a low viscosity; kerosene, turpentine, gasoline, and naphtha have medium viscosities; and tars and jellies have very high viscosities.

- **Clinical presentation** following aspiration includes cough, dyspnea, bronchospasm, cyanosis, tachypnea, hemoptysis, rales, rhonchi, and fever. CNS symptoms are rare, but weakness, dizziness, confusion, depression, excitation, hallucinations, seizures, and coma have been reported. Renal failure and tubular acidosis can also occur.

- **Laboratory studies.** Arterial blood gases should be obtained to document adequate ventilation in symptomatic patients. Chest x-ray abnormalities typically lag behind clinical signs; it may require 6 to 8 hours before findings are demonstrated even in extremely symptomatic patients. Occasionally, abnormalities may be seen within 30 minutes of ingestion. Findings on the chest roentgenogram are bilateral and may include perihilar densities, atelectasias, pulmonary edema, and interstitial and alveolar pneumonitis; pneumothorax, pneumatoceles, pneumomediastinum, and subcutaneous emphysema are also reported.

- The **treatment** of petroleum distillate and turpentine ingestion varies concerning gastric decontamination. Lavage should be considered in alert patients who have ingested high viscosity compounds containing pesticides, heavy metals, or other toxic substances. The most controversial aspect is whether to lavage patients who have ingested large amounts (more than 4–5 mL/kg) of medium-viscosity substances (gasoline, turpentine, naphtha, kerosene). Regional poison control centers should be contacted for advice in patients with large ingestions. Some authorities urge endotracheal intubation before gastric lavage for decontamination. Activated charcoal is used for both high and low viscosity ingestions.

    The treatment of severe pulmonary symptoms includes intubation and use of positive end-expiratory pressure. Bronchospasm is treated with bronchodilators. The use of catecholamines in this setting has been associated with ventricular arrhythmias. Antibiotics and steroids are not recommended.

- **Inhalation** of gasoline produces euphoria within 3 to 5 minutes, which may last up to 3 to 6 hours. It is a relatively common method of drug abuse among young adolescent boys along with the inhalation of other aromatic hydrocarbons. Other effects include nausea, vomiting, ataxia, and excitement, followed by the loss of consciousness, coma, and seizures. Examination may reveal a typical odor on the breath; the pupils may be fixed, dilated and unequal, and nystagmus or dysconjugate gaze may be present. Death may occur suddenly from cardiac arrhythmias or from respiratory depression. In contrast to some of the other inhaled hydrocarbons in which no physical abnormalities are apparent at autopsy, in patients with sudden death, inhalation of gasoline may be associated with cerebral and pulmonary edema. Renal, hepatic, and CNS abnormalities may occur in association with chronic inhalation as well as lead poisoning. Treatment is supportive and is similar to that of the inhaled halogenated hydrocarbons (see "Halogenated Hydrocarbons").

Aromatic Hydrocarbons

Aromatic hydrocarbons include benzene, toluene, and xylene. These compounds are present in solvents, paints, glues, varnishes, paint removers, and gasoline, and they have a variety of other industrial uses.

- **Clinical presentation** varies with acute vs. chronic toxicity. Acute toxicity is caused by inhalation and may result in euphoria, dizziness, weakness, headache, visual blurring, tremors, ataxia, confusion, excitation, seizures, respiratory depression, coma, and death. The chronic effects of benzene are well known and include bone marrow depression, leukemia, and other neoplasms. Toluene is less toxic, but chronic effects include various neuropathies, muscle weakness, and changes in personality. Other chronic toxic effects common to these substances include renal toxicity (proteinuria, hematuria, distal tubular acidosis), abdominal pain, hematemesis, cerebellar dysfunction, and rhabdomyolysis.
- **Treatment** is supportive and is similar to that of the halogenated hydrocarbons (see "Halogenated Hydrocarbons"); the use of catecholamines should be avoided if possible because serious ventricular arrhythmias and sudden death may be precipitated.

Halogenated Hydrocarbons

Carbon tetrachloride, ethyl chloride, chloroform, trichloroethylene, and methylene chloride are examples. Carbon tetrachloride is discussed in "Carbon Tetrachloride" (p. 620). Many of these agents were once used for anesthesia; this use has been largely abandoned because of the high incidence of adverse effects.

- **Clinical presentation** following inhalation include CNS depression, headache, nausea, vomiting, hepatic and renal dysfunction, coma, and sudden death, probably caused by epinephrine-induced ventricular arrhythmias. Acute or chronic exposure to **methylene chloride**, present in some paint removers, results in the endogenous production of **carbon monoxide**.
- **Treatment** involves removing the patient from any contaminated areas and the usual GI decontamination measures, if ingested. Supportive therapy includes adequate ventilation, fluid resuscitation, judicious use of vasopressors (such as dobutamine) for hypotension, and correction of electrolyte abnormalities. Seizures may be treated with diazepam; ventricular arrhythmias are treated in the usual fashion. The use of epinephrine is not recommended. Hemodialysis may be necessary if renal failure ensues. Significant carbon monoxide levels in patients exposed to methylene chloride are treated with oxygen and consideration of hyperbaric oxygen therapy.

Heavy Metals

Iron

Numerous over-the-counter iron preparations are available; these often appear candy-like and are frequently ingested by children. Toxicity depends on the amount of elemental iron ingested; the elemental iron content of the sulfate salt is 20%, the fumarate salt 33%, and the gluconate salt 12%. The potential toxic dose for children younger than 6 years of age is 20 mg/kg.

Iron is absorbed in the duodenum and jejunum in the ferrous form, where it is oxidized to the ferric state and complexed to ferritin. Iron is released from ferritin into the plasma where it is rapidly bound to transferrin. When the transferrin-binding capacity is exceeded, iron freely circulates in the plasma. The metabolism of iron is remarkable for the lack of an excretory route in the event of acute or chronic iron overload.

- **Clinical presentation** occurs in three phases. The **first phase** occurs within the first 2 hours and is predominantly a result of the corrosive effects of iron on the GI tract; gastric and small bowel irritation lead to vomiting and diarrhea, and erosions and ulcerations may produce hematemesis or bloody diarrhea. Hypotension may occur as a result of GI tract bleeding or fluid shifts from the vascular space into the bowel. Lethargy, coma, and seizures may result from a decrease in cerebral perfusion caused by shock or as a direct effect of the free iron. Coagulation abnormalities as a result of early hepatic damage may be present and may contribute to the bleeding diathesis. Ferritin or iron may act directly as a vasodepressant or by the release of histamine and serotonin. Acidosis is common and results from the conversion of ferrous to ferric iron and ferric hydroxides, which result in the release of hydrogen ions, inhibition of the Krebs cycle leading to accumulation of organic acids, and lactic acidosis from reduced tissue perfusion. The **second phase** is seen 2 to 12 hours after ingestion and is marked by apparent clinical improvement. The **third phase** is seen approximately 12 to 48 hours after ingestion and is characterized by severe metabolic acidosis, hepatic and renal necrosis and failure, and often sepsis secondary to bacterial invasion of the damaged intestinal mucosa. Pulmonary edema and hemorrhage may occur as well.

  If the patient recovers from the acute intoxication, intestinal scarring, strictures, obstruction, and gangrenous infarction of the GI tract may be seen approximately 4 weeks after ingestion. Hepatic fibrosis and fatty degeneration may also occur.

- **Diagnostic tests.** Acutely, radiologic evaluation of the abdomen may demonstrate radiopaque pills in the GI tract. Although the serum iron and the total iron binding capacity (TIBC) are diagnostic, they must be drawn 4 to 6 hours after ingestion because iron is rapidly distributed into parenchymal tissue. These results are often difficult to obtain on an emergency basis. The degree of acidosis should be assessed, and blood should be drawn for typing and cross-matching in addition to baseline hepatic and renal function studies.

- **Treatment.** Symptoms that appear within 6 hours suggest toxic amounts of iron, and measures should be taken to empty the stomach along with plans for admission and treatment. Conversely, patients who remain asymptomatic at 6 hours after ingestion are unlikely to have ingested toxic amounts and may be discharged with instructions to return if any symptoms occur. In addition, patients ingesting **greater than 60 mg/kg of elemental iron** should be treated immediately with routine GI decontamination measures and a period of in-hospital observation. Lavage itself may fail to clear bezoars formed by the iron pills. Although charcoal does not bind iron, it should be given if concomitant ingestion of other toxic substances is suspected. Magnesium-containing cathartics should be avoided. Iron concretions may form in the stomach and may require endoscopic removal. Whole-bowel irrigation is the treatment of choice for decontamination of the gut.

  Shock, hemorrhage, and metabolic acidosis are treated with fluids, pressors, transfusions, and IV $NaHCO_3$ as required; fluid balance must be carefully monitored to avoid pulmonary edema. Although vasopressors may be used to treat hypotension and shock, they should be instituted only after fluid resuscitation has failed.

- **Deferoxamine chelation therapy** is indicated for toxic ingestions. Deferoxamine may be given as a diagnostic test in cases of presumptive ingestion when iron and TIBC levels are not quickly available and the patient shows signs of iron toxicity such as acidosis, altered level of consciousness, etc. Deferoxamine, 25 to 50 mg/kg up to a total dose of 1 g, may be given by deep intramuscular injection. The appearance of a characteristic "vin-rosé" color of the urine is diagnostic of iron toxicity. Deferoxamine is a specific chelator of iron in its free and transferrin-bound forms. The deferoxamine-iron complex is rapidly excreted by the kidney. This change in the color of urine is also seen after starting IV deferoxamine. If serum iron levels are rapidly available, treat for ≥350 μg/dL. Intravenous deferoxamine is infused at a rate of 15 mL/kg/h with a maximum rate of 1 g/h. If renal failure is present, the chelated iron may be hemodialyzed. Rapid infusion of deferoxamine may produce hypotension, and idiosyncratic reactions to this agent occur as urticaria, flushing, and intestinal irritation.

Lead

Lead poisoning may present acutely, but exposure is invariably chronic. Distribution is relatively slow, and the elimination half-life of serum lead is estimated to be approximately 2 months. Lead may be ingested as inorganic material (e.g., paint, metallic objects) or inhaled as organic lead (e.g., leaded gasoline).

- **Diagnostic tests.** Acute inorganic lead poisoning may present with nausea, vomiting, abdominal pain, peripheral neuropathies, stupor, convulsions, and coma. Organic lead exposure results in predominant CNS symptoms and occasional bradycardia, hypotension, and increased deep tendon reflexes. "Lead lines" may be noted on examination of the dentition and gingiva in chronic exposure.

- **Laboratory data** in chronic exposure may demonstrate anemia, red cell stippling on the peripheral smear, radiologically noted densities at the ends of long bones and ribs, and radiopaque material within the GI tract. Suspected lead poisoning should be rapidly confirmed by blood lead levels and the erythrocyte protoporphyrin level.

- **Treatment** consists of GI decontamination if ingested material is demonstrated on abdominal roentgenograms or was recently ingested. Seizures should be treated with IV diazepam, followed by phenobarbital or phenytoin. Seizures in patients with acute toxicity or coma indicate increased intracranial pressure (ICP), and mannitol, steroids, and possibly hypothermia should be used to reduce ICP.

Symptomatic patients are given chelation therapy with combined **dimercaprol** (BAL) and **calcium disodium edetate** (calcium EDTA). Dimercaprol is given in a dose of 75 mg/m² by deep intramuscular injection every 4 hours; DMSA (Chemet), a new chelator related to BAL, is an oral agent that can be used in children who are not encephalopathic. Calcium EDTA is begun after the second dose of dimercaprol because EDTA may mobilize more lead than can be excreted, which can, if given before dimercaprol therapy, increase encephalopathy. Calcium EDTA is given in a dose of 12.5 mg/kg intramuscularly every 6 hours in the non-convulsing child and 18.75 mg/kg in the child with seizures up to a total dose of 250 mg. The dose should be mixed with 0.5 mL of 1% lidocaine to reduce pain at the injection site. In the adult, 250 mg IV is given every 6 hours. Urine output should be maintained, because oliguria may result in lead-induced renal tubular damage.

High doses of calcium EDTA may chelate magnesium, zinc, and manganese and result in cardiac arrhythmias. Side effects of dimercaprol include local pain at the injection site, paresthesias, lacrimation, salivation, vomiting, and occasionally neutropenia.

Arsenic

Arsenic is used in industrial and agricultural settings. It may be ingested or inhaled and produce either acute or chronic toxicity. It is commonly used as a wood preservative.

- **Clinical presentation** includes nausea, vomiting, and diarrhea with a burning sensation of the mouth and pharynx. There may be a garlic odor to the breath. Muscular twitches and spasms are seen, followed by cardiac dysrhythmias, QT prolongation, ventricular tachycardia, and hepatic and renal failure. Delirium and coma are common.
- **Laboratory data** show multiple abnormalities of hepatic and renal function. Diagnosis is confirmed by measuring the urinary arsenic level.
- **Treatment includes** fluid and electrolyte correction.
- Specific chelation therapy in acute toxicity is performed with dimercaprol or DMSA (Chemet). Dimercaprol is given 5 mg/kg intramuscular, followed by 2.5 mg/kg every 8 hours for 24 hours and every 12 to 24 hours thereafter for 10 days. Penicillamine may be substituted after 48 hours of dimercaprol treatment (although it should not be given to penicillin-allergic patients) as 25 mg/kg orally every 6 hours for 4 to 8 days. DMSA is given orally at 10 mg/kg three times daily.

Arsine

Arsine gas is produced when arsenic-containing metals are exposed to acids; this results in a severe and rapidly evolving Coombs-negative hemolytic anemia. Signs and symptoms include abdominal pain, nausea, vomiting, hematuria, and progressive hepatic and renal failure. The treatment of acute arsine poisoning is exchange transfusions and hemodialysis for renal failure. Chelation therapy is not effective.

Mercury

Mercury is commonly present in both organic and inorganic forms in the environment, industry, and agricultural settings. Poisoning may occur acutely or chronically by oral ingestion of mercury-containing compounds, by inhalation (which is quite toxic), or as a result of cutaneous exposure. Mercury has a half-life of approximately 40 to 60 days, and excretion is primarily renal. Mercury is avidly attracted and binds to sulfhydryl groups on proteins and enzymes, thereby altering their metabolism and function.

- The **clinical effects** of acute exposure to mercury *vapor* include cough, dyspnea, chest tightness, weakness, nausea, vomiting, diarrhea, and a metallic taste in the mouth. An interstitial pneumonitis may be produced, progressing to a necrotizing bronchiolitis and pulmonary edema. The acute effects of *ingestion* of toxic amounts of mercurial salts are severe nausea, vomiting, diarrhea, hematemesis, and hematochezia, due to mercury's caustic properties. Dehydration, shock, and renal failure may quickly ensue.
- **Diagnostic tests.** The clinical diagnosis of mercury poisoning may be difficult, but blood and urine levels can be measured and monitored to make a diagnosis and guide therapy, respectively.
- The **treatment** of acute mercury poisoning is supportive and involves the use of chelators to decrease the body burden of mercury. GI tract and skin decontamination should be performed early and aggressively when indicated. Charcoal should be administered as well; however, cathartics should be withheld in the presence of diarrhea. Shock and electrolyte abnormalities should be managed with aggressive fluid resuscitation, and transfusions may be required in patients with significant bleeding. Specific therapy involves the administration of dimercaprol (BAL), which is given

initially at a dose of 4 mg/kg intramuscular and then every 4 hours for 7 to 10 days. It may be combined with dialysis for optimal clearance of mercury and treatment of severe electrolyte abnormalities or in patients with renal failure. D-Penicillamine is an alternative to dimercaprol. Once gastroenteritis has resolved, DMSA (Chemet) may be given.

Pesticides and Herbicides

Pesticides and herbicides represent a diverse group of chemicals used as insecticides, herbicides, rodenticides, fungicides, and fumigants. They account for 10% of all deaths caused by ingestion or exposure, and an estimated 100 individuals are poisoned for each death. Approximately 45% of all the pesticides produced in the world are used in the United States; fortunately, the number of pesticides accounting for most human poisonings is small compared with the tens of thousands of available products. The National Pesticide Information Center may be consulted for advice regarding emergency management and information about most pesticides. The telephone number is 1–800–858–7378 and is operational 6:30 AM to 4:30 PM, Pacific Time, daily. Many of the pesticide-producing companies have toxicologists available 24 h/day for emergency consultation.

When treating a specific poisoning, it must be noted that the vehicle (e.g., methyl alcohol, petroleum distillates) may similarly be toxic and may require specific therapy.

Insecticides

- **Organophosphates** are widely used because of their great efficacy. Organophosphate insecticides account for 80% of all hospitalizations for pesticide poisoning. Although all organophosphates should be considered toxic, individual differences in toxicity are significant. The most toxic are used for agricultural purposes (parathion and mevinphos) and the least toxic are available for household use (malathion, dichlorvos).

  Organophosphates are **cholinesterase inhibitors,** acting on acetylcholinesterase in red blood cells and at synapses and on pseudocholinesterase in plasma and in the liver. Inhibition cholinesterase is due to organophosphate-induced phosphorylation; depending on the specific organophosphate, the active enzyme may spontaneously be regenerated within a few hours or irreversibly destroyed.

  Organophosphates may be absorbed through the lungs, GI tract, skin, and conjunctivae. Onset of symptoms usually occurs rapidly with inhalation and within 12 hours of skin contamination.

- **Clinical presentation** results from the accumulation of acetylcholine at cholinergic receptor sites. This initially results in stimulation; however, as acetylcholine accumulates, paralysis or cessation of transmission occurs secondary to persistent depolarization. Receptor sites for acetylcholine are widely distributed throughout the body. Acetylcholine functions as an excitatory mediator at central and peripheral autonomic synapses. Receptors occur in central and parasympathetic nervous systems (both muscarinic) and striated muscle and sympathetic ganglia (both nicotinic).

  The **first signs** and symptoms of organophosphate poisoning are caused by stimulation of muscarinic, parasympathetic receptors and include nausea, vomiting, abdominal cramping, chest pain, dyspnea, wheezing, **miosis,** bradycardia, diaphoresis, blurred vision, bronchorrhea, and the **SLUD** response (*s*alivation, *l*acrimation, *u*rination, *d*iarrhea). **As toxicity increases,** stimulation of nicotinic sites and central muscarinic receptors cause tremors, twitching, weakness, fasciculations, paralysis, **tachycardia,** hypertension, **mydriasis** and pallor. CNS effects include anxiety, restlessness, insomnia, confusion, delirium, agitation headache, weakness, ataxia, tremors, seizures, slurred speech, decreased respirations, hypotension, and coma.

- **Laboratory studies** should include routine admission tests and measurement of arterial blood gases. Confirmation of organophosphate poisoning is based on **depression of red blood cell acetylcholinesterase** activity. Depressions greater than 25% are diagnostic of exposure, greater than 50% associated with symptoms, and greater than 80% to 90% is indicative of severe poisoning. Serum cholinesterase levels should be measured.

- **Treatment** must be promptly initiated before laboratory confirmation of pesticide toxicity; the clinical diagnosis is based on a history compatible with exposure and the expected symptoms. Ingested organophosphates should be removed by the usual GI tract decontamination procedures. Victims of skin contamination or inhalation of organophosphates should undergo skin surface decontamination. Clothing must be removed and placed into plastic bags. The patient's skin and hair are then thoroughly washed with mild soap, followed by copious irrigation; asymptomatic patients may shower. The medical staff must be protected from secondary contamination using appropriate protective equipment. Ocular irrigation with normal saline is indicated for direct exposure. Serum and RBC cholinesterase levels should be obtained.

Atropine reverses the peripheral muscarinic parasympathetic effects as well as many of the central effects. Importantly, atropine will not reverse nicotinic neuromuscular paralysis or other neurologic dysfunction associated with severe poisoning. This is because atropine does not separate the organophosphate from the cholinesterase enzyme. Atropine, 1 to 2 mg IV (0.05 mg/kg IV for children), is given slowly as required; patients with severe symptoms will require 2 to 4 mg up to every 2 to 3 minutes as needed to reverse symptomatic bradycardia, excessive bronchial secretions, and other symptoms. Massive doses, up to 50 mg/day or more, may be required. **Pralidoxime (2-PAM)** is a specific antidote that acts to cleave the organophosphate from the cholinesterase enzyme; it thereby frees the enzyme to hydrolyze excess acetylcholine. Pralidoxime must be given before irreversible phosphorylation has occurred; this agent has the greatest affinity for the phosphorylated enzyme at the nicotinic neuromuscular junction and reverses skeletal muscle paralysis. It does not, however, readily cross the blood–brain barrier and has poor affinity for peripheral muscarinic sites so that coadministration of atropine is always required. Pralidoxime is given intravenously, 1 g in 100 mL of normal saline at a rate not to exceed 500 mg/min. Children should be given 25 to 50 mg/kg (a maximum of 1 g) over 15 to 30 minutes. This dose may be repeated in 20 minutes if muscle strength has not returned and then as needed to maintain strength; up to 0.5 g/h has been required in critically ill patients.

Seizures may be treated with IV diazepam. Several drugs may worsen the toxicity and **should not be given** including β-blockers, quinidine, aminoglycosides, tetracaine, procainamide, morphine, aminophylline, phenothiazines, furosemide, and others. Treatment should be continued until signs of cholinesterase activity return, which is generally within 12 to 24 hours; however, delays of up to 10 days may occur. The patient should be monitored carefully for signs of atropine toxicity—fever, muscle fibrillations, and delirium—and atropine withheld if they occur. The development of rales or bradycardia warrants retreatment with atropine.

- **Carbamates** are reversible cholinesterase inhibitors; they are widely used in agricultural and household settings. The carbamates cause reversible carbamylation of cholinesterase enzymes. Cholinesterase activity commonly reverts to normal levels within minutes to a few hours after exposure. Carbamates are absorbed by all routes, including the skin, inhalation, and ingestion.
  - **Clinical presentation** is similar to the organophosphate insecticides but tends to be milder and less prolonged. Convulsions are rare.
  - **Laboratory data** may be entirely normal. Red blood cell and serum cholinesterase activity may be normal even in symptomatic patients.
  - The **treatment** of symptomatic carbamate poisoning includes skin and GI tract decontamination. **Atropine** is the drug of choice in the management of patients with carbamate poisoning. In adults, the dose is 0.5 to 2.0 mg IV every 15 to 20 minutes as needed to reverse cholinergic effects; children may be given 0.015 to 0.05 mg/kg up to 0.5 to 2.0 mg. Atropine is usually unnecessary after 6 or 12 hours, and large doses are rarely required.

    Several drugs (see "Insecticides" on p. 613) should be avoided in carbamate poisoning. Pralidoxime (2-PAM) is not indicated in carbamate poisoning because the cholinesterase enzyme recovers quickly. Pralidoxime should be used, however, when both a carbamate and an organophosphate are involved and should be used if the clinician is faced with signs of severe anticholinesterase poisoning with an unknown agent.
- **Organochlorines.** The use of organochlorine insecticides (DTT, aldrin, heptachlor, dieldrin, chlordane, kepone, and others) has largely been banned in the United States; however, methoxychlor, Kelthane, and lindane remain available. Lindane in particular is in widespread use as a garden insecticide and is used medically for the control of scabies and lice. Organochlorines are highly lipid soluble and may be absorbed by ingestion or through the skin.
  - **Clinical presentation** results from CNS stimulation and includes apprehension, confusion, paresthesias, nausea, vomiting, muscle tremors, twitching, seizures, coma, dysrhythmias, and respiratory failure. Status epilepticus may occur.
  - **Treatment** is supportive and symptomatic; if ingested, the usual GI tract decontamination measures are employed, but the addition of a resin binder such as cholestyramine should be considered. If poisoning resulted from skin contamination, the skin should be thoroughly washed with soap and irrigated with water. Seizures are managed with the cautious use of diazepam and/or phenobarbital; respiratory compromise is common with the concomitant use of these agents, and intubation and assisted ventilation may be required. Hypotension should be managed with fluids and pressors if necessary. Organochlorines cause myocardial irritability, and epinephrine therefore should be used cautiously. Dialysis and hemoperfusion are not beneficial.
- Botanicals
  - **Pyrethins** are low-toxicity insecticides obtained from refined chrysanthemum flowers. They are used in nearly all household insecticides usually along with the synergist piperonyl butoxide. Severe poisoning is rare, but massive doses may cause vomiting, muscular paralysis, seizures, and respiratory failure. The most frequent problem with the pyrethrins is contact dermatitis and other allergic reactions; 50% of individuals allergic to ragweed will display cross sensitivity. Treatment is symptomatic.

- **Rotenone** is obtained from several plants. It is of low toxicity to humans but highly toxic to birds and fish. Rotenone causes prompt emesis on ingestion and is poorly absorbed through the GI tract. Massive overdose will produce protracted vomiting, respiratory depression, and hypoglycemia. Inhalation of rotenone has caused intense respiratory stimulation progressing to depression and seizures. Treatment is symptomatic and supportive.
- **Nicotine,** extracted from tobacco leaves, is used as a 40% insecticide solution (Black Leaf-40) and is a highly toxic ganglionic stimulant absorbed through the skin, mouth, GI tract, and lungs. It is metabolized in the liver and to a lesser extent in the kidneys and lungs; it is excreted in the urine.
  - **Clinical presentation** mimics acetylcholinesterase poisoning and includes salivation, lacrimation, nausea, sweating, and meiosis. CNS stimulation produces tremors and convulsions. Severe toxicity is associated with mydriasis, hypotension, coma, and respiratory arrest. From the time of ingestion or exposure to respiratory depression is often less than 4 to 5 minutes; death has been reported within 1 hour.
  - **Laboratory data** are usually not helpful.
  - **Treatment** is symptomatic and supportive. GI tract and skin decontamination measures must be rapidly employed to limit further toxicity. Charcoal should be administered when ingestion has occurred. Seizures should be treated with diazepam. Signs of cholinergic excess may be reversed with the use of atropine in low doses. α-Adrenergic blocking agents such as phentolamine may be used in patients who are severely hypertensive.

Herbicides

- **Chlorophenoxy** herbicides (2,4,5-trichlorophenoxyacetic acid [2,4,5-T] and 2,4-dichlorophenoxyacetic acid [2,4-D]) remain widely used. However, 2,4,5-T and its contaminant, dioxin, have been banned since 1969 for use around crops, aquatic areas, and human populations. Agent Orange, a compound used in the Vietnam war, contained high concentrations of 2,4-D and 2,4,5-T, as well as dioxin. Dioxin is a potent teratogen, a possible carcinogen, and one of the most toxic chemicals known to exist; in 1978, the use of 2,4,5-T was totally outlawed, although 2,4-D is much less toxic and remains in widespread use.
  - **Clinical presentation** includes muscular weakness, hypotension, vomiting, diarrhea, abdominal pain, and burning pain in the eyes, nose, throat, and chest. Death may occur secondary to cardiac arrest. Dioxin causes a characteristic dermatitis called chloracne.
  - **Treatment** is symptomatic and supportive. GI tract and skin decontamination should be rapid. The pKa of 2,4-D (2.6) allows for increased excretion by alkaline diuresis.
- **Dipyridyl compounds include paraquat and diquat.** Paraquat is the more toxic, with more than 600 lethal cases of poisoning to date, of which nearly 60% were suicides. The toxic effects of dipyridyl compounds are thought to be caused by superoxide radial formation, its caustic nature, and its aliphatic petroleum solvent. Dermal and inhalational toxicity is low, but ingestion is potentially lethal.
  - **Clinical presentation** is marked by caustic ulcerations of buccal, oral, and esophageal epithelium; corneal ulceration is seen when either compound is splashed into the eyes. Ingestions of greater than 30 mg/kg are associated with multiple organ failure, including hepatic, pulmonary, cardiac, renal, and CNS.

Death typically occurs within hours to days. Paraquat ingestion of more than 4 mg/kg produces reversible renal failure within 24 hours and irreversible pulmonary fibrosis. Myocarditis, epicardial hemorrhage, and adrenal gland injury also occur.

- **Laboratory studies** should be performed to provide baseline values. Serial chest roentgenograms and measurement of arterial blood gases to follow pulmonary function are indicated. Paraquat can be detected by gas and high-pressure liquid chromatography.
- **Treatment** must be aggressive in patients with suspected paraquat poisoning. High supplemental oxygen concentrations should be avoided to minimize superoxide radical formation. GI tract decontamination should be done with activated charcoal. Dialysis is minimally effective; hemoperfusion performed nearly continuously for up to 2 to 3 weeks after ingestion may be useful.

Rodenticides
- **Warfarin** is used universally for rodent control and inhibits the synthesis of vitamin K-dependent clotting factors in the plasma and liver (factors II, VII, IX, and X).
  - **Clinical presentation.** Severe toxicity occurs with repeated doses and is characterized by hemorrhage and anemia; massive single doses (15 g) may also produce severe toxicity.
  - **Treatment.** Patients ingesting large or recent doses of warfarin should be treated with GI tract decontamination if the agent was taken within 1 to 2 hours. In symptomatic patients, or if the ingestion was massive or associated with evidence of bleeding or deranged hemostasis, **phytonadione (vitamin K)** should be administered. If hemorrhage is severe, blood, plasma, or clotting factor transfusions may be required.
- **Phosphorus.** Elemental white (or yellow) phosphorus is a potent rodenticide that is made into a paste and spread onto edible baits. Phosphorus is a protoplasmic poison that interferes with numerous metabolic pathways.
  - **Clinical presentation** is divided into three stages. In **stage 1,** intense nausea, vomiting, diarrhea, and abdominal pain occur. The patient may report a burning mouth, and a **garlic-like odor** may be detected. The **vomitus and stool may be luminescent.** In **stage 2,** lasting for a few hours to days, the patient is asymptomatic. **Stage 3** is the period of systemic toxicity with hepatic and renal failure, convulsions, coma, and death from cardiac arrest or shock. In massive ingestions, death has occurred from intractable cardiac arrhythmias 1 to 12 hours after ingestion.
  - The **treatment** of patients presenting during stage 1 involves measures to neutralize and remove the phosphorus from the GI tract. **Copious gastric lavage** should be performed with a 1:5,000 solution of **potassium permanganate,** which will oxidize phosphorus to inactive phosphate. Gastric lavage is followed by activated charcoal and mineral oil catharsis. Digestible fats, butter, milk, and so on should be avoided. Mineral oil, 30 mL, should be given every 3 hours for the first 48 hours. Treatment is otherwise supportive.
- **Vacor Rat Poison (PNU). PNU is a nicotinamide antagonist** that damages the beta-cells of the pancreas and various autonomic nerves. PNU comes in 39 g cornmeal packets of which 2% is the active ingredient.
  - Symptoms include nausea, vomiting, slurred speech, ataxia, confusion, memory loss, and orthostatic hypotension. It can produce permanent peripheral neuropathy and autonomic dysfunction with permanent orthostatic hypotension. Because

of its effects on beta-cells, it can produce prolonged hypoglycemia followed by insulin-dependent diabetes.

• Treatment: After assuring the ABCs, administer GI decontamination with lavage (if recent ingestion), charcoal, and a cathartic. Nicotinamide should be given, 500 mg IV followed by 10 to 200 mg IV every 4 hours for 12 to 14 days and then 100 mg orally four times daily for 12 to 14 days.

Household Plants

Although a variety of plants may produce symptoms, toxicity is rarely significant, and hospitalization is infrequently required. Attempt to determine the exact species of the plant, the specific parts ingested (e.g., berries, leaves), and if possible an estimate of the amount consumed. In addition, because toxicity varies with the species, sex, and age of the plant, as well as the environmental conditions under which it has grown, a representative sample of the ingested plant should be retained and analyzed for accurate identification; this will frequently require consultation with a poison control center and a botanist. Common names, once a plant has been identified, are imprecise and misleading and should generally be avoided.

Some relatively common plants associated with toxic symptoms are as follows:

Plants Containing Calcium Oxalate Crystals

Plants containing calcium oxalate crystals include *Philodendron* spp., dumbcane (*Dieffenbachia seguine* or *picta*), *Caladium* spp., jack-in-the-pulpit (*Arisaema triphyllum*), elephant's ear (*Colocasia* spp., *Alocasia* spp.), *Spathiphyllum* spp., and calla lily (*Zantedeschia aethiopica*). These plants produce primarily local reactions involving the skin and mucous membranes (burning sensation followed by evidence of inflammation), which is caused by the irritant properties of the needle-like calcium oxalate crystals as well as a possible toxin. Systemic toxicity is not reported. Unless oropharyngeal swelling is significant, outpatient therapy with cool compresses, antihistamines, and soothing agents is all that is required. When swelling is significant, admit for observation.

Plants Containing Cardiac Toxins

Plants containing cardiac toxins include foxglove (*Digitalis purpurea*), lily of the valley (*Convallaria majalis*), oleander (*Nerium oleander*), yellow oleander (*Thevetia perviana*), and star-of-Bethlehem (*Ornithogalum umbellatum*). Minor ingestions of these plants should be considered potentially serious; lavage should be immediately performed, and charcoal and cathartics given. The patient should be hospitalized for continuous monitoring for 24 to 48 hours. GI tract and mucous membrane irritation may occasionally be seen and is treated symptomatically. The administration of digoxin-specific antibody fragments may be indicated in serious foxglove intoxications.

Plants Containing Cyanogenic Compounds

Plants containing cyanogenic compounds include peach, pear, black cherry, apricot, and apple seeds; *Hydrangea* spp.; cassava (*Manihot utilissima*); black elderberry (*Sambucus canadensis, S. pubens*); and certain lima beans (*Phaseolus limensis, P. lunatus*). The roots or seeds of these plants when uncooked and chewed may produce cyanide toxicity. There are numerous reports of cyanide toxicity both in cancer patients who have taken amygdalin (prepared from crushed seeds of the apricot) and from New Guinea as a result of raw, colored lima bean ingestion. Treatment is as for cyanide poisoning (see "Cyanide," p. 601).

Plants Containing Toxic Alkaloids

Plants containing toxic alkaloids include black henbane (*Hyoscyamus niger*), deadly nightshade (*Atropa belladonna*), poison hemlock (*Conium maculatum*), yew (*Taxus baccata, T. canadensis*), daffodil (*Narcissus* spp.), jimson weed (*Datura* spp.), hyacinth (*Hyacinthus orientalis*), Jerusalem cherry (*Solanum pseudocapsicum*), larkspur (*Delphinium ajacis*), Christmas rose (*Helleborus niger*), morning glory (*Ipomoea violacea*), snowdrop (*Galanthus nivalis*), and autumn crocus (*Colchicum autumnale*). These plants contain various alkaloids, which may produce nausea, vomiting, diarrhea, headache, abdominal pain, hypotension, cardiac arrhythmias, CNS and respiratory depression, hallucinations, seizures, and death. Treatment consists of GI tract decontamination in the usual manner and supportive, symptomatic therapy; toxicologic consultation should be sought with respect to the specific ingestion.

Plants Containing Toxic Resins or Phytotoxins

Plants containing toxic resins or phytotoxins include black locust (*Robinia pseudacacia*), holly (*Ilex* spp.), pokeweed (*Phytolacca* spp.), poinsettia (*Euphorbia pulcherrima*), water hemlock (*Cicuta maculata*), chinaberry (*Melia azedarach*), azalea (*Rhododendron* spp.), castor bean (*Ricinus communis*), rosary pea (*Abrus precatorius*), mountain laurel (*Kalmia latifolia, K. angustifolia*), mayapple (*Podophyllum peltatum*), buttercup (*Ranunculus* spp.), mistletoe (*Phoradendron* spp.), and Texas mountain laurel (*Sophora secundiflora*). These plants contain toxic substances that may produce mild GI tract symptoms (e.g., the poinsettia) or severe life-threatening cardiac, respiratory, and CNS symptoms. The castor bean, rosary pea, and water hemlock may be fatal when ingested in small amounts. Treatment consists of the usual GI tract decontamination measures and conservative support; toxicologic consultation should be sought with regard to the specific ingestion.

Rhubarb

Rhubarb (*Rheum rhabarbarum*) contains oxalic acid in the leaf blades, which, when ingested, produces hypocalcemia and intravascular precipitates of calcium oxalate. Symptoms include abdominal pain, vomiting, diarrhea, tetany, seizures, coma, and acute renal failure. GI tract decontamination is indicated, as well as dilution of the gastric contents with milk as a calcium source to precipitate oxalic acid in the bowel and thereby prevent its absorption. Hydration may be helpful in preventing intrarenal deposition of calcium oxalate.

Mushroom Poisoning

Mushroom poisoning causes approximately 100 fatalities and several thousand nonfatal poisonings each year. Mushrooms are categorized into eight groups based on the toxins they contain, and thus the clinical features of the specific mushroom ingestion may indicate the possible species of mushroom ingested, as well as guide treatment. General guidelines in treating patients with mushroom poisoning include obtaining a careful history noting how many types of mushrooms were ingested, the time of ingestion, the exact chronology of symptoms, and whether any other persons ingested similar mushrooms. GI tract decontamination is undertaken in the usual fashion. It is important to save the initial emesis or gastric aspirate for examination and identification of any spores or mushroom fragments by a mycologist if indicated. Supportive measures include airway management and IV fluids and vasopressors as needed.

Group 1: Cyclopeptides

The cyclopeptide-containing mushrooms are responsible for 90% to 95% of all deaths from mushroom ingestion. The toxic agents are *amatoxins,* which cause widespread cellular necrosis resulting in hepatic, renal, and CNS failure. Representative mushrooms of this group include *Amanita phalloides, A. verna, A. virosa, Galerina autumnalus, G. venerata, Lepiota helveola,* and *Conocybe filaris.* The ingestion of one *A. phalloides* mushroom cap may be lethal. The cyclopeptide toxins are not destroyed by heat.

- **Clinical presentation** occurs in three stages. During stage 1, the sudden onset of abdominal pain, nausea, vomiting, and severe diarrhea occurs, usually 6 to 24 hours after ingestion. The diarrhea may contain blood and mucus. Stage 2, which occurs 12 to 48 hours after ingestion, is marked by apparent clinical recovery and rising hepatic enzymes. Stage 3 occurs 24 to 72 hours after ingestion and is characterized by progressive hepatic, cardiac, and renal failure, seizures, coma, coagulopathies, and death.
- **Treatment** is supportive.

Group 2: Muscimol, Ibotenic Acid

This group of mushrooms contains muscimol, a potent hallucinogen, and ibotenic acid, an insecticide. Intoxication becomes apparent within 1 to 2 hours of ingestion with euphoria, ataxia, and hallucinations. Large doses may lead to coma, seizures, or psychosis. Although the mushrooms in this group contain muscarine, a cholinergic agent, most investigators believe that anticholinergic symptoms and findings predominate in serious intoxication. Delirium and coma have been reversed with physostigmine. A careful physical examination is therefore required to assess cholinergic or anticholinergic findings before a particular treatment strategy is chosen. Species of mushrooms in this class include several of the *Amanita* spp., including *A. muscaria.*

Group 3: Monomethylhydrazine

Mushrooms in this group contain monomethylhydrazine, which causes signs and symptoms similar to isoniazid toxicity, as both of these substances **inhibit the synthesis of GABA** in the brain. GABA is an inhibitory neurotransmitter. Symptoms begin 6 to 24 hours after ingestion with vomiting, diarrhea, delirium, seizures, and coma. Toxicity may also result from inhalation of vapors associated with boiling or cooking these mushrooms because monomethylhydrazine is quite volatile. Methemoglobinemia and hemolysis may occur. Treatment consists of administration of IV *pyridoxine* (vitamin B_6), 25 mg/kg initially and repeated as needed until symptoms improve. Methylene blue is administered for methemoglobin levels of more than 30%. Seizures may be treated with diazepam, which acts synergistically with pyridoxine to increase GABA levels. Mushrooms included in this group are the *Gyromitra* spp. (false morels), *Paxina* spp., and *Sarcosphaera coronaria.*

Group 4: Muscarine

Mushrooms in this group produce signs and symptoms of cholinergic poisoning within 1 hour of ingestion. The classic **SLUD** symptoms (i.e., salivation, lacrimation, urination, diarrhea, bronchospasm, bronchorrhea) are found. The cholinergic symptoms are usually mild and treated with IV *atropine* as needed to control pulmonary secretions. Numerous species of *Boletus, Clitocybe,* and *Inocybe* are in this group.

Group 5: Coprine

Coprine-containing mushrooms are nontoxic when consumed alone. Coprine, however, may cause a **disulfiram-like reaction** if alcohol is ingested within 96 hours of eating the mushrooms. Symptoms include flushing, palpitations, dyspnea, chest pain, and diaphoresis. Treatment is supportive and includes the administration of fluids. The reaction is self-limited, usually lasting no more than 3 to 4 hours. This group includes the mushrooms *Coprinus aetramentarius* and *Clitocybe clavipes.*

Group 6: Indoles

The hallucinogenic indole mushrooms contain *psilocin and psilocybin* and have been used for centuries in Native American cultural ceremonies. Symptoms develop within 1 hour of ingestion and include euphoria and hallucinations; physical findings include mydriasis, tachycardia, and paresthesias. Treatment includes gentle reassurance and diazepam if the patient requires sedation. This group of mushrooms includes more than 100 species of the *Psilocybe* genus, *Gymnopilus* spp., *Panaeolus* spp., *Conocybe cyanopus,* and *Stropharis coronilla.*

Group 7: Gastrointestinal Irritants

This group of mushrooms produce mild, self-limited GI irritation; nausea, vomiting, abdominal cramps, and diarrhea occur within 2 hours of ingestion. Antispasmodics should be avoided during treatment. A vast number of mushroom species are in this group.

Group 8: Orellanine (Nephrotoxin)

These toxins manifest symptoms over 24 hours after ingestion. Cortinarius is in this group of mushrooms. It initially produces headache, chills, and a mild gastritis. This is followed by a latent period of 3 to 17 days, after which polydipsia and polyuria are present as renal failure from tubular necrosis develops.

Household Products

Bleach

Bleach is a solution of 3% to 6% sodium hypochlorite in water; the pH is 11, and most often, only very small quantities are ingested. Gastric dilution with water or milk is appropriate when small amounts are ingested. Ingestions of large amounts or high industrial concentrations, however, should be regarded and treated as corrosive exposures, which are discussed in "Corrosives," p. 594. Oral mucous membranes are commonly irritated and may be soothed with cool compresses and demulcents. A period of in-hospital observation is indicated for patients ingesting large amounts or industrial-strength solutions.

Hypochlorite mixed with acids (e.g., some toilet-bowl cleaners) produces chlorine gas. Hypochlorite mixed with solutions containing ammonia produces chloramine gas. Both of these gases are pulmonary irritants with patients manifesting cough, dyspnea, and after prolonged or severe exposure, pulmonary edema.

Carbon Tetrachloride

Although the use of carbon tetrachloride is currently restricted to industrial applications, household ingestions of carbon tetrachloride continue to occur.

- **Clinical presentation** includes nausea, vomiting, abdominal cramping, confusion, dizziness, respiratory depression, and coma. Inhalation may be associated with weakness, dizziness, blurred vision, paresthesias, tremors, and GI tract symptoms. Death is related to hepatic and renal failure and occurs with doses as low as 2 mL.
- **Treatment,** regardless of the amount ingested, must be considered emergent. Gastric lavage, if within 1 hour, and the administration of activated charcoal should be followed by cathartics. Hemodialysis is effective and should be undertaken early.

Soaps and Detergents

Bar soaps, non-dandruff shampoos, fabric softeners, and liquid and granular soaps (excluding automatic dishwashing soap) are relatively nontoxic and usually induce minor GI irritation and emesis. Occasionally, diarrhea may be pronounced and protracted and dehydration ensues. Other than warning the patient about possible fluid and electrolyte losses, and encouraging fluid intake, no specific treatment is indicated.

Soaps intended for use in automatic dishwashing machines are frequently highly alkaline and should be managed as a corrosive exposure (see "Corrosives," p. 594). Severe oropharyngeal and esophageal burns may result.

Mothballs

Mothballs and toilet and diaper-pail deodorants contain naphthalene, an extremely toxic substance, or paradichlorobenzene. Although paradichlorobenzene is used more frequently, exposure to naphthalene continues to occur.

• Patients ingesting **paradichlorobenzene** have mild GI symptoms and require symptomatic treatment only—usually consisting of cool compresses to the mucous membranes of the mouth, which are frequently irritated, and measures to prevent nausea and vomiting.

• Exposure to **naphthalene** warrants aggressive and prompt intervention, particularly in patients with glucose-6-phosphate dehydrogenase deficiency. Intravascular hemolysis is associated with exposure to naphthalene; nausea, vomiting, seizures, coma, progressive jaundice, and oliguria may occur. Treatment includes the immediate lavage followed by activated charcoal and cathartics. Hospitalization is advised when naphthalene exposure has occurred.

Boric Acid

Numerous borate preparations, including borated talc, eyewashes, and roach insecticide powders, are available. Potentially lethal ingestions may occur in association with as little as 5 to 6 g in small children and 30 g in the adult. Toxicity may also result from chronic low-grade exposure. Borate levels of 500 to 1,000 µg/mL are considered toxic. Borates are absorbed from gastrointestinal, mucosal, and abraded skin surfaces.

• **Clinical presentation.** Hemorrhagic gastroenteritis, vomiting (at times with bluegreen emesis), renal failure, seizures, coma, respiratory depression, hypotension, fluid and electrolyte disturbances, and metabolic acidosis occur in severe poisonings. An exfoliative dermatitis, typically beginning on the hands, feet, and buttocks and gradually spreading to involve the entire skin surface may occur.

• **Treatment** includes GI and/or skin decontamination and measures to correct fluid and electrolyte abnormalities, metabolic acidosis, and seizures. Forced diuresis is indicated in patients with mild borate toxicity, whereas dialysis is the treatment of choice in patients with severe poisoning.

Seafood-Related Illness

A variety of pathogenic organisms may be ingested in seawater. These include hepatitis A virus, *Salmonella typhosa,* enterotoxigenic and invasive *Escherichia coli,* and *Vibrio cholerae* and *parahaemolyticus,* which are discussed elsewhere. This chapter discusses illness related to the ingestion of ciguatera and scombroid toxins and contaminated shellfish.

Ciguatera Poisoning

Ciguatera poisoning presents within approximately 24 hours (median 1–6 hours) of ingesting contaminated fish; some patients will develop symptoms within 15 to

30 minutes of ingestion. Barracuda, grouper, amber jack, and red snapper are most often implicated, and the area of highest occurrence is southeastern Florida. Originally produced by dinoflagellates, the toxin, which can be detected by radioimmunoassay, moves up the food chain and is *not* destroyed by cooking or heating.

- **Clinical presentation** includes nausea, vomiting, diarrhea, and abdominal cramping in addition to a variety of nonspecific constitutional symptoms. Symptoms become more specific, however, with the onset of weakness, distal extremity and perioral dysesthesias, photophobia, blurring and occasional loss of vision (which is temporary), hypotension, shock, bradycardia, and **cranial nerve palsies. Respiratory paralysis** and severe hypotension occur rarely.
- **Treatment** includes the administration of activated charcoal and cathartics unless vomiting and diarrhea, respectively, have already occurred. In addition, patients require close observation for the early detection of respiratory or circulatory compromise. Use atropine for bradycardia, and consider using 2-PAM.

Scombroid Poisoning

Patients with scombroid poisoning present acutely within 1 hour (range 1 minute to 3 hours) after ingesting tuna, mackerel, bonito, skipjack, or most commonly the mahi-mahi or dolphinfish.

- **Clinical presentation** occurs approximately 60 minutes after ingestion and **resembles histamine ingestion,** including dry mouth, flushing, oropharyngeal burning, nausea, vomiting, diarrhea, abdominal cramping, pruritus, urticaria; dizziness; and headache. Often dramatic erythema of the face is noted, and bronchospasm may occur.
  The illness results from ingestion of a heat-stable toxin (histamine) produced by the breakdown of histidine by microorganisms infecting the flesh of the fish. Lack of proper refrigeration is thought to be responsible for this process. Contaminated fish sometimes have a metallic or peppery taste.
- **Treatment.** Symptoms are substantially improved with **intravenous diphenhydramine,** 50 mg in adults, and 0.5 to 1 mg/kg in children, and IV H_2 blockers (e.g., Pepcid). If vomiting and diarrhea have not occurred, activated charcoal and cathartics should be considered. Fatalities have not been reported, and most symptoms subside within 6 hours.

Shellfish Poisoning

- **Paralytic and gastroenteric shellfish poisoning.** Aside from true allergic reactions to shellfish, three or four syndromes result from ingestion of contaminated shellfish, most often raw clams, crabs, shrimp, raw oysters, or raw or partially cured fish. **Gastroenteric poisoning** results from the ingestion of contaminated shellfish or water; a variety of organisms can produce gastroenteric symptoms that include diarrhea, cramping, nausea and vomiting, and fever. Onset is usually between 24 and 48 hours. Treatment is supportive. **Diarrheic illness** follows the ingestion of shellfish contaminated with *Dinophysis fortii, D. acuminata,* or *Prorocentrum lima;* these are dinoflagellates that produce toxins whose primary effects are on the intestine. Onset is rapid (within 2 hours), and most patients complain of diarrhea, nausea and vomiting, abdominal pain and cramping, and chills. Treatment is supportive and symptoms subside without treatment in 2 to 3 days.
  Paralytic illness results from ingestion of shellfish contaminated with toxin-producing dinoflagellates; the primary toxin appears to be saxitoxin. Typical species include *Alexandrium* and *Gymnodinium;* these are phytoplankton-like organisms, which

if present in sufficient numbers can discolor the sea, producing the well-known "tide." Depending on the species, red, blue, brown, yellow, or luminescent "tides" or "blooms" are seen. More than 1,000 species of dinoflagellates produce toxins. Symptoms occur within minutes to a few hours after ingestion. Symptoms include perioral paresthesias, which may further involve the arms, followed by a variety of neurologic symptoms (disequilibrium, weakness, lightheadedness, incoordination, incoherence, dysarthria, and nystagmus), nausea and vomiting, headache, diaphoresis, abdominal cramping, and chest pain. Flaccid paralysis, along with respiratory compromise, can occur abruptly, however, with a variable interval after ingestion extending from 2 to 3 hours up to 12 hours. In unassisted individuals, death results from respiratory arrest; children are at increased risk. Patients suspected of the illness should be admitted to the hospital and closely observed for signs of respiratory compromise. If patients present very early, lavage is probably reasonable, plus activated charcoal and sorbitol. Treatment is otherwise supportive. A **neurotoxic illness** follows ingestion of shellfish contaminated with *Ptychodiscus breve,* which produces a toxin causing symptoms similar to those of ciguatera poisoning. These are self-limited and do not include paralysis. Treatment is supportive.

65 Rashes

Most patients with rash presenting to the emergency department are concerned about what is causing the rash, whether it is contagious, and how it can best be treated. The question regarding contagiousness can usually be adequately answered. However, it may be difficult to provide an acceptable answer regarding a specific cause. Angioedematous or urticarial eruptions, for example, may easily be diagnosed, but the actual causative agent responsible is only clearly identified in approximately one fifth of patients. For this reason, it is important to explain to the patient or parent that although it is often difficult to define the exact cause for a specific rash, the particular class of skin reaction may still be defined and adequately treated.

COMMON CAUSES OF RASH

- Acne*
- Candidiasis*
- Carbuncle
- Cellulitis*
- Dermatitis (atopic, contact, seborrheic)*
- Drug-induced*
- Folliculitis*
- Furunculosis*
- Impetigo
- Intertrigo
- Pityriasis rosea*
- Stasis dermatitis*
- Tinea infections (barbae, capitis, corporis, cruris, manum, pedis)*
- Tinea versicolor*
- Urticaria (angioedema)*
- Varicella-zoster*

LESS COMMON CAUSES OF RASH NOT TO BE MISSED

- Erythema multiforme*
- Erythrasma*
- Gonococcemia
- Kaposi sarcoma*
- Meningococcemia*
- Rocky Mountain spotted fever*
- Rubella*

---

*Discussed in this chapter.

- Rubeola*
- Scarlet fever
- Syphilis
- Toxic shock syndrome*

OTHER CAUSES OF RASH

- Actinic keratosis
- Basal cell carcinoma
- Bullous pemphigoid
- Pemphigus vulgaris
- Chancroid
- Collagen vascular disorders (systemic lupus erythematosus, rheumatoid arthritis, dermatomyositis, vasculitis)
- Diaper-related dermatitis
- Erysipelas
- Erythema chronicum migrans (Lyme disease)*
- Erythema infectiosum
- Erythema nodosum
- Henoch-Schönlein purpura
- Herpetic infections
- Insect bites
- Lichen planus
- Lymphogranuloma venereum
- Melanoma
- Mycosis fungoides
- Necrobiosis lipoidica
- Pediculosis*
- Pigmented nevus
- Pretibial myxedema
- Psoriasis
- Roseola infantum
- Sarcoidosis
- Scabies*
- Seabather's eruption*
- Seborrheic keratosis
- Squamous cell carcinoma
- Thrombocytopenia
- Toxic epidermal necrolysis
- Trichophyton infestations
- Verruca (wart)
- Vitiligo
- Xanthelasma/xanthoma

HISTORY

Two important features of the history that are useful in evaluating the cause of rash are a history of contact with or exposure to potential allergens (including drugs, poison ivy, oak, sumac, foods, soaps, perfumes, permanent-press clothing not washed before use) and a history of recent exposure to persons with an infectious illness associated with rash. Other elements of the history useful in distinguishing among causes of rash include any changes in the appearance of the eruption, the manner of progression and distribution of the rash, and the presence of any associated symptoms that may suggest an underlying systemic illness. When severe pruritus confined to the area of skin involvement is the primary complaint, an allergic cause should be strongly considered.

PHYSICAL EXAMINATION

The physical examination is the most important aspect of assessment in the evaluation of rash. All rashes may be characterized according to three distinct factors: specific description of the lesion or lesions, pattern of distribution, and association with fever or other signs of systemic illness. Tables 65-1 to 65-3 classify specific conditions according to these terms.

Table 65-1	Lesion Description

Macules (Circumscribed, Nonpalpable Variations in Skin Color)

Drug eruption
Kaposi sarcoma
Rubeola
Rubella
Seabather's eruption
Varicella (early)
Roseola
Pigmented nevus

Papules (Relatively Small, Raised Lesions of Varying Colors)

Drug eruption
Acne
Rubeola
Rubella
Varicella (early)
Roseola
Seabather eruption
Secondary syphilis
Verruca
Psoriasis
Lichen planus
Kaposi sarcoma

Plaques (Coalescence of Papules; any Raised, Scaling Lesion Larger than 2–3 cm)

Furunculosis
Pityriasis rosea (herald patch)
Intertrigo
Stasis dermatitis
Psoriasis

Table 65-1	Lesion Description (*Continued*)

Basal cell carcinoma
Sarcoidosis
Mycosis fungoides
Erythrasma

Pustules (Circumscribed Collections of Free Pus, Superficial or Relatively Deep in the Skin)

Folliculitis
Impetigo
Candidiasis
Acne
Psoriasis

Scales (Resulting from Acute or Chronic Inflammation; Excessive Superficial, Sloughed Skin Accumulates)

Dermatitis (atopic; contact, including diaper-related; seborrheic)
Psoriasis

Ulcers (Significant Destruction of Skin and Underlying Tissue)

Ischemia
Stasis dermatitis
Pyoderma gangrenosum
Ecthyma gangrenosum

Vesicles and Bullae (Circumscribed Small to Large Collections of Free Fluid in Theskin)

Contact dermatitis (including diaper-related)
Herpetic infections (simplex and zoster)
Erythema multiforme
Drug eruptions
Pemphigus
Pemphigoid

Wheals (Hives; a Special Type of Papule or Plaque Consisting of Pink Edema of the Skin, with or without Surrounding Erythema)

Drug eruptions
Insect bites
Allergic reactions

Linear Eruptions (Eruptions with the Appearance of "Scratch Marks" with Linear, Straight, Sharp Borders)

Contact dermatitis
Scabies
Neurodermatitis

Table 65-2	Distribution Pattern

Face and Scalp

Acne
Atopic dermatitis
Seborrheic dermatitis
Discoid lupus erythematosus
Rubeola (face, then to trunk)
Rubella (face, then to trunk)
Impetigo
Herpetic infections (simplex and zoster)
Xanthelasma

Trunk

Pityriasis rosea
Varicella (trunk, then to neck and face)
Herpes zoster
Roseola (trunk, then to neck and upper extremities)
Tinea versicolor (especially posterior upper thorax)
Acne
Typhus (trunk, then to extremities; centrifugal spread)

Limbs

Psoriasis (extensor surfaces)
Erythema nodosum (extensor surfaces of lower extremities)
Herpes zoster
Lichen planus (flexor surface of wrists, lower legs)
Rocky Mountain spotted fever (extremities, then to trunk; centripetal
   spread)
Stasis dermatitis (lower extremities)
Scarlet fever (especially flexor creases and intertriginous areas and with
   circumoral pallor)
Henoch-Schönlein purpura (petechiae primarily on lower extremities)
Scabies (between fingers, on palms, wrists, axillary folds; almost never on
   face)
Xanthoma (tendinous, palmar, tuberous)
Necrobiosis lipoidica diabeticorum (primarily on lower extremities)

Genitalia

Syphilis (primary and condyloma lata)
Chancroid
Lymphogranuloma venereum
Condyloma acuminata (genital warts)
Psoriasis
Lichen planus
Tinea cruris
Diaper-related dermatitis
Erythrasma
Pediculosis
Herpes simplex

Table 65-3	Rashes with Fever

Seen Primarily in Children

Scarlet fever
Rubeola
Rubella
Varicella
Erythema infectiosum
Roseola
Toxic epidermal necrolysis

Seen Primarily in Adults

Drug-induced
Cellulitis
Erythema multiforme
Rocky Mountain spotted fever
Gonococcemia
Meningococcemia
Herpes zoster (shingles or disseminated zoster)
Erysipelas
Collagen vascular disorders (especially systemic lupus erythematosus, rheumatoid arthritis, and vasculitis)

DIAGNOSTIC TESTS

A complete blood count (CBC) may be useful in patients with suspected systemic infectious causes for rash. The erythrocyte sedimentation rate may be helpful in patients suspected of having a more generalized inflammatory process, such as systemic lupus erythematosus or vasculitis. Bacterial cultures and Gram stain of material obtained from lesions possibly caused by streptococcal, staphylococcal, or gonococcal infection should be obtained. A serologic test for syphilis is recommended for suspicious ulcerative lesions. Potassium hydroxide preparations (10% solution) of scrapings from lesions (primarily those scaling) are useful in identifying fungal infections. Bullae or vesicles should be cultured for herpesvirus infection. Examination of the skin under Wood light may reveal fluorescence of the rash with tinea capitis, tinea corporis, and tinea cruris infections, as well as those with tinea versicolor and erythrasma. Potassium hydroxide preparations of lesions from patients with tinea versicolor infections often reveal the so-called spaghetti-and-meatballs configuration of the fungus.

SPECIFIC DISORDERS

Acne Vulgaris

Acne is a very common, usually self-limited, disorder occurring initially during the teenage years. In these formative years, even a relatively small lesion may have considerable social and interpersonal impact, and decisions regarding therapy and referral must be managed in this context.

Clinical Presentation
- The closed comedo (whitehead) is the initial lesion, after which if the follicular contents extrude, the open comedo (blackhead) develops. Inflammatory papules, pustules, cysts, or abscesses may also evolve. Lesions generally occur on the face and neck but may also involve the back and chest.

Treatment
- Initial therapy in patients with mild (primarily noninflammatory) involvement includes the use of comedolytic or antibiotic agents, including alcohol-based benzoyl peroxide (once or twice per day), retinoic acid, or topical clindamycin (1%–3%) or oral tetracycline or erythromycin (250 mg twice daily or four times daily, depending on severity). Those with severe disease should be referred to a dermatologist.

Cellulitis

Cellulitis may develop secondarily, complicating a preexisting wound or other inflammatory process (e.g., atopic or contact dermatitis), or may occur spontaneously. Cellulitis typically involves the dermis and subcutaneous tissues to varying depths. Common causative agents include group A streptococcus and *Staphylococcus aureus,* as well as a variety of oral-based organisms, such as anaerobic streptococci or *Pasteurella multocida,* any of which may seed wounds after bites or other oral-related trauma. Diabetics are at risk for cellulitis with Enterobacteriaceae and, rarely, clostridia. Pseudomonas causes cellulites when there is a puncture wound and devitalized tissue, and in diabetes.

Clinical Presentation
- **Clinical presentation** is swelling, erythema, and tenderness with or without systemic evidence of infection.

Treatment
- **Treatment** depends on the clinical presentation and whether the immune system is compromised. Patients with temperatures greater than 101°F, other evidence of systemic toxicity (rigors, malaise, or significant leukocytosis), extensive involvement, established lymphangitis, or immune compromise (e.g., diabetes) commonly require hospitalization for the initiation of intravenous antibiotic therapy. Cellulitis due to animal or human bites, particularly when the hand is involved, should routinely be admitted; a culture should be obtained, the wound left open, surgical consultation and intravenous antibiotics instituted early with ampicillin/sulbactam (Unasyn) 1.5 g every 6 hours, or cefoxitin (Mefoxin) 2 g intravenous every 8 hours, cellulitis not associated with bite wounds. Patients who do not appear systemically ill and are not immunocompromised, are treated with oral antibiotics, cephalexin 500 mg every 6 hours for 7 to 10 days or Augmentin 875 mg twice daily for 7 to 10 days. For penicillin-allergic patients, use erythromycin. If MRSA is suspected, clindamycin is indicated. Heat and elevation are useful adjunctive measures. A wound check in 24 to 48 hours should be recommended. Orbital cellulitis can extend into the cavernous sinus, and these patients should be considered for inpatient therapy with a cephalosporin. Children with periorbital cellulitis should be evaluated for sepsis.

Dermatitis
Atopic Dermatitis
- **Atopic dermatitis** (eczema) is a chronic pruritic eruption characterized by itching. Approximately one half of children with atopic dermatitis develop asthma or allergic rhinitis, and approximately two thirds have a positive family history.

Clinical Presentation

- The **clinical presentation** depends on age, with infants demonstrating primary involvement of the chest, face, scalp, neck, and the extensor surface of the extremities with papules, vesicles, oozing lesions, and crusts. In children aged 4 to 10, lesions are less acute, are localized to the flexor folds of the elbows, wrists, and knees, and become progressively lichenified and excoriated. During adolescence and early adulthood, the final phase of the disorder is characterized by densely lichenified, hyperpigmented plaques occurring periorbitally and in the flexor areas.

Treatment

- **Treatment** is symptomatic and involves preventive measures (avoidance of excess humidity and excess bathing), the judicious use of antihistamines, and application of Burow solution to weeping areas for 20 minutes four times daily. In persistent cases, topical corticosteroids, three to six times per day, are used. Only low-potency corticosteroids (i.e., 0.5%–1% hydrocortisone) should be used on the face to minimize steroid-induced atrophic changes in this cosmetically important area.

Contact Dermatitis

- Itching is the most prominent symptom. When erythematous eruptions contain sharp cutoffs, or clearly demarcated borders (often corresponding to protection provided by clothing), or when straight-line or linear lesions are noted, contact dermatitis should be strongly suspected. Environmental irritants or allergic sensitizers are most often responsible for these eruptions. Nickel dermatitis at the site of a watchband on the wrist, hand dermatitis in individuals whose hands are exposed to chemical or abrasive agents in the workplace, and dermatitis about the periphery of the face adjacent to the hairline in response to hair sprays are three common forms of irritant contact dermatitis, all of which respond to avoidance of the irritant agent (if it can be tentatively identified) and topical corticosteroids.

  Allergic contact dermatitis is a form of delayed hypersensitivity and typically produces eczematous skin changes 1 to 3 weeks after initial exposure and 1 to 2 days after rechallenge. Severe pruritus is the hallmark of allergic dermatitis. The poison ivy, oak, and sumac allergic dermatitides are the most common forms. Not all persons are susceptible to these agents; in fact, approximately one third of the population fails to develop dermatitis when exposed to these Rhus species. Eruptions resulting from allergen exposure have an atypical or artificial appearance—sharp borders, straight lines, unusual angles, or a combination. If the area of involvement is well localized and does not include the face or periorbital areas, a topically applied, potent corticosteroid preparation (betamethasone, triamcinolone, or fluocinonide) should be recommended. When involvement is generalized, or when the periorbital area, genitalia, or fingers or toes are significantly involved, a brief course of oral steroids is recommended; prednisone, beginning with 40 mg/day and tapering gradually over 2 to 3 weeks, is advised. Steroid regimens prescribed for less than this interval typically result in recurrence. Antihistamines and emollient baths (oatmeal baths) may also be used as needed during the first several days of treatment.

Diaper Dermatitis

- **Diaper dermatitis** ("diaper rash") is a form of irritant dermatitis and represents a reaction of the skin to chronic maceration, dampness, and the chemical irritation induced by exposure to urine, feces, and any chemical irritants in the diaper. Heat, an increased ambient humidity, a prolonged period between diaper changes, poor cleansing or inadequate drying of the involved area, occlusive diapers or plastic pants, and diarrhea may aggravate this condition.

Clinical Presentation

- **The clinical presentation** of a typical diaper rash (without bacterial or candidal superinfection) shows "raw-appearing" erythema involving the areas of contact. More severe involvement is associated with oozing, shallow erosions, or ulceration. Candidal infection is common and is suggested by the presence of so-called satellite lesions; these are discrete, erythematous papules or pustules occurring outside, but adjacent to, the area of confluent erythema.

    Importantly, diaper-related dermatitis may be a presenting symptom in patients with an atopic or seborrheic diathesis. Because of this, the hands and face should be examined carefully for other evidence of atopy, and the scalp, posteroauricular, and malar areas inspected for coexisting seborrhea.

Treatment

- **Treatment** is based on recognizing and treating any bacterial or candidal superinfection and eliminating the aggravating factors. Factors predisposing to diaper-related dermatitis should be discussed with the parents so that preventive measures can be undertaken after the acute episode has resolved. As much as possible, diapers should be left off to allow the involved areas to dry. Frequent diaper changes (every 1–2 hours) will be more practical and are satisfactory. Occlusive, multilayered diapers and plastic pants should be avoided. After each diaper change, the involved area should be cleansed with warm water; perfumed wipes should be avoided. Advise the parents not to scrub the area and to avoid the use of soaps, no matter how mild. If parents insist on using some type of soap, a superfatted soap, such as Basis or Alpha-Keri, or a soap substitute, such as Aveeno, may be used once per day. All attempts should be made to keep the child's room cool and the humidity as low as possible. In mild cases, a bland ointment or zinc oxide may limit maceration. In patients with evidence of atopic or seborrheic dermatitis, 1% hydrocortisone cream should be recommended and can be applied at diaper changes after cleansing. Patients with significant oozing or eroded areas will benefit from the application of Burow solution three times daily for 2 to 3 days. This agent is available commercially as Domeboro tablets or powder and should be applied with a cool compress for approximately 20 minutes. Mild bacterial superinfection should be treated with an appropriate antibacterial cream.

    Patients with candidal superinfection require treatment with nystatin cream, miconazole, or clotrimazole, three times daily. In patients with severe or refractory involvement, oral nystatin suspension should be prescribed and follow-up arranged for 48 to 72 hours.

Seborrheic Dermatitis

- **Seborrheic dermatitis** is an inflammatory, scaling process that develops in areas with a high density of sebaceous glands, that is, the face, scalp, and trunk.

Clinical Presentation

- **Clinical presentation** includes dandruff and erythematous, greasy, scaling lesions about the eyebrows, eyelids, nasolabial folds, beard, groin, and gluteal areas. Seborrheic blepharitis produces scaling of the lid margins often with a mild associated conjunctivitis.

Treatment

- Selenium sulfide shampoos are indicated for scalp lesions, and topical corticosteroids should be used for other areas. Thick crusts may be removed with a keratolytic gel under overnight occlusion.

Drug-Induced Rashes

Drug-induced rashes may be produced by virtually any pharmacologic agent. Primary offenders include (in order of decreasing frequency) ampicillin, sulfa drugs, semisynthetic penicillins, penicillin, the cephalosporins, quinidine, the barbiturates and the thiazide diuretics. The nature of the skin reactions produced by these agents are varied and include maculopapular eruptions (especially with the penicillins and sulfa drugs), urticaria and angioedema, fixed drug eruptions, acneiform eruptions, psoriatic eruptions, erythema multiforme, and erythema nodosum. Therapy is discontinuation of the drug and symptomatic treatment with antihistamines; more severe drug-associated eruptions, such as erythema multiforme, should be treated as discussed in "Erythema Multiforme", p. 637.

Bacterial Skin Infections

Bacterial skin infections include folliculitis, furunculosis, carbuncles, erythrasma, and impetigo. Folliculitis is a follicular staphylococcal infection from which furuncles or boils may develop; carbuncles or deeper abscesses may evolve. **Impetigo** may be bullous—especially in children, in whom it is caused by bacteriophage group 2 staphylococci—or nonbullous, which is caused by group A streptococcus. Nonbullous impetigo begins as a small erythematous macule, develops into a vesicopustule, and ultimately forms a yellow crust. **Erythrasma** is a mild, superficial bacterial infection of the intertriginous areas caused by *Corynebacterium minutissimum,* which produces sharply demarcated plaques in the inguinal, axillary, or inframammary areas.

- Superficial **folliculitis,** when mild, may be treated with local hygienic measures and topical antibiotics, while more severe or recurrent involvement or folliculitis involving the beard require systemic antistaphylococcal antibiotics.
- Simple **furunculosis** requires only the application of moist heat, whereas lesions associated with surrounding cellulitis should be treated with an antistaphylococcal agent or anti-MRSA agent. Large fluctuant furuncles or carbuncles are treated with incision and drainage.
- **Bullous impetigo** is treated with hexachlorophene washes twice per day and an oral antistaphylococcal agent for 10 days; **nonbullous impetigo** responds to hexachlorophene washes and 10 days of penicillin VK, erythromycin or anti-MRSA agent.
- **Central facial infections** may appear superficial but can lead to a septic thrombophlebitis of the central venous sinuses of the central nervous system (CNS). For this reason, intravenous antibiotic therapy is recommended for all but the most trivial central facial infections. Several regimens are recommended: (1) ceftriaxone 100 mg/kg intravenous every 24 hours plus clindamycin 10 mg/kg intravenous every 6 hours, (2) vancomycin 10 mg/kg intravenous every 6 hours plus aztreonam 30 mg/kg intravenous every 8 hours plus clindamycin 10 mg/kg every 6 hours, or (3) ampicillin/sulbactam (Unasyn) 50 mg/kg intravenous every 6 hours.
- **Erythrasma** is readily treated with a 2-week course of oral erythromycin plus a topical keratolytic agent.

Candidiasis

A moist local environment, pregnancy, diabetes mellitus, chronic corticosteroid use, antibacterial therapy, AIDS, and chronic debility all predispose to candidal infections of the skin, nails, and mucous membranes.

Diagnosis

- Oral or vaginal thrush, paronychial lesions, intertrigo, or perlèche (fissured, erythematous areas at the corners of the mouth) may be the presenting manifestation of this often chronic infection. Scrapings from the lesion stained with potassium hydroxide (10% solution) reveal budding yeast forms with or without hyphae or pseudohyphae.

Treatment

- **Treatment** involves the use of topical drying agents to reduce intertriginous moistness, miconazole, or clotrimazole. Oral thrush may be treated with nystatin oral suspension (400,000–600,000 U four times daily, swish and swallow) or fluconazole, and vaginal involvement with topical miconazole, clotrimazole, fluconazole, or nystatin. Paronychial lesions are notoriously difficult to eradicate and usually require oral antifungal agents. Candidiasis involving the perineal area is particularly common in children and is characterized by so-called satellite lesions (isolated, erythematous pustules or papules occurring outside the primary area of confluent erythema). Severe or refractory mucosal involvement or systemic candidiasis requires treatment with oral fluconazole or intravenous amphotericin B.

Pityriasis Rosea

Pityriasis rosea is a mild, scaling eruption seen primarily in young adults during the spring and autumn months and is believed to have a viral cause.

Clinical Presentation
- The initial lesion is the so-called **herald patch**, which is described as the largest of all the scaling lesions, usually 3 to 6 cm in diameter. Within 1 to 2 weeks of the herald patch, multiple 1- to 2-cm maculopapular lesions with diagnostically significant outer rims of fine scale appear on the trunk and proximal extremities. Lesions often assume a **Christmas tree-like** distribution and typically last for approximately 6 to 8 weeks. Lesions may be mildly pruritic.

Treatment
- **Treatment** is symptomatic, using antihistamines as needed for control of pruritus. Given the similarity of this eruption to that of secondary syphilis, an appropriate screening test for syphilis, such as the RPR, should be obtained.

Stasis Dermatitis

Stasis dermatitis is a chronic, indurated skin change that accompanies the development of venous insufficiency of the lower extremities. Therapy involves protecting the legs from trauma and secondary bacterial infection, elevating the lower extremities whenever possible, and reducing edema with the use of compressive stockings.

Tinea Infections

Dermatophytic fungi (ringworms) are a unique class of organisms that may produce infection of the scalp (tinea capitis), body (tinea corporis), beard and moustache (tinea barbae), groin (tinea cruris), hands (tinea manum), or feet (tinea pedis, or "athlete's foot"). These infections typically occur in the warm months and are spread by fomites. Erythematous, scaling lesions with slightly raised borders are characteristic. Cutaneous lesions are treated with topical miconazole 2% or clotrimazole 1% three times daily for 3 to 6 weeks and 4 to 8 weeks for *T. tonsurans* infections of the scalp, or 4 to 8 weeks for *Microsporum canis* infections of the scalp. Clotrimazole and miconazole are also effective against candidal infections, whereas tolnaftate is effective only against tinea infections. In resistant cases and with onychomycosis, a prolonged course of oral micronized griseofulvin, fluconazole, or terbinafine 250 mg daily for 6 to 12 weeks is necessary.

Tinea Versicolor

Tinea versicolor is a chronic, relatively asymptomatic, superficial fungal infection of the upper trunk caused by *Malassezia furfur* or *Pityrosporum orbiculare*. Lesions are typically described as coalescing tanned macules, which fluoresce under a Wood light. Potassium hydroxide (10% solution) of scrapings from lesions reveals the so-called *spaghetti-and-meatballs* configuration of hyphae and budding yeasts. Treatment consists of fluconazole 400 mg orally in a single dose or ketoconazole 400 mg orally in a single dose. Although the active, scaling macular lesions will resolve, pigmentary changes may take several months to revert to normal or be chronic.

Urticaria and Angioedema

Approximately one fifth of the population will experience urticaria (hives) at some time in their lives. When this reaction involves the deep dermis and subcutaneous tissues with swelling, it is referred to as angioedema. Both reactions are believed to be a manifestation of the release of mast cell-related mediators. The cause of acute urticaria in three fourths of patients defies identification. Causes of urticaria include yeast hypersensitivity, foods, insect bites, drugs (penicillin is the most common), and serum sickness from any cause. Paraimmunologic causes include infections (viral, bacterial, fungal, and especially during the prodrome of hepatitis A or infectious mononucleosis), infestations (most commonly nematodes), endocrinopathies (hypo-thyroidism, hyperthyroidism, diabetes), malignancies (especially Hodgkin disease and non-Hodgkin lymphoma), collagen vascular diseases (systemic lupus erythematosus, juvenile rheumatoid arthritis, and dermatomyositis), and chemicals (especially food additives like sodium benzoate and synthetic food dyes). Nonimmunologic causes include cold, heat, sunlight, trauma, cholinergic urticaria caused by emotional stress and exertion, drugs (morphine, heroin, aspirin, quinine), and emotion.

Despite reviewing common allergens with the patient (including foods such as toma-toes, chocolate, oranges, and nuts; perfumes; new clothing; new soaps), the physician and patient are usually frustrated by the absence of any identifiable environmental cause. The patient should understand that although it is frequently difficult to deter-mine the factor responsible for the eruption, treatment will still be effective.

- **Acute urticarial and anaphylactic reactions** are treated with an oral or parenteral agent, depending on the presentation. In adults with anaphylactic shock or suspected or evolving laryngeal edema, a subcutaneous injection of *epinephrine* (0.3 mL of 1:1,000 dilution) should be administered immediately while intravenous access is established. If shock or laryngeal edema persists, 1 to 2 mL of a 1:10,000 dilution of epinephrine may be administered intravenous over 1 to 2 minutes, followed by intravenous *diphenhydramine,* 25 to 50 mg and intravenous *hydrocortisone,* 100 mg, or an equivalent steroid. When shock or impending upper airway obstruction is not present, adults with significant symptoms (wheezing, extensive or rapidly progressive angioedema or urticaria) may be treated with subcutaneous epinephrine (1:1,000 dilu-tion), 0.3 mL, and IV diphenhydramine. The initial dose of subcutaneous epineph-rine (1:1,000 dilution) in children is 0.01 mL/kg up to 0.3 mL and diphenhydramine is 0.5 to 1.0 mg/kg up to 50 mg. H_2 blockers are typical adjunctive treatment.
- Therapy for **chronic urticaria** remains the antihistamines. Patients may find a par-ticular antihistamine more or less effective than another and, importantly, more or less sedating. For this reason, it may be necessary to change agents until one is found to be effective with minimal drowsiness. Identifying and eliminating the particular environmental factor that causes the chronic lesions, however, is the only effective long-term therapy, and for this reason referral to an allergist is recommended.
- **Rare forms of urticaria/angioedema** include **cholinergic urticaria** (mediated by acetylcholine and not histamine), which may be triggered by exercise or changes in temperature. These lesions are typically smaller and of shorter duration than typical urticaria. The association among **aspirin intolerance,** nasal polyps, and asthma is well recognized and should be considered in patients in whom an urticarial eruption has occurred after the ingestion of aspirin or other nonsteroidal anti-inflammatory agents

or after exposure to tartrazine dye-containing drugs. Urticaria secondary to these agents is often relatively resistant to standard antihistamine therapy. Morphine and its congeners, alcohol, and contrast radiographic dyes degranulate mast cells directly (i.e., not through an immunoglobulin E-mediated reaction) and should be avoided in all patients with urticaria. Finally, **hereditary angioedema,** an autosomal dominant **deficiency of the inhibitor of C1 esterase** in the complement cascade, produces recurrent episodes of cutaneous, laryngeal, or gastrointestinal angioedema, the first of which is usually not pruritic and is often initiated by trauma or surgery. Standard antihistamine or catecholamine therapy is appropriate acutely, but prophylactic therapy involves the use of the androgenic agent *danazol*. Severe symptoms may be treated with fresh frozen plasma, complement 1 esterase inhibitor protein, or kallikrein inhibitor if available.

Varicella-Zoster Infections

Varicella-zoster infections produce chickenpox and shingles. An effective vaccine is available.

- **Chickenpox** or **varicella,** one of the most highly contagious infectious diseases known, is transmitted through the respiratory route, has an average **incubation period of 2 weeks,** and a course of 7 to 10 days. Discrete, erythematous macules and papules develop over the scalp, thorax, and mucous membranes. They progress rapidly to tense, fragile vesicles followed by umbilicated lesions with cloudy, purulent contents, and finally to noninfectious crusts. Generally, lesions occur in three to four crops, and all stages of development may be represented in a given area (in contrast to smallpox in which all lesions are of the same type). The disease is generally mildest in young patients who are treated symptomatically. In adults, pneumonitis is a frequent complication, and those who are immunocompromised benefit from antiviral therapy. Pregnant women with varicella should be admitted for intravenous acyclovir. Children are not routinely treated with acyclovir, and in adults, therapy is most effective if begun within 24 hours of onset of the rash. Children older than age 12 are treated with acyclovir 800 mg orally five times daily for 5 to 7 days. Normal adults can be treated with acyclovir or valacyclovir 1,000 mg orally three times daily for 5 days. Immunocompromised patients, pregnant patients, and those with complications should be treated with acyclovir 10 mg/kg intravenous every 8 hours infused over 1 hour. Pruritus should be treated, because scratching may lead to irreversible scarring and to secondary bacterial infection.
- **Shingles** or **herpes zoster** results from reactivation of latent virus, which is known to be chronically present in the dorsal root ganglion after the initial infection with chickenpox. Most patients are middle-aged or elderly, and many report pain or dysesthesias in the vicinity of the rash before it actually appears. Zoster is self-limited in immunocompetent persons. The lesions first appear posteriorly near the dorsal root ganglion, progressing anteriorly and peripherally; typically, one to three dermatomes are involved, usually contiguously and almost never bilaterally. Erythema, macules, papules, plaques, and ultimately vesicles appear, eventually crusting in 1 to 2 weeks.
  - The treatment of **typical zoster** includes oral antiviral therapy and prevention of bacterial superinfection. Oral antiviral therapy is recommended in the immunocompromised patient; those with disseminated infection or ophthalmic zoster should be treated with IV acyclovir and admitted.
  - **Postherpetic neuralgia** occurs with increasing frequency in the elderly. Postherpetic neuralgia may be chronic. Treatment includes analgesics, gabapentin, and antidepressant.
  - **Zoster involving the first division of the trigeminal nerve** is particularly serious because **blindness may result** from corneal involvement if not treated

immediately. Lesions present near the tip of the nose, "Hutchinson sign," forecast corneal involvement. Corneal involvement is demonstrated by examining the cornea under ultraviolet light after fluorescein staining; a typical branching or fern-like ulcer is diagnostic. Ophthalmologic consultation should be obtained for corneal involvement. Treatment involves analgesia, a cycloplegic, and consideration for admission and IV acyclovir. If close outpatient management is elected, treatment is similar, with oral and ocular antiviral therapy.

- **Varicella-zoster immune globulin (VZIG)** provides effective passive immunity to exposed individuals if administered early in the 2-week incubation period. Exposure may occur in the context of household, playmate or hospital roommate contact. Prophylaxis is recommended in **newborns whose mother had varicella within 4 days** of delivery or 48 hours after delivery. Prophylaxis is also recommended in exposed children and adults with immune compromised conditions and in exposed pregnant women. Exposed patients determined to be antibody positive do not require prophylactic therapy with VZIG.

- **Varicella vaccine** is recommended for children over 12 months of age and adults who are antibody negative. Because it is a live vaccine, it is contraindicated in imunocompromised or pregnant patients **and** their household contacts.

Erythema Multiforme

Erythema multiforme is characterized by the classic "target" lesion. Drugs, various concurrent infections, including herpes simplex, streptococci, and *Mycoplasma,* and underlying malignancies have all been associated with erythema multiforme; however, in one half of patients, no provocative factor can be identified.

Clinical Presentation

- **Clinical presentation** demonstrates symmetric lesions (maculopapular or vesiculobullous) on the extensor surfaces of the limbs and on the palms and soles. The iris or target lesion consists of a central zone of pallor surrounded by a red ring, seen most clearly and frequently on the palms. Malaise, mild fever, myalgias, and arthralgias may occur. In severe cases, widespread mucosal involvement occurs **(Stevens-Johnson syndrome),** and is associated with a high mortality.

Treatment

- **Therapy** consists of treating the suspected underlying infectious process or withdrawing the offending drug as appropriate; antihistamines may be administered. Hospitalization and intravenous corticosteroids are recommended for patients with Stevens-Johnson syndrome.

Meningococcemia

Neisseria meningitidis or the meningococcus is associated with both a presumably benign carrier state and fulminating severe illness. Five to fifteen percent of well persons carry the meningococcus in the nasopharynx. What relationship exists (if any) between the development of clinically important illness, including both meningococcemia and meningococcal meningitis, and the carrier state in these individuals is not understood at present.

Clinical Presentation

- Approximately 40% of patients who have clinically important sequelae as a result of dissemination of the meningococcus from the nasopharynx have meningococcemia without evidence of meningitis. A prodromal illness consisting of cough, sore throat, low-grade fever, and headache is followed by the abrupt onset of high fever, prostration, rigors, muscle aches, arthralgias, and, in a significant majority of patients, a characteristic petechial rash involving the ankles, wrists, and axillae. In some patients, a confluence of petechiae or frank purpura evolves, most often involving the lower extremities, and signals more severe disease. The remainder of patients with clinically important illness secondary to meningococcal dissemination present with meningitis, which may or may not be associated with the rash. **Waterhouse-Friderichsen syndrome** occurs in approximately 15% to 20% of patients and may rapidly progress to death unless diagnosed promptly and treatment instituted. Waterhouse-Friderichsen syndrome is acute adrenal failure due to hemorrhage of the adrenal glands.

Treatment
- The **treatment** of meningococcal disease is based on recovery of the organism from blood or sites other than the nasopharynx or through counterimmunoelectrophoresis of spinal, joint, or other fluid. Scrapings of cutaneous lesions may similarly yield the organism and thereby establish the diagnosis.
- Treatment should be undertaken based on a clinical diagnosis of meningococcal disease and should be done so as early as possible after cultures of blood, spinal fluid, or other appropriate areas are obtained. The treatment of meningococcemia depends on the age and immunologic status of the patient. Accepted treatment regimens are as follows:
  - Neonates 1 week to 2 months old—two-drug therapy: ampicillin 75 mg/kg intravenous every 6 hours plus gentamicin 2.5 mg/kg intravenous every 8 hours
  - Infants and children—two-drug therapy: either cefotaxime 75 mg/kg intravenous every 6 hours or ceftriaxone 50 mg/kg intravenous every 12 hours (up to 2 g per dose) plus vancomycin 15 mg/kg intravenous every 6 hours (up to 1 g per dose)
  - Children with severe penicillin allergy—two-drug therapy: vancomycin 15 mg/kg intravenous every 6 hours (up to 1 g per dose) plus trimethoprim/sulfamethoxazole 5 mg/kg intravenous every 12 hours
  - Adults, normal host—two-drug therapy: ceftriaxone 2 g intravenous every 12 hours plus vancomycin 15 mg/kg intravenous dose (up to 750 mg per dose)
  - Adults older than age 50 or immunocompromised—three-drug therapy: ceftriaxone 2 g intravenous every 12 hours plus ampicillin 2 g intravenous every 4 hours plus vancomycin 15 mg/kg intravenous every 6 hours (up to 750 mg per dose).
  - Adults with severe penicillin allergy—two-drug therapy: vancomycin 15 mg/kg intravenous every 6 hours (up to 750 mg per dose) plus trimethoprim/sulfamethoxazole 5 mg/kg intravenous every 12 hours

Shock must be managed in the usual fashion.

The prophylactic treatment of contacts is discussed in Chapter 42, p. 378.

Gonococcemia

See p. 292.

Kaposi Sarcoma

Classically, Kaposi sarcoma has been a disease of Mediterranean origin, presenting as purple nodules over the distal lower extremities evolving slowly over several years. In contrast, the distinctly more prevalent Kaposi sarcoma seen in patients with AIDS may be seen anywhere on the body (including the oral or rectal mucosa, indicative of gastrointestinal tract involvement) and typically begins as erythematous, violaceous, or rust-colored macules or papules that often enlarge and coalesce. These lesions grow much more rapidly than those associated with classic Kaposi sarcoma. Dermatology consultation is recommended for treatment. Even if untreated, Kaposi sarcoma is rarely the cause of death in patients with AIDS.

Pediculosis

Lice may infest the scalp, body, or pubic areas and typically produce extreme pruritus. As the lice feed, their products of digestion are injected into the skin and result in intense itching. Pyoderma, pruritus, mild inflammation of the scalp or pubic area, or tender cervical or occipital adenopathy without another clear-cut explanation should suggest pediculosis. Adult lice, nits, or both should be searched for, as should linear scratch marks. Permethrin (Nix) is the treatment of choice and is available as a shampoo for pediculosis capitis or pubis and as a cream or lotion for pediculosis corporis. One application is usually sufficient, but occasionally a second treatment may be needed. Persistent pruritus for several days after the initial treatment is expected and should not be attributed to infection. Close friends, family members, and sexual contacts should be screened for involvement and the last prophylactically treated. Bedding, clothing and hairbrushes must be appropriately cleaned.

Rocky Mountain Spotted Fever

Rocky Mountain spotted fever (a true misnomer in that most cases occur on the east coast) is a tick-borne illness caused by *Rickettsia rickettsii;* cases typically cluster from April to September. The incubation period varies between 3 and 12 days, begins with a nonspecific syndrome of headache, malaise, myalgias, and fever, and is followed by the characteristic centripetal rash. The rash is usually delayed until approximately the 4th day of fever; the initial lesions occur on the wrists, ankles, palms, and soles, spreading after 6 to 12 hours to the trunk. Initially, the rash is maculopapular but within 2 to 3 days may become petechial or purpuric. Disseminated intravascular coagulation, thrombocytopenia, periorbital, nonpitting edema, intense headache, myalgias, neurologic complications (neck stiffness, confusion, seizures, hemiparesis), myocarditis, hepatitis, and interstitial pneumonitis may occur. The early institution of therapy is imperative in suspected cases, since the complement fixation and Weil-Felix tests are usually not positive until between the days 8 and 12. Treatment with doxycycline, 100 mg intravenous or, orally every 12 hours for 7 days, is preferred; chloramphenicol, 500 mg intravenous or orally every 6 hours for 7 days, is also effective. Children younger than age 8 and pregnant women should be treated with chloramphenicol 50 mg/kg/day divided into four doses.

Lyme disease

Lyme disease is an Ixodes tick-borne illness caused by a spirochete, *Borrelia burgdorferi.* Three stages are characteristic. In the first stage, which lasts for several weeks, patients can present with the characteristic skin lesion, erythema migrans, beginning at the site of the tick bite. This lesion starts as a red macule or papule that expands to form a large annular lesion with central clearing and bright red borders. The average interval from bite to appearance of the lesion is 7 days; 30% of patients do not have the typical lesion. Other symptoms include severe headache, arthralgias, malaise, generalized lymphadenopathy, splenomegaly, hepatitis, sore throat, iritis, conjunctivitis, and testicular swelling. These early symptoms are often intermittent and evolving. In the second stage, a variety of neurologic abnormalities may develop, including meningitis, encephalitis, and peripheral and cranial neuropathies. Cardiac involvement in this stage may include fluctuating degrees of atrioventricular block and acute myopericarditis. Migratory joint pains may also occur. In the third stage, occurring weeks to 2 years of the initial infection, approximately two thirds of patients have oligoarticular arthritis in the large joints.

Diagnosis

- The **diagnosis** of Lyme disease is difficult to make; it is usually based on epidemiologic and clinical facts and findings. Patients with erythema migrans residing in endemic areas should be presumed to have Lyme disease, and treatment should be initiated. Serologic antibody determination can be helpful in patients with late or disseminated disease (serum antibodies are produced after weeks or months), particularly when cardiac or neurologic symptoms are present, but is negative early in the disease or may be blunted or completely prevented in patients treated with antibiotics. Unfortunately, there is a relatively high incidence of false positives, particularly early and in patients with nonspecific symptoms. Patients with CNS symptoms or signs should have a lumbar puncture with antibody determinations requested, along with the usual other studies and cultures.

Treatment

- **Treatment** for patients with early Lyme disease consists of doxycycline, 100 mg twice daily, or tetracycline, 250 to 500 mg four times daily, for 10 to 21 days in adults; amoxicillin 250 to 500 mg three times daily, for 10 to 21 days is an acceptable alternative in adults and is recommended in children younger than 8 to 10 years of age (25–50 mg/kg/day in three divided doses). Another alternative is cefuroxime axetil 3 g three times daily (90–180 mg/kg/day for children). Patients with more advanced illness, including those with CNS involvement, require parenteral therapy, usually with ceftriaxone 1 to 4 g daily intravenous (for those older than age 12) or penicillin G 20 MU daily.

Rubella (German Measles)

Rubella (German measles) is a viral infection characterized by **fever;** posteroauricular, suboccipital, and posterocervical **lymphadenopathy;** and a generalized *rash.* Most cases occur during the spring and have **a 14- to 21-day incubation period;** patients are contagious from approximately 7 days before to 4 days after the appearance of the rash. Children usually have no prodrome, but adults may have a variety of upper respiratory tract symptoms. Adenopathy usually precedes the rash, which is described as pink and maculopapular, appearing **first on the face,** and **rapidly spreading caudad.** The rash usually lasts only approximately 3 days and may be associated with an enanthem consisting of red spots on the **soft palate (Forchheimer spots).** Complications of rubella are uncommon but may include arthritis, encephalitis, and purpura. Rubella occurring during early pregnancy may result in the congenital rubella syndrome, which includes a wide range of dire complications, including spontaneous abortion, stillbirth, growth retardation, and congenital ear, eye, heart, and brain defects. A vaccine is available and is highly recommended prior to pregnancy in all women for the prevention of this congenital syndrome.

Rubeola (Measles)

Rubeola (measles) is an acute, highly contagious viral infection characterized by fever, a respiratory prodrome, an enanthem (*Koplik spots*—elevated white spots opposite the molars on the buccal mucosa), and a maculopapular rash. The disease, which is seen mostly in children, occurs primarily in the late winter and early spring, has a 10- to

14-day incubation period, and is communicable from 4 days before to 5 days after the onset of rash. The prodrome of **fever, coryza (rhinitis), cough, conjunctivitis,** and Koplik spots occurs 3 to 5 days before the rash. The rash itself is brown-red and appears first on the forehead, behind the ears, and on the **face; it then spreads caudad** over the next 2 to 3 days. Pneumonitis and encephalitis are rare complications of measles, as is bacterial superinfection. Both prevention and treatment of rubeola are possible with human immune globulin, which, if given within 5 days after exposure, will protect against the disease. A live, attenuated measles vaccine is available and is recommended for immunization of all susceptible persons during the second year of life; it will also usually prevent disease if given within 2 days of exposure.

Scabies

Caused by the mite, *Sarcoptes scabiei,* scabies is usually acquired through close or sexual contact and produces a severe pruritus that is presumably caused by an acquired sensitivity to the organism. The characteristic burrow is an S-shaped ridge or dotted line, frequently ending in a vesicle. Lesions are typically located in the interdigital web spaces of the hands, the wrists, antecubital fossae, nipples, umbilicus, genitalia, and gluteal cleft.

Diagnosis

• The **diagnosis** is suggested by the characteristic lesions and their particular pattern of distribution and confirmed by recovering the mite from the burrow after scraping the superficial dermis from the lesion using a sterile needle or number 15 scalpel blade. The organism, which has a characteristic appearance, can then be observed microscopically under low power.

Treatment

• **Treatment** consists of topical permethrin 5% cream, which is applied to the entire body from the neck down at bedtime and removed by shower or bath the next morning. A shampoo is available. Clothing and bed linen should be washed concurrent with treatment. Patients should be told that persistent pruritus should be expected for several days and does not necessarily suggest treatment failure; reapplication at 7 days is occasionally necessary. Family and household contacts should be screened and, if symptomatic, should receive simultaneous treatment, as should all sexual contacts.

Scarlet Fever

See p. 152.

Syphilis

See p. 295.

Toxic Shock Syndrome (TSS)

Toxic shock syndrome (TSS) is an acute, febrile illness with marked systemic manifestations including headache; conjunctival and pharyngeal hyperemia; diffuse myalgias; confusion; a diffuse, macular, erythematous rash, which initially appears "sunburn-like" and may easily be confused with the flush associated with fever; nausea; vomiting; watery diarrhea; renal and hepatic failure; disseminated intravascular coagulation; and vascular collapse. The vaginal examination usually demonstrates hyperemia and tenderness of the external genitalia, punctate ulcerations or pustules involving the vagina, and a scant discharge. The clinical course may be complicated by myocarditis, congestive heart failure, pulmonary infiltrates, and adult respiratory distress syndrome

(ARDS). The rash typically desquamates on the face, trunk, and extremities at 7 to 10 days, whereas peeling involves the palms and soles.

Etiology
- Phage group 1 *Staphylococcus aureus* and groups A, B, C, and G *Streptococcus pyogenes* have been isolated, and an elaborated toxin is responsible for the syndrome. Although the staphylococcal toxin-mediated illness was initially described in young women using vaginal tampons and accounts for most cases, the clinical spectrum of the disease has expanded to include a variety of other settings, including diaphragm use, vaginal infections, pelvic inflammatory disease, the postpartum state, and surgical and nonsurgical infections in either gender. The streptococcal form is usually associated with other conditions such as necrotizing fasciitis, erysipelas, and secondary infections in chickenpox.

Differential Diagnosis
- The **differential diagnosis** includes scarlet fever, Rocky Mountain spotted fever, meningococcemia, erythema multiforme, drug reactions, and leptospirosis. The diagnosis of TSS is entirely a clinical one, and therapy must empirically be initiated.

Laboratory Studies
- **Laboratory studies** include cultures of blood, urine, vagina, and any involved mucous membrane surface. Blood should also be obtained for CBC, BUN, blood glucose, electrolytes, liver function studies, creatinine, prothrombin time, partial thromboplastin time, fibrinogen, and fibrin split products. A urinalysis, electrocardiogram, and chest x-ray should also be requested.

Treatment
- **Treatment** includes aggressive fluid resuscitation, vasopressors, and ICU admission. Parenteral antibiotic therapy (two-drug therapy) is either ceftriaxone 2 g intravenous every 24 hours or vancomycin plus clindamycin 900 mg intravenous every 8 hours. Removal of any vaginal tampons or sponges is also indicated. Methylprednisolone and IV immunoglobulin have shown improvement in some cases. Despite treatment, morbidity and mortality remain high.

Given that the recurrence rate is approximately 30%, all women with TSS must be instructed to permanently avoid the use of tampons. It is also recommended that a follow-up culture be obtained at the completion of therapy to document eradication of the staphylococcal organism from the vagina.

Seabather's Eruption

Seabather's eruption is a pruritic dermatitis that occurs on areas covered by one's swimsuit. Patients report a stinging sensation subsequent to leaving the ocean, followed by the appearance of a pruritic macular or papular, erythematous eruption confined to a swimsuit distribution. Cases have been reported in Florida, the Caribbean, Bermuda, and New York. The cause is the larval stage of organisms belonging to the phylum Cnidaria and, in the northeastern part of the United States, the sea anemone *Edwardsiella lineata.* Symptoms occur when the nematocyst of trapped larvae is activated and toxin is injected into the skin. Interestingly, the larval nematocysts may remain active for several days after exposure, and thus the eruption may recur if a contaminated swimsuit is reused. The eruption subsides over 3 to 7 days; mild systemic symptoms occur in a small percentage of patients with severe reactions. Treatment is symptomatic with oral and topical antipruritic agents; oral glucocorticoids may be helpful in patients with severe symptoms.

PART 13

Psychiatric Emergencies

Evaluation of Psychiatric Patients in the Emergency Department

OVERVIEW

- People come to the emergency department (ED) with a wide variety of psychiatric and emotional concerns, from acute grief to first-break psychosis to medical illness masquerading as psychiatric disease. It is essential that the emergency physician begin with an open mind regarding the range of these possibilities, remain open throughout the process of working with the patient, and create communication that facilitates discussion of the patient's concerns with the doctor.
- As in all other aspects of medicine, a **thorough history** and an **inclusive and accurate differential diagnosis** are most crucial.
- These in turn rest on:
  - **Effective communication, in both directions,** between doctor and patient (and often others **who** are involved)
  - **Thoughtful and thorough history taking, mental status examination, physical examination, and laboratory studies**
  - **Effective use of ancillary sources** of information
  - **Effective negotiation** about what is to be done about the problem

GENERAL APPROACH TO THE PATIENT

- **Preconceptions are almost always dangerous** in the evaluation of psychiatric patients. Individuals with preexisting psychiatric disease often have new, nonpsychiatric problems that are easily overlooked by health professionals; new symptoms should not be attributed to old diagnoses. *New symptoms appearing in the presence of a psychiatric diagnosis are not caused by that diagnosis until proved to be so.*

- Many psychiatric patients have negative perceptions regarding prior experiences in the ED—hours spent waiting, sometimes in restraints; sometimes treated against their will; sometimes treated in a patronizing, or otherwise disrespectful manner—not as adults with the same rights to courtesy and participation in treatment as anyone else. These experiences sometimes color the person's expectations, and they may approach emergency personnel with wariness or hostility. It is wise to expect that anyone with a serious psychiatric disorder, who has had several ED visits, probably has had at least one such negative episode in the past. These perceptions are often accentuated by the physical environment and nature of the ED—lack of privacy, repeated questions, and personal questions asked by strangers.
- The emergency physician should engage the patient in a manner that preserves the patient's dignity and emphasizes the physician's respect for, and empathy with, the individual's current and past problems. The following are simple, commonsense suggestions, but they are worth repeating.
  - Treat the person with at least as much courtesy as you expect in return.
  - Be open, friendly, and candid about your role and what you are doing.
  - Explain what you are doing and why.
  - Use nontechnical language.
  - If there have been undue delays in seeing the patient, or other problems have arisen, apologize—it works wonders.
  - Offer choices whenever possible, for example: Is there anyone you would like us to call, or to call yourself? Have I forgotten anything? Is there anything you would like to add? Anything you would like to ask me? If we need to give you medication, is there anything you prefer that we do or do not use?

PSYCHIATRIC HISTORY AND MENTAL STATUS EXAMINATION

Psychiatric History

General Considerations

- **The history taking comes first, and then the mental status examination,** because most of the mental status examination can be inferred from the history. The function of the history taking, however, is to generate a differential diagnosis.
- **The heart of the history is the history of present illness:** what is wrong now, when did it start, and what has the progress of the problem been to the current time. Frequently, when patients with a known psychiatric illness are evaluated in the ED, this step is skipped entirely, and the evaluation is based on the past psychiatric history. This can be a fatal error.
- Under the time constraints of the ED, with multiple demands on the physician, there is a natural tendency to want to "cut to the chase." This is one of the reasons that doctors so often jump to the conclusion that the current problem is caused by, or related to, psychiatric illness. It also sometimes causes physicians to use a communication style that drastically decreases self-exposure by the patient: rapid use of closed-ended, yes-or-no questions, and the use of symptom checklists (You have been depressed? Is your appetite low? Sleep poor? Suicidal ideas?). These questions may seem to lead rapidly to a ruled-in diagnosis, but they frequently obscure other important elements of the history. For example, the doctor may elicit that the patient is depressed, but not that depression exists now, or has significantly worsened, because of a completely new issue. For the patient to have just learned,

for example, that a spouse has been abusing their child, and it is this fact that has precipitated severe depression, has major significance in regard to prognosis, current treatment, and disposition options.

- **A time-saving, rapport-building suggestion:** In general, it is wise to begin the history by offering to share with the patient what you already know. In doing this, the physician saves time, by obviating the need to repeat information already given; treats the patient in an unusual (and often engaging) way by offering to be the one who first exposes what she or he knows and who offers to share that mysterious document, "the chart"; and very often gives the patient a chance to correct some minor error or misinformation. This last interaction is often very helpful in establishing rapport, because the patient assumes a competent, helpful, and collaborative role—even if only to say he is 32, not 33, for example. This minor interaction validates the importance of the interaction and helps solidify the relationship. It also allows the doctor to demonstrate openness to input and correction, and to convey a respectful, kind, and down-to-earth tone. Even when the patient is in the ED totally against his or her will, this kind of openness and willingness to put the cards on the table on the part of the doctor can be very helpful.

- **After the patient starts to talk, try to be quiet for a minute or two and listen.** On the average, doctors interrupt patients after less than 1 minute of the person's speaking. Strive to hear what the person is saying, from his or her point of view. Then let the first thing you say be a summary of what you have heard so far, for example, "Let me see if I hear what you are saying…" As you summarize what you have heard, use as many of the same words as the patient to describe emotions and other important parts of the history, that is, if the person said he was "freaked out" because his pet died, do not say, "so, you were upset that your pet died." The more exact your repetition, the more the person will feel heard; when you paraphrase or translate, the person tends to hear the difference between what she or he said and what you said, not the similarity. This decreases rapport.

- **The goal of the first part of the history taking is to get the "nod."** The nod is, literally, the person nodding to the doctor as the doctor reflects back what the person seems to be saying. If the doctor gets the nod, then the interview is off to a good and probably fruitful start. If there is no nod, there is almost certainly a communication problem, which the doctor needs to consider. It could be that the patient is so furious about being in the ED that there is nothing the doctor can do to establish rapport, although in such cases sometimes a candid acknowledgment of the person's situation ("I understand that you feel it was a terrible mistake for the police to have brought you here") can break through the person's anger and fear. The lack of the nod could also be because the patient is too psychotic or delirious (a critically important distinction, as is elaborated herein) to communicate with the doctor. In either event, the absence of a nod is an important data point in further history taking and especially in negotiating about what to do.

History of Present Illness

- As one begins to take the history of present illness, listen without interrupting at all in the first minute or so of the patient's discourse; try to step back and take the patient in, as a whole person: the dress, bearing, tone of voice.
- As discussed, **begin the history with general, open-ended questions** that invite elaboration, and then **move gradually to more close-ended, yes-or-no questions about specific symptoms.**
- Be sure to focus on why the person is presenting for care **now.** Do not be misled by an extensive past history into overlooking current problems.

- In interviewing psychiatric patients, **one concern is that one does not want to overlook something that requires immediate action, such as an undisclosed overdose, or a silent serious medical problem.** Pay particular attention to new physical symptoms and reports; these must be adequately explained in the differential. Pay particular attention to recent medication changes, psychiatric and nonpsychiatric.

- **If there is any concern about psychosis or impaired reality testing, be sure that you have established whether the person is delirious.** This is a vitally important differential question. The evaluation of delirium is dealt with more fully below, but the hallmarks of delirium are the following:
  - Confusion about place, person, time, or situation
  - Impaired attention and concentration
  - Hallucinations other than auditory
  - Waxing and waning levels of consciousness
  - Rapid changes in psychiatric symptoms in a setting suggestive of physical or neurologic illness
  - Delirium is a medical emergency, not a psychiatric emergency. The underlying cause of delirium must be established as a priority.

- If there is concern about psychosis or impaired reality testing, and the physician is satisfied that the person is not delirious, it is essential to inquire about **hallucinations** in all sensory modalities. Any hallucination in a nonauditory modality strongly suggests an encephalopathic cause—seizures, poisoning, withdrawal, etc. The differential diagnosis of psychosis is discussed more fully below. The presence of delusions and illusions should similarly be established.

- If there is concern about the presence of **depression**, it is important to establish the time course, whether it is worsening or not, and whether it is accompanied by the so-called neurovegetative signs of depression. These can be remembered by the mnemonic device **SIGECAPS:** disturbances of **s**leep, **i**nterest, **g**uilt, **e**nergy, **c**oncentration, **a**ppetite, **p**sychomotor activity, and **s**uicidal thoughts. The presence or absence of suicidal ideation requires separate consideration as well. This is dealt with more fully below. The number and intensity of the neurovegetative signs of depression are one measure of the intensity of depression and its likely response to pharmacotherapy.

- If the problem concerns mainly relationships with important other people, take note of how the person is describing these people and relationships, to get a sense of how the person copes and what his or her strengths and weaknesses in relationships may be.

- Take into consideration the course of treatment wherever possible—what has been tried and when.

- Note the current, most proximate stressor, "the straw that broke the camel's back," as it were.

- Note all current medications.

Psychiatric History
Note past treatment for conditions similar to the present problem, as well as unrelated psychiatric or substance abuse problems or previous treatment.

Medical History
For all psychiatric patients, it is essential to note the following:
- Surgical history
- Significant past medical problems

- Current medical problems and medications
- Allergies to medications

Family History

A family history of psychiatric illness and substance abuse should be noted.

Social History

Note current living situation (with whom, nature of the relationship); current work or school situation; significant issues in the person's current life.

Mental Status Examination

Overview

Like the history itself, the mental status examination is a process of data gathering attempting to generate and confirm diagnostic hypotheses. Therefore, both positive and negative findings can be significant. As mentioned, most of the mental status examination can be inferred from the history. In practice, it is useful to defer some elements of the mental status examination to a point after the history of present illness has been elaborated. Frequently, these are the portions that are tedious or difficult or may be somewhat off-putting to the patient and could therefore compromise rapport if emphasized earlier. It is wise to generally defer the cognitive aspects of the examination, some questions regarding delusions and other psychotic symptoms, and questions concerning some aspects of sexual practice to this later stage of the interview, for reasons of protecting rapport.

General Appearance

- It is perhaps not too much of an oversimplification to say that a person's appearance is much like a Rorschach test of personality. We manifest our personalities in our fashion, hairstyle, jewelry, and other adornments. Thus, it is worth just taking a moment to see the person.
- From a mental status perspective, one of the most important aspects of the general appearance, apart from this almost universal window into the person's personality, is the presence or absence of incongruities: a foul-smelling man in a three piece suit; an elegant woman with dirt under her finger nails; a reasonably dressed person with the buttons misaligned; these may all signal acute decompensation in psychological functioning—rapid, acute changes that may be associated with nonpsychiatric disease.
- The person's general appearance may offer important clues to his or her physical condition. Whether the skin is pale or red, wet or dry, and whether the pupils are dilated or constricted are all signs that may be assessed by simple observation; these may be important signs of alcohol withdrawal, or anticholinergic delirium, for example.

Level of Consciousness

Level of consciousness may vary from alert and aware to lethargic, stuporous, or comatose.

- **Attention** (the capacity to focus attention on stimuli) may be assessed by observing the patient's responses to the examiner's questions and more formally by requesting that the patient repeat sequences of numbers of increasing length and complexity (normal range is seven digits). If the patient's attention is below this level, the physician should strongly suspect delirium or other causes causing cognitive or neurologic impairment.

Language

- Assessment of the patient's speech should include listening to the rate, rhythm, and coherence of spontaneous speech.

- Rate and rhythm may suggest mania (increased rate, pressured flow); depression (decreased rate, increased latency of speech, impoverished content); psychosis (peculiarities of speech, sudden breaks in the flow of speech); and neurologic conditions.
- Comprehension may be assessed by observing the patient's behavior in the interview and more formally by asking the patient to follow a three-step command.
- Language may also be assessed by asking the patient to
  ○ Name specific objects
  ○ Repeat phrases
  ○ Write a short spontaneous sentence
- Language should be assessed for
  - **Expressive aphasias** (Wernicke aphasia) in which speech is often voluble but incoherent, with many word substitutions and neologistic peculiarities. Expressive aphasias are usually caused by focal defects, but the fluency of the rate and flow of speech may lead to confusion with psychosis or mania.
  - **Receptive aphasias** (Broca aphasia) in which the speech is often very sparse, and in which the latency of speech is increased, leading to confusion with depression and psychosis.
  - Other aphasias of mixed symptomatology. All such aphasias must be explained neurologically, not psychiatrically.

Mood and Affect

- Mood represents the overall state of the person's emotional experience over a sustained period, such as a week. Affect refers to the specific feelings a person is experiencing during a particular time, such as during the evaluation.
- Mood may be inferred by observation but should also be ascertained by asking the person to assess his or her feelings for the previous week. Elevations in mood obviously may connote mania, whereas low mood may be a sign of depression. Less obviously, incongruity of mood between what is observed and reported may be significant (e.g., if the person reports feeling well, but appears depressed, the capacity for denial and ability to participate meaningfully in treatment planning might be suspect).
- Affects (feelings) may similarly be inferred from observation. The nature and intensity of feelings may be of importance, as may be significant absence of emotion (lack of sadness in relating tragic events, or lack of anger in recounting abuse). Similarly, affects that are inappropriate to the material being presented sometimes indicate the presence of psychosis.
- Because of their usefulness in the identification of depressive disorders, the neurovegetative signs of depression may be included in the mental status examination. The presence of four or more of these signs indicates the presence of major depression. They may be handily recalled by the mnemonic SIGECAPS:

Sleep disturbance
Interest disturbance
Guilt
Energy disturbance
Concentration disturbance
Appetite disturbance
Psychomotor retardation/agitation
Suicidal ideation

Thought

- Thought should be assessed for coherence and lucidity. Disjointed, incoherent thought, often seen in psychosis, must be differentiated from the language disorders mentioned. Tangentiality (in which the person veers from subject to subject) may suggest mania, and circumstantiality (in which the person veers away from the subject but by a circuitous route finally returns to it, often with superfluous detail) is associated with a number of conditions, notably obsessive-compulsive disorder and temporal lobe states, among others.

- The content of thought should be assessed for the presence of:
  - **Hallucinations in all sensory modalities.** Hallucinations associated with schizophrenia and bipolar disorders are most commonly auditory in nature. Visual, tactile, olfactory, or gustatory hallucinations strongly suggest an organic encephalopathy.
  - **Delusions** are fixed ideas at odds with reality and may include complex plots and other scenarios but may also include ideas of reference; paranoid ideas; delusions of thought broadcasting or insertion; delusions of feelings being inserted by outside forces; delusions of grandeur, ugliness, odor, or other offensive attributes.
  - **Illusions** are misattributions of actual, real perceptions as opposed to hallucinations; believing that the sprinkler head in the room is an FBI camera is an illusion complicating a delusion.
  - **Obsessions and compulsions** are differentiable from delusions by the fact that the patient recognizes their unreasonableness, even though the behavior cannot be eliminated.
  - **Phobias** are fears of situations, objects, or others.

Suicidal and Homicidal Ideation
See also Chapter 68.
- Suicidal thoughts, impulses, and plans must be explicitly evaluated. These may be inferred from the history or determined directly.
- History of suicidal behavior is also important, including the method, likelihood of rescue, and outcome of previous attempts.
- A family history of attempted or completed suicide is significant and adds to risk.
- The person's ability to acknowledge such feelings when they exist may be a sign of strength if the person can also reliably contract to remain safe, if the person's judgment and reliability are considered adequate, and if adequate social supports exist around the person. This topic is dealt with more fully below.

Cognitive Functions
- **Alertness and level of consciousness** have been described and may range from alert to drowsy to stuporous to comatose.
- **Orientation** refers to the accurate awareness of the person's identity, whereabouts in time and space, and situation. Disorientation may reflect inattention, which may arise in a variety of psychiatric conditions, or may reflect true confusion and inability to register information accurately, which is far more suggestive of delirium and an underlying encephalopathy.
- **Memory** should be tested for immediate recall of three named objects, and then retested at 3 minutes. Remote memory can be ascertained by requesting information available from the chart such as address or date of birth.
- **Calculation** may be tested by asking the person to subtract sevens from one hundred serially (or a similar task appropriate to educational level).
- **Judgment and insight** may be inferred from the interview or may be ascertained by asking hypothetical questions such as what should one do if one discovers a fire in a crowded theater; these questions are of limited diagnostic significance, however.

ENGAGING ANCILLARY RESOURCES

- If the person being evaluated gives permission to do so, conferring with others involved in the person's life can provide invaluable information regarding diagnosis, previous treatment, and assessment of risk.
- Bringing outside individuals such as family or close friends who have accompanied the person to the ED—again, with the person's permission—can save time by gaining access to additional information and by having the benefit of the outside person's perspective in planning what to do next. Oftentimes, if this step is not taken, the doctor and patient may make a plan that the family considers unrealistic, and treatment negotiation has to begin anew.
- For the same reason, safe options may become apparent when the family is included that did not seem possible otherwise; thus, involving the family or other support system may enable the patient to avoid an otherwise necessary hospitalization.
- When the evaluation is at an impasse—such as when the patient is refusing to answer questions or is otherwise displeased with the process—offering to bring in a family member or friend may help the person feel less trapped and may facilitate communication.

PHYSICAL EXAMINATION AND LABORATORY EVALUATION

- The need for detailed physical and neurologic examination depends on the nature of the problem being considered. In cases not involving overdose or medication reactions/interactions, with a sudden onset of new psychiatric symptoms, or when psychiatric symptoms arise in the setting of any new medical or neurologic sign (fever or confusion are important examples), thorough physical and neurologic examinations are essential. In cases in which there are no known active medical problems, no new medical or neurologic symptoms, in which overdose is not suspected, in which the patient's orientation, attention, and concentration are normal, and in which there is no other reason to suspect a "medical masquerader" (see later), no additional examination beyond vital signs and observation is clearly indicated.
- Similarly, laboratory testing depends on the nature of the illness being ruled in or out. There are no appropriate general "screening" tests for psychiatric conditions. Toxic screens and blood alcohol levels accomplish little other than identifying the intoxicant, except in cases of suspected poisoning. If "medical masqueraders" are being ruled in or out, specific tests may be indicated.

MEDICAL MASQUERADERS

A variety of medical and neurologic conditions may be mistaken for psychiatric conditions. Under the right conditions, virtually any medical condition can present with psychiatric symptoms; some of the most common such entities are listed in Table 66-1. These are more likely to present with cognitive or other psychiatric symptoms if the person is otherwise cognitively or emotionally challenged. For example, minor urinary tract infections in the elderly may present with confusion and delirium; small incremental compromises of respiratory function that would not affect a healthy person may substantially impair a person whose functioning is already borderline. These problems, which are primarily medical, and often relatively minor, may, in this specific setting, cause either social or psychiatric decompensation or may worsen or elicit abnormalities of mental status.

Table 66-1	Some Medical Conditions that May Present with Psychiatric Symptoms

Neurologic Diseases

Temporal lobe epilepsy
Huntington disease
Strokes
Multiple sclerosis

Endocrinopathies

Hypothyroidism and hyperthyroidism
Cushing/Addison disease
Hyperglycemia and hypoglycemia

Infectious Diseases

Meningitis
Encephalitis
Human immunodeficiency virus infection

Nutritional Deficiencies

Nicotinamide deficiency (Pellagra)
B_6 deficiency
B_{12} deficiency
Thiamine deficiency

Cardiopulmonary Disease

Hypertensive encephalopathy
Hypoxia
CO_2 narcosis

Gastrointestinal Diseases

Acute pancreatitis
Hepatic encephalopathy

Metabolic Diseases

Acute intermittent porphyria
Wilson disease
Electrolyte and acid/base imbalances
Uremia

Autoimmune Disorders

Systemic lupus erythematosus and others

Exogenous Poisons

Heavy metals
Anticholinergic agents
Drugs of abuse, especially phencyclidine, amphetamines

Neoplastic Diseases

Carcinoma, especially pancreatic carcinoma
Hyperviscosity states
Central nervous system neoplasm

NEGOTIATING THE TREATMENT PLAN

• Having arrived at a reasonable diagnosis, the doctor then faces the challenge of what to do about the problem. Again, under the constraints and pressures of the ED, the temptation is to find a reasonable course of action and dictate it to the patient: for example, return home, call your private doctor in the morning; increase your medication tonight; go to the emergency shelter, and so forth. In practice, such unilateral decision making often backfires. If the patient, or the family, or other support systems find the plan unacceptable or unworkable, it is not likely to be successful, and many patients will subsequently return to the ED. Whenever possible, therefore, involve the patient and the support system in designing the solution to the problem.

• Bear in mind the following parameters when designing solutions:
  • The goals should be ultramodest, basically designed to help the patient manage until the next scheduled or schedulable outpatient appointment.
  • Safety is paramount (see Chapter 68 on suicide evaluation). The patient should be housed in the safest, least restrictive setting available. Sometimes, however, hospitalization is necessary when:
    ○ The patient cannot contract meaningfully for his or her safety or the safety of others
    ○ The patient's judgment is so impaired that the person cannot care for himself or herself outside a protected environment
    ○ The person's care is so complex that it is unmanageable outside an institutional setting, given the nature of the illness and the extent of his or her supports
  • Be wary of making changes to patient's psychopharmacologic regimens without the explicit participation of the primary prescriber.
  • Be cautious about prescribing benzodiazepines, narcotics, or other drugs of dependency or abuse without the explicit participation of the person's primary prescriber. If the patient is not treated by an outpatient clinician, be wary of initiating treatment with these agents in the ED setting.
  • Involve the patient and the support system in finding interim solutions to bridge the interval between the current evaluation and the next scheduled appointment.
  • Do not offer false assurances that things will improve. Instead, consider expressing admiration for the person's coping with his or her difficulties. Empty assurances tend to be experienced as demeaning and patronizing; sincere understanding and appreciation that the patient is dealing with an overwhelming set of circumstances conveys admiration and support and thereby enhances the patient's strength and sense of dignity.

"MEDICAL CLEARANCE" IN THE ED

• **Medical clearance** is the term often applied to the process whereby an emergency physician evaluates a patient before sending the patient to a psychiatric facility, detox center, or other specific disposition, often as determined after an evaluation by a psychiatrist or other mental health professional. This generic process of evaluation has no precise or universally recognized content and varies widely from place to place and practitioner to practitioner. Some patients, unfortunately, receive only the most cursory evaluation. It is therefore often difficult for professionals in receiving facilities to know how carefully patients have been screened. Similarly, it is sometimes difficult for emergency physicians to know what is being asked of them in the evaluation of these patients.

- **The purpose of medical clearance** is to ensure that the patient does not have either a current medical or surgical problem that is causing or substantially contributing to the patient's current behavior or "psychiatric" illness, or a concurrent medical or surgical illness that requires active, concomitant treatment. The process of medical clearance is important because a high percentage of patients presenting with acute psychiatric disease do in fact have significant, concomitant, active medical problems; this has been estimated to be as high as 40% of all psychiatric admissions. Importantly, once a patient has been "medically cleared" and a psychiatric diagnosis made, any developing or subsequent acute symptoms tend to be dismissed as psychogenic in origin. In addition, many psychiatric facilities are not experienced in recognizing or treating subtle or unusual medical/surgical illnesses.
- **Medical clearance in a lucid patient, capable of giving an accurate medical history, is straightforward.** In such a patient, as for all patients, elements of history suggesting an active medical problem point the way to further examination and evaluation, as do abnormalities of vital signs and other elements of the physical examination. In such an individual, with no history of active medical problems and a normal physical examination, no specific laboratory evaluation is indicated (although some specific testing may be required by the receiving facility).
- **"Medical clearance" in a patient with an abnormal mental status or the inability or unwillingness to give a comprehensive history is more complex and demanding.**
  - **An abnormal mental status in the presence of concomitant medical or surgical illness, abnormal physical signs or symptoms, or laboratory abnormalities should be presumed to be causally related to those factors until proved otherwise.** For example, a patient with known diabetes and an abnormal mental status should be evaluated with the presumption that the abnormality of mental status is due in some way to a complication of diabetes, which must be excluded (high or low blood sugar, hyperosmolar nonketotic delirium or coma, sepsis, or any other complication). Similarly, a patient with abnormal mental status and a fever should be presumed to be suffering from an acute encephalopathy (until proved otherwise), which should be excluded; patients with elevated liver function tests and an abnormal mental status should be carefully evaluated for hepatic encephalopathy and for any illness that could be causing both elevated liver function test and an abnormal mental status: acetaminophen toxicity, for example.
  - For this reason, **the history in a patient with an abnormal mental status** needs to focus on:
    - Whether there is a history of a previous or current medical or surgical illness, including trauma, which may have been trivial, that could be contributing to the current situation, including any current medications, or change in medications, that the patient is taking.
    - Whether in the history of the present illness there have been any signs or symptoms suggestive of medical/surgical/neurologic disease other than psychiatric illness. For example, is there a history of headache, neck stiffness, fever?
    - Collateral sources of that information may be essential.
  - For these reasons as well, the **physical examination in patients with an abnormal mental status** needs to include at a minimum:
    - A careful assessment of the patient's vital signs.
    - A complete general examination, including a neurologic assessment, with particular attention to the patient's mental status, including attention, memory, orientation, presence of hallucinations other than auditory, and fluctuations

in consciousness. Are meningeal signs present? Is there cutaneous evidence of hepatic dysfunction (jaundice, ecchymoses, spider angiomata) or evidence of arthritis, suggesting an autoimmune disorder?

- **Laboratory examination in a patient with an abnormal mental status,** who is being referred for psychiatric or detox treatment should include
  - ○ Complete blood count, with platelets
  - ○ Toxic screen to evaluate for undeclared overdose/poisoning
  - ○ Liver function tests
  - ○ BUN, creatinine, blood sugar, and electrolytes
  - ○ Other tests as specifically indicated by history or abnormalities of physical examination, for example, thyroid function studies, B_{12}, folate, erythrocyte sedimentation rate, oxygen saturation, electrocardiogram, chest x-ray, lumbar puncture, computed tomography, etc.
- When a determination as to the etiology of the patient's illness or behavior is unclear, consideration should be given to psychiatric and/or neurologic consultation before a treatment disposition. Any minor medical or surgical problems identified should be discussed with the receiving institution before transfer.

Managing Agitation and Aggression in the Emergency Department

OVERVIEW

- Agitation and the potential for aggression can arise from a number of causes. Some of these stem from the medical or psychiatric condition that brought the person to the emergency department (ED) in the first place, such as PCP intoxication or acute alcohol withdrawal. Some are aggravated by the ED environment, in which people commonly wait a long time, often not knowing what is going to happen next. Additionally, the ED environment can be loud and often not private. Also, in some instances, unfortunately, the person may have been inadvertently shamed or humiliated by ED personnel.

- **The first principle in dealing with aggression and agitation in the ED is to acknowledge the risk and to plan to deal with it proactively**. Cross-functional, multidisciplinary teams including physicians, nurses, security personnel, and others who interact with patients should try to evaluate the experience of patients in the ED setting, to identify potential causes of aggravation, and to have a proactive plan for dealing with aggression and violence when they arise. Each person should have a clear plan for how such situations should be handled.

- **A corollary of such planning is to have well-designed and universally practiced protocols for the ED evaluation and management of psychiatric conditions, especially for drug and alcohol abuse and withdrawal.** These are dealt with separately in Chapter 69.

- In dealing with people who are becoming agitated, certain behaviors and attitudes may help to defuse the situation; some of these are as follows.

- **Be alert that a medical or psychiatric problem is emerging that is inadequately treated.** The most likely culprit is acute withdrawal, which may occur while the medical workup is in progress. It may be necessary to treat withdrawal simultaneously with this evaluation. Remember to consider the diagnosis of **akathisia,** which may be contributing to agitation. Akathisia is severe restlessness, which is most often seen in the first few months of initiating neuroleptic therapy or after an increase in dose; patients wish to be continually pacing or walking around the examining room. Somewhat paradoxically, increasing the patient's medication dose only worsens the symptoms; treatment includes dose adjustment, β-blockers, and benzodiazepines.

- Always remember that **many people have had previous negative experiences in the ED;** these perceptions often include having felt insulted, misunderstood, patronized, or otherwise humiliated. They may therefore come to the ED defensive and expecting the worse. Such people may respond in an exaggerated fashion to minimal or even imagined slights. In dealing with people who have symptoms, it is almost always best to apologize, acknowledge whatever truth there is in the symptom, and try to decrease the person's experience of powerlessness.

- **Be friendly, warm, and polite.** Use the person's name, but be careful to address adults as Mr. or Ms. Explain everything that is being performed, and explain delays wherever possible.
- **Offer food, a blanket, or water as appropriate;** if the person smokes and he or she can safely step outside the ED with family or security personnel, this may go a long way toward calming the situation (this is, of course, subject to the constraints of the individual hospital's smoking policy).
- **Be aware of your posture and tone of voice.** Avoid looking directly into the person's eyes; this is often seen as threatening. It is very effective to look at the person's lips, which conveys that you are interested in what he or she is saying and avoids eliciting the "stare-down" reflex. Similarly, avoid a cross-armed or hands on the hips stance. A slightly stooped posture, standing not directly in front of the person, but turned slightly to the side, is best.
- **Be aware of the person's personal space.** Do not stand too close. In general, exaggerate the social distance, giving the person anywhere from 4 to 8 ft of space around him or her.
- **Be aware of the exits in the situation.** Ideally, both the examiner and the patient should have a sense of ease of egress so neither feels trapped. If one must choose, it is more important for the examiner to be able to get out.
- **Acknowledge the person's situation, clearly and in simple terms, using the same words that the person uses if at all possible**; for example, "I know that the police brought you here, Mr. Jones, and that you do not want to be here. You think you should be able to leave right now. As you said, you are 'extremely angry' about all this. I want to assure you that we will let you leave just as soon as we can. That means we have to know that you are safe, that you do not have any medical condition that would endanger you or anyone else. That is why we want to examine you and do some tests. Is there anything I can do to make this less awful for you?"
- **Offer to call in a third party.** If there is someone the patient trusts, that person can be called and will hopefully facilitate communication, helping the patient to feel less trapped.
- **Warn, do not threaten.** If you anticipate having to use force, for example, and have readied the force to be used, then consider warning the person as follows: "Mr. Jones, I am worried about this situation. I have told you that we cannot let you leave and tried to explain why. You say you are going to leave anyway. I am concerned that if you try to leave it would be necessary to use restraints, which I would really rather avoid. Can you help me avoid them?" This warning is different from a threat, which might sound something like, "If you step toward the door, I am going to have the security guards restrain you." The nonthreatening metaphor is a "heads-up" about what might happen.
- **Help the person save face.** If you can, avoid an audience. If you can, concede something, by breaking the problem up into smaller, manageable pieces.
- **Be prepared to use overwhelming force** and consider allowing the necessary personnel to be within the visual field (but not near the physical space of the individual unless it is needed).
- **Train your personnel thoroughly** in the application of restraints, so they can function smoothly as a team, with a single leader and with clear individual responsibilities. Be extremely clear about how and by whom the decision to initiate the restraint process is made.

- Pharmacologic management of agitation and aggression
  - **Precaution: Be sure that you have accurately and thoroughly identified the underlying cause of agitation.** Aggressively sedating an individual, when a serious underlying medical problem (such as alcohol withdrawal) is responsible for the patient's behavior or contributing to it, is very dangerous.
  - **For most agitated patients, mixture of haloperidol, 5 mg, lorazepam, 1 mg, and benztropine, 1 mg, is effective in calming the patient.** These drugs may be administered orally, intramuscularly, or intravenously (if lorazepam is given intramuscularly, administration in the deltoid muscle promotes greater and smoother absorption). Lorazepam causes less respiratory depression than diazepam. Benztropine (Cogentin) administered in this way protects against the development of dystonic reactions, which are the most likely complication to this regimen. This regimen can be repeated every 30 minutes until the patient is calm. Diphenhydramine, 25 to 50 mg, is an alternative to benztropine to combat dystonia.
  - Alternative regimens for management of agitation and/or aggression include:
    - Olanzapine, 10 mg intramuscularly, is an available substitute for patients who have had an allergy or adverse reaction to haloperidol.
    - Risperidone is available in rapidly dissolving oral tablets. This may be an option for more cooperative patients.

Evaluating the Suicidal Patient in the Emergency Department

OVERVIEW

Scope of the Problem

- **Suicide is a common and profoundly serious problem**, both in patients with identified psychiatric conditions and in people with no previously identified psychiatric disease. Suicide accounts for more than 30,000 deaths per year or 12:1,000 in the general population. But in certain age groups and at-risk groups, the numbers are much higher: Among adolescents and young adults, suicide rates have risen dramatically over the past four decades and now represent the second leading cause of death. Suicide rates climb with age, peaking for women in the seventh decade but continuing to rise steadily for men; hence, elderly men are at four times the risk of the general population, and 25% of all suicides occur in people older than 65 years. Long considered to predominate among whites, with suicide rates for nonwhites approximately half of that of whites, suicide rates have been increasing dramatically among young black men over the past 30 years. Native Americans experience the highest rates among American ethnic groups. Among the elderly and among people with several risk factors, such as chronic illness, social isolation, and substance abuse, suicide is a leading cause of death.
- **Suicide is also an eminently preventable cause of death**. It is estimated that as many as 90% of the people who do complete suicide may have a treatable psychiatric disorder, such as depression. The identification and treatment of these individuals are urgent.
- Not all self-harm is suicidal in intent. Many patients engage in deliberate self-injurious behavior, not to kill themselves but to soothe intolerable psychic pain. Such behavior, which may include cutting, burning with cigarettes, or other auto-erotic painful behavior, is commonly seen in individuals suffering from posttraumatic stress disorder and among victims of sexual abuse. The management of self-injurious behavior is different from that of suicidal behavior.

Obstacles to Successful Management

- Many times **people conceal their suicidal intentions** or the severity of their suicidal wishes. Particularly because suicide is often driven by feelings of shame and inadequacy, it is understandable that many people find these feelings difficult to share with strangers, such as emergency department (ED) personnel.
- The **ED itself is often not conducive to an effective evaluation of patients at risk for suicide**. Noise, intrusions by others, urgency and lack of time, and inadequate privacy make the elicitation and evaluation of subtle or inapparent suicidal intentions very difficult.

- Often, **people who attempt suicide or who harbor self-destructive tendencies elicit negative reactions in caregivers**. These feelings may range from aversion and hostility to overinvolvement and inappropriate rescue actions. These feelings may stem in part from the common experience that many people who come or are brought to the ED following a suicide "attempt" have not really tried to kill themselves; instead, their behavior appears more "manipulative" in an attempt to influence the behavior of others. In a crowded ED filled with people who did nothing to contribute to their suffering or illness, there is a great temptation to blame the person with suicidal behavior. If the practitioner is not aware of these feelings toward the suicidal patient, then he or she runs the risk of expressing them in the treatment of the patient. Such acting out of the doctor's feelings can be manifested as curt treatment, minimizing the patient's difficulties and not appreciating the real risk of death from suicide in the future, particularly if the patient senses that he or she must "up the ante" to be taken seriously.
- **Despite the fact that we can identify numerous risk factors** (see "Risk Factors") **for completed suicide, there is no absolutely reliable way to predict who will complete suicide**. Therefore, we rely on the clinical guidelines outlined here, but we understand the reality that we may underestimate the suicide risk in any given individual.

General Principles of Suicide Evaluation

- Take all suicide attempts seriously.
- Consider occult suicide in all patients who fit high-risk profiles (see "Risk Factors").
- Take enough time and create an adequate space to conduct the evaluation.
- When appropriate, involve outside caregivers, family, and other people in the person's life.
- Seek consultation appropriately.
- Document clearly and carefully.
- The disposition of the person who has been evaluated for suicide must assure his or her safety reasonably, account for the possibility that his or her suicidal tendencies might increase after the completion of the evaluation, and plan accordingly.
- Therefore, everyone in whom suicide is considered even a remote possibility should have a future contact planned with a professional and/or a clear plan and method for accessing help in an emergency.

RISK FACTORS

- **Age.** In general, the risk of suicide increases steadily with age; this is somewhat truer of men than women, whose suicide risk peaks in the sixth decade. Elderly individuals are at extreme risk for suicide. Other peak ages to consider are adolescence and retirement.
- **Sex.** In general, women attempt suicide three times as frequently as men do, but men complete suicide three times more frequently than women do. Therefore, in assessing risk (see below), factor gender into the equation.
- **Race.** In general, Americans of European ethnicity commit suicide with greater frequency than do African Americans. However, Native Americans are at particularly high risk.
- **Concomitant medical illness**. The presence of concomitant medical illness increases suicide risk, particularly if the illness is chronic, or if it involves chronic pain or physical disfigurement.

- **Social isolation**. Human connections are relatively protective against suicide. Married people commit suicide less frequently than people who are not married. Social isolation increases the risk of suicide.
- **Substance abuse**. Active substance abuse dramatically increases the risk of suicide.
- **Family history**. Having a first-degree relative who has completed suicide increases the risk of suicide 35-fold.
- **Previous attempts.** The risk of an individual repeating a suicide attempt is vastly greater than the risk in the general population.
- **Concomitant psychiatric illness** increases the risk of suicide. Suicide is particularly dangerous in individuals with **schizophrenia and other psychotic conditions**, both during the acute phase of illness (especially in the presence of hallucinations "commanding" suicide) and in the depressive aftermath of psychosis. This is especially true for people with "new" diagnoses of psychotic illness, who may be confronting a radical re-evaluation of their life's promise and expectations. Also at grave risk are individuals with **depression with psychotic features, mania with psychotic features, and, particularly, depression that is just starting to improve**, during which time the depressed person may be experiencing more energy to act on suicidal impulses. **All psychiatric conditions are more likely to result in suicide if aggravated by substance abuse**.
- **Method/scenario**. The higher the lethality of means employed or considered, and the lower the likelihood of rescue, the greater the risk of suicide. This principle has been called the **risk-rescue ratio**.
- **Agitation**. The presence of motor restlessness, hyperactivity, hand-wringing, pacing, and a sense of "crawling out of my skin" are all signs of agitation. In the presence of suicidal ideas or impulses, agitation is a grave sign and drastically reduces the person's capacity to remain safe without outside structure.
- **Recent change in job status**. Particularly for men, shame and humiliation seem to be powerful accelerants to suicide.

EVALUATION OF SUICIDE RISK

Approach to the Patient

- **Finding adequate, unhurried time and providing some sense of a private space**, although rare commodities in the ED, are important elements of evaluating a person's potential for suicide. As is true for the psychiatric evaluation as a whole, the evaluation must take place in a friendly and receptive atmosphere. In almost every instance, the issue of suicide must be approached only after a period of building rapport. The issue of suicide is far more easily broached with a person from whom one has gotten the "nod," than with someone with whom such alignment does not exist.
- It is generally wise to address the issue of suicide from a context of feeling bad while **using nonpathological language**, such as "I gather you have been feeling so bad recently that you have been thinking of ending your life." or "I can see you have been feeling horrible lately, and have been dealing with some terrible stress. Has it been so bad that you have thought of death?"
- After the subject has been broached, **encourage the person to say more, leaving the subject open-ended**.
- Only after the person has had a chance to elaborate in this way should the examiner go on to ask more specific questions about the nature of the plan, the reasons for wanting death, and so on, as described.

Evaluating the Current Specific Plan/Situation

• With respect to the current situation, of paramount importance is **the person's attitude toward the issue of suicide**.

  • **Does the person acknowledge suicidal thoughts/feelings/acts?** Failure to acknowledge suicidal thoughts when there is collateral evidence (such as a note or a very suspicious self-inflicted wound) is a worrisome sign and suggests a lack of forthrightness or honesty. The more complete or pervasive the denial, the more the evaluator must assume that suicidal feelings are clear and present, regardless of the person's overt denials, and, therefore, may need to opt for a more secure disposition, such as hospitalization.

  • If there is **independent evidence** of suicidal feelings or behavior (a note, cut wrists, etc.), does the person acknowledge or minimize and rationalize this evidence? Such rationalization similarly bespeaks difficulty in trusting the person's future behavior.

  • If the person does acknowledge suicidal feelings or thoughts, does the person express an **ongoing wish to die**, or does the person express hope for help? The more fixed the suicidal ideas, the more necessary it will be to provide external controls, such as a secure hospital setting.

  • **How does the person assess the issue of suicide?** The more the person can acknowledge realistically the difficulties that he or she is facing and the pain of these difficulties, and still look ahead and ask for help, the more likely it may be that the problem may be handled on an outpatient, voluntary basis.

  • **What does the person think should be done?** This again is an opportunity to assess how realistic the person's perspective is. This inquiry also opens the possibility of finding suggestions or ideas on the patient's part that can be incorporated into the eventual plan. The more that plan builds on the patient's own ideas, the more likely it is to succeed.

• **Evaluate the nature of the specific suicidal behavior that has occurred or is contemplated**

  • **How lethal is the behavior?** Gunshot or hanging is much more lethal than overdoses of small amounts of pills. How likely would rescue be? Was the plan to go far into the woods and overdose, or did the person take pills in front of his or her boyfriend or girlfriend? The higher the ratio of risk to likelihood of rescue, the more ominous the attempt and the more likely it is that a secure treatment setting will be needed.

  • **What seems to be the goal of the suicidal act**—to end unbearable suffering, to avoid shameful humiliation for a specific act that is as yet hidden, to communicate the extent of their pain, to hurt someone by making them suffer the results of the suicide, or to force someone to behave in a desired way? The more suicide arises as an escape from insurmountable internal pain, as opposed to arising in the context of an ongoing relationship, the more difficult it may be to design an outpatient intervention plan that is safe and effective.

  • Does the suicidal behavior arise in the context of an ongoing relationship with another person? If so, consider getting the patient's consent to contact that individual to participate in the evaluation. If the person is in such a relationship, what is the current status of that relationship?

• **Evaluate the psychiatric context of the suicidal behavior**

  • **Is the person in current treatment for a psychiatric disorder?** If so, can the treating clinician be contacted to participate in the evaluation? If the person is in treatment, what is the status of that treatment—have there been recent medication changes, disruptions or problems in therapy, etc.? It may be that if there are acute difficulties in the treatment relationship, the consultation of the ED visit may help to stabilize the situation, particularly if the treating clinician can be contacted and his or her perspective on treatment taken into account.

- **Is the person currently psychotic**, and if so, **does the suicidal ideation or behavior seem driven by the psychosis**, for example, by command hallucinations? If so, such command hallucinations are powerful indicators for a secure treatment setting.
- **Does the person currently suffer from a major affective disorder, psychotic disorder, or anxiety disorder, and is his or her treatment adequate?**

Evaluating the Risk Factors

- Consider the age, sex, race, and ethnicity of the individual.
- Consider the presence of concomitant medical illness, especially chronic illness or conditions producing chronic pain or disability.
- Consider the presence of substance abuse and, in particular, whether the person was intoxicated at the time of the attempt and whether the person is intoxicated at the time of the evaluation. If so, seek a safe way to let time pass for the person to sober up before making a definitive disposition.
- Consider the social connectedness of the person, and the stability and availability of these connections. Have there been recent losses/problems in these relationships?
- Consider the history of suicide attempts in this individual. What was the degree of risk and likelihood of rescue in previous attempts? What was the outcome and why? Did the person seek help or was he or she accidentally discovered? What were the circumstances of past suicide attempts and do they shed any light on the current situation, for example, anniversaries of important events or losses of a similar nature?
- Consider the family history, with respect to suicide and to psychiatric illness.

Evaluating Strengths and Resources

- Consider the **positive attributes of the person**—virtually everyone has them. These may include tenacity, persistence, a capacity to survive, intelligence, verbal skills, or religious faith. Consider how these might or might not be useful in coping with the current crisis.
- Consider **interpersonal resources and supports** available to the individual. Consider who matters to them and to whom they matter. How available are these important individuals and relationships now?
- Are there other **mitigating factors** that should be considered? For example, a person might be very highly motivated to get back to work or school; if sufficient support exists around him or her, and if other factors do not suggest a different course of action, helping him or her return rapidly to these normative behaviors may be very constructive.

Evaluating the Overall Psychiatric Picture

Based on all of the information, does the person appear to be in effective treatment for the problems they are facing?

Evaluating Options

- The range of options includes
  - Hospitalize involuntarily
  - Hospitalize voluntarily

- Admit to an observation facility or acute residential facility, if available
- Hold in the ED for a period of time and re-evaluate, for example, if the person is intoxicated
- Discharge from the ED with specific follow-up
- **Involuntary hospitalization** statutes vary from state to state. In general, involuntary hospitalization will be necessary if the person continues to pose a serious risk of harm to self or others on the basis of a mental illness and if no less restrictive setting is appropriate or available. In practice, if the person continues to manifest suicidal ideation directly, or if the examiner suspects that a serious degree of such ideation persists despite the person's denials, and if no adequate alternative setting exists, then involuntary admission will probably be necessary. For example, in a borderline case, if the patient has an extended, involved, and committed family who agrees to watch the person constantly until he or she can meet with his or her own doctor the next day, and if the patient can meaningfully commit to cooperate with the family in this way, then discharge to the family's care might be an option. In this case, the family and patient should be encouraged to call or return to the ED immediately if the situation deteriorates.
- **Voluntary hospitalization** and admission to acute residential facilities usually require that the person be able to give meaningful assurances of his or her own safety to be admitted. Thus, the evaluator in the ED must conclude that the person is safe enough to manage in such a relatively unstructured setting.
- **Discharge from the ED** to follow-up on an outpatient basis requires that the evaluator establishes the following:
  - The person does not pose a substantial, immediate threat to himself or herself or to anyone else on the basis of mental illness.
  - An adequate plan is in place such that the person can, and will, be able to access emergency services if suicidal ideation worsens.
  - A reasonable plan for follow-up services is either in place or, in the event that it is impossible to make these arrangements from the ED, the person and support system are aware of how to make such arrangements.

Consultation

When a risk of suicide is suspected, the ED physician may wish to obtain consultation from a psychiatrist. In the event that a psychiatrist is unavailable, it may be wise to ask a colleague to participate in the patient's evaluation and to review the decisions regarding suicide risk, management, and disposition. The consulting physician should document concurrence with the plan in the medical record.

Documentation

Clearly document exactly what your findings are and why you are making the decision you are making. If the person is allowed to leave the ED despite the presence of suicidal ideation or behavior on admission, it is essential to document that the physician is aware of this behavior, has thoughtfully assessed this behavior as part of the overall evaluation of the patient, and is of the opinion that the patient currently does not pose a substantial risk of harm to self or others as well as to document the plan for obtaining services for the patient after the discharge, scheduled outpatient follow-up, and how to access emergency services.

Negotiating the Outcome

- As is true for psychiatric evaluations generally, **the outcome of the evaluation is usually better if there is substantial buy-in from the patient and family with**

the proposed outcome. This is more likely to occur if the patient and family are actively involved from the outset of the evaluation and if they participate actively in evaluating options.

- Nonetheless, **sometimes it is necessary to recommend or to implement a plan that the patient and/or family disagrees with, such as hospitalizing the patient against his or her own will.** In the event that this is necessary, it is very desirable to obtain consultation and to permit (or invite) the family to have their own doctor participate in the decision making. To the extent possible, it is wise to give the patient and family a voice and a role in choosing some aspects of care, for example, to which specific hospital the patient will be committed or who may accompany the patient. It is also generally wise to clearly explain to the patient and family what you are doing and why, how you have arrived at your decision, and to ask if you have overlooked any important information. In these difficult situations, consider stressing that you are doing what you believe you are professionally and ethically bound to do and that you are sincerely providing the care that you would want for a loved one in the same circumstances. Acknowledge the patient's and the family's distress and perspective, and take it seriously.

- **Whenever a person is being discharged from the ED after an encounter that involves a suicide evaluation, follow-up is always indicated**. The knowledge that there is a proximal scheduled appointment is very reassuring to the patient; optimally, this will be with the patient's therapist, with an individual providing direct care to the patient during the current crisis, or with a consulting therapist. A clear means of contacting a caregiver can be an important lifeline for the patient if suicidal ideation returns or increases. All patients should feel comfortable returning to the ED, if necessary.

Evaluation and Management of Drug and Alcohol Problems in the Emergency Department

EVALUATION OF THE PATIENT WITH DRUG OR ALCOHOL ABUSE

Introduction

Evaluating patients with drug or alcohol abuse poses significant challenges in the emergency department. Belligerence and disinhibition may make patients demanding, difficult, and dangerous. Obnoxious behavior may alienate medical personnel and interfere with appropriate and methodical evaluation and treatment. The symptoms of intoxication and withdrawal may mask or mimic other potentially life-threatening conditions.

Evaluating Intoxicated Patients

- Paramount concerns in the evaluation of intoxicated patients are:
  - to guarantee the safety of the patient and the medical staff
  - to conduct a sufficiently exhaustive examination to rule out potentially life-threatening entities in the differential diagnosis
  - to identify the substance abuse problem accurately
  - to lay the foundation for effective management and referral.
- The signs and symptoms of intoxication vary with the intoxicating substance, of course, but they often share the common characteristics of disinhibition, such as impaired judgment and emotional lability, any varying degrees of slurred speech, confusion regarding time, place, and/or situation, and ataxia
- The differential diagnosis of such a presentation includes the following:
  - Alcohol intoxication
  - Sedative-hypnotic intoxication
  - Anticholinergic poisoning from medication toxicity or overdose
  - Hypoglycemia/hyperglycemia/ketoacidosis/hyperosmolar states
  - Hepatic encephalopathy
  - Postictal confusion
  - Acute cerebrovascular events, including subdural hematoma, subarachnoid bleeds, transient ischemic attacks, etc.
  - Encephalitis/meningitis
  - Alcohol or sedative-hypnotic withdrawal, which may occur in a setting suggestive of ongoing intoxication, for example, alcohol on the breath, elevated blood alcohol levels
  - Other causes of delirium (hypertensive encephalopathy, hypoxia, sepsis, etc.).

- **Evaluation of the intoxicated individual** should include:
  - An adequate **history,** including:
    - substance abuse and psychiatric history
    - last substance ingested, including amount and time since ingestion
    - previous history of withdrawal complications, especially seizures
    - medical history, including currently active medical problems and symptoms
    - current medications that the patient is taking or to which the patient has access
    - collateral information from family, friends and other observers
  - **Physical examination,** which is admittedly difficult in some belligerent individuals, should include at a minimum:
    - Careful observation of the patient, to determine spontaneous and symmetric movement of all extremities, and for signs of ataxia, orientation in space, and any indication that the person is responding to visual, auditory, or tactile hallucinations, as well as for any signs of head injury and any ictal phenomena.
    - Vital signs
    - Evaluation of skin color, moisture, and temperature
    - Pupillary size and presence of nystagmus and ophthalmoplegia
    - Abnormalities in any of these may necessitate a more thorough examination, even if restraint or sedation is necessary. In the absence of elevated pulse or fever and in the absence of any obvious neurologic impairment in an individual who is oriented to place and situation, further intrusive or invasive examination is probably not necessary, at least initially.
  - **Mental status examination.** The mental status examination of intoxicated individuals focuses on:
    - Cognitive functions, including orientation to space, time, person, and situation; attention; concentration; and memory
    - Fluctuations in the level of consciousness
    - The presence or absence of hallucinations, especially visual, tactile, olfactory, or auditory; other disorders of thought content or form
    - Flow, rate, prosody, and content of speech
    - Suicidal or homicidal ideation and impulses
    - Other psychiatric signs and symptoms
  - **Laboratory evaluation.** Laboratory evaluation should be directed by clinical suspicion for specific organic disease processes, and may include: a urine toxic screen to identify any intoxicant or concomitant intoxicants in addition to an obvious one (e.g., undeclared drug use in an individual obviously intoxicated with alcohol); a complete blood count (CBC), blood urea nitrogen (BUN), serum glucose, electrolytes, liver function tests, calcium, and magnesium. Blood alcohol levels are of little clinical usefulness, other than to identify alcohol as an intoxicating agent.
- The evaluation of intoxicated individuals should permit the physician to determine:
  - Whether there is a **significant collateral medical or surgical condition requiring immediate management**, for example, acute poisoning, stroke, sepsis
  - Whether there are **acute complications of the intoxication** requiring immediate management, for example, respiratory depression, cardiac arrhythmias, hepatic toxicity, etc
  - Whether there is evidence of **current or imminent withdrawal** that requires management
  - Whether there is **concomitant psychiatric illness** that requires acute management, for example, suicidal ideation

Management of the Intoxicated Patient

- Management of intoxicated behavior depends on maintaining control of the situation, avoiding needless struggles with the patient, vigorous and appropriate treatment of withdrawal, and recognizing and treating concomitant conditions.
- **Maintaining control of the situation**
  - It is important to have a **proactive policy, developed with the various disciplines involved, as to how intoxicated patients will be managed.** This involves decisions about:
    - Where in the emergency department such patients should be seen; how and by whom they should be triaged
    - What the initial workup will consist of
    - When, why, and how to treat signs of withdrawal
    - When and whom to consult and for what
    - The role of security officers, including specific guidelines for initiating and continuously reviewing the necessity for restraint
    - The expectations and requirements of the facilities to which intoxicated individuals are to be referred
- **The more these issues can be resolved in advance, by a multidisciplinary team, the less likely it will be that intoxicated individuals will unduly disrupt their own and others' care.**
- Intoxicated people are often offensive, and they therefore can elicit defensive, sarcastic, or abrupt behavior from their caregivers. These responses often inflame the situation. It is imperative to have a **welcoming, calm, and nonjudgmental attitude toward intoxicated patients.** Offering water, coffee, a blanket, or other concrete comforts can reassure intoxicated people that they are welcome and do not need to be aggressive to get their needs met. Letting the person know what to expect and how long waits are likely to be as well as keeping the person informed as the process unfolds can avoid some difficulties.
- However, it is **pointless and counterproductive to argue with an intoxicated person. Friendly, nondefensive firmness is best.**
- It is imperative to **know in advance, as described above, the parameters for detaining and even restraining individuals who are intoxicated.** In general, patients who are suspected of posing a significant risk to themselves or others, by virtue of a mental illness, or whose judgment is so impaired by intoxication that they may pose an immediate risk to themselves or to the public if they were to leave the emergency department, should be detained and restrained if necessary. The legal issues involved in such decisions vary from state to state; consult legal counsel in your jurisdiction to be clear about these issues.
- Having **made the decision to detain, and if necessary restrain, such an individual, it is imperative to have adequate, overwhelming force available to the emergency department staff to achieve this end.**
- **Pharmacologic approach to management of belligerent intoxicated individuals.**
  - In the event that the nonpharmacologic approaches outlined fail to help the patient calm down and cooperate with care, or if the person's behavior is significantly compromising his or her evaluation and treatment, or that of other patients in the emergency department, it may be necessary to provide sedation, even to intoxicated patients. In such instances, **haloperidol (2.0–5.0 mg) with benztropine (1.0 mg) and lorazepam (1.0 mg) administered orally or intramuscularly, will usually result in sedation without placing the patient at undue risk.** Alternatives are available as discussed in Chapter 67.

ALCOHOL-RELATED EMERGENCIES

Overview

Dimensions of the Problem

Alcohol is by far the most common drug of abuse encountered in most emergency departments. It is estimated that 13.6% of the general population suffers from alcohol abuse or dependence, and 100,000 deaths per year are attributable to alcohol. Of special importance in the emergency department, it is estimated that 25% of all suicides involve alcohol.

Diagnostic Issues

Alcohol-Related Diagnoses

- **Acute alcohol intoxication** is not subtle. At low blood levels, patients generally experience euphoria, disinhibition, and impulsiveness; at increasingly higher blood levels one sees irritability, hostility, belligerence, slurred speech, incoordination, unsteady gait, nystagmus, impaired attention and concentration, and eventually sedation, respiratory depression, and coma.
- **Alcohol abuse** is defined as at least 1 month of impaired social and occupational functioning associated with alcohol use. The person may use alcohol in dangerous circumstances and despite negative consequences. When tolerance to alcohol develops and increasing amounts are consumed, the appropriate diagnosis is **alcohol dependence.**
- **Alcohol withdrawal** is characterized by autonomic hyperactivity in the setting of alcohol cessation; this often produces tremor, insomnia, nausea/vomiting, anxiety, agitation, and sometimes transient visual, tactile, or auditory hallucinations, and seizures.
- When the hallucinations are not transient and are accompanied by disturbances of consciousness (with reduced ability to focus or attend), or in the face of other cognitive impairments such as decreased awareness of the environment, the diagnosis of **alcohol-induced delirium** should be considered. In a setting of alcohol cessation and falling (even if absolutely elevated) alcohol levels, this clinical picture suggests alcohol withdrawal delirium. In less than 5% of cases, such alcohol withdrawal delirium may proceed to **delirium tremens,** a potentially lethal syndrome of alcohol withdrawal requiring vigorous treatment.
- Hallucinations or delusions in the presence of ongoing alcohol use, but without any impairment of consciousness (i.e., the person is oriented to person, place, and time, without impairments of memory, attention, or concentration) characterize the syndrome of **alcohol-induced psychotic disorder (formerly called alcoholic hallucinosis).**
- Impairments in memory without impairments in concentration suggest the possibility of **Wernicke-Korsakoff syndrome**.

Differential Diagnosis

- Except at toxic levels (blood levels generally above 400 mg/dL), alcohol intoxication in itself does not pose serious medical problems. It is important to remember, however, that serious medical conditions frequently accompany prolonged or "binge" alcohol abuse and these may easily be mistaken for, or attributed to, alcohol intoxication and therefore overlooked.
- The **differential diagnosis of alcohol intoxication** includes the following:
  - Alcohol intoxication and poisoning
  - Sedative-hypnotic intoxication

- Anticholinergic poisoning from medication toxicity or overdose
- Hypoglycemia/hyperglycemia/ketoacidosis/hyperosmolar states
- Hepatic encephalopathy
- Postictal confusion
- Acute cerebrovascular events, including subdural hematoma, subarachnoid bleeds, transient ischemic attacks, and other acute strokes.
- Encephalitis/meningitis
- Alcohol or sedative-hypnotic withdrawal, which may occur in a setting suggestive of ongoing intoxication, for example, alcohol on the breath, elevated blood alcohol levels
- Other causes of delirium (hypertensive encephalopathy, hypoxia, sepsis, etc.)

Evaluation of the Patient with Established or Suspected Alcohol Abuse

History
- Determining whether a person merits a diagnosis of alcohol abuse or dependence is often difficult, since patients tend to deny and minimize the extent of drinking and its consequences. When the person is intoxicated, this history can usually be obtained only after the person becomes sober.
- The history taking at the time of initial evaluation must **address the issue of whether there are other problems aside from the intoxication that may need to be the focus of the emergency evaluation.** In particular, has the person taken any other drugs or medications? Is there any evidence to suggest a suicide attempt? Is there evidence of other medical or surgical conditions that may need to be a focus of evaluation?
- The **drinking history** should include the amount most recently consumed, the time of the last drink, the average daily consumption, the pattern of consumption, consequences of consumption, previous attempts at sobriety, and family history of alcohol and drug abuse.
- The history should also determine whether seizures, blackouts, hematemesis, hematochezia, head trauma, etc., have occurred.
- The history should also include **psychiatric symptoms**, especially depression, anxiety, and suicidal ideation.

Physical Evaluation
The physical examination should include careful monitoring of vital signs to detect early signs of withdrawal; signs of autonomic hyperactivity, nystagmus, and ophthalmoplegia (the last two suggestive of Wernicke encephalopathy); also, the details of the routine physical examination should be noted.

Mental Evaluation
The mental status examination must evaluate the person's level of consciousness, ability to attend and concentrate, orientation, presence of hallucinations or delusions, mood, and potential for suicide or violence.

Laboratory Evaluation
- A **blood alcohol level has little clinical usefulness** other than establishing that the person has consumed alcohol, except at toxic levels, usually more than 400 mg/dL. A blood alcohol level, however, may have other uses, such as determining whether an individual can drive on leaving the emergency department, or whether some facilities will accept the patient for inpatient treatment.

- **Other laboratory investigations** may not be necessary but may be useful depending on clinical suspicion of other disease entities. These include a urine and blood screen for other substances and a CBC, which may serve to alert the examiner to nutritional deficiencies, infections, and other conditions; serum glucose, electrolytes, transaminase levels, BUN/creatinine, and calcium and magnesium levels may also be useful.

Management of Alcohol-Related Problems

Acute Management of the Alcoholic Patient

Acute Withdrawal

Manifestations

- Alcohol withdrawal may be precipitated by a number of factors, voluntary and involuntary, including illness or accident that interrupts the supply of alcohol. In general, withdrawal symptoms begin within 8 hours of the discontinuation of drinking, but the onset of withdrawal may be delayed for as long as 14 days, particularly in individuals who may be using other central nervous system (CNS) depressants, such as benzodiazepines.
- **Symptoms of alcohol withdrawal** include autonomic hyperactivity, tremor, insomnia, nausea and/or vomiting, transient tactile, visual, or auditory hallucinations, anxiety, and seizures.

Emergency Department Management

- The **patient will probably need medical admission in the presence of:**
  - Delirium
  - Hallucinations
  - Fever above 101°F
  - Recurrent seizures
  - Significant autonomic instability not rapidly reversed by benzodiazepines
  - An inability to take fluids.

Patients with unstable support systems, suicidal ideation, or poor judgment may similarly require inpatient treatment.

- **Benzodiazepine protocols** are directed at reversing autonomic instability, providing sedation, and preventing seizures.

  For patients without liver disease, the long-acting benzodiazepines may be more convenient and safe, given their long half-lives. **Diazepam,** for example, or **chlordiazepoxide** will provide smooth, slow descents in blood levels with subsequently less problematic withdrawal. **A reasonable protocol for such a patient would be to administer 10 mg of diazepam or 50 mg of chlordiazepoxide, orally, and reevaluate the patient in 1 hour, with repeated dosing every 1 to 2 hours until symptomatic improvement is achieved.**

  For patients with compromised hepatic function, **oxazepam** (30–60 mg as an initial dose) or **lorazepam** (1–2 mg as an initial dose) **may be used. Lorazepam has the additional advantage of smooth and reliable intramuscular absorption, particularly from the deltoid muscle.**

  In the presence of delirium, more aggressive regimens may be needed, with administration of intravenous benzodiazepines every 10 to 15 minutes as necessary to gain control of symptoms.

- Other drugs sometimes used in the treatment of alcohol withdrawal include **carbamazepine (Tegretol),** which has been found to be effective in treating autonomic hyperactivity in alcohol withdrawal, and **propranolol,** which may be effective in treating autonomic hyperactivity, but which does not prevent hallucinations, confusion, or withdrawal seizures. **Phenobarbital** can be effectively used in the management of alcohol withdrawal when the patient is dependent on both alcohol and barbiturates.

Nonpharmacologic Management

- **Vitamin replacement.** Because of the risk of **thiamine** deficiency and consequent Wernicke-Korsakoff syndrome, thiamine 100 mg intramuscular or intravenous should be administered in the emergency department.
- **Fluid and electrolyte management.** Patients who are withdrawing from alcohol are not always fluid depleted; some are overhydrated. In the presence of fever, diarrhea, or vomiting, however, significant volume depletion may be present and should be considered.

Delirium Tremens
Diagnosis

Delirium tremens is a late-appearing withdrawal syndrome (usually presenting 24–72 hours after abstinence), with the same signs and symptoms as those described for alcohol withdrawal, but with intense autonomic hyperactivity, fever, waxing and waning consciousness, confusion, often with visual and tactile hallucinations, and agitation.

Management

- General principles of treatment are the same as for alcohol withdrawal, but with more aggressive therapy and closer monitoring. Patients often require treatment in the intensive care unit.
- **Benzodiazepine protocols** are the same as above, but may need to be administered every 15 minutes, and sometimes in very large doses.
- **Haloperidol,** 5 mg orally, intramuscular, or intravenous, given every 1 hour for 1 to 2 doses if needed, may substantially alleviate some psychotic symptoms if used concomitantly with benzodiazepines.
- Fluid, electrolyte, and vitamin replacement are as noted. In the presence of fever and agitation, fluid losses may be substantial.
- Most patients diagnosed with delirium tremens will require admission to an intensive care setting for agitation control, vital sign monitoring, and seizure precautions.

Alcoholic Coma

Alcoholic coma should be managed as a medical emergency, with the usual approach to coma (establishment and maintenance of an effective airway, rapid prophylactic treatment of the reversible cause of coma, administration of intravenous thiamine, 100 mg, followed by 50% intravenous dextrose, and intravenous naloxone), support of blood pressure initially with isotonic intravenous fluids, if needed, etc. A toxic screen for illicit substances should also be obtained.

Seizures

Alcohol abuse is one of the most common causes of adult-onset seizures; approximately 10% of adults experiencing alcohol withdrawal will have a seizure. Ninety-five percent of such seizures are generalized, and sixty percent are recurrent, with eighty-five percent of subsequent seizures occurring within 6 hours of the first.

- Phenytoin does **not** prevent alcohol withdrawal seizures.
- Magnesium sulfate does not reduce seizure frequency, even in patients with low serum magnesium levels.
- **Lorazepam, 2 mg intravenous, after the index seizure, significantly reduces the risk of recurrent seizures in alcohol withdrawal and is the preferred treatment.**

Referral for Treatment

- **Treatment planning.** Emergency department encounters provide potentially fruitful opportunities to confront the consequences of excessive drinking. This is an ideal time to educate the patient and family about the nature of alcoholism and its treatment.
- **Treatment options** include referral to inpatient detoxification; partial hospital (day treatment) programs; 12-step programs; and referral to individual practitioners.

Other Alcohol-Related Problems
Wernicke-Korsakoff Syndrome

This is a syndrome of ophthalmoplegia, memory impairment, and ataxia caused by acute thiamine deficiency. Properly identified and treated, its symptoms may be entirely reversible; improperly identified and untreated, its consequences may be cognitively devastating and irreversible.

- **Clinical manifestations:**
  - Nystagmus
  - Ophthalmoplegia (sixth nerve palsy)
  - Ataxia
  - Anterograde amnesia
  - Confabulation
  - Inattention
- Treatment consists of **rapid thiamine replacement** (100 mg intravenous and then 100 mg/day orally). Additional intravenous thiamine may be required and should be titrated to reverse ophthalmoplegia if possible. Magnesium replacement should also be considered. Fluvoxamine may be useful in treating residual memory impairment.

Disulfiram-Alcohol Syndrome

The **disulfiram-alcohol syndrome** occurs within 10 minutes of the ingestion of alcohol in patients currently taking antabuse (disulfiram, a medication used as a relapse deterrent). It is characterized by facial flushing, headache, vomiting, chest pain, hypotension, syncope, confusion, vertigo, and severe distress. The syndrome may last up to several hours. Rarely, complications include arrhythmias, hypotension, and seizures.

SEDATIVE-HYPNOTICS

General Considerations

By far the most commonly prescribed sedative-hypnotics are now the **benzodiazepines,** which have almost entirely replaced the barbiturates and other older sedative agents. Most benzodiazepine prescriptions and use are appropriate and do not constitute abuse. For certain anxiety disorders, long-term benzodiazepine use is medically indicated. Under these conditions, tolerance is rarely a problem, and escalating dose or frequency is rare. Withdrawal may be precipitated by an intervening medical illness or by (sometimes well-intentioned) practitioners attempting to "detoxify" patients from appropriate medications. Benzodiazepine abuse in the context of other drug abuse, however, such as stimulants or heroin, tends to escalate.

Clinical Manifestations

- The symptoms of sedative-hypnotic withdrawal depend on the half-life of the drug being used. Short-acting benzodiazepines, such as **alprazolam,** may

cause withdrawal syndromes within 6 hours of the last dose; long-acting agents such as diazepam cause withdrawal syndromes as late as 7 to 14 days after discontinuation.
- **Symptoms of sedative-hypnotic withdrawal** include anxiety, tremor, nightmares, insomnia, anorexia, nausea, vomiting, orthostatic hypotension, seizures, delirium, and fever.

Differential Diagnosis
Differential diagnosis is the same as for alcohol withdrawal.

Principles of Treatment
Principles of treatment include the following:
- **The treatment of acute withdrawal** begins **with reintroducing the agent of dependence.**
- **Slow, gradual tapering of the agent** of dependence is employed if withdrawal is appropriate (i.e., if the agent is not being used for a legitimate medical purpose).
- If discontinuation of the agent is indicated, **substitution of a long-acting agent for a short-acting one,** with gradual reduction of dose is recommended. Particularly on an outpatient basis, such reduction should be extremely slow, for example, not faster than 25% per week.

OPIOIDS

Overview
- Intoxication from opiates—**heroin, morphine, methadone, hydromorphone, and codeine**—causes euphoria, sedation, and sleepiness. Physical symptoms include pupillary constriction and, dangerously, respiratory depression and arrest in overdose.
- The signs and symptoms of withdrawal from opiates begin 8 to 12 hours after the last use, with the period of withdrawal lasting 5 to 7 days. Methadone generally has a later onset of withdrawal and a longer period of symptoms. **Symptoms of withdrawal** include:
  - Gastrointestinal distress, including diarrhea, nausea, and vomiting.
  - Pain, including arthralgias, myalgias, and abdominal cramping.
  - Anxiety.
  - Insomnia.
  - Rhinorrhea, lacrimation, piloerection, restlessness, and anorexia.

Treatment Options for Withdrawal
Treatment options for withdrawal include

Clonidine
- Clonidine alleviates some symptoms of opioid withdrawal but not myalgia, insomnia, or drug craving.
- An appropriate protocol is 0.1 to 0.2 mg orally every 4 to 6 hours.
- A transdermal patch may be used.
- Hold for blood pressure below 90/60.

Methadone
- Be aware of legal considerations regarding the dispensing of methadone.

- Reversal of withdrawal depends on titrating methadone against objective measures, such as two or more of the following:
  - Pulse greater than 90 in the absence of known tachycardia
  - Blood pressure greater than 160/90 in the absence of known hypertension
  - Dilated pupils
  - Gooseflesh, sweating, rhinorrhea, or lacrimation
- If patients meet these criteria, administer methadone 10 mg orally and reevaluate in 1 hour; if symptoms are not improved, repeat dose and reevaluate. Only rarely should an individual require more than 40 mg/day in the first day.
- Give the total dose for day 1 in two divided doses on day 2.
- Beginning with day 3, taper the dose by 5 mg/day.
- This protocol would be best initiated in the emergency department with input from a consulting opiate addiction specialty service, in part to assure patient follow-up in the setting of outpatient treatment.

Buprenorphine

Buprenorphine is a mixed opioid agonist-antagonist approved by the Food and Drug Administration for the treatment of pain, and recently for the treatment of opioid dependence. Its effectiveness is characterized by:

- Less euphoria and dependence
- Lower potential for misuse
- Ceiling on opioid effects
- Relatively milder withdrawal profile.

It must be prescribed by a practitioner with specialized training in treating addiction and with a special DEA number allowing its prescription and dispensing. It is available alone or in combination with naloxone (Suboxone).

Symptomatic Treatment

- Antiemetics, such as prochlorperazine or trimethobenzamide.
- Antidiarrheals, such as loperamide.

STIMULANTS

Cocaine

General Considerations

Cocaine intoxication and poisoning frequently produce behaviors or complications that precipitate emergency department visits. Acute intoxication and poisoning may follow intravenous injection, insufflation, or smoking.

Intoxication States

- **Cocaine intoxication** produces CNS and cardiopulmonary stimulation. CNS effects include euphoria, increased energy, social disinhibition, impulsivity, and a sense of often unrealistic strength and mental capacity. Non-CNS effects include increased blood pressure, pulse and temperature, bruxism, and dilated pupils. At higher doses and/or more protracted periods of intoxication, stereotyped behaviors, dysphoria, paranoid delusions, anxiety and panic, and visual, auditory, or tactile hallucinations may emerge.
- **Cocaine poisoning** may involve the symptoms of severe intoxication, but may also lead to severe tachycardia, ventricular irritability, hyperthermia, seizures and status epilepticus, and respiratory arrest.

- **Low-dose cocaine intoxication requires no treatment except** reducing stimulation and reassurance. Typically, symptoms clear in a matter of hours.
- **Severe cocaine poisoning is a medical emergency** and requires vigorous treatment.
  - Stimulation should be reduced.
  - Seizures may be treated with intravenous diazepam, using the usual precautions against respiratory depression/arrest.
  - Psychotic symptoms may be treated with haloperidol (5 mg), lorazepam (1.0 mg), and benztropine (1.0 mg); these can be given intravenously, intramuscularly, or orally.
  - Fever should be reduced by external cooling.

Withdrawal
The withdrawal syndrome from cocaine involves profound yearning for the drug and drug-seeking behavior; other symptoms may include agitation, anxiety, fatigue, hypersomnia, and depression. These symptoms, apart from depression, usually require no medical treatment and clear spontaneously over 5 to 7 days. Depression, with suicidal ideation, may emerge as a serious complication, requiring pharmacologic management. Noradrenergic antidepressants such as **desipramine** and the dopamine agonist **amantadine** have been found to decrease cocaine craving in some individuals.

Amphetamines
General Considerations
Perhaps because of reduced availability and less intensity of effect when taken by most routes, the rate of amphetamine abuse is generally lower than that of cocaine. There is, however, a rising prevalence of amphetamine use in the form of crystal methamphetamine.

Intoxication States
- Amphetamines produce a syndrome of alertness, a sense of well-being, talkativeness, confidence, and concentration, which gradually at higher doses evolve into dysphoria, tension, anxiety, agitation, tremor, confusion, and emotional lability.
- **Prolonged, high-dose abuse may cause paranoia, visual, tactile, or auditory hallucinations, and extreme irritability, which may erupt into unpredictable violence.**
- The physical signs of intoxication may include tachycardia, headache, chills, vomiting, dry mouth, hyperpyrexia, and seizures.
- The **treatment** of severe amphetamine toxicity is the same as described above for cocaine toxicity, with the additional caveat that excretion of the drug can be accelerated by acidification of the urine, achieved in the absence of renal or hepatic abnormalities by administering ammonium chloride 500 mg orally every 4 hours.

Withdrawal from Amphetamines
Withdrawal from amphetamines involves drug craving, dysphoria, anxiety, fatigue, insomnia/hypersomnia, agitation, and, often, depression, which may warrant pharmacologic and other treatment. Amphetamines may be stopped abruptly.

HALLUCINOGENS

General Considerations
Hallucinogens include LSD, mescaline, psilocybin, dimethyltyramine (DMT), and 3,4 methylenedioxymethamphetamine (MDMA).

Intoxication States

- Hallucinogens produce states of altered awareness affecting both external stimuli and internal sensations. Sensory phenomena may be heightened, and imbued with a sense of enhanced importance and significance. The distortion of sensory input and conflation of sensory experiences, together with the sense of expanded time, can be pleasurable or frightening.
- The physical signs of intoxication are variable, but tachycardia, increased blood pressure and temperature, and pupillary dilation are often seen. Peak effects of LSD occur in 2 to 3 hours, and abate after 8 to 10 hours.
- **Hallucinogen intoxication generally requires no treatment.** Panic reactions that occur often respond to simple reassurance. **Benzodiazepines** can sometimes be calming. In general, **drugs with anticholinergic activity should be avoided.**

Withdrawal States

There is no significant withdrawal from hallucinogens. Residual effects, however, may include recurrent sensory disorders, usually involving visual distortions or hallucinations. These "flashbacks" may persist for years, and generally respond poorly to treatment.

MARIJUANA

Intoxication States

- Intoxication from marijuana involves feelings of well-being, relaxation, and a general sense that time passes slowly. Physical signs of intoxication are few but may include tachycardia and conjunctival injection. Peak activity occurs within an hour and dissipates over approximately 3 to 5 hours, depending on whether the drug has been smoked or taken orally.
- **Marijuana may be adulterated with other more potent drugs,** thereby producing unexpected effects, often without the user's knowledge. Particularly troublesome in this regard is adulteration with **phencyclidine,** which may cause panic and a psychotic-like state (see later).

Withdrawal States

Marijuana does not cause physically significant withdrawal. In chronic users of high dosages, interruption of use may cause irritability, insomnia, dysphoria, and gastrointestinal distress. No treatment is necessary.

PHENCYCLIDINE

General Considerations

Phencyclidine, **PCP, is a particularly dangerous drug** because of the intensity of negative reactions it often engenders; these include **an unexpected or uncharacteristic propensity toward extreme violence,** often because many individuals use it unknowingly, when it has been used to adulterate other drugs, such as marijuana, cocaine, or hallucinogens. The drug can be ingested by smoking or insufflation or taken orally. Effects peak in 30 to 45 minutes, but despite a short half-life, in overdose the drug may be present in clinically significant amounts for days because of its distribution in adipose tissue and the brain.

Intoxication States

- Intoxication may cause euphoria, feelings of unreasonable strength and capability, grandiosity, and invulnerability, as well as panic, perceptual distortions, and a severe paranoid psychosis, with hallucinations in all modalities; these seem to be aggravated by stimuli of all kinds. Physical signs include nystagmus, hypertension, ataxia, dysarthria, fever, posturing, and drooling.
- The psychotic state induced by PCP can sometimes persist for weeks after ingestion.
- **Intoxicated patients are at severe risk for disinhibited behavior, particularly violence.**
- The treatment of the toxic state, as well as PCP psychosis, involves the following:
  - Destimulate the patient by placing him/her in a quiet room with dim lighting. Do not try verbally to reassure or "talk down" the patient.
  - Try to calm the patient with **benzodiazepines,** for example, diazepam (5–10 mg orally) or lorazepam (2 mg orally or intramuscularly).
  - Psychotic symptoms may be alleviated **with haloperidol 5 mg orally or intramuscularly every 1 to 2 hours as needed.**
  - Excretion of the drug may be enhanced by acidification of the urine, in the absence of hepatic or renal disease.

Withdrawal States

PCP does not induce dependence or withdrawal.

INHALANTS

General Considerations

Abuse of solvents is common, particularly among latency-age children and teenagers. Substances of abuse include paint thinners, lighter fluid, aerosols, cleaning fluids, and gasoline.

Intoxication

Intoxication involves mild euphoria, confusion, disorientation, and ataxia. Toxic effects may include psychosis, seizures, and coma. Other toxic effects, depending on the solvent used, may include cardiac arrhythmias and renal toxicity.

Withdrawal

Tolerance to the solvents develops quickly, as does psychological dependence. Withdrawal may be accompanied by dysphoria, tremulousness, tachycardia, disorientation, hallucinations, and abdominal pain. These symptoms should be treated symptomatically with a close eye to underlying damage to the kidneys, liver, bone marrow, and heart.

Index